Fou

AMSSM Sports Medicine CAQ Study Guide

- A resource for testing sports medicine knowledge
- Exam questions from previous AMSSM In-Training Exams
- Two complete 200-question tests with up-to-date critiques and references
- Modeled after the ABFM Sports Medicine CAQ exams
- Featuring a keyword index with question numbers and page numbers
- Including case studies (complete with images) that are coordinated with the content of the exam questions to augment learning
- With more images in this edition

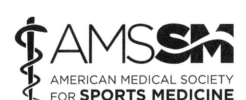

Editors:
Stephen R. Paul, MD
Leah Concannon, MD
Morteza Khodaee, MD
Michael Henehan, DO

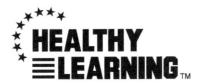

AMSSM Executive Director: Jim Griffith, MBA, CAE

©2019 Healthy Learning. Fourth edition. All rights reserved. Printed in the United States.

No part of this book may be reproduced, stored in a retrieval system, or transmitted in any form or by any means, electronic, mechanical, photocopying, recording, or otherwise, without the prior permission of Healthy Learning. Throughout this book, the masculine shall be deemed to include the feminine and vice versa.

ISBN: 978-1-60679-463-0
Library of Congress Control Number: 2019937423
Cover design: Cheery Sugabo and Rachel Ronan, Kiwi Creative
Book layout: Cheery Sugabo
Front cover illustration: Hemera/Thinkstock

Healthy Learning
P.O. Box 1828
Monterey, CA 93942
www.healthylearning.com

Acknowledgments

As with the previous editions, this book would not have been possible without the tremendous contribution of the volunteer AMSSM members who wrote and edited the questions and cases. Additionally, we asked collaborators and members to help provide images used in this edition. Without the dedication of the individuals who actually write new questions for the In-Training Exam (ITE) every year, we would not have the exams, and we would not have the basic content for this edition. Each year, we ask volunteer faculty to write questions to be used on each new exam. We also rely on a group of editors who review each question for the test every year. Finally, I work with Scott Rand, Mark Stovak, Irfan Asif, and Leah Concannon to write the actual ITE tests we use.

Leah Concannon oversees the AMSSM ITE program, coordinating the volunteer question writers and editors. She supervises the writing of the test each year. Dr. Concannon was invaluable in the final edits, helping proof the rewrites and last-minute changes. She and Morteza Khodaee, who assists her, have put in a tremendous amount of volunteer time every year with the ITE program, making sure all questions are submitted and properly edited on time.

For this edition, we have spent immense time reviewing each of the questions used, verifying and updating all the references to current standards. We also verified each image for quality and copyright. New to this edition, we are adding case studies, based on the content of the two tests used in the book. Michael Henehan, who initiated and has overseen the AMSSM Case Studies Library, contributed to this edition. He collected and reviewed each case, as well as updating the format and images, tracked down the authors and editors, and updated all of the information. I would like to acknowledge the case editors listed in the contributor section.

Again, we needed assistance finding quality images—free of copyrights—for this edition. I would like to thank the following contributors for their assistance in submitting images used in this edition: Irfan Asif, MD; Donna G. Blankenbaker, MD; Susannah M. Briskin MD; Alison Brooks, MD; Kirkland W. Davis, MD; Arie DeGrio, MD; Jonathan Drezner, MD; Matthew Grady, MD; Barry E. Kenneally, MD; Morteza Khodaee, MD; Stephen R. Paul, MD; Jeff Roberts, MD; Darren Willius, DO; and Eliot J. Young, MD.

I would like to thank the following people at AMSSM: Jim Griffith, executive director; Jody Gold, director of operations; Michele Lane, information technology, registration, and design manager; and the board of directors. I would like to thank Jim Peterson, owner of Healthy Learning, who has always been supportive of this project since the early days (the first edition was the first joint publication between Healthy Learning and AMSSM). Finally, I would like to thank Kristi Huelsing of Healthy Learning, who assisted with oversight in editing this and the previous three editions.

Leah, Morteza, Mike, and I have agreed in summary to thank our families and friends who have supported us in this project, allowing us the necessary time to spend on it and encouraging our work. Thank you.

—Stephen R. Paul, MD

Foreword

The American Medical Society for Sports Medicine exists to provide a forum to foster professional relationships among sports medicine physicians to advance the discipline of sports medicine through education, research, advocacy, and excellence in patient care. Education continues to be a major focus of our organization and of our leadership, and our members continue to be world leaders in this area.

AMSSM is excited once again to partner with Healthy Learning to bring the *AMSSM Sports Medicine CAQ Study Guide* (Fourth Edition)—an invaluable educational and training resource—to sports medicine physicians certifying or recertifying for their specialty CAQ examination. This manual will also be a valuable resource for others who wish to assess or increase their knowledge levels, as it covers a wide breadth of sports medicine topics.

The first three editions of the *AMSSM Sports Medicine CAQ Study Guide* proved to be a unique, high-quality, go-to, ready reference for many fellows taking their first CAQ exam successfully, and for sports medicine physicians seeking recertification. The editorial team of Stephen Paul, Leah Concannon, Morteza Khodaee, and Michael Henehan have done an outstanding job of building on these previous editions to bring us the best study guide yet. The guide continues to provide up-to-date discussion of answers with references so interested readers can delve further into a topic as desired. AMSSM congratulates them and the rest of the outstanding contributors on another successful edition.

AMSSM is proud to make this must-read guide available to anyone who endeavors to become more knowledgeable in the field of sports medicine, whether taking the CAQ exam or not. And AMSSM is privileged to have our talented editors and content authors call AMSSM their professional home while we firmly stand behind the quality of this important resource.

Chad Asplund, MD, MPH
President, American Medical Society for Sports Medicine 2018-2019

Contents

Acknowledgments 3
Foreword 5
Preface 8
Introduction 9

Chapter 1: Test 1 Questions 11
Chapter 2: Test 2 Questions 91
Chapter 3: Test 1 Answers, Critiques, and References 171
Chapter 4: Test 2 Answers, Critiques, and References 397

Appendix: Case Studies 621
About the Editors 685
About the Contributors 687
About the Case Study Contributors 701
Index 705
Answer Sheets 717

Preface

This edition represents the actual questions used in the AMSSM In-Training Exam for the sports medicine CAQ. It is divided into four sections. Two sections each have a 200-question test, assembled from the recently given In-Training Exams. Two additional sections contain the same questions along with the correct answers, critiques, and up-to-date references. New to this edition, we have added select case studies from the AMSSM Case Study catalogue to augment study for the CAQ. They were selected by topic, and edited, as well as formatted, for inclusion in this edition. An index is included again to aid referencing questions by subject matter based on the topics from the ABFM blueprint for the CAQ. Many are cross-referenced for ease of use.

We have again maintained the format of the ITE and CAQ exams. We provide up-to-date, easy-to-find references, mostly online and mostly for free. The editors have reviewed each question and verified each reference to be sure they are up to date and reflect the best evidence-based practice. Please note, as with all "board-type" exams, the questions must be chosen on the best evidence-based practice that is accepted and available at the time of writing the question. Similar to the CAQ exam, there always needs to be a delay of one to two years for dissemination of current evidence, as well as verification of new practice standards and research, before a quality test question can be written and a majority of the audience will have access to the information. So, this text reflects accepted practice standards, which may not always be *the* most recent.

This book is published in e-book and paper formats to provide the optimum study tool based on the user's preference. Included are answer sheets for taking the tests on paper.

The intention of the book is to be an invaluable companion to study for the sports medicine CAQ. Additionally, it should prove useful to anyone wishing to test and seek further understanding of their sports medicine knowledge, whether in medical school, residency programs, or fellowships in primary care or orthopedic sports medicine.

Introduction

The first edition of this book was co-edited by the original leaders of the AMSSM Sports Medicine CAQ ITE program, Scott Rand and Mark Stovak, along with Marc Hilgers, who also served as an original editor. Irfan Asif successfully took over the AMSSM In-Training Exam test project in 2013, and through tireless diligence and commitment, he moved the program forward with many improvements. He and I teamed up for the second edition of the study guide. The ITE program leadership passed to Leah Concannon, with significant assistance from Morteza Khodaee, in 2015. The ITE program has continued to grow. We have increased the ranks of question writers, and with each year, the quality of the written questions has improved.

We strive to improve each new edition. With the second edition, we added an index with the intent to assist studying by specific topic and to also aid in teaching sports medicine learners by having questions available by topic. With this edition, we are adding case studies with the help of Michael Henehan, who developed and oversees the AMSSM Case Studies Library. This provides another tool for study, validation of clinical case knowledge, and most importantly, an opportunity to publish the work of contributors to the AMSSM Case Studies Library. We have also strived again to eliminate all duplicate questions, and to add images where appropriate.

Consistent with previous editions, the tests used in this edition are modeled after the ABFM Sports Medicine CAQ exam and are from recent ITE exams. We re-edit each question, as well as verify and update each reference. We further attempt to make all of the references available from online and/or for-free resources of high quality. The layout of the book is organized so readers can initially see the questions in test format, without correct answers or critiques, to simulate a test-taking environment. (Answer sheets to score practice tests are provided at the end of the book.) Subsequent chapters include the same test questions along with the correct answers, critiques, and references. The critique that follows each question gives good background explanation for why the answer provided is correct and why the other answer options are incorrect. Finally, the appendix includes selected case studies that reflect the content of the exams and are intended as another way to test and add to an individual's knowledge base.

As noted with the previous editions, this book represents the culmination of the success of the AMSSM ITE program, since its beginning in 2006. Again, as in previous editions, I feel it is important to recognize the key people who assisted in getting this program started in 2005–2006. This includes previous board members Kim Harmon, Sean Bryan, and Mark Lavallee. From the ABFM, president Jim Puffer, Roger Fain (senior editor), and Jason Rinaldo (psychometrician). From AMSSM, Michele Lane, Jody Gold, and Jim Griffith, and original pioneers, editors, and test writers Mark Stovak and Scott Rand. From Healthy Learning, Jim Peterson and Kristi Huelsing.

Finally, I would like to thank every volunteer test question writer and editor. Without their commitment to writing new questions every year, this program could not exist. Please take a moment when you see or chat with a contributor (from any of the editions) to thank them for their commitment.

Thank you,

Stephen R. Paul, MD

Test 1 Questions

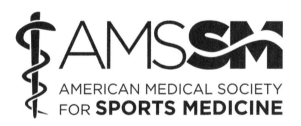

1. A 17-year-old female cross-country athlete presents to your office with one month of left-sided groin pain made worse with running. She now has some pain with walking and increased pain with stairs. Hip x-rays demonstrate a non-displaced lateral (tension-side) stress fracture of the femoral neck (see images). What is the most appropriate management of this injury?

   A. Non-weight-bearing with crutches for two weeks, followed by a gradual return to running protocol
   B. Discontinue running for one month and begin supplementation with calcium and vitamin D
   C. Patient is made non-weight-bearing immediately and referred to orthopedic surgery for potential surgical procedure
   D. Avoid running but may continue weight-bearing while MRI is ordered

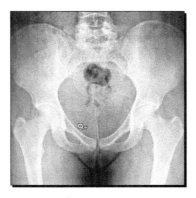

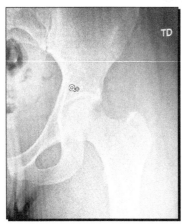
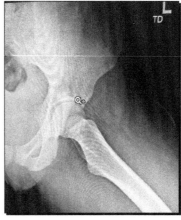

2. The sleeper stretch addresses which specific part of the shoulder?

   A. Inferior glenohumeral ligament
   B. Anterior inferior labrum
   C. Posterior capsule
   D. Rotator interval

3. A 15-year-old high school crew athlete with no prior orthopedic history presents to you with two months of progressive low back pain. The pain was originally intermittent, but now is persistent, both with rest and activity, particularly when her back is in a maximally extended position (the "drive" position). Initial x-rays, including standing AP, lateral views, and oblique views are unremarkable. What is the next appropriate imaging study that may help clarify the diagnosis?

   A. Bone scan with SPECT study
   B. CT scan of the lumbar spine, with thin cut scan through the area of concern
   C. MRI of the lumbar spine
   D. DEXA scan

4. A 13-year-old female soccer player presents to the office with bilateral anterior knee pain. Physical examination is notable for lateral patella facet pain, ankle dorsiflexion 10 degrees, hamstring popliteal angle complement 10 degrees, and knees going into slight valgus with single-leg squat. The single most important part of physical therapy for this patient is?

   A. Strengthen VMO
   B. Strengthen gluteus medius
   C. Stretch hamstrings
   D. Stretch gastrocnemius

5. A 55-year-old male presents to your office with right posterior heel pain of eight months duration. The patient notes a stabbing pain with ascending stairs as well as running, particularly uphill. Up to this point, the patient has attempted a home stretching program, as well as intermittent NSAIDs, with minimal benefit. On examination, the patient has localized pain to the Achilles insertion with palpation, single-leg raises, as well as passive ankle dorsi-flexion. In reference to the treatment of chronic insertional Achilles tendinopathy, which of the following statements is true?

    A. Full range of motion eccentric therapy programs provide greater patient satisfaction than floor-level eccentric therapy programs
    B. Low-energy shock wave therapy provides superior recovery (return to normal activity), compared to full range of motion eccentric loading therapy programs
    C. Concentric therapy programs provide superior pain relief, compared to full range of motion eccentric therapy programs
    D. Injectable therapies (including hyperosmolar dextrose and polidocanol) have been shown to be ineffective in significantly decreasing VAS pain scores

6. With regard to eccentric rehabilitation of hamstring strains, which of the following statements is true?

    A. Should only be performed in the shortened position to prevent re-injury
    B. Can begin as early as day two post-injury, without adversely affecting healing
    C. Has never been proven to prevent recurrent hamstring strains
    D. Can only be performed on special equipment
    E. Should have the load determined by 1RM

7. A 35-year-old female presents with three months of anterior knee pain, made worse with running, squatting, and using stairs. She originally presented to her primary care physician and was told she had runner's knee. She was given a referral to physical therapy, but she did not go, because of time and cost. Six months ago, she had started training for an upcoming 5 km race but had to stop due to the knee pain. She still aspires to run the race and is looking for Answers on how to return to running without knee pain. Which of the following recommendations is true with regard to patellofemoral pain?

   A. Prefabricated foot orthoses improve patellofemoral pain at three months and one year
   B. Bracing the patella has not been shown to be effective for pain reduction in the short term
   C. Taping has no role in patellofemoral pain rehabilitation
   D. A physical therapy program, consisting of quadriceps and gluteal strengthening, stretching, and patellar taping, has a moderate therapeutic effect within three months

8. Which of the following are common sites of compression of the ulnar nerve?

   A. Cubital tunnel and Guyon's canal
   B. Cubital tunnel and pronator teres muscle
   C. Pronator teres muscle and Guyon's canal
   D. Radial tunnel and Guyon's canal

9. You are covering a high school football game when a player comes out of the game after a helmet-to-helmet tackle. When evaluating him for concussion, which of the following symptoms warrants prompt referral to the emergency department?

   A. Headache
   B. Nausea
   C. Photophobia
   D. Lethargy
   E. Retrograde amnesia

10. A sophomore college football player sustains a burner during a game. Which is true regarding his neurologic examination, when determining if he is safe to return to the game?

   A. He can be cleared to return to play after experiencing bilateral numbness in both small fingers as long as his strength has returned and he is asymptomatic
   B. C6 nerve root is tested by checking the strength of the wrist extensors
   C. C7 can easily be tested by checking forearm flexion
   D. C5 innervates the triceps so it can easily be checked by forearm extension

11. You evaluate an 18-year-old defensive tackle for the local college football team for a preparticipation physical evaluation. He reports that in his senior season in high school, he suffered two neck injuries, both while making a tackle. The first injury involved mild neck pain, as well as burning and numbness to his left arm that lasted for 30 minutes and completely resolved. He returned to practice and play several days later. Three weeks following that injury, he experienced another hit that left him with bilateral arm and leg tingling and mild weakness lasting two days. He was hospitalized until his symptoms resolved and missed the final two games of the season. His examination today is completely normal. Regarding these two injuries, what are the most appropriate recommendations for this athlete?

   A. Clear him for full return to play, as long as he remains symptom free
   B. Clear him for full play, but refer to a neurosurgeon for further workup
   C. Disqualify him from any collision sports immediately
   D. Hold him from lifting or contact activities, obtain an MRI, and consider referral

12. A softball pitcher continues to have precordial pain and complains of palpitations after a softball hit her in the chest. A 12-lead ECG performed by EMS at the softball park is normal. Which of the following statements is true?

   A. A normal ECG after the incident rules out a cardiac contusion
   B. A normal concentration of cardiac troponin I or T eight hours after the incident rules out cardiac damage and consequently minimizes the risk of cardiac complications
   C. Transthoracic echocardiography will detect aortic injury or isolated myocardial edema without wall motion abnormality
   D. Chronic dilated cardiac dysfunction and constrictive pericarditis can both be early complications of a cardiac contusion

13. What items would a sports medicine physician want in the game bag to help emergently reduce a symptomatic posterior sternoclaviclar dislocation in the field?

    A. Trainer's Angel
    B. Towel roll
    C. Towel clamp
    D. Sling and swathe

14. A 15-year-old male soccer player is following up in clinic four days after being involved in a moderate-speed traffic accident. He was evaluated in the emergency department and found to have a pulmonary contusion of the right lower lobe by CT. No abnormalities were seen on chest x-ray. No other injuries were reported, and he was discharged home after a 24-hour observation in the hospital. At the present time, he states that he is a little short of breath and was sweating a lot last night while trying to sleep. Despite performing incentive spirometry as instructed, he has developed a cough. Which of the following is the next best step in the management of this patient?

    A. Repeat chest x-rays
    B. Perform a CT of the chest with IV contrast (pulmonary embolism protocol)
    C. Perform a non-contrast CT of the chest
    D. Perform a V-Q scan
    E. Start the patient on low molecular weight heparin

15. A 35-year-old male aerobics instructor is seen in your clinic because he has had several months of lower abdominal and groin pain. He reports that over the past two months, the pain has increased, exacerbated by coughing or laughing. He reports no acute injury and no prior muscle strains. He stopped all physical activity for the past four weeks. An inguinal hernia is not appreciated on physical examination. X-rays, MRI, and bone scan do not show any bony abnormalities. What would be considered the best initial treatment plan for this athlete?

    A. Corticosteriod injection to the conjoined tendon sheath
    B. Reassurance and rest
    C. Non-weight-bearing and crutches for six weeks, given the patient may have occult stress fracture
    D. Conservative treatment with a comprehensive rehabilitation program to improve core strengthening and posterior abdominal wall weakness

16. A 21-year-old senior female softball player presents to the clinic with left-sided abdominal pain. She says she first noticed the pain after hitting a double and sliding head-first into second base in last night's game. She was able to finish the inning, but felt like she had trouble taking a deep breath and removed herself from the game. Today, she says she is breathing okay, but still has pain with deep inspiration. She has pain with trunk rotation and bending, and bruising in the anterolateral abdomen of the left side. She has bilateral breath sounds equal in nature and is tender to palpation along her ribs and abdominal wall of the left side. A chest x-ray and vital signs are normal. Her pain has likely resulted from which of the following?

    A. Rib fracture
    B. Costochondritis
    C. Internal oblique strain
    D. Splenic hematoma

17. Over the past weekend, an 18-year-old male was playing tackle football with his dormitory buddies. At one point, he was running down the field for a touchdown, when another person tackled him to the ground, falling onto his chest and abdomen. He felt an immediate pain in his right upper quadrant. The pain worsened very quickly, and he was taken to the emergency room. Which of the following statements addresses the management of this patient?

    A. A negative history and physical examination reliably excludes liver injury
    B. Physical findings sensitive and specific for liver injury include right upper quadrant or generalized abdominal tenderness, as well as abdominal wall contusion or hematoma
    C. Immediate assessment with ultrasound has replaced diagnostic peritoneal lavage and CT as the gold standard
    D. Operative management (laparotomy) remains the preferred treatment in stable patients

18. A high school soccer player is struck in the abdomen with an opponent's knee while contesting a corner kick. She experiences immediate abdominal discomfort, sitting down immediately on standing. Vital signs are within normal limits on the field, but she experiences increasing discomfort and cannot return to play. Following blunt abdominal trauma in sports, which of the following is true?

    A. While rare, bowel perforation is the most frequent cause of death
    B. She can be watched at home without concern for serious injury
    C. Radiation of pain isn't helpful during assessment of need for transport
    D. Splenic rupture is the most common catastrophic injury

19. You are evaluating an athlete with recurrent low back pain, with negative provocative testing for discogenic causes and negative imaging. You suspect a lumbar strain. In addition to the transversus abdominis, what muscle has been shown to have increased fatigability and a delayed onset of activity in sufferers of recurrent low back strains?

    A. Lumbar multifidus
    B. External oblique
    C. Iliocostalis
    D. Longissimus
    E. Psoas major

20. A 68-year-old female, a retired nursing assistant, comes in with eight months of worsening low back pain. She denies any previous injuries or surgeries and does not recall an inciting event. X-rays of her lumbosacral spine revealed degenerative spondylolisthesis of L4-L5. What is this condition usually associated with?

    A. Peripheral neuropathy
    B. Multiple myeloma
    C. Previous scoliosis during adolescence
    D. Solitary plasmacytoma
    E. Spinal stenosis

21. A 12-year-old girl tennis player and former gymnast comes to your office complaining of six months of low back pain that appears when only she serves while playing tennis. She quit gymnastics about a year ago but does not remember any issues when she was in gymnastics. Off and on, she has been taking ibuprofen as needed for pain. What is the most appropriate examination maneuver for evaluating your suspected diagnosis?

    A. Stork test
    B. Straight-leg raise test
    C. FABER test
    D. FADIR test

22. Regarding the management of low back pain, which of the following statements is true?

    A. In patients with acute low back pain, imaging results, physical examination findings, and type of injury usually correlate with chronicity or severity of symptoms
    B. Acetaminophen, antidepressants, skeletal muscle relaxants, and lidocaine patches appear more effective than placebo for chronic low back pain
    C. Topiramate (Topamax), select opioids, and NSAIDs appear more effective than placebo in the short-term treatment of chronic non-specific low back pain
    D. Few randomized trials suggest that there is some advantage of bed rest for patients with sciatica

23. A 16-year-old female cheerleader presents to you with insidious onset of progressive lumbar back pain. She denies neurologic symptoms, and examination is normal, except for reproducible pain on extension. Your evaluation produces a diagnosis of unilateral spondylolysis at the L5 level. Which one of the following statements is correct?

    A. Surgery is indicated at this time, in order to keep her active in her sport
    B. She will likely never play sports again, due to risk for neurologic complications
    C. She should wear tight-fitting clothing for support under her uniform
    D. While no consensus exists to guide treatment in all cases, some period of rest is recommended, with or without bracing

24. You suspect a patient of yours has quadrilateral space syndrome and order an electromyography (EMG) study to confirm your diagnosis. In the event that your diagnosis is correct, you would anticipate seeing neurogenic changes in which of the following muscles?

    A. Supraspinatus
    B. Infraspinatus
    C. Subscapularis
    D. Teres minor

25. A 25-year-old female with no past medical history presents with a one-day history of severe right-sided shoulder girdle pain. Her pain is unremitting, regardless of position, and radiates into her forearm with associated paresthesias. She does not attribute the pain to injury, although she is a front-door greeter at your hospital, and she occasionally helps patients into wheelchairs. Her pain was the most severe last night, as she was unable to sleep. Of note, she is recovering from an upper respiratory tract infection. What is the best test to help confirm the diagnosis?

    A. MRI
    B. EMG
    C. Laboratory analysis to include CMP, CBC, and an ESR
    D. X-ray of the shoulder

26. What is the most common complication found in anterior shoulder dislocations (beyond typical Hill-Sachs and Bankart lesions)?

    A. Rotator cuff tears
    B. Axillary nerve injury
    C. Greater tuberosity fractures
    D. Lesser tuberosity fracture

27. A 25-year-old right-handed man has a six-month history of right shoulder pain. He denies any specific injury, but works out regularly at the gym. His pain resolves if he takes a week off. The pain is worse with weight-bearing and loading activities, such as the shoulder press and chest press. His MRI arthrogram is shown below. What is his diagnosis?

   A. Rotator cuff tear
   B. Clavicular osteolysis
   C. Labral tear
   D. Subacromial bursitis

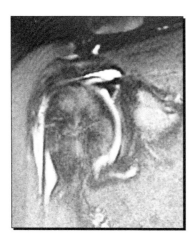
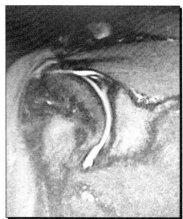

28. A six-year-old boy is brought into the emergency room with left elbow pain and swelling, after a fall on his outstretched arm, with his elbow in extension. Despite being left-handed, he is now only using his right arm. On lateral elbow x-ray views, the anterior humeral line does not transect the capitellum. Which of the following, if also injured, could mask a developing compartment syndrome?

   A. Ulnar nerve
   B. Distal radius
   C. Radial nerve
   D. Scaphoid
   E. Median nerve

29. A 33-year-old female recreational golfer presents with three months of right lateral elbow pain. She has tried a counter-force elbow brace and naproxen with no improvement. On physical examination, she has tenderness in the extensor mass, 3 cm distal from the epicondyle, and pain with resisted extension of the middle finger. No sensory or motor deficits are noted on examination. What is the most common site of nerve compression associated with this patient's diagnosis?

   A. Supinator edge
   B. Arcade of Frohse
   C. ERCB edge
   D. Radial artery recurrent leash of Henry

30. A 30-year-old elite male swimmer presents with posteromedial elbow pain, especially when the elbow reaches terminal extension during the breaststroke. He denies numbness or tingling. He has tenderness to palpation to the posteromedial elbow. He has a negative milking maneuver, with 30 to 100 degrees of flexion. There is no pain with resisted flexion of the elbow, resisted extension of the elbow, resisted pronation of the forearm, resisted wrist dorsiflexion, or resisted third-finger extension. His strength is normal in the distal extremity. Small irregular loose bodies are seen posteriorly on radiograph. What is the most likely diagnosis?

   A. Triceps tendinosis
   B. Osteochondral lesion of the radial head
   C. Medial epicondylosis
   D. Valgus extension overload

31. In the evaluation and management of ulnar collateral ligament (UCL) injury, which one of the following is correct?

   A. Point tenderness is produced at the medial epicondyle
   B. All partial tears respond well to conservative non-surgical care
   C. Varus stress is applied to the elbow in extension and shoulder abduction and external rotation
   D. MRI has 100% specificity for ulnar collateral ligament tears
   E. MR Arthrogram adds no additional benefit to the evaluation of ulnar collateral ligament tears

32. An 18-year-old soccer player misses a potential game winning goal and punches the ground in frustration. He comes to the sideline holding his right hand and subsequently develops ecchymosis and swelling of over the dorsal aspect of his hand. There is focal tenderness over the distal fifth metacarpal, without associated lacerations or dermal injury. Plain radiographs demonstrate a fifth metacarpal neck fracture, with 20 degrees of apex dorsal angulation. (see image) What is the most appropriate next step in management?

   A. Sugar tong splint, with follow-up in 7 to 10 days
   B. Orthopedic referral for operative management
   C. Ulnar gutter splint, with follow-up in 7 to 10 days
   D. Volar splint, with follow-up in 7 to 10 days

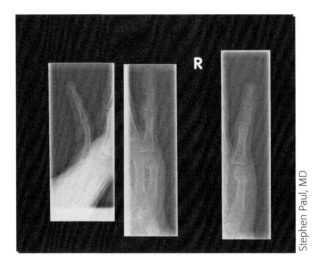

33. A 30-year-old female sustained a fall onto the outstretched hand (FOOSH) while snowboarding. X-rays show a non-displaced Colles' fracture. You treated her fracture appropriately and she presents to your office four weeks after her injury and complains that she cannot move her thumb towards the back of her hand. On examination, you ask her to place her hand flat onto the table, with her palm down, and she is unable to lift her thumb off of the surface. In which dorsal wrist compartment does her ruptured tendon reside?

   A. First compartment
   B. Second compartment
   C. Third compartment
   D. Fourth compartment

34. A 17-year-old basketball player presents with second finger pain after "jamming" it catching a pass. Examination reveals difficulty with active extension at the DIP joint, but normal passive extension. X-ray shows no evidence of bony injury. What are the treatment components of this condition?

   A. Radial gutter cast for six weeks, followed by removable custom hand splint for six weeks
   B. Urgent referral to orthopedic hand surgeon for surgical repair
   C. Buddy tape to third finger for four to six weeks, then as needed with activity for four to six weeks
   D. Splint DIP in full extension for six to eight weeks continuously

35. A 33-year-old male drummer presents with pain and swelling in the dorsoradial aspect of his left wrist for eight weeks. He denies any acute injury, but reports more drumming over the past four months. His symptoms, however, have impaired his ability to practice and perform, and he is very eager to return to drumming with his band. On physical examination, you note an area of soft tissue swelling, tenderness, and crepitus with active wrist movements in an area about 6 cm proximal of Lister's tubercle. You decide to include an ultrasound-guided corticosteroid injection as part of his treatment plan. Which of the following injection targets most closely approximates the locus of this patient's pathology?

   A. Between the compartment with the abductor pollicis longus and extensor pollicis brevis, and the bony surface of the distal radius
   B. Between the compartment with the extensor pollicis longus, and the bony surface of the distal radius
   C. Between the compartment with the extensor carpi radialis longus and extensor carpi radialis brevis, and the compartment with the extensor pollicis longus
   D. Between the compartment with the extensor carpi radialis longus and extensor carpi radialis brevis, and the compartment with the abductor pollicis longus and extensor pollicis brevis

36. Which of the following strategies is helpful in counseling families of youth athletes in preventing overuse injuries from early sports specialization?

    A. Keep hourly average weekly training volumes lower than their age in years
    B. Spend less than six months participating in one sport each year
    C. Begin sports specialization after puberty
    D. Try to participate in cross-training activities during off-season training

37. Your athletic director comes to you to schedule preparticipation evaluations for the incoming fall athletes. She would like them scheduled as close as possible to the start of school, so the athletes won't have to come to town too early. When would you recommend the physicals are optimally be done?

    A. At least one day prior to the start of the activity
    B. At least one week prior to the start of the activity
    C. At least four weeks prior to the start of the activity
    D. At least six weeks prior to the start of the activity

38. A 16-year-old high school swimmer presents for her preparticipation physical evaluation at the local high school. She denies any chest pain, syncope, pre-syncope, shortness of breath, or any significant family history of sudden cardiac death prior to the age of 50, Marfan syndrome, long QT syndrome, or hypertrophic cardiomyopathy. She denies history of asthma, seizures, or diabetes. She denies taking any medications and did not drink coffee or energy drinks today. She did not exercise or practice prior to this examination. She is not anxious and denies previous history of anxiety, hypertension, or murmurs. On examination, you find her blood pressure to be 160/110. Her examination was otherwise normal. Which three factors must you consider in order to diagnose the patient with stage 2 hypertension?

    A. Age, height, weight
    B. Age, weight, gender
    C. Height, weight, gender
    D. Age, height, gender

39. After performing a preparticipation physical evaluation on an 18-year-old male with a seizure disorder, you counsel him on activity participation. Which of the following recommendations is correct?

    A. Scuba diving, skydiving, and swimming are strictly forbidden
    B. Contact sports should be avoided, since head trauma may provoke seizures
    C. Swimming is considered safe if directly supervised by trained individuals and personal flotation devices are used appropriately
    D. Exercise is detrimental, because the associated physiologic stress will often exacerbate an underlying seizure disorder
    E. Physical fitness confers no benefit to the individual with a seizure disorder

40. An 18-year-old female swimmer presents to you for a preparticipation physical evaluation (PPE). In the fall, she will be attending and swimming for a NCAA Division I college, for which you are the team physician. Her history is unremarkable, except for a past medical history of Ehlers-Danlos syndrome. She has no records with her, but assures you that she has been followed by a specialist in her hometown and that she has had no issues with her illness. Other than having hypermobility, her physical examination is unremarkable. What is the next best course of action?

    A. Full clearance and participation without restriction
    B. Disqualify from competitive activity, as Ehlers-Danlos syndrome poses a significant cardiac risk
    C. Clearance deferred, pending review of medical records
    D. Cleared for participation limited to low to moderate static and dynamic activity

41. A 16-year-old right-handed high school athlete presents for a preparticipation physical evaluation in order to play club sports. On physical examination, he was found to have visual acuity of 20/30 in the right eye and 20/60 in the left eye. He does not wear glasses. Which sport is not recommended for him?

    A. Gymnastics
    B. Track and field
    C. Swimming
    D. Boxing

42. An 18-year-old male presents to clinic for a preparticipation physical evaluation so that he can be cleared to try out for his local college's football team. He has no significant past medical history, no medically related complaints, and normal vital signs. He has a normal physical examination, with the exception of an enlarged spleen palpated on his abdominal examination. What is the most appropriate next step in his management?

    A. This is an incidental finding, and he should be cleared for all sports without restrictions
    B. If the spleen is acutely enlarged, all sports should be avoided, due to risk of rupture
    C. If the spleen is chronically enlarged, no further workup is necessary
    D. He may be cleared for all noncontact activities, but all contact/collision and limited contact sports should be avoided

43. Which of the following is not a mental health predictor of injury and illness in student athletes?

    A. Post-traumatic stress disorder
    B. Substance abuse
    C. Reactive depression
    D. Burnout

44. The preparticipation physical evaluation (PPE) is utilized in several sports. Regarding each specific population, which of the following is true?

    A. 75% of patients with hypertrophic cardiomyopathy with left ventricular outflow obstruction have a murmur on physical examination
    B. Geriatric patients undergoing PPE should have a physical examination, including postural vital signs, heart murmur, femoral pulses, and screening for Marfan disease
    C. Female athletes should not be asked about their menstrual cycles, as it may lead to distrust between the physician and the athlete
    D. Athletes with intellectual disabilities do not need PPE, as they have lower reported injury rates than physically disabled and general population athletes

45. Individuals with Down syndrome have an increased risk of atlantoaxial instability and are required to have screening neck radiographs prior to sports participation. Those identified as having atlantoaxial instability are excluded from which of the following Special Olympic sports, unless the athlete and guardian grant written consent and obtain signatures from two independent medical professionals prior to participation?

    A. Tennis
    B. Gymnastics
    C. Figure skating
    D. Athletes with atlantoaxial instability are automatically disqualified from high-risk and contact sports

46. When training for an endurance event, which of the following is the most critical factor to consider when planning a training regimen?

    A. Frequency
    B. Intensity
    C. Time
    D. Technique
    E. Recovery

47. Which of the following is a credible theory for why stretching may hinder athletic performance and potentially lead to injury?

    A. Increased joint stability
    B. Decreased joint-movement efficiency
    C. Increased ability of the tendon and muscle to absorb energy
    D. Decreased pain tolerance
    E. Increased strength before the recovery phase of training

48. A 10-year-old male comes into your office. He would like to start weight training for football. Which of the following statements is correct regarding weight/resistance training in pediatric athletes?

    A. Weight training will help gain size and strength
    B. Weight training may be preferable for overweight children and adolescents compared to aerobic activity
    C. Weight training should be done with standard (adult-sized) equipment
    D. Weight training is associated with growth plate injuries in skeletally immature athletes

49. A 45-year-old patient comes to your office interested in learning more about training for a marathon that will be run at high altitude (about 6,000 feet or 1,829 meters above sea level). He is concerned because he lives only 500 feet or 152 meters above sea level and does not travel frequently to locations considered high altitude. He is a generally healthy person and exercises regularly. Which of the following statements gives him the best opportunity to safely and effectively participate in this marathon?

    A. Endurance events are not affected as much as sprint events, therefore his training does not need to be modified
    B. Illness related to altitude (acute mountain sickness, high altitude cerebral edema) only affects those individuals who are at a high altitude longer than 72 hours
    C. Acclimatization has not been shown to improve performance for races run within three days of reaching altitude
    D. The effect of altitude on $\dot{V}O_2$max is greater on those who perform endurance events
    E. High-intensity training (i.e., hard sprints to improve speed and other interval training) is best performed at high altitude as this improves training velocity and $\dot{V}O_2$max

50. Which type of training program provides the greatest improvement in cardiorespiratory fitness?

    A. Moderate-intensity continuous training
    B. High-intensity interval training
    C. Strength training
    D. Long aerobic workout

51. A 33-year-old female runner returns to your clinic to follow up for patellofemoral syndrome of the left knee. As you are about to leave the room after her visit, she asks for your opinion on vitamin C supplementation in athletes to help with immune function. Which of the following is the most appropriate response?

    A. Vitamin C is an essential component to the diet, and athletes should try to consume at least 1 g per day to optimize performance
    B. Vitamin C is not an essential component to the diet, and athletes should avoid supplementation for optimal performance
    C. Vitamin C is an essential component to the diet, and athletes should try to consume approximately 200 mg per day for optimal performance
    D. Vitamin C is an essential component to the diet, and athletes should try to consume under 100 mg per day to optimize performance

52. Which one of the following is correct about vitamin D in athletes?

    A. Supplementation for an athlete with a vitamin D level below 20 ng/ml is achieved with 2000 IU of vitamin D2 daily
    B. Maximum sports health benefit is achieved at a vitamin D level of 50 ng/ml
    C. Screening athletes for vitamin D deficiency includes obtaining a serum (1,25) dihydroxyvitamin D level
    D. Dietary supplementation with vitamin D2 is more advantageous than cutaneous synthesis of vitamin D

53. What is the evidence-based proportion of fat in a typical diet for natural bodybuilders?

    A. 15% to 30 %
    B. 10% to 15%
    C. 15% to 20%
    D. 30% to 40%

54. Which of the following patients would you advise further evaluation prior to initiation of an exercise program?

    A. Patient with stable CAD wanting to restart their moderate exercise regimen
    B. COPD patient with dyspnea at rest
    C. A young, well-controlled hypertensive patient without risk factors and no evidence of organ damage
    D. A well-controlled patient with epilepsy wanting to take up running for exercise

55. A 30-year-old male with T6 paraplegia presents to the office with a desire to begin a wheelchair exercise program. He has been gaining weight, due to a lack of activity since the injury several years ago. He wants your advice on how to safely begin an exercise program. Along with advising proper equipment, carrying water, and avoiding hot or humid days, you also advise which of the following?

   A. Wear tight leg straps to increase sympathetic tone
   B. Take 10 g of carbohydrates every 30 minutes during exercise
   C. Empty his bladder and bowels before each workout
   D. Have cervical x-rays to rule out atlantoaxial instability

56. An obese patient (BMI > 30 kg/m2) without other comorbidities presents to your office. To improve compliance, one strategy for the patient's exercise prescription could include which of the following?

   A. Incorporating high-impact aerobic activities
   B. Emphasizing exercising after their morning (am) meal
   C. Strict cardiovascular prescription at 85% maximum HR for at least 30 minutes five times per week
   D. Increasing weight-bearing activities very rapidly to increase metabolism
   E. Start with non-weight-bearing activities, such as swimming and recumbent bike

57. Which of the following is true regarding exercise among patients with type 2 diabetes?

   A. Muscular contractions stimulate blood glucose transport via an additive mechanism not impaired by insulin resistance or type 2 diabetes
   B. Blood glucose remains stable during physical activity, due to an increased reliance on fat to fuel muscular activity as intensity increases
   C. There is little risk of hypoglycemia with moderate aerobic exercise, even in patients using exogenous insulin or insulin secretagogues
   D. Persons with type 2 diabetes should undertake no more than 120 minutes per week of moderate to vigorous aerobic exercise, spread out during at least three days during the week

58. A pregnant woman wants to learn more about what activities she can participate in during pregnancy. Which of the following activities should be avoided during pregnancy?

    A. Swimming
    B. Elliptical machine
    C. Cycling
    D. Light exercise, including weight training

59. Which of the following is true of exercise in patients with osteoporosis?

    A. In postmenopausal women, impact exercises can increase BMD in the hip and spine
    B. Weight-bearing exercises are more beneficial than non-weight-bearing, high-force exercises in preventing bone loss and fractures in post-menopausal women
    C. Swimming can improve BMD in postmenopausal women
    D. Smoking cessation will improve overall health but will not reduce risk of osteoporosis

60. Which of the following statements is true regarding athletic equipment and the prevention of injury?

    A. Ankle bracing is better than taping in prevention of recurrent ankle sprains
    B. Mouthpieces help prevent concussion
    C. Soccer headgear helps prevent concussion
    D. Knee bracing helps prevent ACL injury

61. You are the medical director for a marathon race, and you review the epidemiologic data on the common causes of mortality among marathon runners. What is the most common cause of death during a marathon in the United States?

    A. Coronary artery disease (CAD)
    B. Hypertrophic cardiomyopathy
    C. Exercise-associated hyponatremia (EAH)
    D. Cardiac arrhythmias

62. In the planning and preparation for a large mass participation international sporting event, there are many factors that should be considered. One environmental consideration is that of severe inclement weather. Which of the following should be part of the planning for such an occurrence?

    A. Appropriate number of medical supplies should be monitored
    B. Lead medical physicians should have good communication with local weather reporters
    C. A safe area must be designated for athletes and spectator protection, in the event evacuation is required due to inclement weather
    D. Environmental planning should be managed by local authorities, not the medical personnel

63. You are responding as part of the medical team to athletes and spectators who have been victims of a mass casualty in a sports arena due to an active shooter. Local authorities have cleared the area to begin medical treatment. There are multiple victims with extremity, as well as chest, wounds. Which of the following is the best course of action?

    A. Begin CPR on any patient without a pulse
    B. Apply tourniquets to all extremity wounds high and tight and label the time, and move on to the next patient
    C. Apply pressure to chest wounds in sight only
    D. Begin CPR on any patients without a pulse and look for an AED

64. Which of the following is true regarding children and sports activity?

    A. Preteen athletes most commonly injure lower limbs, whereas teenagers injure upper limbs
    B. Salter-Harris II fractures generally require surgical intervention
    C. Joint dislocations and ligamentous injuries are more common than buckle and other types of fractures
    D. Physes close on average at 14.5 years of age in girls and 16.5 years of age in boys
    E. Non-union of fractures are common in the immature skeleton

65. The parents of a young female soccer player solicit your advice regarding general injury prevention strategies during an office visit. In providing recommendations, which of the following injury prevention methods has been proven effective?

    A. Neck strengthening programs for concussion
    B. Mouthguards for concussion
    C. Bracing for anterior cruciate ligament injury
    D. Neuromuscular training programs for anterior cruciate ligament injury
    E. Stretching programs for groin injury

66. Which of the following is true regarding sports participation in the athlete with a solitary kidney?

    A. Before clearing an athlete with a solitary kidney for sports, testing should be undertaken to ensure normal kidney function
    B. Kidney injuries are a common occurrence in sports
    C. Traumatic kidney injuries in sports usually warrant urgent surgery and have high potential to be catastrophic
    D. Athletes with one kidney should be discouraged from participation in contact or collision sports
    E. Specialized padding has been proven to be beneficial in protecting a solitary kidney from injury

67. You are performing a preparticipation physical evaluation (PPE) on the new college quarterback. It is noted in his history that he has cystic fibrosis. Prior to matriculating at the school, he played a full four years of high school football without a problem. Which of the following recommendations would you make as team physician?

    A. The athlete is not cleared because he has cystic fibrosis
    B. The athlete is cleared for full participation without further testing
    C. The athlete is required to have pulmonary function testing prior to clearance to evaluate lung capacity
    D. The athlete is required to have an exercise treadmill test prior to clearance to evaluate oxygen saturation during exercise
    E. The athlete is required to have an induced sputum culture to see if he needs prophylactic antibiotics during play

68. Which of the following statements regarding participation in competitive sports is most accurate in a patient with aortic stenosis (AS)?

    A. Patients with mild AS may participate in all sports and require no follow-up after initial testing
    B. Patients with moderate AS are allowed to participate in moderate-intensity static sports if an exercise tolerance test demonstrates satisfactory exercise capacity without symptoms or ECG changes, and the patient has a normal blood pressure response to exercise
    C. Patients with asymptomatic severe AS may participate in low-static- and low-dynamic-intensity competitive sports
    D. Patients with symptomatic moderate AS may participate in low-static- and low-dynamic-intensity sports with serial evaluations of AS severity on at least an annual basis
    E. Patients with severe AS should not engage in a low-intensity recreational walking program after being excluded from competitive sports, due to increased risk for syncope

69. A 25-year-old male Italian soccer player presents to you for his preparticipation physical evaluation. He complains of some shortness of breath with exercise. His family history is significant for an older brother who died from a heart-related issue while training in the military. Physical examination was within normal limits. Because of his family history, you decide to order a 12-lead ECG. The ECG shows T wave inversion in leads V1 to V3. A terminal notch in the QRS complex is noted (see image). You refer your patient to the cardiologist, where he undergoes a two-dimensional echocardiogram, which shows an enlarged, hypokinetic right ventricle, with a thin RV free wall. Your patient undergoes a cardiac biopsy, and several days later, you get a pathology report which reads "fibro-fatty infiltration of right ventricular free wall." What is your diagnosis based on the above?

A. Hypertrophic cardiomyopathy
B. Arrythmogenic right ventricular dysplasia
C. Anomalous coronary artery
D. Prolonged QT syndrome

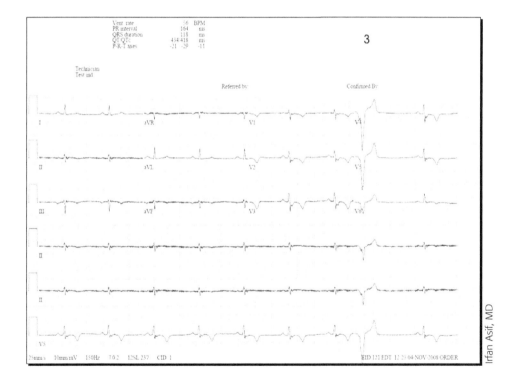

70. As part of a preparticipation physical evaluation, a 20-year-old previously healthy, asymptomatic African-American male college long distance runner has an ECG performed. Which of the following ECG findings is abnormal in athletes and warrants additional testing?

    A. Sinus arrhythmia
    B. Incomplete right bundle branch block
    C. Mobitz type II second degree AV block
    D. QRS voltage criteria for LVH

71. During the athletic preparticipation physical evaluation, which of the following findings would be concerning for hypertrophic cardiomyopathy?

    A. Normal auscultation findings
    B. Widening of second heart sound
    C. Midsystolic murmur that gets louder with standing or Valsalva maneuver
    D. Systolic ejection murmur at the upper right sternal border

72. During the preparticipation physical evaluation for athletes, you should look for non-cardiac signs of cardiovascular disease. Which of the following is a physical finding of Marfan syndrome?

    A. Thumb sign
    B. Elbow hyperextension
    C. Fibrillin-1 mutation
    D. Pes cavus

73. While evaluating a child for a preparticipation physical evaluation, you auscultate a murmur at the upper left sternal border. It is a crescendo-decrescendo murmur, and you are debating between a pathological murmur and an innocent murmur. Which of the following is true?

   A. An atrial septal defect (ASD) would have a murmur that has a normal S2 split and moves with respiration
   B. Pulmonic stenosis would present as a quiet murmur that can also be confused with an innocent murmur
   C. Patients with an ASD may also have a diastolic murmur that sounds like a rumble across the tricuspid valve area
   D. This murmur may be the initial finding in a patient with aortic stenosis
   E. If this murmur decreases in intensity when the patient stands, it could be a finding of hypertrophic cardiomyopathy

74. A 13-year-old male middle school soccer player presents for a preparticipation physical evaluation (PPE). He is asymptomatic, has a normal physical examination, and his family history is negative for cardiovascular disease. His PPE should include?

   A. An electrocardiogram, because he is male
   B. An electrocardiogram, because he plays soccer
   C. An electrocardiogram, because he is 13 years old
   D. An electrocardiogram is not routinely indicated

75. Which of the following statements regarding endurance and fluid replacement exercise is true?

   A. Older athletes have increased thirst sensitivity when dehydrated
   B. Prehydration has not been proven to help prevent dehydration during exercise
   C. Hydration plans should have a goal of preventing > 2% weight loss from water deficit
   D. Body size and speed should be disregarded when developing hydration plans

76. A 15-year-old female soccer player complains of right hip pain. Her pain began one week ago, after running sprints at soccer practice. Lifting her leg, flexing her hip, and running make the pain worse. On exam, she is focally tender over the anterior superior iliac spine (ASIS). Pelvic x-rays reveal that she is skeletally immature. You diagnose her with ASIS apophysitis. Which muscle originates at the location of her injury?

   A. Sartorius
   B. Rectus femoris
   C. Biceps femoris, long head
   D. Gracilis

77. Which of the following statements is true of congenital coronary artery anomalies?

   A. Diagnosis is based on abnormalities on 12-lead electrocardiogram
   B. Coronary artery anomalies are the most common cause of sudden cardiac death in athletes
   C. The most common anomaly is a single right coronary artery, with an absent left coronary artery
   D. All athletes with anomalous coronary arteries will experience symptoms (e.g., chest pain, syncope) at some point in time
   E. Blood flow may be compromised during exertion, resulting in ischemia and fatal arrhythmia

78. Which of the following is true of hypertrophic cardiomyopathy (HCM)?

   A. HCM is a genetic disorder with an autosomal recessive pattern of inheritance
   B. HCM is characterized by right ventricular wall thickness of > 5 mm
   C. The murmur associated with HCM is exacerbated by the Valsalva maneuver
   D. Most patients have detectible signs of HCM before sudden death
   E. Gold standard for diagnosis is cardiac CT

79. A 15-year-old male comes to you for his preparticipation physical evaluation. He has a positive family history of Marfan syndrome in an older sibling, who has been restricted from collision sports. By history, this young man denies any ocular, cardiovascular, or pulmonary concerns. On examination, he is found to have positive wrist and thumb signs, pes planus, minor pectus carinatum, joint hypermobility, and a high arched palate. You find no skin or cardiopulmonary abnormalities on examination. Which statement is correct for further assessment of this child?

   A. Although he has positive family history and skeletal findings, there is no evidence for involvement of a third system, therefore no additional workup is needed
   B. Send for ophthalmology evaluation and transesophageal echocardiogram
   C. Get a one-time normal radiograph of the lumbar spine and both hips to rule out protrusio acetabulae and scoliosis and, if normal, no additional workup is needed
   D. No additional workup is needed; simply ban the child from contact or collision sports, as a precaution

80. A 19-year-old male college lacrosse player complains of a "racing and pounding" heart beat intermittently during lacrosse practice for the past two weeks. It lasts for a few minutes and then resolves. He denies any chest pain, syncope, radiation, nausea, or difficulty breathing. He is otherwise healthy and has no family history of cardiac disease or unexplained sudden death. You obtain an ECG (see image), which shows normal sinus rhythm, with a delta wave and a shortened PR interval. To determine if the patient has the antidromic or orthodromic form of this condition, what would you do next to test for this?

   A. Signal averaged ECG
   B. Transesophageal echocardiogram
   C. Cardiac MRI
   D. Electrophysiology study
   E. 12 lead ECG treadmill stress test

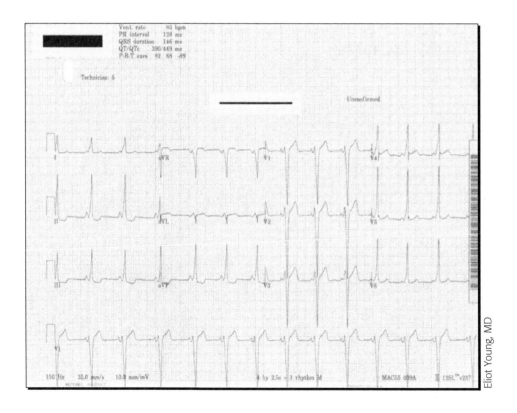

81. Which of the following is correct?

    A. Congenital sensorineural deafness is associated with long QT syndrome
    B. Albuterol should be encouraged in patients with suspected congenital prolonged QT interval
    C. Taking ciprofloxacin does not prolong the QT interval
    D. Athletes with known prolonged QT can be cleared to run the 110 meter hurdles, but not to run the 1500 meters in track and field

82. Which of the following test results is considered the most sensitive test for diagnosing exercise-induced bronchospasm in athletes?

    A. A decrease of FEV1 by 10% in a field-exercise challenge test
    B. A drop of FEV1 of 10% from baseline in an eucapnic voluntary hyperventilation test
    C. A decrease of 20% of FEV1 from baseline on a methacholine challenge test
    D. An elevation of exhaled nitric oxide greater than 15 ppb
    E. All of the above

83. A 25-year-old very competitive female track athlete notes that she develops throat tightness, dyspnea, and an audible inspiratory stridor while running during competition. Her symptoms seem to resolve within five minutes of stopping her event. The symptoms seem to be very mild or be absent during her routine training and practice. What is her most likely diagnosis?

    A. Asthma
    B. Exercise-induced bronchospasm
    C. Vocal cord dysfunction
    D. Malingering

84. A 30-year-old male presents with worsening hip pain over the past six months. He points to the area of the groin as the area of maximal pain and demonstrates a "C sign." He recalls stepping funny in a pothole a few years ago while running, but no other trauma or injury. He reports pain is worst with internal rotation of the hip in yoga. He reports catching without locking. You suspect a labral tear, with possible femoral acetabular impingement (FAI). Which of the following clinical tests will be most helpful to confirm your suspected diagnosis?

    A. FABER (flexion abduction external rotation) test
    B. Impingement test (internal rotation of the hip while flexed to 90 degrees)
    C. Thomas test (flexion of the unaffected hip causing concomitant flexion of the affected hip)
    D. Ober's test

85. While working as the team physician for a local high school football team, you are approached by the parents of one of the junior linebackers. Recently, after his second episode of transient quadriparesis, the player had an MRI showing severe cervical spinal stenosis and cord compression. He was advised by the neurosurgical specialist to no longer play football or other contact sports. He now exhibits no neurologic signs or symptoms. Both the player and his parents voice understanding of the risk of catastrophic injury, yet desire for him to continue playing, so that he can "hopefully get a college scholarship and possibly play professionally one day." What is the best course of action to protect yourself legally if the player were to resume playing football?

    A. Have the player complete an "exculpatory waiver" or "risk release," releasing the physician and the activity sponsor from any liability
    B. Have the player and his parents complete an "exculpatory waiver" or "risk release," releasing the physician and the activity sponsor from any liability
    C. Have the player and his parents hand-write and sign a letter indicating their understanding of the risks of continued participation
    D. Complete a standard waiver indicating the risks of continued participation and have it signed by the player and his parents, and then allow the athlete to return, since both the player and the parents voiced understanding of the risks

86. A 35-year-old female long distance runner who is training for a marathon by running 50-70 miles per week presents with a one-month history of right anterior hip and groin pain. The pain develops after two miles of running and is alleviated by stopping. Her examination demonstrates right anterior groin tenderness to palpation over the pubic ramus, as well as pain with hopping on the affected leg. Which of the following statements is correct with regard to the diagnosis of a pubic ramus stress fracture?

   A. Men are more susceptible to pubic rami stress fractures than women
   B. A positive radionuclide bone scan definitively confirms the diagnosis of a pubic ramus stress fracture
   C. A small avulsion fracture off the inferior pubic ramus is pathognemonic of a pubic ramus stress fracture
   D. Pubic rami stress fractures are caused by the adductor and gracilus muscles pulling on the lateral aspect of the pubic ramus

87. Which of the following is considered a significant risk for hamstring strain injury?

   A. Previous hamstring strain
   B. Young age (adolescent)
   C. Female gender
   D. Hamstring to quadriceps ratio of 0.6

88. You move to a rural area, where you are the only sports physician in town. You want to set up a relationship with the local high school to become their team physician. This high school, however, only has one athletic trainer and has never had a team physician before. They ask you what your role will be. Which of the following is a role of the team physician?

   A. Provide for appropriate education and counseling regarding nutrition, strength and conditioning, ergogenic aids, substance abuse, and other medical problems that could affect the athlete
   B. Provide medical advice for the teachers and the custodian
   C. Ask the high school athletic director to establish a chain of command for injury and illness management
   D. Dismiss the need for proper documentation and medical record keeping

89. A 16-year-old cross country skier presents with her mother for management of her exercise-induced bronchospasm. She has not been diagnosed with asthma, and has been managed with an inhaled beta-2 agonist prior to exercise, along with a proper warm-up. Unfortunately, she is still experiencing chest tightness and wheezing when racing, which is affecting her participation. Her mother wants to know what else can be done. Which of the following is the next best step in management?

    A. Add an inhaled corticosteroid 15 minutes prior to exercise
    B. Add a diet high in omega-3 fatty acids
    C. Add an oral beta-2 agonist, along with methylxanthines, 15 minutes prior to exercise
    D. Add inhaled cromolyn sodium 15 minutes prior to exercise

90. A 32-year-old female has been training for a marathon for four months. She complains of right lateral knee pain, exacerbated with running, climbing stairs, and riding a bicycle. The pain is reproducible to palpation along the lateral knee, 2 cm superior to joint line. Range of motion is pain-free and normal. There is no joint effusion. She has decreased her mileage over the last two weeks and has tried local ice application and oral anti-inflammatory medications, which have provided temporary improvement. What should be the next consideration in treatment?

    A. Stop training
    B. Physical therapy
    C. Corticosteroid injection
    D. Referral to orthopaedic surgeon

91. A fit 58-year-old male with bright red rectal bleeding and known hemorrhoids presents to your office following a rowing marathon. Which one of the following is appropriate?

   A. Treat his hemorrhoids conservatively, avoid constipation, and watch for further bleeding
   B. Ask to see him in the office for a rectal examination and guaiac assessment, and follow his case clinically if the guaiac test is negative
   C. Ask him to call the office if the bleeding recurs, otherwise, no other assessment is needed
   D. A colonoscopy should be recommended

92. Regarding strength training in children and adolescents, which of the following is true?

   A. There is no minimal age requirement for participation in strength training, but each participant should have the maturity to accept and follow directions
   B. Strength training does not improve performance or reduce the risk of injury in children and adolescents
   C. Strength training does not increase strength in children, because they do not have enough testosterone
   D. Strength training is unsafe and stunts growth

93. A 10-year-old male soccer player comes to the office complaining of two weeks of right knee pain. He reports the pain began after he struck the ball really hard when trying to shoot the ball. Since then, he has had persistent pain with running and kicking the ball. The pain is located at the inferior aspect of his patella. He denies any popping, swelling, or locking. His parents report that he usually will begin to limp after 30 minutes of playing soccer. He reports pain associated with running around playing in the backyard, as well as while using stairs. On examination, he has full active range of motion of both knees, with no extension lag. He is tender at the inferior pole of the patella on the right, and no effusion is present. He has pain with resisted knee extension test on the affected side. He has a mildly antalgic gait. You obtain the x-ray shown below. What is the diagnosis?

A. Patellar sleeve fracture
B. Osgood-Schlatter disease
C. Tibial tubercle avulsion fracture
D. Sinding-Larsen-Johannson syndrome
E. Patellar tendonitis

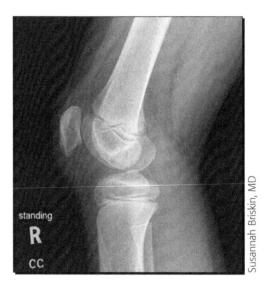

94. An 18-year-old female recreational athlete reports insidious onset of left-sided knee pain. The pain is pressure-like, behind the patella and worse with prolonged sitting. She denies any injury, swelling, locking, or instability. You find a tight lateral retinaculum on examination. Which of the examination findings suggest a tight retinaculum that can be seen with this condition?

    A. Decreased patella glide
    B. Positive single-leg squat
    C. Positive patella compression
    D. Positive patella apprehension

95. A 17-year-old football player complains of a six-month chronic history of vague knee pain in the anteromedial aspect of the knee. The pain is worsened with activities such as squatting, lunging, and going up and down stairs. It is relieved with icing and ibuprofen. There is no history of trauma. His knee examination is unremarkable, with the exception of a tender cord-like structure on the anteromedial aspect of the knee that reproduces a popping sensation and pain with extension from a flexed position. A diagnosis of plica syndrome is made. Which of the following is the mainstay of treatment for this condition?

    A. Activity modification, ice, scheduled anti-inflammatories, and physical therapy
    B. Immobilization with a straight leg brace for four weeks
    C. Orthopedic surgical referral for removal
    D. Medial heel wedges and a corticosteroid injection

96. Which of the following drugs is a risk factor for exertional rhabdomyolysis?

    A. Ibuprofen
    B. Sertraline
    C. Fexofenadine
    D. Lisinopril
    E. Methylphenidate

97. A football player is seeing you for a knee injury sustained in a recent game. Following the game, he noticed his left knee did not feel right. He played the entire game, but the left knee felt like it was going to give out when he was running and planting. As you examine the player, you are concerned that he may have suffered an injury to his posterior cruciate ligament. Which of the following is true regarding injury to the posterior cruciate ligament (PCL) in sport?

    A. Injury to the PCL in sport is common and accounts for the majority of knee-ligament injuries in sport
    B. The pivot shift test is the most sensitive and specific physical examination test for PCL injury
    C. A common mechanism for injury to the PCL in sport is a fall onto a flexed knee
    D. Most PCL injuries require surgery in order to allow athletes to return to sport

98. Avulsion of the iliotibial band off of Gerdy's tubercle, biceps femoris avulsion off of the fibular head, and popliteus avulsion are most like associated with which of the following knee injuries?

    A. Posterolateral complex injury
    B. Patellar dislocation
    C. Medial collateral ligament sprain
    D. Lateral meniscal tear

99. An athlete you see in clinic had 3+ proteinuria on a routine dipstick a week ago on his checkup. As per protocol, 48 hours later, abstaining from heavy exercise, you obtain a morning urinalysis (UA) in which the protein persists at 2+. There is no personal or family history of renal disease, anemia, hypertension, or medication usage (e.g., protein powder supplements, NSAIDs, antibiotics) that would suggest organic disease. What is the best next step in your workup of proteinuria?

    A. Referral for kidney biopsy
    B. Order a CBC, renal function, including full metabolic panel, fasting blood glucose
    C. 24-hour urine collection test
    D. Refer to nephrologist
    E. CT scan with thin cuts through renal, ureter and bladder

100. A 35-year-old male long distance recreational cyclist presents to your office with acute perineal pain and numbness. He is riding his bicycle several days per week. His genitourinary and neurologic examination is normal, and you offer a diagnosis of pudendal neuropathy. What is the most appropriate initial step in management?

   A. Medical management with gabapentin
   B. Physical therapy to address pelvic stabilization
   C. Ultrasound-guided nerve block
   D. Attention to bicycle fit and saddle adjustment
   E. Permanent cessation of bicycling

101. You are at the finish line medical aid station of a 161 km (100 miles) ultramarathon race in Arizona in April. You see a runner with fatigue and mild dizziness, who has completed the race in 25 hours. Otherwise, he is able to drink fluids. He has been urinating regularly and provides you his urine sample, which is bright yellow. His dizziness improves significantly after drinking some fluids. You decide to check him with a blood analyzer, and you note his creatinine (Cr) is 1.4 mg/dL (reference range 0.6 to 1.3 mg/dL) and his creatine kinase (CK) is 1,400 U/L (reference range 30 to 223 U/L). What would you do next?

   A. Advise him to keep drinking fluid and follow up only if he develops worsening of symptoms or his urine turns to dark color
   B. Give a bolus of 1 l of intravenous (IV) normal saline and recheck his creatinine and creatine kinase
   C. Treat his rhabdomyolysis with acidification of urine
   D. Refer him to a nearby hospital

102. A 37-year-old female triathlete presents with left lower extremity pain. She has been training for a marathon and has been increasing the intensity of her workout over the past month. On her examination, she has point tenderness over her mid-tibia and has a positive tuning fork sign. X-ray is negative for a fracture, but you order a bone scan that reveals a posterior mid-shaft tibial stress fracture. She is adamant about being able to compete in her marathon next month. What is the best option in this situation?

   A. Instruct her to continue her training and complete her race
   B. Refer her to physical therapy
   C. Put her in a pneumatic brace, with activity modification
   D. Refer her to orthopedic surgery for immediate surgery

103. Which of the following is the correct relationship of the median nerve of the wrist?

    A. Radial side of the palmaris longus tendon
    B. Ulnar side of the palmaris longus tendon
    C. Anterior to the palmaris longus tendon
    D. Posterior to the flexor pollicis longus tendon

104. Which of the following statements is true regarding nail disorders in athletes?

    A. The risk of ingrown toenails can be minimized by having the athlete wear shoes that are snug and minimize the sliding of the foot inside the shoe
    B. Trimming the toenails in a curved arc just distal to the free edge will minimize the risk of ingrown toenails
    C. Any collections of dark fluid beneath the nail bed should be immediately drained with a red-hot paper clip
    D. The persistence of a linear black band or streak running the length of the nail warrants further evaluation
    E. The treatment of choice for onychomycosis is a topical antifungal

105. You see a high school football player in the training room for an injury which occurred yesterday morning. He says his dog bit him on the arm. On examination, there is a 4-cm long laceration. The wound is fairly deep, but you see no injury to bone, muscle, or tendon. There is minimal erythema or swelling. He believes he had a tetanus shot within the last five years. What is the best initial management to prevent infection?

    A. Suture the wound
    B. Use a cyanoacrylate tissue adhesive to close the wound
    C. Irrigate and debride
    D. Give a Td booster

106. A 13-year-old male presents at your clinic after sustaining an injury during skiing. His lower left leg was cut by his ski blade (see image below). His past medical and social histories are unremarkable. What would be the best management option after irrigating the wound?

    A. A referral to an orthopedic surgeon
    B. Wound closure with tissue adhesives (e.g., Dermabond)
    C. Wound closure with 4/0 silk
    D. Wound closure with 4/0 monofilament nylon
    E. Wound closure with 4/0 polyglycolic acid sutures (e.g., Vicryl)

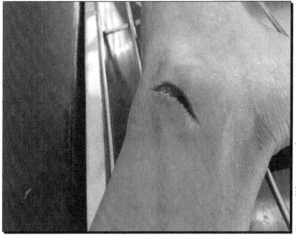

107. In relation to exercise and its effects on the immune system, which of the following is correct?

    A. Exercising while acutely ill leads to enhancement of the immune system called the open window
    B. Moderate, short bouts of exercise can increase circulating IgA levels, leading to a decreased risk of infection
    C. High-intensity exercise stimulates T-cell proliferation, leading to a decreased risk of a viral infection
    D. Endurance running for longer than 60 minutes leads to a decreased rate of infection

108. A 25-year-old soccer athlete presents to your office for further evaluation of bilateral lower extremity pain associated with numbness of the first web space of the foot. The onset of symptoms typically begins after running for 10 minutes and ceases immediately after rest. Which of the following describes the pathophysiology?

   A. An abnormal increase in muscle compartment pressure interferes with tissue circulation, causing temporary ischemia and neurological deficits
   B. During exercise, muscles are perfused, but neurologic structures are compressed
   C. Compartment pressures increase, due to hyperperfusion
   D. Improved muscle blood flow during exercise results in ischemic pain and impaired muscle function

109. A 43-year-old female runner presents to clinic with medial ankle and foot pain. She states the pain has been present for three months and is gradually getting worse. She reports no specific injury or trauma. She has taken ibuprofen, rested, and used ice, with some improvement. However, the pain recurs when she resumes running. Her examination is remarkable for tenderness and mild swelling posterior and inferior to the medial malleolus. Subtle weakness is appreciated with resisted plantarflexion and inversion of the foot compared to the opposite side. With weight-bearing inspection, a mild pes deformity is present. What is the most appropriate treatment option?

   A. Tenosynovectomy with tendon debridement
   B. Orthotic with rehabilitation exercises
   C. Corticosteroid injection within the posterior tibialis tendon sheath
   D. Rigid foot-ankle brace with activity

110. A wrestler comes in during his preseason training with concerns of localized hair loss of his posterior scalp. This is associated with about six weeks of pruritis and an occasional burning sensation. On examination, you observe mild erythema over a well-demarcated patch of alopecia, with small black dots noted flush to the surface of the skin. He has a single, moderately tender, enlarged occipital lymph node, but otherwise his dermatological and remaining examination is negative. Which of the following is true regarding this condition?

   A. Precautions for avoiding sharing of hats and combs is not necessary
   B. Monitoring liver function is recommended, with medicines required for treatment
   C. This condition responds well to topical medication
   D. A minimum of 72 hours of treatment is required by NCAA prior to return to competition

111. While in the athletic training room on a Tuesday, you are asked to see a 17-year-old high school wrestler with a rash on his arm. On examination, there are two raised, scaly, ring-shaped lesions, with irregular erythematous borders on the volar aspect of his left arm (see image). He asks if he can wrestle in the upcoming regional championships the coming Saturday. In addition to recommending an appropriate occlusive covering on the affected site, what would you advise him?

    A. May compete without further restriction
    B. May compete if he has a minimum of 72 hours of treatment with an oral antiviral
    C. May compete if he has a minimum of 120 hours of treatment with an oral antifungal
    D. May compete if he has a minimum of 72 hours of treatment with a topical or oral antifungal

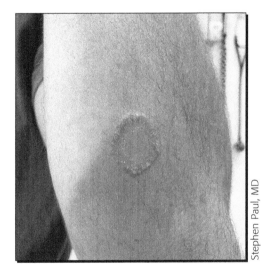

112. A 15-year-old male lacrosse player presents with a three-month history of left shin pain. He was diagnosed with a stress fracture and has been wearing a fracture boot for six weeks without improvement. The pain, which is worse at night, is relieved by ibuprofen. His imaging is below. What is the most appropriate next step?

   A. Strict non-weight-bearing
   B. Continue the fracture boot for six weeks
   C. Radiofrequency ablation
   D. Bone scan

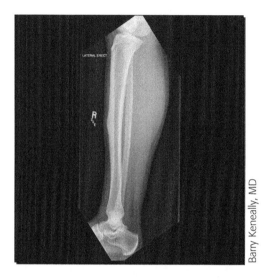

113. During knee flexion, the primary restraints to medial and lateral translation of the patella change. When the knee is in 30 to 60 degrees of flexion, what is the primary restraint?

   A. Vastus medialis oblique (VMO)
   B. Medial patellofemoral ligament (MPFL)
   C. Femoral trochlear groove
   D. Lateral retinaculum

114. Which of the following nerves innervates the skin of the first dorsal web space of the foot?

    A. Sural nerve
    B. Saphenous nerve
    C. Lateral plantar nerve
    D. Deep peroneal nerve

115. A 17-year-old high school wrestler with a prior history of herpes skin outbreaks presents to you with a "typical outbreak" for him—a vesicular rash, with some surrounding erythema to his left anterior chest. There is no evidence of drainage or axillary lymphadenopathy. His examination is otherwise normal. He is hoping to compete tomorrow. Which is the most appropriate choice for treatment and return-to-play recommendations?

    A. Begin acyclovir, hold him from wrestling or other contact sports, and reevaluate in five days
    B. Cover the area with a sterile dressing, and allow the patient to participate tomorrow
    C. Begin acyclovir, hold from wrestling for two days
    D. Begin acyclovir, cover the area, and allow the patient to participate tomorrow

116. A Division I wrestler comes in for evaluation of a non-itchy skin breakout on his trunk. He states that he is feeling well, without fever, malaise, or other systemic symptoms. Within a 1 cm region, there are three small, firm, shiny, dome-shaped papules, each approximately 3 mm in size. On closer examination, these lesions have a shallow indentation and sit on a non-erythematous base (see image). He has a tournament in six days and wants to compete. According to NCAA regulations, which option for management will give him the best chance for participating?

    A. Acyclovir 800 mg orally twice daily for five days, and no new lesions for 72 hours prior to competition
    B. Mupirocin 2% ointment applied three times daily, without new lesions for 48 hours prior to competition
    C. Terbinafine 250 mg orally daily for at least 72 hours prior to competition
    D. Curettage and cover the area with a gas-permeable membrane with tape

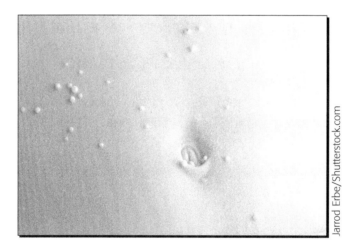

117. A 38-year-old female presents to your clinic with foot pain that began six weeks ago. She is an avid runner, but states that she has not made any changes to her training program or changed her shoes or running surface recently. She describes the pain as a burning sensation that radiates to her toes. What is the most common location for the lesion causing her pain?

    A. Between the second and third metatarsals
    B. Between the third and fourth metatarsals
    C. Between the fourth and fifth metatarsals
    D. Between the first and second metatarsals

118. You are providing skin checks at your high school's wrestling tournament. Upon close inspection, you notice that one wrestler has a scabbed-over lesion, with a small amount of discharge (see image below). He appears surprised, stating that he did not notice the lesion until just now. What would be your recommendations?

    A. He is allowed to participate today, as long as the lesion remains covered
    B. He is not allowed to participate until the lesion is dry, he has no new skin lesions for 48 hours, and he has completed 48 hours of directed antibiotics
    C. He is not allowed to participate until the lesion is dry, he has no new skin lesions for 24 hours, and he has completed 24 hours of directed antibiotics
    D. He is not allowed to participate until the lesion is dry, he has no new skin lesions for 48 hours, and he has completed 72 hours of directed antibiotics

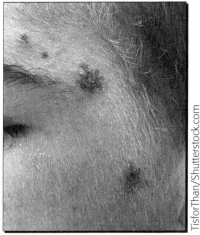

119. Which of following is a true statement with respect to adolescent idiopathic scoliosis?

    A. The less ossification there is at the iliac apophysis, the greater the potential for curve progression
    B. Tanner-Whitehouse methods of assessment use the epiphyses of the small bones in the foot to stage skeletal maturity
    C. The Risser grade is a measure of vertebral apophyseal fusion
    D. The majority of idiopathic scoliosis cases have a curvature that is convex to the left side

120. You have been treating a 36-year-old male runner for chronic recalcitrant right plantar fasciitis for several months. His pain has been consistently located at the plantar aspect of the calcaneus around the medial calcaneal tuberosity, without other bony tenderness, and worsens from the morning throughout the day while walking for his job. He denies numbness or paresthesias and has 5/5 strength in his foot, although he notes occasional discomfort when flexing or abducting his toes. He has had only limited response to treatments, including rest, night splinting, direct and indirect fascial massage and flexibility, oral medications, and a trial of booting and orthotics. Ultrasound imaging two months prior demonstrated a calcaneal osteophyte at the insertion of the plantar fascia and a mild thickening of the fascia itself, without evidence of degeneration. Due to his pain, limitations, and the chronicity of the problem, you decide to obtain an MRI. What would you expect to find on the MRI?

    A. Rupture of the plantar fascia
    B. Edema within the abductor digiti minimi
    C. Calcaneal stress fracture
    D. Tenosynovitis of the flexor digitorum longus

121. A 20-year-old college football player sustained an ankle injury in the first quarter of a game while being tackled. You evaluate him at halftime. He is able to partially bear weight on his injured ankle. He recalls his ankle being in a dorsiflexed position while sustaining an eversion injury. Which of the following would most likely suggest a syndesmotic ankle injury?

    A. Pain to palpation over the anterior talofibular ligament
    B. Pain along the anterior ankle when an external rotation force is placed on the ankle with the proximal leg stabilized and the ankle dorsiflexed
    C. Pain along the mid-calf level, with compression of the proximal fibula and tibia
    D. Decreased range of motion with plantarflexion

122. Which of the following is true concerning iron deficiency anemia?

    A. Males are more commonly affected than females
    B. Risk factors include chronic illness, heavy menstrual blood loss, and obesity
    C. Athletic performance is never affected by iron deficiency anemia
    D. Ferritin levels remain normal until the late stages of iron deficiency anemia

123. Which is the most common associated findings in athletic pseudo-anemia due to exercise?

    A. Normal hemoglobin; low MCV; low ferritin
    B. Low hemoglobin; normal MCV; normal/low ferritin
    C. Low hemoglobin; low MCV; elevated/normal ferritin
    D. Low hemoglobin; high MCV; normal/low ferritin

124. A 14-year-old soccer player kicked the soccer ball during an abrupt pass and felt intense pain in the anterior groin. She was unable to return to play. Which of the following supports the diagnosis of a pelvic avulsion fracture at the origin of the rectus femoris?

    A. Pain at the pubic tubercle
    B. Pain at the anterior margin of the iliac crest
    C. Pain at the anterior superior iliac spine
    D. Pain at the anterior inferior iliac spine

125. A 15-year-old female swimmer presents to your office with a complaint of mild neck stiffness for the last week. She has a past medical history significant for polyarticular juvenile idiopathic arthritis (JIA), which she has had since she was eight years old. It primarily involves the joints in her hands. She has been stable on her disease-modifying antirheumatic drugs prescribed by her rheumatologist. On examination, she is noted to have mild decreased extension of her cervical spine, but no tenderness, however. Given her past medical history, x-rays of her cervical spine are ordered. What is the most likely finding to be seen on these x-rays?

    A. Cervical spine fusion
    B. Normal x-rays
    C. Spinal stenosis
    D. Spondylolysis

126. A 12-year-old male baseball pitcher presents to the office with four months of experiencing mild intermittent right groin pain. Pain is an intermittent dull ache. It does not prevent him from playing. He reports running normally in his baseball games with no pain. He is the star pitcher on his all-star team, and is looking forward to playing this weekend. On physical examination, he has mild pain with right hip internal rotation, but full ROM compared to the left. Bilateral hip strength is normal. Gait is normal. Hamstrings and iliopsoas hip flexors are tight (the popliteal angle is 45 degrees bilaterally), a positive Thomas test. X-rays of the pelvis are shown below. What is the next best step in management?

   A. Follow up with orthopedic surgeon next week, do not play in baseball game this weekend
   B. Okay to play in baseball game, follow up if the pain increases
   C. Immediate transport to the emergency department for urgent orthopedic evaluation
   D. Referral to physical therapy to stretch hamstrings and hip flexors and follow up in four weeks

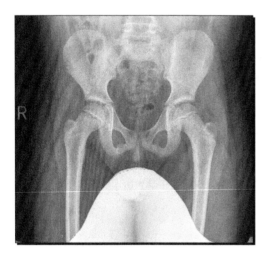
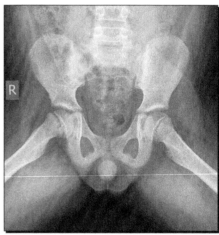

127. A 20-year-old male collegiate wrestler sustained a severe injury to his right shoulder during the beginning of the wrestling season. He required surgery, which precluded him from participating for the remainder of the season. He is in his junior year, and during his sophomore year, achieved multiple All-Conference honors, and was anticipated to be an All-American this year. His surgery and initial post-operative rehabilitation with his athletic trainer were unremarkable, and he was progressing on schedule. About six weeks post-op, he began having more trouble with rehabilitation. He described severe pain, became very angry, and stopped reporting for therapy, stating that it was painful and a waste of his time. A thorough evaluation by his surgeon did not reveal any structural reason for the setback. His friends disclose that he has been more withdrawn and angry, and he also recently broke up with his long-time girlfriend. Which is the best approach in the continuing treatment of this athlete?

   A. Modify the rehabilitation protocol to allow for more recovery time and a less strenuous schedule
   B. Prescribe pain medications to be taken prior to rehabilitation, as the pain response is most likely responsible for his set-back
   C. Report to the coaches that he is now non-compliant with his treatment
   D. Discuss and implement techniques for coping with stress and other psychological factors involved in injury recovery of a high-level athlete
   E. Recommend transfer of care to a physical therapist instead of the athletic trainer currently overseeing the rehabilitation process

128. A 13-year-old male presents with medial anterior knee pain. No knee effusion is present. X-rays and subsequent MRI show an osteochondritis dissecans lesion in the medial femoral condyle. The articular cartilage surface is intact; the physis is open. What is the next most appropriate step in management?

   A. Physical therapy
   B. Activity modification
   C. Surgery
   D. Observation

129. Although exercise is one form of treatment for a patient with depression, patients seen in a sports medicine setting are not immune to depression. Second-generation antidepressants, most commonly selective serotonin reuptake inhibitors (SSRIs), have been shown to be an effective pharmacological treatment for depression. How soon should a patient be seen after initiating pharmacological treatment for depression?

    A. Within one month
    B. Within two weeks
    C. Within two months
    D. In six months

130. A 10-year-old right-handed baseball catcher presents to your clinic with one month of right shoulder pain. He denies any acute injury to the shoulder, but states that his pain has progressively worsened over time. When the pain first started, he was pitching and decided to switch to catcher to give his arm a rest. Despite this switch, his pain has persisted. He has noticed that his accuracy and velocity have significantly decreased in the last week. Your examination is unhelpful, since the patient has diffuse tenderness to palpation, and most of your special tests are positive. You are suspicious the patient has Little League shoulder, so you order shoulder x-rays. You review the films with the patient and his father. Given that the x-rays look within normal limits, the father insists that he continues to play baseball and take ibuprofen for pain before his games. What is your next best step?

    A. Provide the family reassurance and encourage them to monitor their son for any worsening pain
    B. Consider obtaining an x-ray of the contralateral shoulder to compare with his opposite shoulder
    C. Allow the patient to continue to play catcher, but not pitch, while you start him in physical therapy
    D. Order an MRI to help definitively diagnose the etiology of the patient's pain

131. The following question refers to noninstitutionalized or community-dwelling asymptomatic adults without a history of fractures (defined as not residing in an assisted living facility, nursing home, or other institutional care setting). Which of the following statements is true regarding vitamin D supplementation and the prevention of fractures in adults without a history of osteoporosis or vitamin D deficiency?

    A. In community-dwelling, postmenopausal women, daily supplementation with ≤ 400 IU of vitamin D3 and ≤ 1,000 mg of calcium has no net benefit for the primary prevention of fractures
    B. There is clear evidence regarding the benefit of daily vitamin D and calcium supplementation for the primary prevention of fractures
    C. There are no risks to supplementation with 400 IU or less of vitamin D3 and 1,000 mg or less of calcium
    D. The USPSTF recommends against vitamin D supplementation to prevent falls in community-dwelling adults 65 years or older who are at increased risk of falls because of a history of recent falls or vitamin D deficiency

132. A high school freshman who normally throws the shotput comes into the office with severe hip pain that started yesterday after he ran the relay the last day of track practice. He was sprinting around the track and felt a pop. He fell and could not continue running. He was helped off the field and given crutches by his athletic trainer. On examination, he is tender to palpation over the anterior hip and cannot flex the hip more than a few degrees without significant pain. An x-ray in the office confirms your diagnosis of minimally displaced avulsion of the anterior superior iliac spine. Which of the following is true?

   A. The ASIS avulsion is due to a forceful contraction of the rectus femoris during sprinting
   B. You call your orthopedic partner to get the patient on the schedule for ORIF
   C. This type of injury may be misdiagnosed as an acute muscle strain
   D. CT scan is never helpful if this is a possible diagnosis on your differential

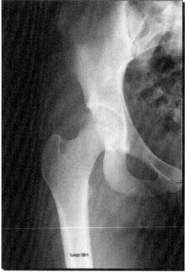

133. What is the medication class that is least likely to cause hypoglycemia during exercise?

   A. Insulin
   B. Sulfonylurea
   C. Biguanide
   D. Meglitinides

134. A thin 26-year-old male runner presents to your office with complaints of intermittent numbness and tingling over the distal anterolateral right lower leg and the dorsum of the right foot, sparing the web space of the first two toes. Upon further questioning, he reveals that this only occurs when he sits with his right leg crossed over his left leg, with the lateral aspect of his right lower leg approximately 8 cm proximal to the lateral malleolus resting on his contralateral knee. It will resolve quickly over a period of about 15 seconds after uncrossing the leg. The patient obliges to demonstrate his seated position. You examine him after he is able to recreate his symptoms and note normal vascular status on examination. You advise the patient to stop sitting in this fashion. Compressing of what structure is likely leading to his complaints?

   A. Deep peroneal nerve
   B. Popliteal artery
   C. Superficial peroneal nerve
   D. Lateral tibialis nerve
   E. L5 nerve root

135. A 20-year-old athlete comes into your office for counseling on a recent diagnosis of HIV. The athlete wants to know if they can exercise and take part in their sport. What advice do you give the athlete?

   A. Per NCAA regulations, an athlete with HIV cannot participate in an NCAA sport
   B. It is detrimental to the health of an HIV positive patient to participate in exercise
   C. Research has shown a high risk of HIV transmission in athletics
   D. HIV transmission risk is rare in athletics, although the risk is higher in some contact sports

136. A seven-year-old male presents to your clinic with a limp of recent onset. He has difficulty localizing his pain, but states that he did fall off his skateboard onto his knee several weeks ago, before his limp started. He has no other medical problems or significant past medical history. He denies any recent illnesses or fevers. He plays soccer and baseball. His parents have noticed the limp has gotten worse, but it has not kept him from playing his sports. What is your next course of action?

    A. Full knee examination with four view knee x-rays, and if negative, prescribe RICE and close observation
    B. AP and frog-leg lateral hip x-rays to rule-out slipped capital femoral epiphysis
    C. Complete examination of bilateral lower extremities with x-rays, and if negative, consider advanced imaging of the hip
    D. Provide parental reassurance, given that this is likely benign growing pains that should respond to rest, ice, and NSAIDs

137. A 42-year-old female runner presents to your office with a history of multiple joint pain that started after her return from a sprint distance triathlon in Michigan last week. Her diet, menses, and weight are unchanged. She runs about 15 to 20 miles a week, swims three miles per week and bikes 50 miles a week. She denies a fever but does feel flushed at times. No history of autoimmune condition exists in her family. Her vitals are normal and afebrile. She has a normal musculoskeletal examination outside of subjective joint soreness. Her skin examination shows the following lesion on her abdomen. The test you would most likely order FIRST is?

    A. CBC
    B. Lyme titre
    C. ANA
    D. Rheumatoid factor
    E. Thyroid stimulating hormone

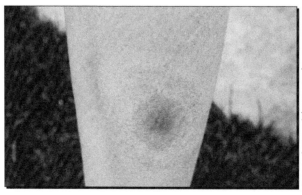

138. A 20-year-old military recruit comes into your office, concerned because he has been unable to run more than three or four miles at a time, due to right-leg cramping and weakness. Eventually, the pain forces him to stop running. He has been following a training plan without major increases in distance or time. His past medical history includes a left wrist fracture from a fall as a teenager. On examination, his pelvis is symmetrical without rashes. Palpation reveals moderate tightness of both lower extremities, right more than left. His distal pulses are 2+, with normal capillary refill. Reflex testing reveals 2+ patellar and Achilles reflexes. Proprioception is normal, although you find diminished sensation on the plantar surface of his right foot. With strength testing, he is weak with toe flexion and foot inversion. Compartment syndrome is highest on your differential, but which compartment is most likely affected?

    A. Anterior compartment
    B. Deep posterior compartment
    C. Lateral compartment
    D. Superficial posterior compartment

139. A six-year-old male presents to his primary care physician, complaining of a one-month history of progressive heel pain that worsens with increased activity. The pain initially started when he began kindergarten, which his parents attributed to him being more active. They have now noticed that he will intermittently limp and is complaining of pain on a daily basis. They have not tried any interventions up to this point in time. His mom feels that he limits his daytime activities to minimize pain. On examination, he is tender to palpation overlying the calcaneus primarily on the plantar and medial and lateral aspects. He has full range of motion of ankles, knees, and hips, without effusion. There is no swelling, and he is not limping in clinic today. He hops on his toes on the involved side to minimize pain. What do you do next?

    A. Recommend conservative treatment for Sever's disease
    B. Obtain radiographs of the patient's foot to evaluate for the appearance of the calcaneal apophysis
    C. Provide mom with reassurance that this is most likely related to his growth and will spontaneously resolve
    D. Recommend further evaluation with a CBC, ESR, CRP, and rheumatologic panel

140. What are the four structures that form the boundaries of the quadrilateral space?

    A. Teres major, teres minor, humeral neck, long head of triceps
    B. Infraspinatus, teres minor, humeral neck, long head of triceps
    C. Infraspinatus, teres minor, deltoid, long head of the triceps
    D. Teres major, teres minor, deltoid, humeral neck

141. A 16-year-old female basketball player presents with five days of sore throat, fever, and fatigue. On examination, she has an exudative pharyngitis and posterior cervical lymphadenopathy. She has a playoff game scheduled for the weekend and wants to know if she can play. Which of the following tests is the most sensitive and could assist with the decision to allow the athlete to play?

    A. Heterophile antibody-latex agglutination (Monospot)
    B. Viral capsid antigen IgM
    C. Viral capsid antigen IgG
    D. Complete blood count

142. A 16-year-old male competitive soccer player competes year-round on his high school team, as well as on a club team. He has displayed declining performance, despite intense training. His grades have been worsening at school over the past six months, and he has recently lost weight, due to decreased appetite. He reports achy calf muscles. What is the best diagnosis?

    A. Iron deficiency
    B. Overtraining
    C. Mononucleosis
    D. Somatization

143. Which of the following muscle fiber types is most often associated with early fatigue and predominately anaerobic activity?

    A. Type I
    B. Type Iα
    C. Type IIA
    D. Type IIB

144. A 10-year-old gymnast reports acute onset right buttock pain after doing the splits. Examination reveals tenderness to palpation over the right ischium. She has difficulty actively extending the hip and increased pain with passive hip flexion. Based on the history and physical examination, what would you recommend?

   A. X-rays to evaluate for apophyseal avulsion fracture
   B. Rest for treatment of a hamstring strain
   C. Rehabilitation for treatment of piriformis syndrome
   D. Oral steroid course for treatment of a lumbar radiculopathy

145. A 16-year-old male presents to your office for a preparticipation physical evaluation. He is a competitive high-school wrestler, and has previously missed several competitions due to herpes simplex infections. Upon further questioning, he admits to six episodes during the last year, with no episodes prior to that. His father, who is also his wrestling coach, would like to have him started on suppression therapy during the season. He is asymptomatic today. What would you recommend?

   A. No medication, until you can verify active lesions
   B. Acyclovir 400 mg five times daily during wrestling season
   C. HSV serology testing to confirm the diagnosis, and valacyclovir 1 g daily during wrestling season
   D. Griseofulvin 500 mg daily during wrestling season

146. You are the physician covering a mid-summer track and field meet, conducted at a local college for middle school athletes. It is already 90 degrees Fahrenheit (32.2 degrees Celsius) at 9 o'clock in the morning, and local weather forecasts are predicting record highs with 80% humidity. You are extremely concerned for heat illness in the athletes. Which of the following is true regarding pediatric athletes?

   A. Children have a smaller body-surface-to-body-mass ratio than adults, making children more likely to gain heat from the environment
   B. Children have decreased heat production per kilogram of body mass when compared to adults, leading to slower increases in body temperature in warm weather
   C. The sweating rate in children is lower than in adults, making it harder for children to dissipate heat through sweat evaporation
   D. When dehydrated, the body temperature in children rises slower than in an adult

147. A 12-year-old male baseball pitcher presents to the office with medial elbow pain that began gradually. On examination, he is Tanner stage 2, with pain over the medial epicondyle area, mild pain with valgus stress, negative Tinel's over medial elbow. He has normal elbow and wrist strength. What is his most likely diagnosis?

    A. Medial epicondylitis
    B. Ulnar collateral ligament strain
    C. Medial epicondyle apophysitis
    D. Medial epicondyle avulsion fracture

148. In a patient diagnosed with a C6 cervical radiculopathy on the right-hand side, what would you expect to find?

    A. Pain radiating from the neck to the lateral arm and the right thumb, weak biceps and wrist extensors, decreased sensation along the lateral forearm and thumb, and an altered brachioradialis reflex compared to the contralateral side
    B. Pain radiating into the shoulder and right lateral arm, decreased sensation along the right lateral arm, and an altered biceps reflex on the right side
    C. Pain in the lower neck and trapezius region, as well as a sensory deficit in a cape distribution
    D. Pain in the ulnar region of the right forearm, weakness in the right intrinsic finger muscles, and a decreased sensation on the right ulnar aspect of the forearm

149. You are evaluating a 27-year-old recreational tennis player. She felt some searing chest wall pain on her dominant side while extending for a forehand shot three days ago. On her examination today, you notice substantial bruising along the anterior chest wall, suggesting some soft-tissue injury. You begin by palpating the pectoralis major muscle. Of the following points, which one is least helpful when trying to palpate the pectoralis major?

    A. Sternum
    B. Clavicle
    C. Second to sixth ribs
    D. Humerus
    E. Coracoid process

150. Which of the following statements is true concerning the respiratory system during pregnancy?

   A. Tidal volume decreases
   B. Vital capacity is unchanged
   C. Minute ventilation is unchanged
   D. Reserve volumes increase

151. A 21-year-old male presents to your clinic with lower back pain that began suddenly after performing a squatting exercise at the campus recreation center four weeks ago. He has been resting and taking ibuprofen, but the pain is not improving. Which examination findings support the diagnosis of an L3/L4 disc herniation?

   A. Numbness along the lateral aspect of the foot
   B. An absent patellar reflex
   C. Weakness with plantarflexion of the foot
   D. Weakness with extension of the great toe

152. A 25-year-old male who is preparing to travel to high altitude requests a prescription for acetazolamide. He denies prior altitude illness. He has no underlying chronic disease. Which statement is true of this medication?

   A. Masks the symptoms of acute mountain sickness
   B. Causes decreased urination
   C. Will cause a dry cough and increasing dyspnea at increasing altitude
   D. Could cause paresthesias of hands, feet, and periorbital region

153. A 24-year-old female patient presents to your office with right ear pain and decreased hearing. It started three days ago while she was ascending from scuba diving. She denies recent illness. She denies any discharge from the ear. Her examination shows a bloody infiltrate in the middle ear. How should this be treated?

   A. Symptomatic relief
   B. Tympanotomy
   C. Typmanostomy tube
   D. Antibiotics

154. Which of the following statements is true regarding innervation of the hamstring?

    A. The hamstring musculotendinous unit is solely innervated by the tibial branch of the sciatic nerve
    B. The hamstring musculotendinous unit is solely innervated by the peroneal branch of the sciatic nerve
    C. The biceps femoris is innervated by both the peroneal branch and the tibial branch of the sciatic nerve
    D. The semimembranosus is innervated by both the peroneal branch and the tibial branch of the sciatic nerve

155. A 15-year-old female who plays soccer presents to your clinic with a two-month history of anteromedial knee pain. She denies any injury, and her pain comes and goes. The pain is worse with the knee in flexion, and she complains of some painful popping as well. Her examination shows tenderness to palpation just medial to the patellofemoral joint, with palpation of a rope-like structure and some localized swelling to the same area. There is no joint effusion. Ligaments are intact on examination. McMurray's and Thessaly's tests are negative. What is your suspected diagnosis and what imaging would you order to confirm your diagnosis?

    A. Medial plica syndrome; MRI
    B. Medial meniscal tear; MRI
    C. Medial plica syndrome; no imaging
    D. Pes anserine bursitis; ultrasound

156. A 12-year-old female soccer player presents to your sports medicine clinic with a right wrist injury. She was playing soccer yesterday, when she fell onto her right arm. After developing pain and swelling, she was taken to a local emergency room, where x-rays revealed a Salter-Harris type II fracture of the right distal radius. Which one of the following statements regarding Salter-Harris type II fracture is correct?

    A. The most common type of Salter-Harris fracture
    B. A fracture through the physis and epiphysis
    C. An intra-articular fracture at risk for chronic disability
    D. Best visualized with diagnostic ultrasound

157. What is the best treatment for an athlete with a tarsal navicular stress fracture?

    A. Minimum of four weeks of non-weight-bearing cast immobilization
    B. Minimum of six weeks of non-weight-bearing cast immobilization
    C. Weight-bearing-boot immobilization for four to six weeks, followed by rehabilitation and progression based on symptoms
    D. Surgical intervention to return the athlete to sport sooner

158. A collegiate distance runner has been seeing you for chronic exertional lower leg pain for over six months. She has tried a period of rest, medication, and physical therapy. Testing to date has been normal, including plain radiographs, bone scan, intra-compartmental pressure measurement, and EMG/NCS. You decide to proceed with yet another study to evaluate this young runner's leg pain. What is an important consideration in ordering your next imaging study or test?

    A. Perform the study with the foot in neutral, passive dorsiflexion, and maximum active plantarflexion
    B. Add contrast to the study for better visualization
    C. Have the patient rest for several weeks, before performing the next study
    D. Ensure the patient is fasting after midnight the day before

159. A 45-year-old ultramarathon runner presents to your office two days after his most recent ultramarathon complaining of anterior ankle pain. He reports no pain during the race, but significant anterior ankle pain starting the morning after the race. He is able to bear weight on the ankle, but has pain with walking and has not yet attempted running. There is mild swelling and no ecchymosis. On examination, there is crepitus as you palpate over a tendon closer to the medial aspect of the anterior ankle. He has pain with resisted dorsiflexion and inversion, and he has no pain with resisted great toe extension. Which muscle tendon is the source of his symptoms?

    A. Extensor hallucis longus
    B. Extensor digitorum longus
    C. Fibularis (peroneus) tertius
    D. Tibialis anterior

160. The most accurate test for a posterior cruciate ligament (PCL) injury is which of the following?

    A. Posterior sag test
    B. Quadriceps active test
    C. Posterior drawer test
    D. Reverse pivot-shift test
    E. Pivot-shift test

161. A 40-year-old male runner presents to your clinic with right lateral knee pain. This has been going on for the past six months and worsened with running or walking downhill. On palpation, the pain is localized to the lateral femoral condyle. Ober's test and Noble's test are equivocal. McMurray's test is normal, and hyperflexion of his knee does not reproduce his pain. Varus stress test of the knee is normal. The pain is reproduced with resisted active internal rotation of the tibia with the patient lying prone and his knee flexed to 30 degrees. X-rays of the knee are normal. The patient has been in physical therapy for the past four months, without any improvement of his pain. What is your diagnosis?

    A. Iliotibial band syndrome
    B. Lateral meniscus tear
    C. Lateral collateral ligament sprain
    D. Popliteus tendinopathy

162. A 16-year-old male pitcher is pitching in the high school playoffs. Being a sports medicine physician, you are interested in watching his biomechanics. Which of the following events in the pitching motion best describes the late cocking phase?

    A. Starting with initial movement of the contralateral lower extremity and ending with the elevation of the lead leg to its highest point and the ball being removed from the glove
    B. Starting when the lead leg reaches its maximum height and the ball is removed from the glove and ending when the lead foot contacts the pitching mound
    C. Starting with lead foot contact and ending with the point of maximal external rotation of the throwing shoulder
    D. Starting with maximal external rotation of the throwing shoulder and ending with ball release
    E. Starting with ball release and ending with maximal humeral internal rotation and elbow extension

163. Tibial plateau fractures are uncommon, occurring in less than 1% of all fractures. What are the indications for surgery for tibial plateau fracture?

   A. Athletes wishing for faster return to play
   B. Osteoporosis, age over 65 years, or other co-morbidities
   C. Lateral margin location
   D. Displaced fracture, compartment syndrome, neurovascular compromise, or knee laxity or instability

164. While performing an examination on a patient who presented to your clinic for hand weakness, you notice that she is unable to hold her fingers in abduction against resistance on the right, but is able to on the left. Sensation is intact over both upper extremities, as is her strength in extension and flexion of the wrist and fingers. Her Hoffman's sign is negative bilaterally. Which of the following would most likely explain these physical examination findings?

   A. A spinal cord lesion causing myelopathy at the level of C5
   B. A disc bulge at C4 causing central cord compression
   C. Compression of the deep branch of the ulnar nerve at the wrist
   D. Compression of the superficial branch of the ulnar nerve at the wrist
   E. Compression of the inferior trunk of the brachial plexus

165. You saw a 32-year-old male in your office seven days ago, and you diagnosed him with lumbar radiculopathy. As part of the treatment plan, you place him on a two-week course of naproxen 500mg twice daily. He returns to your office today complaining of epigastric pain. You diagnose him with NSAID-induced gastritis. The patient questions you on other possible adverse reactions to taking NSAIDs. Which of the following is true regarding adverse reactions to NSAIDs?

   A. NSAID-induced gastritis is due to a lack of gastric mucosa, protective leukotriene production inhibited by NSAIDs
   B. Interstitial nephritis is a prostaglandin mediated kidney injury seen in patients taking NSAIDs
   C. Celecoxib, a COX-2 inhibitor, has an increased incidence of clotting dysfunction compared to nonselective NSAIDs, because of inhibition of COX-2's synthesis of thromboxane
   D. Side effects of NSAIDs are due to the pharmacologic action of the drug itself or an Ig-E mediated drug hypersensitivity reaction
   E. NSAIDs irreversibly bind to platelets, leading to increases in bleeding time

166. Creatine enhances athletic performance by which mechanism?

   A. Decreasing lactate threshold
   B. Increasing muscle phosphocreatine concentration
   C. Decreasing calcium uptake in sarcoplasmic reticulum
   D. Earlier muscle glycogen use

167. Which of the following diagnostic tests is most likely to help confirm the diagnosis of piriformis syndrome?

   A. Straight leg raise
   B. Freiburg sign
   C. X-ray pelvis
   D. MRI pelvis
   E. EMG

168. Physiologic and performance effects of human growth hormone (hGH) include which of the following?

   A. Increases muscle strength
   B. Decreases heart rate
   C. Increases lean body mass
   D. Increases workload capacity

169. A 73-year-old female presents to your office because she heard that flexibility exercises are important for older individuals. Her goal is to be able to maintain her activities of daily living, like dressing and walking. She wants to know how often and when to stretch. Which of the following best summarizes the current recommendations regarding stretching?

   A. Flexibility exercises should be performed at least twice a week for at least 10 minutes and be done when the body is warmed up
   B. Flexibility exercises should be performed daily, but held for 10 seconds or less due to age-related tendinopathy
   C. Flexibility exercises should be performed at least twice a week for 10 minutes at the beginning of the workout
   D. Flexibility exercises should not be performed after age 65

170. A 33-year-old white female presents with a 14-month history of pelvic pain following the birth of her son. She has abnormal x-rays of the pelvis. She had improved with rest, but experienced aggravation of her pain with return to running. Diagnosis of osteitis pubis was confirmed by examination and MRI of pelvis. She was successfully treated with injection of the pubic symphysis with steroid, sacroiliac stabilization belt, and physical therapy. Which of the following is a true statement about osteitis pubis?

    A. Osteitis pubis is generally a surgical problem
    B. Osteitis pubis is generally treatable with rest and rehabilitation
    C. Osteitis pubis is rarely seen in running athletes
    D. Osteitis pubis is best imaged by radiograph of the pelvis

171. Which of the following is a physiologic adaptation to ascent to high altitude?

    A. A decrease in cardiac output
    B. An increase in pulmonary artery pressure
    C. Worsening ventilation-perfusion matching
    D. A decrease in alveolar ventilation

172. What is the maximal lactate steady state (MLSS) during exercise testing?

    A. Refers to the exercise intensity at which blood lactate removal is surpassed by lactate production, and lactate begins to accumulate above baseline levels
    B. Refers to the highest exercise intensity at which no significant rise in blood lactate occurs with continued exercise over time
    C. Refers to when blood lactate concentration rises by 1 mmol/L above exercise baseline
    D. Occurs during exercise at a respiratory exchange ratio (RER or R) of 0.85

173. What is the correct physiological adaptation of the respiratory system to exercise?

    A. Mean arterial PCO_2 decreases, due to increased ventilatory rate
    B. Ventilation to perfusion ratios (V/Q) become more uneven throughout the lung tissues
    C. Increase in arterial pH, due to rapid renal buffering
    D. Increase in pulmonary blood flow as a percentage of cardiac output

174. A 16-year-old male volleyball player presented to your office six weeks ago with the complaint of vague posterior right shoulder pain and no history of trauma. He was referred to physical therapy for rotator cuff and periscapular strengthening, with little success. Unfortunately, his symptoms have continued, and he is unable to play volleyball, secondary to pain and weakness. He denies any numbness or tingling. On examination, he demonstrates supraspinatus and infraspinatus weakness. X-rays of the right shoulder are unremarkable. An MRI of the right shoulder demonstrates supraspinatous and infraspinatous muscle edema, but no evidence of bursitis, tendinopathy, or a tearing of the rotator cuff. You suspect a neuropathy. Given the information about this patient, what is the most likely diagnosis?

    A. Compression of the seventh cervical nerve root
    B. Suprascapular neuropathy, with compression at the transverse scapular ligament
    C. Suprascapular neuropathy, with compression at the spinoglenoid ligament
    D. Axillary nerve injury

175. Which of the following is associated with barefoot running?

    A. Rearfoot landing
    B. Increased stride length
    C. Increased cadence
    D. Increased foot eversion moment
    E. Decreased proprioception

176. Which of the following best describes the anatomy and/or function of the posterolateral corner structures of the knee?

   A. The fibular collateral ligament is the primary dynamic restraint to varus stress
   B. The popliteus tendon is a static stabilizer against varus stress
   C. The popliteofibular ligament is an important stabilizer of tibial external rotation
   D. The anterior cruciate ligament is a major restraint to tibial internal and external rotation
   E. The posterior cruciate ligament is the primary static restraint to varus stress

177. In the clinical evaluation of anterior hip and groin pain, which of the following pain generators is most correctly paired with its correlating finding on physical examination?

   A. Tensor fascia lata tendon—tenderness to palpation between femoral pulse and the pubic symphysis
   B. Adductor longus muscle—tenderness to palpation between femoral pulse and the anterior superior iliac spine
   C. Pectineus muscle—tenderness to palpation over femoral pulse
   D. Rectus femoris tendon—tenderness to palpation over the anterior superior iliac spine

178. Which of the following best describes the relationship of the structures implicated in intersection syndrome?

   A. The abductor pollicis longus (APL) and extensor pollicis brevis (EPB) cross over extensor carpi radialis longus (ECRL) and extensor carpi radialis brevis (ECRB)
   B. The abductor pollicis longus (APL) and abductor pollicis brevis (APB) cross over extensor carpi radialis longus (ECRL) and extensor carpi radialis brevis (ECRB)
   C. The extensor carpi radialis longus (ECRL) and extensor carpi radialis brevis (ECRB) cross over abductor pollicis longus (APL) and extensor pollicis brevis (EPB)
   D. The extensor carpi radialis longus (ECRL) and extensor carpi radialis brevis (ECRB) cross over abductor pollicis brevis (APB) and extensor pollicis longus (EPL)

179. Atlantoaxial instability can be an acquired or existing condition that places a young athlete at risk for spinal cord injury. Which ligament is the primary stabilizer of the atlantoaxial joint?

    A. The transverse atlantal ligament
    B. The alar ligament
    C. The posterior longitudinal ligament
    D. The anterior longitudinal ligament

180. As the head team physician for a Division I college, you have been caring for the starting center for the football team. You have seen him weekly in the training room for the last three weeks. His blood pressure, on these three separate training room visits, has been determined to be in the stage 2 hypertension range. A thorough workup has been performed, without identifying any secondary causes for the elevated blood pressure or evidence of end organ damage. In addition to lifestyle modifications that have failed to this point, you determine that the athlete will need to be treated with medication to control the blood pressure. The patient has no known medication allergies. Which would be the best medication to initiate treatment?

    A. Hydrochlorothiazide
    B. Metoprolol XL
    C. Diltiazem
    D. Lisinopril

181. When performing a palpation landmark-guided injection of the carpal tunnel, which of the following observations indicate that the needle tip is in an acceptable position for introducing the injectant?

    A. Resistance is encountered when initially depressing the plunger
    B. The patient reports numbness, tingling, and burning upon placing the needle bevel at the target
    C. A small amount of blood enters the barrel upon initially drawing the plunger
    D. The needle shaft does not move with voluntary finger movements

182. With proper skin cleansing and the use of aseptic technique, the risk of introducing infection into a sterile joint via knee aspiration can be reduced. What is this reduced risk?

    A. 1:100
    B. 1:1,000
    C. 1:10,000
    D. 1:100,000

183. You are moonlighting in an urgent care clinic when a 23-year-old male presents with a right shoulder injury he sustained while playing football with some friends. After thoroughly examining the patient, you obtain shoulder x-rays that confirm an anterior shoulder dislocation (see image). As soon as you touch the patient to attempt your reduction, he screams in pain and demands you give him pain medication. What is your best next step?

    A. Provide the patient intravenous sedation and reattempt your reduction using an external rotation technique
    B. Continue with your reduction, despite his requests to avoid muscle spasm
    C. Inject a small amount of intra-articular lidocaine using a posterior glenohumeral approach, and then re-attempt your reduction using a scapular manipulation technique
    D. Provide the pain medication he prefers and reattempt your reduction, starting with the Milch technique

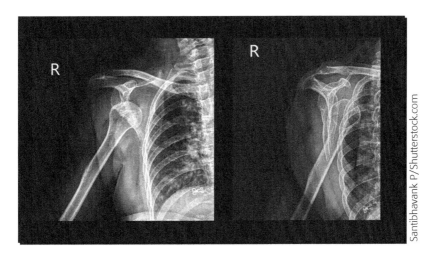

184. A 37-year-old, right-hand-dominant female who is an avid golfer complains of right dorsal forearm pain with activity for three months. She does not recall any trauma. On physical examination, there is tenderness over the radial head with minimal wrist extensor weakness and pain, with resisted supination of an extended forearm with wrist flexion. Radiographs are negative. She has tried icing, an elbow sleeve, oral NSAIDs, and occupational therapy for lateral epicondylitis, without significant improvement. What other diagnosis should be considered at this time?

    A. Radial tunnel syndrome
    B. Cubital tunnel syndrome
    C. Lateral epicondylitis
    D. Medial epicondylitis

185. A 16-year-old male presents to your clinic for follow-up from the emergency department. He was seen three days ago for a fracture. On review of his discharge paperwork, you notice he was diagnosed with a non-displaced, bicortical distal radial metaphysis fracture. There was no reduction performed in the emergency department. He has pain with pronation and supination and is tender to palpation over the fracture site. You repeat radiographs in the clinic and confirm that the fracture has not moved since initial presentation. You decide to treat this fracture with an appropriately molded cast and not refer for surgery. Which is the most correct application of the cast for the treatment of this fracture?

    A. Placement of a short-arm cast with the wrist in flexion and ulnar deviation
    B. Placement of a long-arm cast with the wrist in flexion and ulnar deviation, the forearm in neutral position, and the elbow flexed at 90 degrees
    C. Placement of a long-arm cast with the wrist in mild extension and ulnar deviation, the forearm in neutral position, and the elbow flexed at 90 degrees
    D. Placement of a long-arm cast with the wrist in mild extension and ulnar deviation, the forearm in supination, and the elbow flexed at 90 degrees
    E. Placement of a long-arm cast with the wrist in mild extension and ulnar deviation, the forearm in pronation, and the elbow flexed at 90 degrees

186. You are seeing a 16-year-old soccer player with the eye injury noted in the picture. Which of the following statements is true?

    A. This injury, which is often caused by sneezing, should be treated with topical antibiotics and followed up in your office within 24 to 48 hours
    B. This is an uncommon injury in sports, as it is mostly seen in motor vehicle trauma
    C. This injury can be associated with sickle cell disease, hemophilia, and Von Willebrand's disease
    D. This is usually an isolated injury to the posterior chamber of the eye

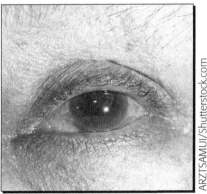

187. What is an important physical finding in head trauma?

    A. Battle's sign
    B. Castell's sign
    C. Kehr's sign
    D. Tactile fremitus

188. Your last patient of the day is a 17-year-old male soccer player complaining of progressive left-sided scrotal pain over the past eight hours. He reports a kick to the scrotum and groin during a collision with another player in a game earlier this morning. He has developed nausea and vomiting in the past hour. On physical examination, his left testicle is elevated and oriented transversely compared to the right testicle. What is the next step in management of this athlete?

    A. Manual detorsion, followed by ice pack and compression to the scrotum
    B. Referral to the emergency department for an emergent evaluation by urology
    C. Schedule for urgent ultrasound within 24 to 48 hours
    D. Urinalysis and CBC with differential

189. You are the physician at the finish line tent of a large marathon when a 44-year-old female runner collapses 100 meters before the finish line. The athlete is confused, sweating profusely, and cannot walk. A rectal temperature is obtained, revealing a temperature of 103 degrees Fahrenheit (39.4 degrees Celsius). Which of the following methods is the most effective treatment?

    A. Help the athlete walk it off
    B. Continuous spraying of cool water
    C. Apply ice to the neck, axilla, and groin
    D. Ice water immersion

190. Which of the following statements is correct regarding an epidural and subdural hematoma?

    A. Only subdural hematomas can be monitored by CT scan and managed non-operatively
    B. Subdural hematomas more commonly exhibit a higher Glasgow Coma Score (GCS) on admission to the emergency department
    C. An epidural hematoma is normally due to a bleeding middle meningeal artery, caused by a temporal skull fracture
    D. A subdural hematoma on CT scan demonstrates localized bleeding between the dura and skull
    E. If treated early, prognosis for subdural hematoma is better than that for epidural hematoma

191. A 22-year-old male soccer player is stung by a bee on the practice field. He approaches you on the sideline and is quickly noted to have pronounced wheezing. You run for your medical bag and when you return moments later his wheeze is less audible but he is still in respiratory distress. You notice that his lips are beginning to swell, and he is increasingly panicked. After telling the athletic trainer at your side to call 911, what is your first action?

    A. Establish intravenous access
    B. Administer 0.5 mL of Epinephrine (1:1,000) intramuscularly
    C. Administer 0.3 mL of Epinephrine (1:100,000) subcutaneously
    D. Give the patient 50 mg of diphenhydramine, monitor closely, and repeat every four hours as needed

192. What sign helps to differentiate a simple pneumothorax from a tension pneumothorax?

   A. Tracheal deviation away from the affected side
   B. Unilateral chest pain
   C. Dyspnea
   D. Open wound to the chest

193. A 32-year-old male soccer player suffered a contusion of his left lower leg against the goal post while playing. He developed swelling and tenderness over his left tibia. He is taken to the emergency room after the game finished. X-rays showed a non-displaced tibial shaft fracture (see images). He is immobilized with a cast and sent home. Five hours later, he comes back to the hospital, complaining of terrible pain that is worsening and does not respond to prescribed narcotics. On arrival, he starts complaining of tingling of the left lower extremity that he did not have when he came to the emergency room before. He has normal sensation and normal peripheral pulses of lower extremities. He is given IV narcotics, but pain is not going away. What is the most appropriate next step in the management of this case?

   A. Admit him to the hospital for observation, keep his leg in the cast with constant elevation, and consult orthopedics the next day
   B. Remove the cast and place a splint instead, discharge him from the hospital, and tell him to keep ice and elevation at all times when resting and to follow up with orthopedics as an outpatient
   C. Consult the neurologist on call immediately
   D. Remove the cast and immediately consult the foot and ankle orthopedist on call

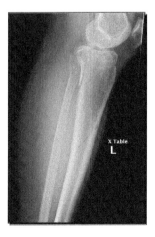
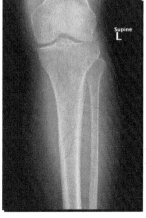

194. A 44-year-old male travels from Florida to a ski resort in Colorado at an altitude of 9,600 feet (2,926 m) in one day for a ski vacation. He has been there before and had no problems during that trip. One day after arriving, he began complaining of a headache and some minor nausea, with trouble sleeping. His mental status was normal. Which of the following is true?

    A. This patient has early HACE, as a result of the altitude change in one day
    B. This patient would likely benefit from acetazolamide
    C. This patient would likely benefit from sildenafil
    D. This patient would likely benefit from using over-the-counter Ginkgo biloba

195. According to the most recent AMSSM position stand on concussion management (based on 2012 statement), which of the following is correct in the immediate assessment of a suspected concussion injury?

    A. Standard sideline tests are reliable across age, ethnic, and sports groups
    B. Neuroimaging should be ordered for all athletes
    C. There should be no same-day return to play for any athlete diagnosed with a concussion
    D. Only physicians should be allowed to make the diagnosis of a concussion injury
    E. Balance disturbance is both a sensitive and specific indicator of concussion injury

196. An 18-year-old male rugby player is involved in a high-velocity collision during a match. He falls to the ground, clutching his left knee, saying he felt a "big pop." Your on-field examination shows marked laxity, with varus and valgus stress of the knee in full extension and a positive Lachman's maneuver. Palpation of the dorsalis pedis and posterior tibialis pulses are diminished in left leg. What is the next appropriate step for management?

    A. Reassure the athlete that he has suffered a sprain
    B. Arrange for an MRI for suspected anterior cruciate ligament (ACL) tear
    C. Emergent transportation to a local ED for an angiogram to evaluate for popliteal artery injury
    D. Keep the athlete on the sideline and check serial ankle brachial indexes (ABI), watching for worsening signs of ischemia

197. Which of the following is true regarding commotio cordis?

    A. Little League Baseball now requires the batter to wear chest protectors for prevention in children under 12 years of age
    B. The apparent mechanism for death is ventricular fibrillation, induced by an abrupt blunt precordial blow during a specific time in the cardiac cycle
    C. Baseballs thrown at 20 mph, a blow in the left area of the heart, and blunt impacts are associated with more deadly outcomes in commotio cordis
    D. With rapid defibrillation, cardiac support, and AED maneuvers, greater than 25% of individuals may survive commotio cordis
    E. Impact must occur within the QRS of the cardiac cycle in order for ventricular fibrillation to occur and cause commotio cordis

198. A 26-year-old male triathlete presents to your clinic with a right shoulder injury after a crash during the bike stage of a race three days prior. He reports that he was 10 miles into the stage when he felt slightly dizzy for a split second. The next thing he remembered was that he was on the ground. He was taken to the emergency department, where shoulder x-rays were negative. He also had a normal ECG and normal head CT. He denies any symptoms other than mild pain to his right shoulder. His examination is normal except for abrasion (road rash) to his right upper arm. He is hoping for clearance to participate in an event next weekend. What is the best management plan for this patient?

    A. Provide wound care instructions, and clear the patient to participate as tolerated
    B. Obtain a repeat ECG and an echocardiogram. If both tests are normal, clear him to participate
    C. Refer him to cardiology and only clear him for running (not cycling or swimming) until further assessment
    D. Hold him from any athletic participation and refer him to cardiology

199. You are covering a high school football game when one of the players goes in for a tackle with his head down and does not immediately get up off the field. You suspect an acute cervical spine injury. Which of the following pieces of equipment should be removed while you maintain in-line cervical stabilization and await emergency transport?

   A. Facemask
   B. Helmet
   C. Shoulder pads
   D. Remove no equipment

200. A 45-year-old female with type 2 diabetes mellitus on oral medications and insulin has recently started an exercise program after speaking with you for recommendations. She often finds herself unable to complete the one-hour exercise class, as she is diaphoretic and weak. She reports mild dizziness and increased thirst, as well as a fast pulse. A trainer finds her blood sugar to be 45 mg/dL. What recommendation is true regarding her situation?

   A. She should try to exercise in the evening, because hypoglycemia is more likely in the morning than the evening due to diurnal variation in growth hormone and cortisol
   B. She has exercise-induced hypoglycemia and should always check her blood sugar 30 minutes before exercise, with goals in the range of 150 to 200 mg/dL
   C. If her blood sugar is higher than 250 mg/dL, she is safe to exercise, as hyperglycemic numbers are safer than hypoglycemic numbers during exercise
   D. In order to prevent these episodes, she should exercise before meals, instead of afterwards, and keep her pre-meal insulin and medications the same
   E. Since her class is only one hour long, she needs adequate hydration, rather than extra carbohydrate snacks to avoid hypoglycemia

Test 2 Questions

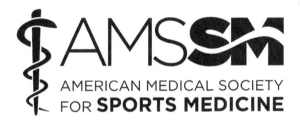

1. A 20-year-old collegiate soccer player presents to the training room with a complaint of groin pain that radiates to the testicle, a situation that has been going on for about four months. He cannot identify an acute injury as a cause. The pain is worse after practices or games, and has been increasing in intensity. He has not lost any weight, and there has been no recent increase in his level of training. He does not complain of any lumps in the groin. On exam, the testicle is normal in size, and no masses are present. No hernia, provocation, or bulge is palpated, even with Valsalva maneuvers. You elicit pain with resisted hip flexion, and with palpation of the posterior inguinal wall and pubic tubercle. The single-leg hop test does not elicit pain. What is the most likely diagnosis?

    A. Acute adductor strain
    B. Sports hernia
    C. Femoral neck stress fracture
    D. Inguinal hernia

2. A 20-year-old ballet dancer presents with sudden proximal posterior thigh pain after practice yesterday. He had been practicing for a performance, when he felt a pop during his grande jeté. Which of the following would limit his return to participation?

    A. Full concentric strength
    B. Injury involving the proximal free tendon
    C. Active straight leg raise deficit
    D. Pain-free range of motion

3. Which of the following has a significant association with the risk of future ankle sprains?

    A. Current ankle taping
    B. Previous contralateral ankle injury
    C. Positive single-leg balance test
    D. Current ankle bracing

4. Which of the following has evidence-based support for use in the rehabilitation of acute ankle sprains?

    A. Electrical stimulation
    B. External ankle supports
    C. Acupuncture
    D. Therapeutic ultrasound

5. The men's soccer athletic trainer at the university you cover asks for your opinion on an athlete. One of the starting players was home in Ecuador for the summer and tore his Achilles tendon. He had surgery, and the coach wants to know the fastest way for him to get back to playing. Following an acute Achilles tendon rupture and subsequent surgical repair, which of the following postoperative rehabilitation protocols is safe, and associated with earlier return to function and significantly higher subjective patient outcomes (patient satisfaction)?

   A. Non-weight-bearing in a rigid cast for at least six weeks
   B. Early, dynamic postoperative ankle motion and weight-bearing in a brace
   C. Early loading with eccentric exercises using heavy weights
   D. Stair-climbing protocol, with multiple, prolonged sessions per week
   E. Isometric stretching using a fixed weight

6. A 42-year-old male baseball pitcher player presents to your office with a history of shoulder impingement and corresponding signs on physical exam. Which of the following conditions has the most relevance for successful rehabilitation of this problem?

   A. Scapulothoracic dyskinesis
   B. Prominence of the lateral border of the scapula
   C. Increased internal, compared to external, range of motion of the shoulder
   D. Mild pain and limited weakness of the rotator cuff immediately after pitching

7. A 14-year-old female soccer player presents to the office with a two-week history of right anterior knee pain, without a preceding injury. Physical examination shows full range of motion, no effusion, and intact ligaments. She has pain over the lateral patella facet. Hamstring and iliotibial band flexibility are normal. Her knee goes into valgus with one-leg squat. X-rays are normal. What is the most appropriate initial management of this condition?

   A. MRI knee
   B. Physical therapy, with an emphasis on hip strengthening
   C. Patella-stabilizing brace
   D. Physical therapy, with an emphasis on vastus medialis strengthening

8. A 19-year-old female soccer goalie receives a direct blow to the face from blocking a shot on goal. She develops pain and blurred vision in the right eye, and is removed from the field. On exam, you see a collection of blood in the anterior chamber of the right eye and diagnose her with a hyphema. Appropriate management includes which of the following?

   A. Since the hyphema collection covers less than 25% of anterior chamber, she may continue playing with the use of protective eyewear
   B. Advise patient to rest, safely apply ice, take anti-inflammatory as needed for pain, and follow up with her ophthalmologist within the next one to two days
   C. Start antibiotic ointment immediately, as there is a high likelihood of developing associated bacterial infection
   D. Refer to ophthalmologist for prompt evaluation

9. A 15-year-old lacrosse player presents for concussion assessment from an injury suffered the previous day. His parents say he was hit from behind and think the opponent's stick or elbow hit the back of his skull. The player and his parents are concerned about his headache, dizziness, and bruising to the right mastoid area. He reports ongoing symptoms that have not improved, including headache, sleep disturbance, dizziness, and neck pain. On exam, the patient has moderate tenderness along his occiput, his temporal bones, and ecchymoses superficial to his mastoid area. You remember reading about "Battle's sign" describing ecchymoses along the mastoid area. This exam finding is suspicious for?

   A. Vestibular problem
   B. Cervical spine injury
   C. Skull fracture
   D. Tumor

10. When it comes to concussions, which of the following has less evidence to support it as a risk factor for an athlete to suffer a concussion?

    A. Prior concussion
    B. Participation in collision sports
    C. Female gender
    D. Participation in women's lacrosse

11. During a karate tournament, an eight-year-old male has a primary tooth knocked out. After a thorough examination, it was found to be a complete avulsion, with no fracture. No swelling of his gum line is noted, and there are no concerns for airway obstruction. What do you do with the tooth?

    A. Stop the bleeding and do nothing with the tooth
    B. Place the tooth in Hank's Balanced Salt Solution
    C. Place the tooth in normal saline solution
    D. Place the tooth in his mouth next to his buccal mucosa
    E. Place the tooth in room-temperature tap water

12. A 20-year-old elite rower presents to your office complaining of worsening pain over her right chest wall for the past few weeks. Recently, she has developed point tenderness over the sixth rib. After examining her, you are concerned about a possible stress fracture. Which of the following is true regarding stress fractures of the ribs?

    A. Stress fractures tend to have acute onset and are often associated with obvious deformity at the fracture site
    B. Chronic stress of upper body muscles, which attach to the ribs, can result in stress fractures of the ribs
    C. Increased shortness of breath, pain, cyanosis, and subcutaneous emphysema are commonly seen with stress fractures of the ribs
    D. Serial rib series radiographs would be used in this athlete to diagnose her stress fracture and to monitor healing

13. A 19-year-old female presents to the campus health service with anterior shin pain, ongoing now for three weeks. She denies any trauma, disordered eating, or infrequent menstrual periods. She is on the Ultimate Frisbee team and they are a month into the season. Her pain now starts with practice, and on long practice days or game days her shins stay sore afterwards. She noted recently it hurts to walk—but resting does not relieve the pain; it is residual. Also, she reports the area of pain on the shin is much more localized than before. There is no numbness or tingling. What is the most likely diagnosis?

    A. Chronic exertional compartment syndrome (CECS)
    B. Shin splints (medial stress syndrome)
    C. Common peroneal nerve entrapment
    D. Stress reaction to the tibia
    E. Popliteal artery entrapment

14. Which of the following is true regarding adolescent idiopathic scoliosis management?

    A. Scoliosis screening is recommended by the United States Preventive Services Task Force (USPSTF)
    B. Initial evaluation includes MRI of the thoracolumbar spine to measure the Cobb angle
    C. Individuals with adolescent idiopathic scoliosis often need more than observation alone
    D. Apex right curves (dextroscoliosis) are most common in patients with idiopathic scoliosis. Back pain and left curves (levoscoliosis) should prompt concern for other spinal disease, such as tumor
    E. Indications for surgery are largely functional and should use the Cobb angle as the sole criteria for intervention

15. Which of the following statements is true regarding proximal humeral epiphysiolysis (Little League shoulder)?

    A. It typically occurs in pitchers aged 8 to 10 years old
    B. A widened proximal humeral physis on plain radiograph clinches the diagnosis
    C. The athlete is usually pain-free until the acute onset of pain
    D. It is caused by repetitive loading of the shoulder with both torque and distraction forces

16. A 21-year-old, right-hand-dominant collegiate starting pitcher has been struggling with progressive, intermittent soreness in his right shoulder that is relieved with rest and worsens with continued pitching. Despite normal x-rays, rotator cuff sports ultrasound, and appropriate physical therapy, he continues to struggle and is moved to the bullpen to decrease his workload. Over the weekend, he goes rope-swinging at the local river with his teammates, and accidentally falls hard onto the lateral right shoulder. He has immediate severe pain, but the x-rays at the local ER are normal. A CT scan shows a one-part anatomical neck fracture of the proximal humerus. What is the best treatment option for this patient at this time?

    A. Routine icing with a shoulder sling and swathe, and allow the fracture to heal non-operatively over the next six to eight weeks
    B. Let him know his pitching career is in jeopardy and treat the fracture conservatively over the next six to eight weeks with early functional rehabilitation
    C. Refer to the orthopedic surgeon for ORIF, due to potential disruption of the blood supply and risk of avascular necrosis of the humeral head
    D. Obtain an MRI to evaluate the rotator cuff tendon for a potential supraspinatus tear that occurred with the fracture in order to expedite a recovery program

17. You are asked by a colleague for assistance in interpreting a right-shoulder MRI arthrogram following injury. You make note of a tear of the posteroinferior labrum and an impaction fracture of the antero-medial humeral head. Which of the following most accurately describes the mechanism of injury?

    A. Acute strike to the right shoulder from a posteroinferior direction
    B. Repetitive overuse
    C. Trauma sustained during a tonic-clonic seizure
    D. Trauma sustained from improper technique tackling in football

18. A 40-year-old, right-handed male presents with increasing right shoulder pain with overhead activities. He denies trauma but recently returned to playing softball. The pain is located over the lateral deltoid, is aching in nature, and disrupts sleeping on the right side. He presents with an MRI demonstrating supraspinatus tendinopathy. Which physical exam finding is most likely to be present in this patient?

    A. Pain with hornblower's test
    B. Pain with empty can test
    C. Pain with lift-off test
    D. Pain with resisted external rotation

19. A 40-year-old gentleman presents to his primary care physician for severe right shoulder pain. He awoke with pain three days ago, and has not improved with over-the-counter analgesics. Now, he is unable to reach overhead with his right arm. Which of the following advice is most appropriate for this patient?

    A. An electromyography should be performed immediately to evaluate his shoulder and neck
    B. Strenuous exercise and/or infections or immune triggers can predispose individuals to this condition
    C. Urgent orthopedic surgery referral is recommended, as surgery is usually necessary
    D. The loss of passive range of motion is usually the cause of the impaired shoulder function

20. Which of the following is required for a diagnosis of shoulder impingement?

    A. History and physical exam of the shoulder
    B. MRI of the shoulder with gadolinium contrast
    C. MRI of the shoulder without contrast
    D. X-rays of the shoulder

21. A seven-year-old male presents to your clinic after falling off the monkey bars at his school playground. He cannot remember how he landed on the ground, but is complaining of forearm pain. On clinical examination, you notice a bowed deformity to the forearm, but a normal elbow and wrist exam. You obtain a radiograph that reveals no obvious fracture, but you do see bowing of the radius that was apparent on exam. Using the Schemitsch and Richards method, you measure the bowing of the radius to be 25 degrees. What is your next step in treatment?

    A. This abnormality is called a plastic deformity and should be reduced to an acceptable angle of less than 20 degrees
    B. Since there is no fracture, you reassure the parents and do not provide any further treatment
    C. This abnormality is called a plastic deformity, but you do not need to reduce this injury, because the patient is less than 12 years old
    D. You send him to the radiology department for a stat CT scan, because that will assist you to create a treatment plan

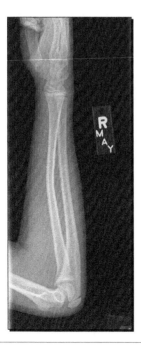
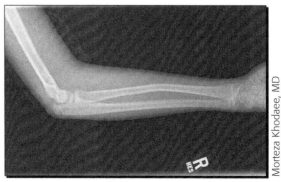

Morteza Khodaee, MD

22. You are finishing clinic for the day when a mom comes in with her two-year-old child. She relates that they were holding hands and about to cross the street when her son stepped forward toward traffic and she pulled him back by his right hand. Since then, he has refused to use his right arm and cries when his mother tries to move it. After an exam that confirms the most likely diagnosis, what is the most appropriate next step?

    A. X-ray of the elbow
    B. Surgical consult
    C. Long-arm cast
    D. Hyperpronation reduction

23. Which one of the following statements is correct regarding medial epicondylitis?

    A. The magnitude of grip strength impairment is greater than that seen in lateral epicondylitis
    B. Examination findings include pain with resisted wrist flexion, wrist pronation, and valgus stress testing
    C. Corticosteroid injections were shown to improve symptoms at six weeks, but showed no difference when compared with controls at three and 12 months
    D. Medial epicondylitis is more common than lateral epicondylitis in the general population

24. Which of the following statements is true regarding ulnar neuropathy in throwing athletes?

    A. Athletes with laxity of the ulnar collateral ligament are at increased risk for stretching the nerve
    B. The most common location of impingement is Guyon's canal
    C. These injuries may be treated by having the athlete wear braces that keep the elbow maximally flexed while sleeping
    D. Athletes often have a positive pronator compression test in which compression over the pronator teres reproduces symptoms

25. A 16-year-old high school football player impacts his right forearm against an opponent's helmet while tackling. He complains of pain over the point of impact at the dorsal lateral aspect of the proximal right forearm. He subsequently notes weakness with right wrist extension and finger extension, but no pain or tingling in his hand. His exam is remarkable for tenderness over the proximal edge of the supinator muscle, and diminished strength (4/5), with wrist extension and thumb and finger extension at metacarpal-phalangeal (MCP) joints. Diminished strength with forearm supination is also noted. Sensation is intact to light touch over radial and median distribution. X-ray of the right radius and ulna showed no fractures or dislocation. His most likely diagnosis is?

    A. Extensor tendon rupture
    B. Wartenberg syndrome
    C. Anterior interosseous nerve syndrome
    D. Posterior interosseous nerve syndrome

26. During the preparticipation physical exam, an athlete has 20/20 vision in his left eye and 20/80 vision in his right eye. When is an athlete considered functionally monocular?

    A. When the best corrected vision in one eye is less than 20/40
    B. When the best uncorrected vision in one eye is less than 20/40
    C. When the best corrected vision in one eye is less than 20/80
    D. When the best uncorrected vision in one eye is less than 20/100

27. A six-month-old child is brought to your office because he refuses to use his right hand. The child seems drowsy, but his mother states that she just gave him an OTC antihistamine/decongestant for an upper respiratory infection. The child weighs eight pounds, and his head circumference is 40 cm. He is sleepy, but awakens easily, and is non-toxic in appearance. His right wrist is swollen. You radiograph his right upper extremity and find a fracture, along with a partially calcified scaphoid bone. What is the most important next step?

    A. Reassure the child's mother that this type of fracture heals very well in a child of this age
    B. Immobilize the child's arm and wrist with a long-thumb spica cast
    C. Radiograph the opposite extremity and ask the child's mother some more questions about the mechanism of injury and any other injuries or illnesses that the child may have
    D. Consult an orthopedic surgeon comfortable treating patients in this age group

28. A 15-year-old female basketball player comes to the clinic after jamming her index finger trying to catch a basketball. On examination, she is tender at the DIP joint, and isolation of the DIP joint reveals an inability to actively extend the distal phalanx. Passive extension is intact. X-ray reveals a fracture of the proximal dorsal aspect of the distal phalanx. What is the proper treatment for this condition?

    A. Surgical referral within seven days
    B. Splinting the DIP joint in extension for eight weeks, followed by one month of night splinting
    C. Buddy taping the index finger to the middle finger
    D. Splinting the DIP joint with a clam-shell splint, with motion at DIP beginning after two to three weeks

29. A 35-year-old, right-hand-dominant police officer presents to the emergency room after falling off his horse on an outstretched hand. He complains of severe pain in his wrist and numbness in his index finger and thumb. Radiographs reveal that he has a perilunate disassociation, Mayfield Classification Stage III. Which of the following is true?

    A. An emergent MRI arthrogram is required to confirm the diagnosis
    B. This patient requires immediate operative treatment of this condition
    C. The numbness in his hand is due to injury of the radial artery
    D. This condition is best treated by emergent closed reduction, followed by open reduction, ligament repair, fixation, and carpal tunnel release

30. A 20-year-old discus thrower presents to clinic after dropping the discus onto his left middle finger. On exam, he has diffuse swelling and pain of the distal aspect of his finger, with a large subungal hematoma involving the entire nail bed. The nail is still attached. He is neurovascularly intact, and the tendon function of his finger is intact. What is the most appropriate intervention at this time?

    A. Place him in an aluminum splint with a compression dressing and prescribe RICE therapy
    B. Trephinate the hematoma
    C. Obtain radiographs, and if no evidence of fracture, offer trephination
    D. Obtain radiographs, and if no evidence of fracture, removal of nail and drainage of hematoma

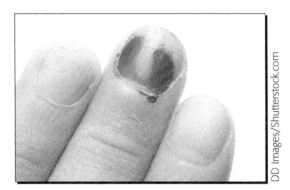

31. Which of the following is true regarding carpal tunnel syndrome?

    A. Patients have a positive Froment's sign
    B. Patients have numbness and tingling over the ulnar side of the ring finger and the fifth digit
    C. Nerve conduction studies are not helpful with diagnosis
    D. Patients typically complain of numbness and tingling affecting the first three digits and the radial side of the ring finger

32. A 33-year-old, right-hand-dominant male presents with complaint of right wrist pain. He is a competitive racquetball player and reports falling on his wrist during a match yesterday. He states the pain is worst over the ulnar side of the wrist, and he is especially concerned that he may have a fracture, because he has a "clicking" sensation when he moves his wrist. On physical exam, there is tenderness to palpation in the area between the ulnar styloid and pisiform. He has no tenderness with palpation of the hand or fingers. The pain is worsened with ulnar deviation of the wrist, as well as resisted pronation and supination. Patient is unable to lift the exam table with his wrist supinated, due to worsening pain. Given the physical exam findings, what is the most likely diagnosis?

   A. Ulnar styloid fracture
   B. Extensor carpi ulnaris tendinopathy
   C. Triangular fibrocartilage complex injury
   D. Scapholunate ligament disruption

33. An 18-year-old male college freshman presents to your training room with right dorsal wrist pain. He denies any trauma or new activities. He is rowing in the freshman boat and is training for his spring racing season. The pain is located on the dorsal surface of his wrist, on the radial side, just proximal to the proximal carpal row. He states the pain is worse when he extends his wrist while he is feathering his oar. You diagnose him with intersection syndrome and place him in a thumb spica wrist splint. What does the second dorsal compartment of the wrist contain?

   A. Extensor pollicis longus and abductor pollicis longus
   B. Extensor pollicis brevis and abductor pollicis longus
   C. Extensor carpi radialis brevis and extensor carpi radialis longus
   D. Extensor carpi radialis brevis and extensor pollicis longus

34. Which of the following is true of De Quervain's tenosynovitis?

   A. The two tendons involved are the abductor pollicis brevis and the extensor pollicis longus
   B. The grind test is the most sensitive test for diagnosis
   C. A corticosteroid injection into the tendon sheath of the second dorsal compartment has been shown to alleviate symptoms.
   D. Splinting of the thumb and wrist can relieve symptoms

35. You are working at a ski resort in Colorado when a skier comes in complaining of pain in his thumb after a fall. Following your examination, you suspect that he has suffered a gamekeeper's thumb or skier's thumb, without evidence of dislocation. What x-ray finding would prompt you to refer this patient to an orthopedic surgeon?

   A. Stener lesion
   B. Bankart lesion
   C. Segond fracture
   D. Bennett fracture

36. A 45-year-old man presents with sudden onset of severe right hip pain. His pain is mainly with weight-bearing. He denies any trauma or systemic symptoms. He had a similar episode of severe pain in his left hip three years ago, which resolved after several months. He did not have surgery. He has no risk factors for avascular necrosis. On examination, the patient is in distress and using crutches. He has preserved hip range of motion. His x-ray is below. What is his most likely diagnosis?

   A. Osteomyelitis
   B. Lumbar radiculopathy
   C. Avascular necrosis
   D. Transient osteoporosis of the hip
   E. Femoral neck fracture

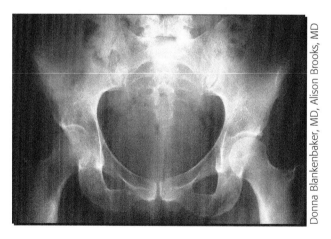

Donna Blankenbaker, MD, Alison Brooks, MD

37. Following hip replacement surgery, your patient was found to have an iatrogenic injury of the obturator nerve. Which of the following is true?

    A. Obturator nerve injury can be associated with quadriceps muscle weakness
    B. It innervates the adductor longus and brevis
    C. It originates from L5 and S1 nerve roots
    D. It innervates the vastus lateralis and the vastus intermedius

38. An active 24-year-old female presents complaining of right hip pain associated with episodes of painful snapping. Which of the following is true about internal snapping hip?

    A. Physical therapy is not indicated
    B. Hip snapping is reproduced with extension of the hip from a flexed position
    C. A hip radiograph often confirms the diagnosis
    D. NSAIDs can be used for treatment, but corticosteroid injections are contraindicated

39. A 31-year-old man presents with a several month history of right knee pain and swelling. His pain has become severe with weight-bearing. There was no injury. He denies any other joint issues or any constitutional symptoms. On exam, his distal femur is tender and there is minimal soft tissue swelling. His x-ray reveals a cystic lesion in the distal femur, abutting the joint. His x-ray and MRI are below. What is the most likely diagnosis?

A. Enchondroma
B. Giant cell tumor of bone
C. Nonossifying fibroma
D. Intramedullary bone infarct

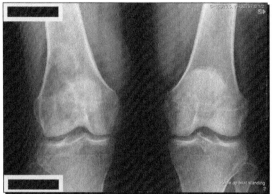

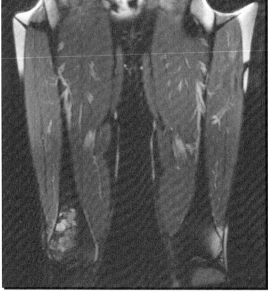

Test 2 Questions

40. A seven-year-old female soccer player presents to your office with pain in her left knee. The pain began during a soccer practice, and she was unable to walk after onset. On examination, she is acutely tender on the inferior aspect of her patella. She is unable to perform a straight-leg raise. What is the most likely diagnosis?

    A. Traction apophysitis of the tibial tubercle (Osgood-Schlatter's disease)
    B. Traction apophysitis of the distal patellar pole (Sindig-Larsen-Johansson disease)
    C. Patellofemoral dysfunction
    D. Patellar sleeve fracture

41. Which of the following is a dynamic stabilizer of the posterolateral corner of the knee?

    A. Fibular collateral ligament
    B. Popliteofibular ligament
    C. Popliteus tendon
    D. Arcuate ligament

42. A 25-year-old male runner presents with bilateral lower extremity throbbing pain and numbness in the first web space of his feet that begins consistently after 10 minutes of intense exercise and is completely relieved with rest. He reports symptoms are brought on the following day in about half the time. What is the most likely explanation for this?

    A. His muscles are increasingly fatigued
    B. He has chronic exertional compartment syndrome and now has acute compartment syndrome
    C. He has increased muscle damage and necrosis, due to intense exercise
    D. He is experiencing the second-day phenomenon

43. A 15-year-old tennis player presents to your office with an injury that has been present for two months. After examining him, you diagnose him with an overuse injury. He tells you that he has played tennis year-round for the last five years and trains at an elite tennis academy. He participates in weekly resistance training with a certified trainer while at the academy. You recall that you treated him successfully for a similar overuse injury one year ago. On chart review, you note that he has grown three inches in the last six months. Which of the following is true with regard to his risk factors for an overuse injury?

    A. Sport specialization at a young age has been shown to decrease injuries
    B. Resistance training leads to increased injuries in pediatric populations
    C. A history of a prior injury is an established risk factor for overuse injuries
    D. Injuries rarely occur during adolescent growth

44. You are conducting preparticipation examinations for your local high school team. A 16-year-old female cross-country runner reports that her last menstrual period was approximately four months ago. Her menarche was at age 13, and her periods were regular until four months ago. She is not sexually active. She does not take any medications. There is no history of stress fractures, but she did see the athletic trainer for "shin splints" during both track and cross-country seasons last year. Body weight has been stable in the past year. Her BMI is 19. She follows a vegetarian diet but does not follow any other restrictions. The rest of her physical examination is normal. What is the next best step in management of this athlete?

    A. Refer for a DEXA
    B. Obtain more information regarding her diet history, exercise habits, and life stressors
    C. Initiate oral contraceptive pills to restore menses
    D. Order labs including beta HCG, complete blood count, basic chemistry, thyroid function tests, serum FSH, LH, and prolactin levels
    E. Instruct the athlete to add lean meats to her diet

45. Which corticosteroid is most likely to cause hypopigmentation and subcutaneous fat atrophy when used for a soft-tissue injection?

    A. Betamethasone
    B. Triamcinolone
    C. Dexamethasone
    D. Hydrocortisone

46. While performing percutaneous needle aspiration of a knee effusion, which of the following best describes findings suggestive of an intra-articular fracture?

    A. Thin, turbid, serosanguinous fluid, with small white flecks of debris
    B. Thin, opaque, bloody fluid, with no discernible debris
    C. Thin, turbid, serosanguinous fluid, with white-cheesy clumps of debris
    D. Thin, opaque, bloody fluid, with greasy sheen or oil globules

47. Which of the following confirms the diagnosis of chronic exertional compartment syndrome (CECS)?

    A. One-minute post-exercise pressure of 28 mm Hg
    B. Pre-exercise pressure of 19 mm Hg
    C. Pre-exercise pressure of 14 mm Hg
    D. Five-minute post exercise pressure of 17 mm Hg

48. You are the team physician for a youth club lacrosse team. One of the 15-year-old boys was struck in in the upper left abdominal area with an opponent's stick. Onfield evaluation demonstrates that he is hemodynamically stable, with point tenderness and early bruising to the left upper abdomen. He is also complaining of left shoulder pain. It is difficult to determine if he has true rebound tenderness on exam, although guarding is present. Given this scenario, if he remains hemodynamically stable, what is the next most important follow-up test/action?

    A. Laboratory tests: liver function and pancreatic enzymes
    B. Radiographs: plain upright films, KUB
    C. If he remains hemodynamically stable, no further study/exam is necessary other than serial observation and exams
    D. Ultrasound can reliably be used to determine free intraperitoneal blood

49. Which of the following is true regarding laryngotracheal (LT) injury?

    A. Stridor is the earliest symptom of LT injury
    B. MRI is the preferred diagnostic study for LT injury
    C. Flexible fiberoptic laryngoscopy should be performed immediately if the airway is unstable
    D. Intubation is essential to establish a secure airway in all suspected cases of LT injury
    E. The initial manifestations of LT injury may be subtle

50. A 20-year-old female basketball player presents by EMS transport to the emergency department in respiratory distress that began acutely while scrimmaging at the end of basketball practice. She first started noticing intense urticaria of her upper torso and arms as the team started doing full-court drills. A few minutes later, one of her teammates noticed red raised wheals on both of her arms. She continued to play, and while they were scrimmaging, she started wheezing and had to stop due to severe difficulty breathing. EMS was then contacted, and she was taken to the nearest hospital. En route, she was placed into a partially reclined position, which was the position of comfort for her, and she was placed on oxygen. She was hypotensive with a blood pressure of 95/60, and therefore she was given a fluid bolus. She was also given a dose of epinephrine, which relieved her shortness of breath, and the wheals on her skin began clearing as well. Based on the most likely diagnosis for this athlete, what recommendations should be made for her long-term treatment?

    A. Always exercise with a partner who is trained in administering epinephrine and basic life support, and carry an epinephrine auto-injector
    B. Recommend athlete refrain from all exercise in the future to prevent another episode
    C. Allergy testing should be performed; if athlete avoids any identified allergens, no further episodes should occur, and no other intervention is needed
    D. Recommend taking a daily antihistamine to prevent future episodes

51. A 17-year-old male comes to your office complaining of severe left lower quadrant pain that appeared six hours ago, which he believes is the result of strenuous physical activity before the symptoms started. Pain is described as achy and constant, with associated nausea and vomiting. He denies any other associated signs or symptoms or any positive medical, family, or surgical history. Vitals are within normal limits. On abdominal exam, you find that he has normal bowel sounds. The abdomen is soft, non-tender, and there is no rebound. All special tests for intraabdominal and abdominal wall conditions are negative too. What is your next step?

    A. Prescribe him a 10-day course of Ciprofloxacin and Metronidazole, with follow-up in one week
    B. Prescribe oral Tramadol prn pain and Promethazine prn nausea or vomiting, with follow-up in two days
    C. Order STAT complete blood count (CBC), comprehensive metabolic panel (CMP), Urinalysis UA), and a CT scan of the abdomen and pelvis
    D. Perform a testicular exam immediately

52. You are covering a high school track and field event. During one of the longer runs, you notice a thin young male who is suddenly slowing down, holding the right side of his chest. He keeps walking to finish the round, but when he arrives at the medical tent, he is pale and diaphoretic, complaining of right-sided chest pain and problems breathing. When you examine him, you notice a left deviation of his trachea, normal breath sounds over the left lung, and no breath sounds over the right lung. Hypertympany with percussion is noted over the right chest. You quickly make the diagnosis of spontaneous tension pneumothorax. Prior to the definite treatment of inserting a chest tube, which of the following would be the location of next best intervention?

    A. Fourth intercostal space, anterior axillary line
    B. Second intercostal space, midclavicular line
    C. Fifth intercostal space, anterior axillary line
    D. Fifth intercostal space, midaxillary line

53. Which intravenous (IV) solution is usually preferred over other solutions for fluid resuscitation in anaphylaxis?

    A. Normal saline
    B. Lactated Ringer's
    C. Dextrose
    D. Colloid solutions

54. A 14-year-old male with Down syndrome presents with his parents, complaining of axial neck pain after falling one day prior on the tennis court. Pain is worsened with end ranges of flexion and extension. He denies any numbness, tingling, or weakness in his upper extremities. On exam, he has mild tenderness of his cervical paraspinal muscles. His range of motion is full in all directions, with pain at end ranges of flexion, extension, and bilateral rotation. His neurologic exam is intact. What condition must he be immediately evaluated for?

    A. Cervical stenosis
    B. Atlantoaxial (AA) instability
    C. Herniated disc
    D. Degenerative disc disease (DDD)

55. Commotio cordis is the term used to describe ventricular fibrillation triggered by chest wall impact most commonly over what structure?

    A. Right atrium
    B. Right ventricle
    C. Left atrium
    D. Left ventricle

56. A professional basketball player comes off the court complaining of right-sided pleuritic chest pain and shortness of breath. He denies any injury. After a brief rest, his respiratory rate is 16 breaths per minute. He has slightly diminished breath sounds and absent tactile fremitus in his upper right lung field. A chest x-ray reveals a right-sided pneumothorax (PTX), with a 2 cm apex-cupola distance. What is the most appropriate action?

    A. Place a chest tube
    B. Send him home with his team, as long as he flies in a pressurized cabin
    C. Take him out of the game and repeat the x-ray in three hours
    D. Allow him back on the court, as long as his oxygenation is normal

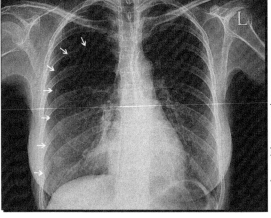

57. A 23-year-old college football player is taken off the field during practice on a hot and humid summer day after appearing to be confused and disoriented. He seems to be warm to the touch and is sweating profusely. You obtain a core rectal temperature that measures 105 degrees Fahrenheit (40.5 degrees Celsius). What is the most effective cooling method?

   A. Spray water over him while using a fan to cool him down
   B. Immediately give oral acetaminophen to bring his core temperature down below 102 degrees Fahrenheit (38.8 degrees Celsius)
   C. Place him in a bath of ice water
   D. Use cold packs at the neck, groin, and axillae

58. While fielding a ground ball at second base, a 16-year-old African-American female softball player sustains a right eye injury when the ball bounces up and strikes her at the right orbital region. The patient complains of right periorbital pain, photophobia, and diminished visual acuity. Right eye exam reveals an intact globe, no enophthalmos or ptosis, and mild periorbital edema. Pen light exam shows blood at the inferior third of the anterior chamber. Initial medical treatment should include which of the following?

   A. Topical cycloplegic (atropine 1%), systemic and/or topical corticosteroid, rigid eye shield, reevaluate in three days
   B. Topical cycloplegic (atropine 1%), systemic and/or topical corticosteroid, rigid eye shield, restrict activities, and immediate referral to ophthalmology
   C. Topical cycloplegic (atropine 1%), systemic and/or topical corticosteroid, rigid eye shield, and return to play
   D. Topical cycloplegic (atropine 1%), systemic and/or topical corticosteroid, and may return to play if normal visual acuity

59. You are evaluating a 20-year-old patient for a suspected concussion one hour ago during soccer practice. As part of your evaluation, you measure the near point convergence (NPC). What distance would be considered a normal NPC?

   A. 3 cm
   B. 6 cm
   C. 8 cm
   D. 10 cm

60. A 37-year-old male is carried into the emergency department by his wife immediately after completing a marathon in Key West. He complains of severe muscle cramps in his legs. He reports that he drank fluids during the race, but probably not enough, and admits he hasn't urinated since before the race. His wife thinks he's running a temperature. On physical exam, his calves and thighs are in muscle spasms. Glascow Coma Scale score is 15, no loss of consciousness during or after race. Vitals normal, except temperature 100.1 degrees Fahrenheit (37.8 degrees Celsius). ECG shows peaked T waves. The blood work will likely show which of the following abnormalities?

    A. Increased serum creatinine kinase, increased serum potassium, increased serum lactate dehydrogenase, decreased serum calcium
    B. Increased serum creatinine kinase, increased serum potassium, decreased serum lactate dehydrogenase, increased serum calcium
    C. Increased serum creatinine kinase, decreased serum potassium, increased serum lactate dehydrogenase, increased serum calcium
    D. Decreased serum creatinine kinase, increased serum potassium, increased serum lactate dehydrogenase, increased serum calcium

61. During a football game you are asked to evaluate a running back for a knee injury on the field. While running the ball, he states his foot was planted on the ground while a defender was holding his leg. As he tried to spin out of the tackle, a defensive lineman dove to tackle his legs, causing a heavy valgus load on the knee. He felt immediate pain and was unable to get up to walk off the field. On examination, you note normal alignment of the knee. However, he is unable to straighten it. There is a positive posterior sag sign. Both anterior and posterior drawer tests are grossly abnormal, and valgus stress reveals no endpoint. There appears to be an effusion forming, and all exam maneuvers are painful. Which of the following is true regarding the treatment of this patient?

    A. The patient should be made non-weight-bearing to avoid completing an attached bucket handle tear of the medial meniscus
    B. A majority of patellar dislocations are medial
    C. Popliteal artery damage is the most serious complication of this injury
    D. An intact knee extensor mechanism rules out an injury requiring emergent surgical repair
    E. Peroneal nerve injury in this condition is rare, occurring in less than 5% of those affected

62. A 25-year-old male presents to the emergency department with blunt ocular trauma after he was struck in the face with a baseball. Which of the following exam findings is associated with an ophthalmologic emergency requiring the most immediate attention?

    A. Restricted upgaze
    B. Proptosis
    C. Hyphema
    D. Constricted pupil

63. You serve as a college team physician. While you do not receive any financial compensation for this position, you serve a formal role with regard to game coverage and return-to-play decisions. Which of the following statements best reflects how you manage this position?

    A. Due to competing pressures from other parties, this will alter how you counsel an athlete, since care is managed differently than the typical patient in the community
    B. Despite not receiving financial compensation from the team, Good Samaritan laws do not provide protection from malpractice litigation
    C. Since return-to-play decisions affect both the athlete and the team, the usual principles of informed consent and patient autonomy do not apply
    D. This position should be used as a significant part of marketing your practice

64. As part of your duties as team physician for a local NCAA Division II university, you perform a preparticipation examination on a 22-year-old defensive back, who is transferring to the university to play football. He informs you that 16 months ago, he had a surgical fusion of his fifth and sixth cervical vertebrae. He provides a letter, from a neurosurgeon at a prominent referral center, that states he can return to football without restrictions. You order a cervical MRI study and review the findings with the radiologist and the team neurosurgeon. The MRI findings demonstrate degenerative changes and disc space narrowing at the levels above and below his fusion. After extensive discussion with the athletic training staff, the team neurosurgeon, the athletic director, and the Vice President for Student Affairs, you decide not to clear this athlete to play football, because you and your team believe he is at high risk for another cervical spine injury. The athlete and his family are irate and threaten legal action against you and the university. Which of the following is the correct response to this situation?

    A. The athlete should be allowed to play football, because he received clearance from a specialist at a highly regarded tertiary referral center
    B. The university should have a standard waiver form for these situations that would allow athletes and parents to absolve the university of any responsibility for athletic participation
    C. You and the university have the legal right to restrict this athlete from participation in football, as long as the decision is individualized and demonstrates sound medical judgment
    D. The physician's risk is negligible is this situation, because Good Samaritan Laws protect physicians from liability in the performance of preparticipation physical examinations

65. A 25-year-old female cyclist is training for her first century (100 miles) bicycle ride. She has been increasing her training mileage over the past two weeks. She complains of volar right ring finger and right little finger pain and tingling after her 20-mile bicycle ride. She also notes weakness with extension of her right ring finger. The examination of her right hand shows no atrophy. Mild weakness with extension of right ring finger and right little finger are noted. Decreased sensation to light touch is noted at the ulnar aspect of right ring finger and at right little finger compared to left side. Tinel's test over Guyon's canal is positive. Tinel's over flexor retinaculum at wrist and Phalen's test are negative. What is the most likely diagnosis?

    A. Wartenberg syndrome
    B. Carpal tunnel syndrome
    C. Radial tunnel syndrome
    D. Ulnar tunnel syndrome

66. Which injury can be associated with electrodiagnostic findings of denervation of the infraspinatus muscle?

    A. Quadrilateral space syndrome
    B. Posterior glenoid labral tear
    C. C7 radiculopathy
    D. Grade I AC joint separation

67. When evaluating the cardiovascular risks of a certain sport, the sports medicine physician must consider both the static and dynamic demands of the sport. What is an example of a sport with both high static and high dynamic demands?

    A. Rowing
    B. Long distance running
    C. Sprinting
    D. Baseball
    E. American football

68. Which of the following is true regarding complex regional pain syndrome (CRPS)?

    A. MRI scans can demonstrate soft tissue changes in CRPS with high specificity but low sensitivity
    B. Three-phase bone scintigraphy can provide valuable information during the first year and is useful in differentiating CRPS from other pain syndromes
    C. Elevated ESR can confirm the diagnosis of CRPS
    D. A negative EMG can rule out the possible diagnosis of CRPS

69. Which of the following is true with regard to strength training for pediatric athletes?

    A. Emerging evidence confirms that strength training in childhood is detrimental to bone health
    B. Although not contraindicated, pediatric athletes less than 10 years of age should be discouraged from strength training to minimize risk of injury
    C. To minimize the risk of growth or development disturbance, pediatric athletes should adhere to pediatric protocols based on one repetition maximum lifts
    D. There is no evidence-based minimum age for participation in a supervised strength training program

70. According to the NCAA Drug Testing Program, every Division I athlete will be drug tested for performance-enhancing drugs at least once each academic year. If an athlete tests positive for a banned substance, without a previous offense, what is the penalty?

    A. Ineligibility for athletic competition for the remainder of the competition season, including the post-season
    B. Ineligibility for athletic competition for the remainder of the academic year
    C. Ineligibility for athletic competition for one calendar year from the date of notification
    D. Ineligibility for athletic competition for the remainder of their NCAA athletic career

71. An 18-year-old, right-hand-dominant offensive lineman complains of right wrist pain for several weeks. He denies any particular injury, just that it is getting worse. He denies numbness in the hand, but says when he tries to grab things, do pushups, or perform lineman drills, the pain gets worse. The pain is located in the middle of the wrist and does not radiate. An x-ray of the wrist, including clenched-fist views, is read as negative. An MRI of the wrist demonstrates a decrease in T1 weighted signal in the lunate. Which of the following is the most likely diagnosis?

    A. Scapholunate ligament disruption
    B. Lunate dislocation
    C. Disruption of the distal radial-ulnar joint
    D. Dietrich disease
    E. Kienbock's disease

72. Neuromuscular training that strengthens hip abductors and core strength, and that which improves knee control, has been an effective intervention in reducing anterior cruciate ligament injuries in female athletes. By increasing the frequency and duration of the neuromuscular training exercises, what has happened to the rate of anterior cruciate ligament injuries?

    A. Doubled
    B. Remained the same
    C. Increased
    D. Decreased

73. A nine-year-old pitcher comes to the office after pitching in a select tournament two weeks ago for one team, as well as pitching for his league team the next day. He complains of lateral elbow pain that did not occur on one pitch, but hurts only when he throws. He is having trouble completely extending the elbow. What is the most likely diagnosis?

    A. Osteochondritis dissecans of the capitellum
    B. Lateral epicondylitis
    C. Osteochondrosis of the capitellum (Panner's disease)
    D. Radial nerve entrapment at the arcade of Frohse
    E. Radial head fracture

74. Which of the following statements is true regarding the biomechanics of throwing?

    A. The primary generators of force in the throwing athlete are the shoulder girdle muscles
    B. Throwing athletes with open growth plates are at greater risk for ulnar collateral ligament tears, because with the smaller muscle mass, these athletes are unable to effectively dissipate the stress across the elbow
    C. In general, the biomechanics of youth pitchers are different from adult pitchers, due to the differences in lever arm length and muscle mass
    D. In theory, any pitch thrown at 80 miles/hour (130 km/hour) or faster has the potential to injure the ulnar collateral ligament

75. A patient presents with chronic forearm pain that she describes as a "deep ache" and associated with some weakness, but no loss of sensation. The pain is worse at night, and she points to an area distal to the lateral epicondyle. On physical exam, she has normal sensation, but the pain is reproduced with wrist extension and finger extension. You suspect a compression neuropathy, which of the following anatomical structures is the most likely source?

    A. Arcade of Frohse
    B. Arcade of Struthers
    C. Guyon's canal
    D. Two heads of pronator teres

76. A 13-year-old cross country runner complains of right anterior knee pain. He denies any trauma to the knee or specific injury. Pain worsens with running and prolonged walking, and improves with rest and ice. He denies locking or popping sensation. An x-ray of the right knee demonstrates a well-circumscribed, nondisplaced fragment of subchondral bone on the articular surface of the patella and no loose bodies. What is the next step in treatment of this condition?

   A. Obtain an MRI
   B. Stop running for six weeks and undergo rehab
   C. Stop running and undergo eccentric strengthening of the quadriceps
   D. Straight leg brace for two weeks

77. What is the structure labeled on the sagittal and transverse imaging of the shoulder?

   A. Ulnar nerve
   B. Supraspinatus tendon
   C. Tendon of the long head of the biceps brachii
   D. Tendon of the short head of the biceps brachii
   E. Axillary nerve

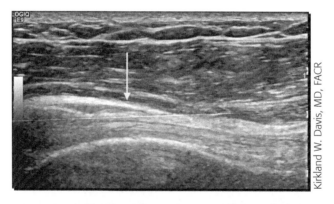
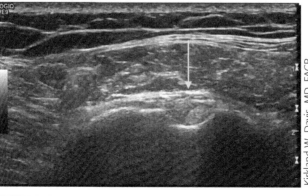

78. A 12-year-old baseball player complains of worsening pain and swelling on the lateral aspect of his left foot for the past three to four weeks. He states that he notices it the most after he has played in a full baseball game or practice, or if he has just been very active that day. It generally has improved by the time he wakes up in the morning. He also states that his baseball cleats and other tight shoes cause pain. He has been wearing flip-flop-type shoes for relief. There is no known trauma to the area, and he has never had this before. Upon further questioning, his mother states that he has been growing quite a bit over the last few months. He has no other complaints of lower limb pain. Physical exam reveals tenderness to palpation directly over the base of the fifth metatarsal of the left foot and swelling at the same level on the lateral aspect of both feet. Below is a radiograph of the left foot. What is the diagnosis?

   A. Stress fracture
   B. Jones fracture
   C. Iselin's disease
   D. Kohler's disease

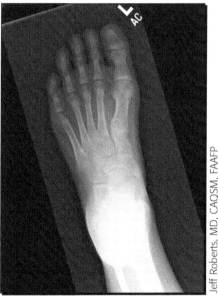

79. During knee flexion, the primary restraints to medial and lateral translation of the patella change. When the knee is in 30 to 60 degrees of flexion, what is the primary restraint?

    A. Vastus medialis oblique (VMO)
    B. Medial patellofemoral ligament (MPFL)
    C. Femoral trochlear groove
    D. Lateral retinaculum

80. Exercise has been found to be beneficial for those living with HIV. Which of the following measures is not a result of moderate exercise (aerobic and resistance training) in those infected with HIV?

    A. Increase in strength
    B. Decrease in resting heart rate
    C. Improved insulin sensitivity
    D. Decrease in lean tissue mass

81. A nine-year-old male fell on an outstretched left arm while skateboarding. He immediately had pain and a noticeable deformity of his left wrist. Radiographs show a displaced fracture of his distal radial metaphysis. He is in pain, but neurovascularly intact. Which of the following is true?

   A. He will need to be followed closely over the next few years for growth arrest of the radius
   B. He should be splinted and follow-up with orthopedic surgery in two weeks for further management
   C. He should undergo open reduction and immobilization
   D. Secondary to a significant degree of remodeling, incomplete reduction of distal radial metaphyseal fractures may yield successful outcomes in children

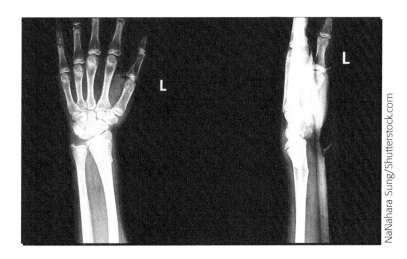

82. You are working in a medical tent of a marathon in September. The wet bulb globe temperature on race day is 80 degrees Fahrenheit (26.7 degrees Celsius), and many runners are experiencing heat-related symptoms. A 42-year-old woman presents to your tent with vomiting, altered mental status, and cramping. On examination, her skin is hot and dry. Her rectal temperature is found to be 104 degrees Fahrenheit (40 degrees Celsius). You quickly treat her with cold water immersion in the medical tent. What concept of thermoregulation occurs during cold water immersion?

    A. Radiation
    B. Evaporation
    C. Convection
    D. Conduction

83. An 11-year-old male presents in clinic with his mother because he's complaining of pain in his right heel after basketball practice and games. At the end of games and practices, he appears to limp and continues to limp for the next hour or so afterwards. On inspection, he has no swelling about the foot or ankle, and normal appearance of both feet, with normal arches. He has tenderness to palpation at the posterior aspect of his calcaneus. Radiographs of both feet show no asymmetry, fracture, or bone cysts. What is the most likely diagnosis?

    A. Calcaneal apophysitis
    B. Os trigonum syndrome
    C. Freiberg's disease
    D. Köhler disease

84. Normal growth and regeneration of muscle tissue in response to training or injury is controlled by satellite cells. Which of the following activates these satellite cells?

    A. Myosin
    B. Insulin-like growth factor-1 (IGF-1)
    C. Interleukin-7 (IL-7)
    D. Interleukin-3 (IL-3)

85. A 16-year-old male football defensive end presents with left knee pain. He was rushing the quarterback at practice and felt a pop in his left knee. He has been unable to weight-bear. He reports no previous knee pain. Physical exam is notable for pain with knee flexion, and he cannot do a normal straight-leg raise against gravity. There is swelling over the tibial tubercle and across the proximal medial and lateral tibia. There does not appear to be a significant knee effusion. Ligament testing is deferred. X-rays are ordered. Based on this description, which of the following is the most likely injury?

    A. Osgood-Schlatter apophysitis
    B. Patellar tendon tear
    C. Patellar sleeve fracture
    D. Tibial tubercle avulsion fracture

86. What is the major contributor to the increased cardiac output in response to an acute bout of aerobic exercise in a well-trained athlete?

    A. Increase in heart rate
    B. Increase in stroke volume
    C. Increase in peripheral resistance
    D. Increase in the systolic blood pressure

87. A high school freshman baseball player presents to your office with the complaint of right elbow pain for two weeks. He describes sudden onset of pain on the medial aspect of the right elbow while throwing. Which of the following is the most likely injury in this patient?

    A. Golfer's elbow
    B. Ulnar collateral ligament (UCL) tear
    C. Medial epicondyle avulsion fracture
    D. Medial epicondyle apophysitis

88. When using ultrasound to evaluate lateral hip pain, it is important to identify tendon insertions on bony landmarks. Which muscular groups have attachment sites on the greater trochanter of the femur?

    A. There are no muscles that attach to the greater trochanter of the femur
    B. The gluteus medius and gluteus maximus have attachment sites on the greater trochanter of the femur
    C. The gluteus medius and gluteus minimus have attachment sites on the greater trochanter of the femur
    D. The gluteus medius, gluteus minimus, and gluteus maxiumus have attachment sites on the greater trochanter of the femur

89. Which is true regarding vascular supply to the knee?

    A. With knee dislocations, the main concern is possible injury to the middle genicular artery
    B. The main blood supply to the ACL is from the superior medial genicular artery
    C. Regarding OCD in the knee, the medial femoral condyle is more often involved compared to the lateral femoral condyle, due to its relatively poor blood supply
    D. Regarding OCD in the knee, the lateral femoral condyle is more often involved compared to the medial femoral condyle, due to relatively poor blood supply

90. Which of the following muscles is correctly paired with the lower leg compartment in which it is found?

    A. Anterior compartment—extensor hallucis longus muscle
    B. Lateral compartment—flexor hallucis longus muscle
    C. Deep posterior compartment—soleus muscle
    D. Superficial posterior compartment—tibialis posterior muscle

91. Your patient is a 32-year-old professional baseball player. He is African-American and had failed conservative management for uncomplicated hypertension. His BP is 145/98 mm Hg. What is the most appropriate first line drug choice?

    A. Amlodipine
    B. Valsartan
    C. Enalapril
    D. Hydrochlorothiazide

92. An aspiring bodybuilder inquires about anaerobic exercises in order to promote strength, speed, and power. Currently, he is more involved in doing aerobic exercises, and wishes to know more about what exercises lead to anaerobic energy expenditure, and what there is to expect once he starts doing more anaerobic exercises regularly. Which of the following is correct?

    A. Considerable anaerobic energy expenditure can be obtained with intense exercise, such as in a 10-mile race
    B. Greater performance in short-duration, high-intensity activities, lasting from seconds to about two minutes, has been observed in muscle energy systems trained using anaerobic exercise
    C. Recruitment of slow-twitch muscle fibers leads to increased anaerobic energy expenditure, as these operate using anaerobic metabolic systems
    D. The anaerobic system does not enable muscles to recover for the next burst in sports that require repeated short bursts of exercise
    E. The by-product of anaerobic glycolysis, lactate, may be detrimental to muscle function, and elevated muscle and blood lactate concentrations can be avoided by doing aerobic exercises in between, as these do not lead to lactate production

93. A 55-year-old male presents for evaluation of numbness and tingling in the thumb and radial aspect of the left hand. He is a mechanic and has known degenerative disc disease in his neck from previous radiographs. For further evaluation of his symptoms, an EMG/NCV test was performed that indicated the source of his symptoms was coming from his cervical spine. The nerve root likely being compressed exits between which two vertebrae?

    A. C4-5
    B. C5-6
    C. C6-7
    D. C7-T1

94. An 18-year-old male baseball pitcher presents to your office with a six-month history of medial-sided elbow pain aggravated by throwing. He has pain and some laxity when testing his ulnar collateral ligament. The transverse ligament (Cooper's ligament) contributes what percentage of ligamentous stability to valgus stress of the elbow?

    A. 0%
    B. 10%
    C. 25%
    D. 33%

95. A 10-year-old girl, level 8 gymnast, presents to your clinic with right greater than left wrist pain. She grew two inches in the past three months. Her 16-year-old sister, who is also a gymnast, presents with the same pain. Why might the younger gymnast's growth spurt put her at increased risk for physeal injury as compared to her older sister?

    A. Decreased physeal strength
    B. Increased bone mineralization
    C. Decreased muscle-tendon tightness
    D. Decreased strength of surrounding fibrous tissue

96. A 26-year-old male endurance athlete complains of weakness with pushing off with the toes of his left foot, as he tries to return to recreational running. Weakness is also noted with plantarflexion and inversion with running for the last few years, as well as slight numbness of the posterior calcaneus. In college, he recalls having lower leg pain with long runs that resulted in having a fasciotomy for chronic exertional compartment syndrome. What nerve may have been injured in the procedure?

    A. Deep peroneal nerve
    B. Superficial peroneal nerve
    C. Sural nerve
    D. Tibial nerve

97. Which of the following fractures involves only the physis and epiphysis, using the Salter-Harris fracture classification system?

    A. I
    B. II
    C. III
    D. IV
    E. V

98. A 33-year-old triathlete comes to your office to discuss his training for the upcoming triathlon season. He is trying to lose weight, but wants to ensure optimal performance as he continues to increase his aerobic endurance. He is interested in a ketogenic diet to help him meet his goals. How would you best describe a ketogenic diet?

    A. High in protein, low in carbohydrates
    B. Low in protein, high in carbohydrates
    C. High in fat, high in carbohydrates
    D. High in fat, low in carbohydrates

99. A 24-year-old male is deep scuba diving with his friends. He starts swimming off course. His friends go after him, and he is not responding to them appropriately. They swim him to the surface. Within a few minutes, he is back to normal. Which gas is responsible for this reaction?

    A. Nitrogen
    B. Helium
    C. Oxygen
    D. Xenon

100. Which of the following statements is true regarding exertional headache?

    A. Factors associated with increased risk of exertional headaches include hot weather and high altitude
    B. Exertional headaches are always benign
    C. Exertional headaches most commonly occur in young women
    D. The typical duration of exertional headaches is seconds to minutes

101. A 31-year-old competitive triathlete training for the Ironman Triathlon presents with severe bilateral quadricep pain and swelling three days after completing an intense hill workout. Which of the following is the correct advice to give him regarding his training?

    A. Discontinue exercise and have lactic acid measurement performed
    B. Discontinue exercise until muscle soreness has been alleviated
    C. Continue exercise, with an intense warm-up
    D. Continue exercise, with pre- and post-exercise stretching

102. In comparison to adult bone, how does pediatric bone differ?

    A. Pediatric bone is more dense
    B. Pediatric periosteum is thinner, and therefore more susceptible to fracture
    C. Pediatric bone is metabolically less active
    D. Pediatric bone is more cartilaginous

103. A 12-year-old female presents to your clinic with a two-month history of generalized right foot pain and limping. The patient says her left foot hurts on occasion, as well. She cannot recall a specific injury, but this pain has started to make basketball practice somewhat difficult. On exam, you notice that she has rigid flat feet. You obtain bilateral, standing-foot radiographs and note an abnormality consistent with tarsal coalition. Which of the following is most true regarding the diagnosis and evaluation of tarsal coalition?

    A. On radiographs, beaking of the talar neck and widening of the talonavicular joint may be associated with tarsal coalition
    B. If a tarsal coalition is present, a radiograph should always be diagnostic, and a CT is rarely needed for diagnosis
    C. It would be unusual for this patient to have a tarsal coalition, as this condition typically presents around five years old
    D. Her right foot may have a tarsal coalition, but it is unlikely her left foot also has a tarsal coalition, because bilateral occurrence is extremely rare

104. A 45-year-old female presents to the office with chronic plantar heel pain. In considering a differential diagnosis, which of the following statements best describes tarsal tunnel syndrome?

   A. Tarsal tunnel syndrome does not co-exist with plantar fasciitis
   B. Tarsal tunnel syndrome causes "first-step" pain when rising from a resting position, and remits promptly with walking
   C. Tarsal tunnel syndrome causes pain with walking and gradually remits with rest
   D. Tarsal tunnel syndrome is associated with lateral ankle pain

105. A 50-year-old female patient presents to your office with exertional pain in her right calf. She has noted the pain during exercise for the past several weeks. Which of the following historical and physical findings would you expect with a diagnosis of popliteal artery entrapment syndrome?

   A. Diminished foot pulses at rest
   B. Pain more closely associated with volume of exercise, rather than intensity of exercise
   C. Slow resolution of symptoms at conclusion of exercise
   D. Patients may have normal pulses that disappear or decrease with plantarflexion or dorsiflexion of the ankle
   E. Markedly elevated compartment pressure

106. A 15-year-old gymnast presents to the office with back pain that has been present for several months, but she has not wanted to address the problem until the end of her competitive season. Her parents are very concerned that she has been complaining daily of back pain with all flipping skills, but became more concerned when she started having pain while lying supine. She has pain on extension of her back, but otherwise her exam is normal. You order x-rays, which are below. What would you tell her family?

   A. This is a normal back x-ray and she can take over-the-counter medications for pain. It will go away with time
   B. This is a vertebral crush injury and needs to be monitored very carefully, especially with the dynamics of gymnastics
   C. She needs an MRI, because this x-ray is non-diagnostic, and an MRI will give you the detail needed to appropriately address her findings
   D. She has a pars interarticularis fracture that has slipped forward (spondylolisthesis) and will need prolonged rest before a slow return to sport

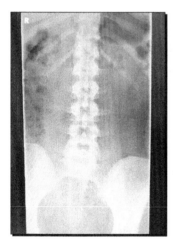
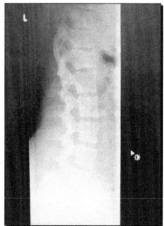
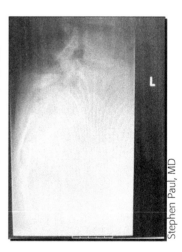

107. A 35-year-old Paralympian with a T4 spinal cord injury is competing in wheelchair basketball at the national level when he is accused of "boosting." When evaluated just prior to the game, his heart rate is regular at 55 and his blood pressure is 195/100. By what mechanism is this patient able to achieve these parameters to improve his performance?

    A. Autonomic dysreflexia
    B. Amphetamine abuse
    C. Epogen injections
    D. Parasympathetic response

108. Which athlete with type 1 diabetes mellitus is at the most risk for developing hyperglycemia from a bout of exercise?

    A. 22-year-old cyclist racing in his first 150-mile event, with good glycemic control, who gave himself a pre-race bolus of regular insulin
    B. 18-year-old multi-event sprinter in the Texas state championship track meet, with elevated fasting blood sugars prior to the event, who pre-medicated with Lantus (insulin glargine)
    C. 19-year-old soccer player participating in early spring conditioning at 75% of her maximal heart rate, with hypoglycemia in the days leading up to her training
    D. 20-year-old rower performing drills in practice, who gave herself a pre-practice bolus of regular insulin, despite not eating that morning

109. An incoming freshman lacrosse player at an NCAA Division I university reports for his preparticipation evaluation. He is an asthmatic and uses an albuterol inhaler prior to exercise and as a rescue medication. He also uses an inhaled corticosteroid in the winter, as his symptoms tend to increase in cold weather. Which of the following statements is most accurate regarding his use of beta-2 agonists?

    A. He should switch to a long-acting beta agonist, given that short-acting beta agonists are banned by the NCAA
    B. He should switch to an inhaled corticosteroid year-round to avoid using a banned substance
    C. The NCAA should be notified of his use of a banned substance for therapeutic use
    D. Proper documentation of the verification of his diagnosis, treatment plan, and medication dose, as well as need for treatment, are sufficient for participation
    E. A request for exception to use a banned substance should be submitted to the NCAA

110. A 16-year-old female Junior Olympic javelin thrower presents with her father for her yearly sports physical. Her weight is 60 kg, she is feeling well, and her exam is normal. She has an international Junior Olympics competition coming up, and her father is concerned that she is drinking so much coffee that it would be considered illegal. The patient reports drinking an eight-ounce mug of regular coffee in the morning, and usually another in the mid-afternoon after school and before her workout. Regarding her caffeine intake, what is the most appropriate recommendations for this patient?

    A. She is consuming too much caffeine to legally compete in international competition, and should abstain from caffeine
    B. She should limit her coffee intake to eight ounces of regular coffee daily in order to avoid disqualification
    C. Inform them that caffeine is a legal performance enhancer, and intake is not enforced by the International Olympic Committee
    D. Inform them that her current intake is acceptable, but that caffeine is considered a performance-enhancing agent at high doses

111. Which of the following is seen as an important aspect in the biomechanics of patellofemoral dysfunction that can respond to conservative treatments?

    A. Internal rotation of the femur at foot strike
    B. External rotation of the femur at foot strike
    C. Trochlear dysplasia
    D. Laterally displaced tibial tuberosity

112. The diagnosis of arrhythmogenic right ventricular cardiomyopathy (ARVC) can be challenging. Which of the following criteria suggest true ARVC, rather than changes that may occur within the normal athletic heart?

    A. Incomplete right bundle branch block
    B. Inverted T waves within the precordial leads
    C. Occasional premature ventricular complexes (two or less per 10 seconds)
    D. Bulging of the right ventricle or systolic dysfunction

113. A 40-year-old Caucasian male was admitted to the hospital after an episode of syncope that occurred while he was jogging. Witnesses reported that the patient began to swerve off of the jogging path into the adjacent bike lane, where he then passed out. In the emergency room, a 12-lead electrocardiogram was completely normal. A trans-thoracic echocardiogram was also completely normal. A two-hour postprandial glucose test was normal. An MRI of the brain was normal. Due to concerns about shortness of breath at the time of the incident, a ventilation-perfusion scan was performed, results: normal. A stress test (Bruce protocol) lasted 15 minutes, achieved 17 METs, a maximum blood pressure of 180/70 mm Hg, and a maximum heart rate of 184 beats per minute (100% of the maximal predicted value for age). A signal-averaged ECG revealed no abnormalities. After being released from the hospital, he had another pre-syncopal episode on a Holter monitor, which did not record any abnormalities. He said that his peripheral vision turned dark, and he became dizzy and experienced chest pressure. The patient reported that the Bruce protocol did not achieve the level of exertion necessary to produce his symptoms. Which of the following is your number one suspicion for his symptoms?

    A. Hypertrophic cardiomyopathy
    B. Acute myocarditis
    C. Cardiac aneurysm
    D. Coronary artery abnormality

114. A 35-year-old Hispanic male cyclist presents to your clinic with continued concerns after being evaluated by cardiology. He was originally referred to cardiology after findings of sinus bradycardia of 45 bpm on ECG, as well as mild cardiomegaly on chest x-ray during a pre-operative evaluation prior to right knee arthroscopy. He has recovered from his knee surgery, but is now concerned that he is at risk for heart disease and asks your opinion on whether he should continue to cycle. You review his echocardiogram from three months ago. Which of the following is the most accurate recommendation?

   A. You recommend the patient should continue to cycle, because his findings of eccentric LV wall hypertrophy of 11 mm and left atrial enlargement are not uncommon findings with his sport and age
   B. You recommend the patient should continue to cycle, because isometric exercises can cause normal physiological changes to his heart, and he should not be concerned with a left ventricular hypertrophy of 16 mm, given the expected increase with exercise
   C. You recommend the patient should not continue to cycle, because the increase in his cardiac mass, along with the left ventricular end diastolic diameter of 55 mm, is consistent with cardiomyopathy
   D. You recommend the patient should not continue to cycle, because a second echo demonstrated decreasing cardiac mass, as well as decreasing left ventricular hypertrophy from 12 mm to 10 mm

115. Which of the following findings on a preparticipation cardiovascular exam would be suspicious for a pathologic murmur and require further follow-up with a cardiologist prior to clearance?

   A. Crescendo-decrescendo murmur
   B. Murmur heard best over the pulmonic area
   C. Murmur that becomes louder with squatting
   D. Murmur that becomes louder with standing from a squatting position
   E. Murmur with musical or vibratory quality

116. Which of the following findings on an ECG would NOT be considered a normal physiological adaptation to training in an athlete?

   A. Sinus bradycardia greater than or equal to 30 beats per minute
   B. QTc of 490 ms
   C. First degree AV block
   D. Incomplete right bundle branch block

117. With regard to Brugada syndrome, which of the following statements is true?

    A. It is prompted by structural changes in the right ventricle, causing ventricular fibrillation and sudden death
    B. It is the same as early repolarization,.
    C. It is a channelopathy, characterized by a susceptibility to sudden death and associated with incomplete right bundle branch block and precordial ST elevations
    D. It is another name for short QT syndrome
    E. It cannot be identified on a preparticipation ECG

118. Which of the following is associated with the onset of shoulder adhesive capsulitis?

    A. Lumbar spondylolisthesis
    B. Aortic stenosis
    C. Renal disease
    D. Parkinson disease

119. A 15-year-old male athlete comes into your office for a sports physical. He appears to be in good shape. During the encounter, the patient's mother asks about a prior incident, in which the patient had passed out while playing basketball. The patient reports that during the incident he became very lightheaded and had tunnel vision just prior to syncope. Upon recovering, the patient experienced no confusion. Mom states the patient's older brother experienced this at a young age and was advised to stop intense physical activity. Upon examination, cardiac auscultation reveals a systolic ejection murmur at the left lower sternal border. The murmur associated with hypertrophic cardiomyopathy would be expected to increase with which of the following?

    A. Increased venous return
    B. Decreased venous return
    C. Increased systemic vascular resistance
    D. Increased afterload

120. A 17-year-old female volleyball player presents for her first college preparticipation exam. You note that she is 6'4" with long thin limbs, arachnodactyly, scoliosis, and a pectus excavatum. Which of the following would be considered a major eye criteria in assisting in making the clinical diagnosis of Marfan syndrome?

    A. Ectopia lentis
    B. Flat cornea
    C. Myopia
    D. Retinal detachment

121. Morphologic adaptations of athlete's heart can closely resemble cardiovascular disease. Which of the following findings on ECG is abnormal and would be concerning in an athlete?

    A. First-degree AV block
    B. Early repolarization
    C. Incomplete RBBB
    D. Left-axis deviation

122. An 18-year-old female lacrosse player presents for her annual preparticipation examination. In her history, she relates several episodes of "heart racing," accompanied by slight shortness of breath. Her physical examination, including vital signs, is normal. ECG testing was ordered and appears below. Which is true regarding her ECG?

   A. She has delta waves and a shortened PR interval, consistent with ventricular pre-excitation. She should be withheld from athletic participation and referred to a cardiologist for a diagnosis of Wolff-Parkinson-White syndrome
   B. She has atrial fibrillation and should be placed on anticoagulation after consultation with a cardiologist. She should be withheld from participation
   C. She has findings consistent with the athletic heart, and should be allowed full participation
   D. Normal ECG examination. Allow full participation

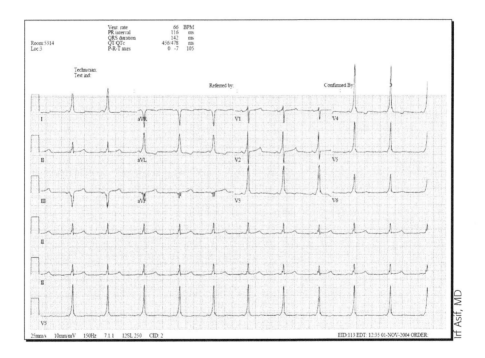

123. A 22-year-old female rower presents with the complaint of recurrent episodes of respiratory distress. These episodes are associated with inspiratory stridor, cough, choking sensations, and throat tightness. You suspect the diagnosis of vocal cord dysfunctions. Which of the following is a mainstay in the treatment of vocal cord dysfunction?

    A. Inhaled albuterol
    B. Speech therapy
    C. Inhaled corticosteroids
    D. Immediate administration of intramuscular epinephrine

124. A 15-year-old tennis player presents with wheezing and shortness of breath while playing. Criteria for moderate persistent asthma includes which of the following?

    A. Symptoms two to three times a week
    B. FEV1 of > 60% and < 80% of predicted
    C. Nighttime awakening three to four times per month
    D. Using short-acting beta agonist two to three times per day for symptoms control
    E. Minor limitation with normal activity

125. A female athlete comes to you for her NCAA preparticipation physical prior to her freshman year of college. She has had a successful career running cross country in high school, and was only held out for a period of weeks to allow for a tibial stress fracture to heal last year. She has since resumed running and is increasing her mileage in anticipation of the upcoming rigorous training schedule. She currently runs daily, approximately 55 miles weekly. Her only other notable finding on history is that she has missed her period for 16 months. When asked about this, she shrugs and states that she expected this due to her athletics. Menarche was at age 13. Vitals: BP: 110/62, pulse rate: 56, respirations: 11, BMI: 17.2 Kg/m2. You diagnose her with female athlete triad. What is the most successful intervention to reverse this condition?

    A. Prescribe oral contraceptives to regulate the menstrual cycle
    B. Prescribe 800 IU Vitamin D and 1200 mg Ca
    C. Refer her to sports psychology to manage the condition, as this is their specialty
    D. Referral to a nutritionist to develop a plan for a well-balanced diet ensuring sufficient caloric intake

126. You have volunteered to help cover the local Paralympic training facility in town. You have heard that several players on the wheelchair basketball team have been clamping their urinary catheters (boosting) to gain a competitive advantage. What mechanism is giving them this advantage?

    A. Increased blood pressure from unopposed sympathetic discharge
    B. Decreased blood pressure from unopposed sympathetic discharge
    C. Increased blood pressure from unopposed parasympathetic discharge
    D. Decreased blood pressure from unopposed parasympathetic discharge

127. Which antidepressant is an activating agent and is on the World Anti-Doping Agency's (WADA) monitoring program list?

    A. Nortriptyline
    B. Venlafaxine
    C. Paroxetine
    D. Bupropion

128. A 13-year-old male track and field athlete presents to clinic with a two-month history of decreased energy and anterior knee pain. His parents are concerned, because he seems depressed and tired all the time. He participates on his school's cross country and track team, and six months ago, he joined a community running team to help prepare for his first marathon. He used to be a member of the soccer and baseball teams but gave these up so that he could focus on becoming a better runner. Which statement is true regarding this athlete?

    A. He should not participate in endurance events like marathons because they may lead to overuse injuries
    B. He should avoid resistance training, as it may further increase his risk of injury
    C. He should avoid multi-sport participation, since he is already suffering from an overuse injury at the age of 13
    D. He is at risk of injury to his growth cartilage

129. A 45-year-old man from Colorado with no significant past medical history went with his friends to climb Pikes Peak (> 14,000 feet). He exercises regularly, without symptoms. He does not take any medications and is a non-smoker. After climbing to over 4000 m (13,000 feet) in one day, he developed headache, fatigue, nausea, and vomiting after setting up camp for the night. Upon closer examination, he appears slightly lethargic. His blood pressure is 138/72, pulse is 90/min, and respiratory rate is 20/min. The remainder of the general and neurological physical exam is unremarkable. The problem has slowly worsened overnight. What is the most appropriate next step?

    A. Ibuprofen and ondansetron
    B. Acetazolamide
    C. Dexamethasone
    D. Immediate descent

130. A patient is brought into your clinic, accompanied by his friend, complaining of worsening generalized muscle and joint pains, shortness of breath, and dry cough upon return from a scuba diving excursion a few hours ago. The patient is a new diver, and his experienced friend is concerned he may have ascended too rapidly. You astutely diagnose the patient with decompression sickness (DCS) and begin treatment by giving 100% oxygen via NRB mask. Despite treatment, the patient shows no improvement, and you decide to treat with recompression therapy via a hyperbaric oxygen chamber. Which of the following accurately describes this mechanism of treatment?

    A. Compression of oxygen gas bubbles that caused the symptoms of DCS to diffuse into tissues and replacing them with oxygen
    B. Compression of nitrogen gas bubbles that caused the symptoms of DCS to diffuse into tissues and replacing them with oxygen
    C. Compression of nitrogen gas bubbles that caused the symptoms of DCS to diffuse into tissues and replacing them with nitrogen
    D. Compression of oxygen has bubbles that caused the symptoms of DCS to diffuse into tissues and replacing them with nitrogen

131. Exertional heat stroke (EHS) is the most severe form of heat illness. Which one of the following statements is true?

    A. Lowering the core body temperature to less than 104 degrees Fahrenheit (40 degrees Celsius) within 30 minutes should be the primary goal of EHS treatment
    B. Cool towels over the patient's head are sufficient to reduce the hyperthermia
    C. A body temperature of < 102.2 degrees Fahrenheit (39 degrees Celsius) by an oral thermometer can rule out EHS
    D. Altered mental status needs to be present to make the diagnosis of EHS

132. A 23-year-old cross country runner is complaining of a generalized papular itchy rash that occurs only during exercise. What would you recommend?

    A. Use sunscreen with PABA (para-aminobenzoic acid) at least 20 minutes prior to exercise
    B. Use topical steroids on the rash during exercise
    C. Take a hot shower the night before a long run or try an antihistamine tablet one hour prior to exercise.
    D. Desensitize with PUVA (Psoralen + UVA)

133. In 2008, the United States Department of Health and Human Services recommended comprehensive guidelines on physical activity for pregnant women. For healthy women (non-exercisers and moderate exercisers), what is the minimum recommended time per week of moderate-intensity aerobic activity during pregnancy?

    A. 90 minutes
    B. 150 minutes
    C. 300 minutes
    D. 225 minutes
    E. Only mild-intensity exercise is advised during pregnancy

134. Which sport reports the highest incidence of urinary incontinence during participation among women?

   A. Softball
   B. Gymnastics
   C. Golf
   D. Swimming
   E. Cross country running

135. A 17-year-old soccer player was diagnosed with infectious mononucleosis (IM) at an urgent care center 10 days ago. Her symptoms began approximately four days prior to diagnosis, so she is now two weeks from her onset of illness. She presents to you for follow-up regarding her return to play. She is no longer febrile, her pharyngitis has resolved, and she is well hydrated, but has continued complaints of fatigue. She is a starter for her high school team. Since they are in the middle of their competitive season, she is anxious to return to play. Which of the following is true regarding her return to contact sports?

   A. A short course of corticosteroids would be useful in helping her symptoms resolve and hastening her return to play
   B. Absence of splenomegaly on physical exam would allow for a safe return to contact sports
   C. In light of her persistent symptoms, she ought to be quarantined from her team to help prevent a spread to her teammates
   D. The athlete should to be afebrile, well hydrated, and asymptomatic before a return to play is considered

136. A three-year-old male presents to your office with pain in his right hip and an inability to bear weight. His parents deny any acute injury or previous similar symptoms. Upon exam, he is febrile and appears acutely ill. He will not allow you to passively move his hip, which is held in flexion, abduction, and external rotation. Which of the following is the most likely diagnosis?

   A. Legg-Calve-Perthes Disease
   B. Juvenile rheumatoid arthritis
   C. Septic arthritis
   D. Leukemia

137. Which of the following statements is true with respect to type 1 diabetic adults and exercise sessions of greater than one hour (endurance exercise)?

    A. Insulin increases are recommended prior to initiation of exercise
    B. Capillary glucose monitoring is only helpful in athletes who are using insulin pumps
    C. Glucagon is the recommended choice to reverse exercise-induced mild hypoglycemia that may occur with exercise
    D. Late-onset hypoglycemia related to prior exercise can be prevented by increasing carbohydrate intake and lowering longer-acting insulin dosages

138. A 12-year-old boy and his mother present to clinic for a preparticipation examination. The boy is healthy, but is known to have sickle cell trait. He has never played organized sports, but engages in active play on most days of the week. He is interested in trying out for various sports teams in his junior high school this year. His mother is concerned about any potential risks associated with his sickle cell trait. How do you counsel her?

    A. Her son should continue to be active and engage in moderate-intensity daily activity, but avoid competitive sports, where he may be subjected to high levels of physical exertion
    B. It is safe for her son to participate in sports characterized by intermittent bursts of intense exertion, but he should avoid sports that emphasize endurance or sustained activity
    C. It is safe for her son to participate in any sports of his choosing, as long as he follows universal precautions regarding hydration, acclimation to heat or altitude, and appropriate progression of exercise intensity
    D. Recommend hemoglobin electrophoresis testing for her son to determine the percentage of HbS, as this will determine if he can participate in sports

139. A 25-year-old female long distance runner presents to your office complaining of fatigue and poor performance. Her history and physical exam are consistent with anemia. Almost all lab work, including peripheral smear and serum iron and total iron binding capacity, are consistent with iron deficient anemia. The one exception is that the ferritin level is normal. What is the most likely explanation for a normal ferritin level in this athlete?

A. Sickle cell trait
B. Vitamin D malabsorption
C. Hepatitis
D. Volume depletion
E. Malaria

140. You are starting a new position in the state of Colorado as a high school team physician. Towards the end of the first football practice of the year, during conditioning drills, an African-American football player collapses to the turf. He complains of severe pain in his bilateral quads and tells you that he is cramping. As the new team physician, you don't know the players yet. You ask the trainer about his medical history, and his response is that this athlete is a recent transfer student from Alabama, and he doesn't know him well. The athlete doesn't know any of his past medical history, other than to say that he's pretty healthy and doesn't know any of his family history. On exam, his muscles are soft, and there is no spasm. The cramps are spreading. He denies any new medications or drug use. He is lucid, alert, and oriented. What should your working diagnosis be, and what is your next step?

A. Cramping from dehydration—start an IV or give him oral fluids
B. Sickle cell trait—atart high flow oxygen and call 911
C. Heat stroke—get him in a tub of cold water and call 911
D. Not in shape—give him some water and let him sit on the sideline until he recovers, then let him go back to practice

141. A 19-year-old male Division I collegiate wrestler presented to you with a complaint of a painful rash on the right upper arm for the last day. Upon further inspection, it appears to look like a cluster of vesicles, with an erythematous base. You decide to withhold him from practice and treat the lesion. When can he resume participation in wrestling?

    A. He can return to play, as long as the lesion is covered with a non-permeable dressing and stretch tape
    B. After the lesion is treated with a topical steroid cream, and he has not developed any new lesions in the last 48 hours
    C. He has not developed any new lesions in the last 72 hours, all the lesions have a firm crust, and he has been on antiviral therapy for 120 hours
    D. He has no new lesions for 48 hours before a meet, has completed 72 hours of antibiotic therapy, and has no moist or draining lesions prior to competition
    E. The lesion has been treated with both topical therapy for 72 hours and a minimum of two weeks of oral therapy, and all lesions are adequately covered

142. A 16-year-old high school football player comes to see you with a tender, red nodule on his leg. It is hot and swollen, and has been worsening for four days. There is some weeping of purulent fluid from the wound surface. Several members of his team have recently been diagnosed with methicillin-resistant staphylococcus aureus infections. Your exam shows a fluctuant area. See image below. What is the most appropriate treatment?

    A. Trimethoprim/sulfamethoxazole orally
    B. Amoxicillin orally
    C. Bactroban topically to the lesion
    D. Trimethoprim/sulfamethoxazole orally, with incision and drainage of the lesion
    E. Rifampin orally, with incision and drainage of the lesion

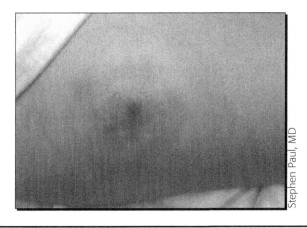

143. Which of the following is true regarding testicular torsion?

    A. Surgical detorsion and orchiopexy should be done within four to six hours of presentation
    B. Manual detorsion should be attempted, followed by observation if the color of the scrotum returns to normal
    C. Scrotal Doppler ultrasound is the test of choice and should be done before treatment is considered
    D. Testicular torsion is a problem seen only in adolescence

144. Gastroesophageal reflux disease (GERD) is a common diagnosis for runners who experience heartburn-type symptoms during activity. Which of the following is true?

    A. GERD symptoms occur because of the relaxation of the upper esophageal sphincter with activity
    B. Eating a large meal right before running will help relieve symptoms
    C. Certain foods, such as tomato sauce or orange juice, may exacerbate symptoms, while other foods, such as yogurt, may help decrease symptoms
    D. Over-the-counter and prescription treatments will provide no relief, and the only option is stopping all physical activity

145. Which of the following is not likely to be beneficial for osteoarthritis (OA) of the knee, based on available evidence-based literature?

    A. Physical therapy
    B. Taping of the knee
    C. Lateral wedge insoles for medial compartment OA
    D. Tai chi
    E. Exercise

146. A healthy appearing 36-year-old white female runner presents to your office with a three-week history of left-sided sinus pain. She has been taking ibuprofen and pseudoephedrine for symptom relief. She continues with intermittent headache, despite the medications, which have given temporary relief of pain. Her pain is slightly increased with running and is mildly improved after running. Past medical history includes hospitalization for the birth of each of her three children. She has no other past medical problems. She takes estrogen/progesterone oral birth control pills, multivitamins, and fish oil. She has a family history of hypertension, CAD, and depression. On exam, her vital signs are as follows: height 5'4", weight 155 pounds, pulse 62, and blood pressure 170/100 mm Hg. She is awake and alert, with no significant distress. Heart and lung exam are within normal limits. What is the best initial choice for treating hypertension in this runner?

   A. Lisinopril
   B. Metoprolol
   C. Hydrochlorothiazide
   D. Lifestyle modification of weight loss, decreased alcohol intake, and decreased caffeine intake
   E. Discontinuation of birth control pills, ibuprofen, and pseudoephedrine

147. The athletic heart syndrome includes which adaptive changes to exercise?

   A. Left ventricular wall thickness greater 15 mm
   B. Left ventricular cavity end diastolic diameter less than 45 mm
   C. Impaired left ventricular filling
   D. Interventricular septum to left ventricular posterior wall thickness ratio less than 1.3

148. A 26-year-old male marathon runner presents with a three-week history of progressive fatigue and exercise intolerance after a flu-like illness. His evaluation leads you to make the diagnosis of viral myocarditis. Per the 36th Bethesda guidelines, you recommend that he withdraw from competitive sports and undergo a prudent convalescent period of approximately?

   A. One month
   B. Three months
   C. Six months
   D. The athlete should never return to competitive sports

149. A 19-year-old female Division I collegiate cross-country athlete presents to the training room with complaints of fatigue and decreased performance. She is concerned she is anemic. Her BMI is 15 kg/m2. You ordered some labs, and her ferritin was 36 ng/ml with a hemoglobin of 12 g/dl. Upon further questioning, she reveals she hasn't had a menstrual period in four months, but she reports this is normal for her, since she rarely has one when she's in-season. Her first menstrual period was at 16 years of age. What is the recommended goal of treatment?

   A. Increase energy availability to 25 kcal/kg FFM
   B. Increase energy availability to 35 kcal/kg FFM
   C. Increase energy availability to 45 kcal/kg FFM
   D. Decrease energy availability, so that she can lose three to five pounds, which puts her at a better running weight

150. A 20-year-old college basketball player injures her knee while landing after pulling down a rebound. Her Lachman's test is positive, and there is concern that she tore her anterior cruciate ligament (ACL). Which of the following is thought to have made her more susceptible to this injury as compared to her male counterparts?

   A. Decreased femoral anteversion
   B. Smaller Q angle
   C. Greater amount of knee flexion while landing
   D. Greater quadriceps activation prior to landing

151. What is the most common cause of sudden death in older athletes (> 35 years old) while running the marathon?

   A. Exercise-associated hyponatremia
   B. Neurocardiogenic syncope
   C. Coronary artery disease
   D. Hypertrophic cardiomyopathy
   E. Cerebral vascular accident

152. Which of the following is the most effective preventative measure for Lyme disease in athletes who spend a significant amount of time outdoors?

   A. Avoiding areas of high tick burdens
   B. Careful removal of ticks within 72 hours
   C. Immunization for those in high-risk or endemic areas
   D. Prophylaxis with amoxicillin for those who cannot take doxycycline

153. Which of the following is false regarding hepatitis B infection?

   A. Concurrent hepatitis D (delta) virus infection increases risk of fulminant infection
   B. Patients with positive HBsAb need immunization against hepatitis B virus
   C. Sexual contact increases the risk of transmission
   D. HBeAg positive status is of concern for possible transmission
   E. Symptoms begin two to four months post-exposure

154. A 24-year-old professional soccer player came off the field during an exhibition match due to laceration to the scalp (see image below). There was head-to-head contact, and the opposing player left the field holding his mouth—no missing or loose teeth or blood noted. You bring the player with a scalp laceration to the training room. Which is the preferred treatment option?

   A. Irrigate with hydrogen peroxide, primary closure with hair apposition and adhesives (e.g., Dermabond)
   B. Irrigate with sterile saline, primary closure with tissue adhesives (e.g., Dermabond)
   C. Irrigate with sterile saline, primary closure with running suture
   D. Irrigate with tap water, allow secondary, delayed closure
   E. Irrigate with tap water, primary closure with staples

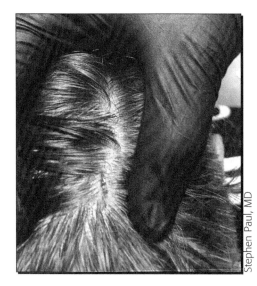

155. A 67-year-old woman presents to your clinic with a persistent foot drop, after sustaining a fibular head fracture two years ago. What type of orthotic would you prescribe?

   A. Metatarsal bar
   B. Ankle foot orthosis (AFO)
   C. UCBL (University of CA Berkeley Lab) shoe insert
   D. Hinged knee brace
   E. Hip-knee-ankle-foot orthoses (HKAFO)

156. In addition to descent, which of the following therapies is advised for the initial treatment of acute mountain sickness?

    A. Rest, ibuprofen, and magnesium sulfate
    B. Increased fluid intake and acetazolamide
    C. Alcohol in small amounts, hydrochlorothiazide, and propoxyphene
    D. Loop diuretics, beta-blockers, and calcium antagonists
    E. Oxygen, acetaminophen, and IV fluids

157. You are evaluating a 35-year-old soccer player with known HIV. His physical exam is normal. His HIV was discovered during an evaluation for penile discharge two years ago. Appropriate recommendations about clearance to play include which of the following?

    A. He may play without restriction as long as his CD4 count is > 200 cells/mm3
    B. He may play as long as his viral load is < 1000 IU/ml
    C. He may play without restriction for an abrasion as long as it can be covered
    D. He may not play unless he discloses his status to the team ATC

158. A 25-year-old female presents to your office with the chief complaint of left thigh pain. She is not doing anything unusual, e.g.. training or workouts. She primarily does low-impact workouts, but did increase the frequency of them. She denies weight training. She denies any trauma. No pain at rest. Prior to her initial visit with you, she went to the ED and had negative radiographs. Your initial exam was unremarkable—no pain with IR, scour compression. A week later, she did a workout with weighted lunges and jump squats. On exam, she notes a bruise, as well as some pain to walk, causing a limp. She now has pain with figure 4, scour, IR, and compression, in addition to some pain with FADIR. She points to the lateral hip as the source of her pain. Palpation of the left thigh reveals a poorly localized area of pain in the midshaft of the femur. There is no difference in circumferential measurement of the right and left thighs. Strength testing of the right quadricep with resisted straight-leg raise does not exacerbate her pain. Radiographs performed in the office of the right hip and femur are negative (see below). What is the most likely diagnosis?

   A. Quadriceps tear
   B. Anterior superior iliac spine avulsion fracture
   C. Femoral stress fracture
   D. Myositis ossificans

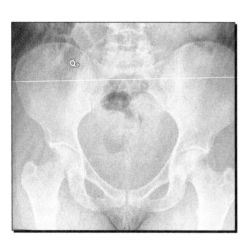
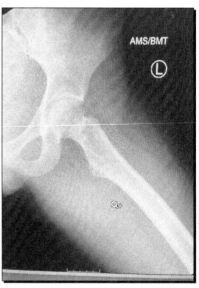

159. A 15-year-old male football player presents to the sports medicine clinic complaining of left posterior thigh pain. Yesterday, he felt a pop at the posterior thigh while running, and this morning, he woke up with a stiff-legged gait and ecchymosis. What is the mechanism of action of this injury?

    A. Knee flexion and knee abduction/concentric contraction
    B. Hip flexion and knee extension/eccentric contraction
    C. Knee flexion and hip flexion/eccentric contraction
    D. Hip internal rotation and knee extension/pylometric contraction

160. Which of the following statements is true regarding hip flexor injury?

    A. In adolescents with the possible diagnosis of hip flexor pain and tenderness over the ischial tuberosity should have an x-ray to rule-out hip flexor origin avulsion
    B. A hop test with pain in the ipsilateral groin is indicative of a hip flexor strain
    C. Patients with large, palpable defects in the rectus femoris rarely need surgery
    D. Hip flexor strains are commonly accompanied by a tingling sensation in the anterior thigh because of irritation of the lateral femoral cutaneous nerve
    E. Significant weakness is usually seen on exam with hip flexor strains

161. A young female soccer player presents with hip pain and clicking. X-rays of the hip are negative, with no evidence of femoral acetabular impingement. What is the appropriate next step?

    A. Order a plain MRI of the hip
    B. Injection of the hip with corticosteroids
    C. Refer for arthroscopy
    D. Order an MR arthrogram of the hip

162. An 18-year-old female freshman college soccer player presents to clinic with a two-month history of pubic and groin pain that began intermittently with activity and has progressively worsened. She originally noted some pubic and medial groin pain on her right side towards the end of practice. It gradually became more frequent, occurring when she kicked the ball or made a sudden twisting movement. Now, even jogging can trigger pain. Over the last six weeks, she has been treated by her trainer for a muscle strain with no benefit. On exam, her vitals are age-appropriate. She has pain with pelvic compression and tenderness to palpation of her pubic symphysis. There is no tenderness to palpation of the inguinal ligament or asymmetry in her musculature. Range of motion is slightly decreased on her right side, with pain noted on resisted hip flexion and adduction. No bulging is noted with Valsalva maneuvers. Thomas test is negative. She has difficulty standing on her right leg. Radiographs (see below) reveal widening of the pubic symphysis and some periarticular sclerosis. What is her most likely diagnosis?

A. Osteitis pubis
B. Adductor strain
C. Iliopsoas strain
D. Stress fracture of the pubic bone
E. Right indirect hernia

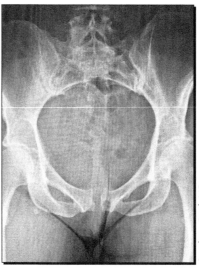

163. A 17-year-old male high school football player injured his right knee after cutting while running. As he pivoted with the football, he stopped abruptly, hyperextended his right knee, and felt a "pop." He then felt excruciating pain in the anterior knee, as well as at the posterior lateral joint line. He rapidly developed an effusion and is now in your sports medicine clinic for rapid assessment of this injury. Examination of the patient is limited, secondary to pain and effusion. However, he does not appear to have an endpoint with anterior drawer. He does have a solid endpoint with posterior drawer, and a positive pivot shift test, and is stable to both valgus and varus stress. His dial test was negative. An x-ray taken in clinic of the right knee demonstrates a small avulsion fracture. Where is this fracture most likely located?

   A. The medial tibial plateau
   B. The medial aspect of the lateral femoral condyle
   C. The medial aspect of the medial femoral condyle
   D. The lateral tibial plateau

164. A high school basketball athlete presents to the emergency department after sustaining a knee injury. He went up for a rebound and landed awkwardly on his right leg, while an opposing player fell into the lateral side of his knee, causing it to buckle. There was a gross deformity to the right knee. EMS states there was no dorsalis pedis pulse present initially at the scene, but after transferring the patient into the ambulance, the DP pulse returned, and the knee did not appear as deformed as before. The patient is complaining of severe pain. X-rays are taken and do not reveal any acute fracture. After adequate analgesia, you exam the knee and find significant laxity with Lachman test, posterior drawer test, and valgus stress test at 0 and 30 degrees of flexion. You are able to palpate a strong dorsalis pedis pulse and popliteal pulse on the right. The peroneal nerve appears intact. What is the next best step in the management of this injury?

   A. Place the knee in a knee immobilizer and discharge
   B. Place the knee in a hinged brace locked at 30 degrees, and discharge
   C. Place the knee in a long-leg posterior splint and discharge with crutches
   D. Measure compartment pressures in the lower leg
   E. Perform ankle-brachial index

165. A 27-year-old female training for a 5K race presents with progressively worsening left lateral knee pain, ongoing for six weeks. She has steadily increased her mileage and has been running on the treadmill, as well as on pavement. Symptoms are exacerbated with running, climbing stairs, and squats. She denies any injury or prior knee problems. On exam, there is no joint effusion, normal and pain free range of motion, and no joint line tenderness or mechanical symptoms. Which of the following should be considered as initial treatment?

    A. Icing, stretching program, activity modification
    B. Referral to orthopaedic sports surgeon
    C. Corticosteroid injection
    D. Physical therapy

166. A 15-year-old female field hockey player cuts laterally to avoid an opponent and falls to the ground. She sits up, but cannot stand, and other players wave you onto the field. She has an obvious deformity to her anterior knee, and she states something "popped." Her knee is stable on testing, no effusion is present, and the neurovascular status of the leg is intact. Which of the following statements is correct regarding the athlete's injury?

    A. Reduce the injury, with the patient sitting, and send her to the hospital for angiography
    B. Reduction is best performed with the patient supine and hip extended
    C. Patients with genu valgum and increased Q angle are predisposed to this injury
    D. Sport specific activity should be continued in a couple of days to prevent deconditioning

167. A 33-year-old male runner presents to your office with complaints of anterior right knee pain, worsening over the past month. He has just recently started training for a marathon that will take place in four months. On physical exam of the right knee, you find mild effusion, vague tenderness over the medial femoral condyle, and some swelling, just medial to the patellar border. With the patient in supine position, you apply pressure with the thumb over the inferior and medial aspect of the patellofemoral joint, and passively flex and extend the knee. The patient reports pain between 30 and 45 degrees, as well as a clicking sensation. Plain radiographs of both knees are unremarkable. What is the most likely cause of this patient's symptoms?

    A. Medial meniscal tear
    B. Osteoarthritis
    C. Patellofemoral pain syndrome
    D. Plica syndrome
    E. Pes anserinus pain syndrome

168. A 62-year-old female presents to your office with increased right medial knee discomfort for one week, with no apparent injury. She has no swelling, and reports no locking or giving way episodes. She has had mild knee discomfort for 10 years. She has had no relief with anti-inflammatories. On exam, she has complete range of motion and no effusion, but does report medial joint line pain with palpation, and discomfort with McMurray's test. In-office x-rays performed show Kellgren-Lawrence grade III changes in the medial compartment. What is the next management step?

    A. MRI to confirm diagnosis
    B. Surgical referral for arthroscopy
    C. Surgical referral for total knee replacement
    D. Acetaminophen and physical therapy

169. A 21-year-old comes in for evaluation after an ankle injury. Using the Weber classification for lateral malleolus fractures, which of the following demonstrates a need for immediate evaluation?

    A. Weber A
    B. Weber B
    C. Weber C
    D. Both Weber A and B require consideration for surgical treatment

170. A 45-year-old overweight male presents with a complaint of pain in the left great toe. Recently, he started jogging two miles a day due to a desire to lose weight, but has not changed his diet. Patient reports drinking four cans of beer every night. The pain has developed over the last two weeks and is increased after running. Exam demonstrates a normal foot with tenderness and swelling of the medial plantar aspect of the left first metatarsophalangeal joint. Passive dorsiflexion of the toe causes pain in that area. Plantarflexion produces no discomfort, and no numbness can be appreciated. Which of the following is most likely his diagnosis?

    A. Cellulitis
    B. Gout
    C. Morton's neuroma
    D. Sesamoid fracture

171. A 34-year-old male runner presents to your office with pain in the left Achilles region for the past six months. His pain has been worse over the past six weeks. He has had difficulty performing his six-mile runs, and yesterday, he could not run at all. Which of the following is true regarding Achilles tendinopathy?

    A. Achilles tendinopathy is a degenerative, as opposed to an inflammatory, condition
    B. Most patients fail non-operative measures, even if the condition is treated early
    C. Surgery is required in most cases involving decompression of the tendon by tenotomy and aggressive measures to improve the local circulation
    D. Surgery is recommended after non-operative methods of management have been tried for at least three months

172. Which of the following statements is true regarding seizures and participation in water sports?

    A. Individuals with uncontrolled seizures should only be cleared for swimming activities when undertaken in the presence of a lifeguard
    B. Individuals with uncontrolled seizures may be cleared for non-swimming water sports with no restrictions
    C. Individuals who have been seizure-free for five years and are not taking anti-seizure medications may be allowed to participate in watersports
    D. Individuals with a history of epilepsy who are cleared for water sports should hyperventilate before entering the water, since this reduces the chance of seizures

173. What is the most common cause of weakness in entrapment syndromes?

    A. Neurapraxia
    B. Denervation
    C. Axonotmesis
    D. Neurotmesis
    E. Disuse atrophy

174. You are consulted on a female track athlete with a known seizure disorder. Her favorite events are the middle distances, and she has never had a seizure training or in competition. She has not had a seizure in three years and has not changed medications. The school is concerned about whether she should be allowed to compete, due to her medical condition. Refraining from which of the following sports may be considered for this patient?

    A. Track
    B. Cycling
    C. Singles ice skating
    D. Football
    E. Swimming

175. Which of the following is an absolute contraindication to collision-sports participation?

    A. Torg-Pavlov Ratio < 0.8
    B. Recurrent cervical cord neuropraxia/transient quadriparesis
    C. Healed, non-displaced, stable fracture of C3-C4 at posterior ring
    D. Clay shoveler's fracture
    E. Healed cervical herniated disc

176. You are performing preparticipation physical exams at a local high school prior to the fall sports season. You examine a freshman male going out for football for the first time. His paperwork indicates that he is missing one of his testicles. After a little bit of questioning, he tells you his left testicle never came down and had to be surgically removed while he was a young child. You perform a physical exam and confirm the presence of only one testicle, which is on the right side. Which of the following is the best course of action for this young athlete?

    A. Do not clear him for football, pending further evaluation by a urologist to determine if he can safely play
    B. Restrict this athlete from playing football, but recommend trying out for golf or cross country as alternative sports for participation
    C. Clear the athlete to play football without restriction, since studies have demonstrated there is a low risk of testicular injury in sports
    D. Have a discussion with the athlete and his parents regarding the risk of injury to the lone testicle and review the use of protective equipment

177. Which of the following is correct regarding preparticipation decisions?

    A. An athlete with one congenitally missing kidney, who also has a polycystic remaining kidney, should be allowed to participate in football, as long as he has regular blood pressure monitoring and uses a kidney guard pad during practice and games
    B. An athlete with one testicle does not need to be counseled regarding the risk of losing his fertility during play if sport participants routinely use a protective cup (e.g., baseball and football)
    C. When an athlete has only one functional eye (with less than 20/40 corrected visual acuity), further evaluation by an ophthalmologist is recommended
    D. Athletes with only one functional eye can participate in boxing if the functional eye is ipsilateral to their dominant hand

178. A 14-year-old male with known solitary kidney, which is located in its normal anatomical location, presents to you for his preparticipation physical evaluation. He has played football for several years and wants to join his high school team this year. He and his parents report no known problems, hospitalizations, or concerns related to the kidney. His exam is normal. Which of the following recommendations best fits this athlete's clearance to play?

   A. This athlete should be cleared to play non-contact sports only
   B. This athlete may be cleared to play collision sports with a qualified yes, meaning that protective equipment must be worn
   C. This athlete may be cleared to play non-contact and limited contact sports only, but absolutely no collision sports
   D. This athlete should be cleared to play any sport without further recommendation

179. A 30-year-old female computer worker presents with occupation-related forearm pain for several months. On physical exam, weakness is noted in the extensor carpi ulnaris and the distal extensors of the hand, but no sensory deficit is noted. You suspect which nerve syndrome?

   A. Posterior interosseus nerve syndrome
   B. Anterior interosseus nerve syndrome
   C. Carpal tunnel syndrome
   D. Tarsal tunnel syndrome
   E. Ulnar neuropathy

180. A 200-pound, first-string NCAA Division I quarterback reports to football camp after being diagnosed both clinically and by laboratory tests with mononucleosis three weeks ago. He is in excellent health, feels great, and brings with him a note from his internist that he is cleared for full contact. What facts can you count on when determining his return-safely-to-play status?

   A. There is no good evidence that return to play after clinical recovery from mononucleosis is particularly dangerous, but the risk is not zero
   B. His primary physician already signed off, and your exam is normal. This player is at no risk for splenic rupture now
   C. You have recently attended point-of-care ultrasound training. You ultrasound his abdomen. Because his spleen is not enlarged, you determine there is no risk for splenic rupture
   D. The patient and his family will sign a waiver exempting the medical staff and the university from any liability if he returns to play

181. In order to prevent exercise-induced bronchospasm (EIB) during competition, athletes with documented asthma would benefit from which of the following treatments?

    A. Pre-medicate with beta-adrenergic agonist
    B. Pre-medicate with corticosteroids
    C. Pre-medicate with inhaled corticosteroids
    D. Pre-medicate with anti-histamines
    E. Pre-medicate with nasal steroids

182. A 17-year-old senior high school cross country runner with a history of two femoral neck stress fractures presents to your sports medicine clinic for persistent amenorrhea in the setting of decreased performance. She has not had her menstrual period for at least one year and also appears thin and frail. Her performance at recent track meets has suffered, as she was all-county last year, but has not even placed at her meets in quite some time. She says she feels a great deal of pressure as she applies for college, and badly wants an athletic scholarship. Which of the following is not a prudent next step in managing this patient?

    A. Educating the patient, her parents, and her coaches about the health risks of her diagnosis
    B. Supplementation with calcium/vitamin D and increasing caloric intake
    C. Limiting the time she spends running at her practice sessions
    D. Starting an oral contraceptive

183. A 17-year-old female notes on her preparticipation physical that she has had regular menstrual periods over the past four years, until the last 10 months. During the last 10 months, she has had no menstrual periods. Her history reveals no obvious causes for this, other than her participation in cross-country and track. Her physical exam is unremarkable. Which of the following statements is the best statement that reflects her condition?

    A. She is suffering from exercise-related amenorrhea and should be counseled about starting on calcitonin to prevent osteoporosis
    B. She is suffering from oligomenorrhea and should be counseled to gain weight so that her menstrual cycles return to normal
    C. She is normal for her age and should wait one year to see if her menstrual cycle returns to normal
    D. She is suffering from an eating disorder and should be counseled to seek a mental health consultation
    E. She is suffering from amenorrhea and should be counseled to have laboratory testing to determine the cause

184. A defensive player on a collegiate football team has just come off the field after making a tackle. He tells the athletic trainer that the left side of his neck hurts, and he feels tingling and burning in his left shoulder. Sideline examination reveals decreased sensation over the lateral deltoid and weakness with abduction and elbow flexion. Spurling's maneuver is negative. After halftime, the symptoms abate. Of note, the player had one previous episode with similar symptoms two weeks prior. What is the next step in management of this player?

    A. Studies show that neck rolls and cowboy collars successfully prevent this type of injury
    B. He should not return to play and will need further imaging workup
    C. He should not return to play and requires an urgent nerve conduction study
    D. He should not return to play and should be withheld for the remainder of the season, since he has now had two injuries

185. You are working at a clinic in the Key West Florida and are asked to evaluate a group of scuba divers. They are planning to get certified for scuba diving and would like preparticipation clearance. Which one of the following patients has an absolute contraindication to scuba dive?

    A. 23-year-old female type 1 diabetic, who has been on an insulin pump for 12 years. She is a high-level triathlete. No recent episodes of ketoacidosis and no evidence of end organ damage. Her hemoglobin A1C is less than 7.5
    B. 28-year-old female with a recent past medical history of concussion while playing volleyball eight weeks ago. She completed her return-to-play protocol. She is thinking about getting pregnant
    C. 62-year-old male, former Navy diver, with a 12-year history of type 2 diabetes, who is on metformin. He was recently diagnosed with peripheral neuropathy and impaired low-glucose awareness. His last A1C was 9.1
    D. 22-year-old male with asthma. An albuterol inhaler is his only medication, and his last FEV1 was greater than 80% of predicted normal

186. A mother brings her 13-year-old boy with Down syndrome to your office for medical clearance to participate in Special Olympics. Which of the following statements is true regarding sports participation in this athlete?

   A. Athletes with Down syndrome should never participate in sports such as equestrian, diving, high jump, or alpine skiing
   B. There is a congenital absence or laxity of the transverse atlas ligament in 10% to 30 % of patients with Down syndrome
   C. Cervical spine manipulation is frequently recommended for patients with Down syndrome
   D. Routine yearly x-rays are recommended to evaluate for atlantoaxial instability

187. A 15-year-old male with Down syndrome presents to your clinic for his preparticipation examination. He will be participating in judo. Per Special Olympics guidelines, the patient will require a lateral cervical spine x-ray, with flexion and extension views, to rule out atlantoaxial instability (AAI). These x-rays will be used to assess the atlanto-dens interval (ADI), which is the space between the posterior aspect of the anterior arch of the atlas and the odontoid. Which measurement of the atlanto-dens interval (ADI) would disqualify the athlete from competing in a high-risk sport such as judo?

   A. Greater than 1.5 mm
   B. Greater than 2.5 mm
   C. Greater than 3.5 mm
   D. Greater than 4.5 mm

188. A 26-year-old male soccer player consults with you about groin injuries. He has had a number of groin injuries in the course of sports participation, usually diagnosed as "groin strains" by his team's athletic trainers. His last injury was about eight months ago, and while he is currently asymptomatic, he asks you if there was any way to potentially prevent recurrence of this injury, while still allowing him to participate in soccer. His physical examination shows no areas of tenderness to palpation, full normal range-of-motion, and roughly equal adductor and abductor muscle strength bilaterally. What do you recommend as part of a training strategy to prevent athletic groin strains?

   A. Strengthen the hip adductors to increase the adductor: abductor strength ratio
   B. Strengthen the hip abductors to increase the abductor: adductor strength ratio
   C. Strengthen the hip flexors to increase the flexor: extensor strength ratio
   D. Strengthen the hip extensors to increase the extensor: flexor strength ratio

189. Overtraining syndrome (OTS) is a poorly understood condition characterized by the following symptoms: mood changes, fatigue, and decreased performance, accompanied by increased achiness and more frequent injuries. What is the best explanation of the pathophysiology?

   A. Branched-chain amino acid (BCAA) deficiency
   B. Glycogen depletion
   C. Cytokine overload
   D. Hypothalamic dysregulation
   E. Overtraining syndrome involves a complex, poorly understood pathophysiology, likely involving multiple pathways

190. A 28-year-old male endurance runner complains of symptoms of fatigue as he increases his training runs in preparation for an upcoming marathon. He also mentions that his mile split times have worsened, which is causing him a lot of anxiety. His wife is concerned that he has grown more irritable and has not been eating well lately. What do you recommend?

   A. Start a selective serotonin reuptake inhibitor (SSRI)
   B. Try drinking a caffeinated beverage 30 minutes to an hour prior to his training runs
   C. Take a break from running until his symptoms resolve
   D. Start iron and vitamin C supplementation
   E. Be sure to plan for carbohydrate ingestion (either a carbohydrate-electrolyte solution or sports gel containing glucose and fructose) during his longer training runs

191. A 15-year-old female elite figure skater presents to your clinic with her sixth injury in six months. Review of history reveals fatigue, loss of appetite, decrease in athletic performance, sleep disturbance, and worsening school grades. In addition to treating her current injury, you diagnose her with overtraining and burnout. One strategy for preventing overtraining/burnout is periodization. What is periodization?

   A. A process of slowly progressing workout intensity and workload
   B. A process of periodically evaluating an athlete for symptoms and signs of overtraining
   C. A process of emphasizing proper technique and mechanics to prevent chronic or acute injuries
   D. A process of cyclically varying the training stimulus in phases throughout the calendar year

192. A running group that is currently developing their training regimen for an upcoming marathon in six months has asked you to speak to them about the effects of altitude training on running performance. Which of the following is the most appropriate general recommendation?

    A. Training at altitude does not seem to improve performance in endurance events and is generally not thought to be effective
    B. Best available evidence suggests that living at moderate altitude then training and competing at low altitude does improve performance in endurance events
    C. Current recommendation is to live and train at high altitude as often as possible, regardless of the altitude of the competition site
    D. Encourage the participants to live at low altitude and train at high altitude to maximize performance

193. You are the medical director for a large youth soccer tournament that will be played in hot weather. Which of the following is correct about pediatric patients exercising in hot weather?

    A. Pediatric patients who are well hydrated and acclimated to heat are able to exercise in the heat at no greater risk than adult patients
    B. Pediatric patients have similar sweat volumes compared to adults
    C. Pediatric patients have the same number of sweat glands compared to adults
    D. Pediatric patients have a similar body surface area-to-mass ratio and a similar heat gain from the environment compared to adults

194. Which of the following is true of resistance training in the pediatric population?

    A. Resistance training can result in increased strength without muscle hypertrophy or changes in body composition
    B. Strength gains are not lost during detraining
    C. Resistance training is generally discouraged in children and adolescents, due to safety concerns
    D. Growth in height and weight of preadolescents can be influenced by resistance training

195. You are one of several first responders on the scene of an unresponsive 17-year-old female with witnessed collapsed during basketball practice. CPR is begun, EMS activated, and the AED placed. Shock is advised. What is the next step?

    A. Give three consecutive shocks, followed by resumption of CPR
    B. Give one shock, and then check pulse/rhythm and immediately reshock if advised
    C. Give one shock, and then resume CPR for five cycles before rechecking rhythm
    D. Give two rescue breaths and five cycles of CPR before proceeding with shock

196. Which of the following is a correct statement about burnout and overtraining in youth sports?

    A. Most young athletes who drop out of sports are burned out
    B. Most youth who discontinue a sport do so as a result of poor coaching
    C. To reduce the likelihood of burnout, an emphasis should be placed on competition more than skill development
    D. Symptoms may include fatigue, lack of enthusiasm about practice or competition, or difficulty with successfully completing usual routines

197. A 14-year-old male patient presents to your office for a preparticipation physical exam. The patient's mother and brother have Marfan syndrome. The family has been tested for the genetic mutation for Marfan syndrome. This patient was found to be negative and cleared for all sports in the past. What is the mutation that is tested for?

    A. Prothrombin gene mutation
    B. Trisomy 21
    C. Sarcomeric mutation
    D. BRCA1 gene
    E. Fibrillin 1 mutation

198. A 14-year-old football player at the 25th percentile for height and 100th percentile for weight has a persistent blood pressure of 145/80 mm Hg during his preparticipation physical, with an otherwise normal cardiovascular exam. Which of the following is true regarding sports clearance for this athlete?

    A. Clearance for sports with no further evaluation required
    B. Clearance for sports with recommendation of repeat blood pressure measurement in six months
    C. Clearance for sports after the athlete has lost 10% of his extra weight
    D. Clearance for sports after blood pressure is controlled

199. Which of the following is a current American Heart Association (AHA) recommendation regarding cardiac evaluation during the preparticipation exam?

    A. Auscultate for heart murmur during provocative maneuvers
    B. Palpate bilateral brachial pulses
    C. Obtain bilateral brachial blood pressure with the athlete standing
    D. Perform electrocardiogram on all athletes

200. A 16-year-old male presents for his preparticipation physical evaluation. On exam, he is found to have corrected right eye visual acuity of 20/20, but corrected left eye visual acuity of only 20/200. Mom explains that the left eye vision loss was due to a childhood injury at age two. He has just recently been seen for his yearly eye exam with an eyecare professional, who did not suggest any change in his correction or any eye protection for this athlete's sports of choice, which are football, wrestling, sprinting events, and full-contact martial arts. Which of the following is the correct protective eyewear recommendation for the associated activity for this athlete?

    A. Track: normal street-wear frames with 2 mm polycarbonate lenses
    B. Football: helmet with wire face mask
    C. Baseball: normal street-wear frames with 2 mm polycarbonate lenses
    D. Full-contact martial arts: custom made sport goggles

Test 1 Answers, Critiques, and References

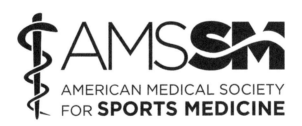

1. A 17-year-old female cross-country athlete presents to your office with one month of left-sided groin pain made worse with running. She now has some pain with walking and increased pain with stairs. Hip x-rays demonstrate a non-displaced lateral (tension-side) stress fracture of the femoral neck (see images). What is the most appropriate management of this injury?

    A. Non-weight-bearing with crutches for two weeks, followed by a gradual return to running protocol
    B. Discontinue running for one month and begin supplementation with calcium and vitamin D
    C. Patient is made non-weight-bearing immediately and referred to orthopedic surgery for potential surgical procedure
    D. Avoid running but may continue weight-bearing while MRI is ordered

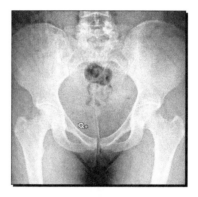

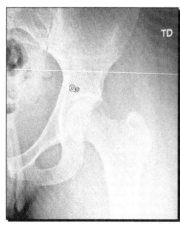
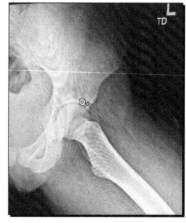

Correct Answer: C. Patient is made non-weight-bearing immediately and referred to orthopedic surgery for potential surgical procedure

Tension-sided femoral neck stress fractures are unstable and have a significant risk of major complications, including fracture displacement, AVN of the femoral head, and hip replacement. Answers A and B are incorrect, because the time frame is too short to return an athlete to running with this fracture, there is no mention of follow-up, and no consideration of surgical intervention. Answer D is incorrect because this patient should be made non-weight-bearing immediately. If suspicion is high for a femoral neck stress fracture, and radiographs are negative, the patient should be made non-weight-bearing until MRI is obtained. Compression-sided femoral neck stress fractures that comprise greater than 50% of the neck width may also require surgery.

1. DeFranco MJ, Recht M, Schils J, Parker RD. Stress fractures of the femur in athletes. Clin Sports Med 2006 Jan;25(1):89-103, ix.
2. Finn T. Femoral neck stress fracture. Medscape. Accessed May 12, 2014 at http://emedicine.medscape.com/article/86808-overview.
3. Jacobs JM, Cameron KL, Bojescul JA. Lower extremity stress fractures in the military. Clin Sports Med 2014 Oct;33(4):591-613.

2. The sleeper stretch addresses which specific part of the shoulder?

    A. Inferior glenohumeral ligament
    B. Anterior inferior labrum
    C. Posterior capsule
    D. Rotator interval

Correct Answer: C. Posterior capsule

The sleeper stretch is a self-directed stretch of the posterior capsule of the shoulder. With the patient in a side-lying position and a roll under the axilla, the opposite extremity forces the flexed elbow in a downward direction, thereby internally rotating the shoulder and stretching the posterior capsule. This can be an especially useful stretch for the overhead throwing athlete. None of the other Answer choices are targeted with the sleeper stretch.

1. Tyler TF, Nicholas SJ, Lee SJ, Mullaney M, McHugh MP. Correction of posterior shoulder tightness is associated with symptom resolution in patients with internal impingement. Am J Sports Med 2010;38:114-119.
2. Reinold MM, Gill TJ, Wilk KE, Andrews JR. Current concepts in the evaluation and treatment of the shoulder in overhead throwing athletes, part 2: injury prevention and treatment. Sports Health 2010 Mar;2(2):101-115.

3. A 15-year-old high school crew athlete with no prior orthopedic history presents to you with two months of progressive low back pain. The pain was originally intermittent, but now is persistent, both with rest and activity, particularly when her back is in a maximally extended position (the "drive" position). Initial x-rays, including standing AP, lateral views, and oblique views are unremarkable. What is the next appropriate imaging study that may help clarify the diagnosis?

   A. Bone scan with SPECT study
   B. CT scan of the lumbar spine, with thin cut scan through the area of concern
   C. MRI of the lumbar spine
   D. DEXA scan

Correct Answer: A. Bone scan with SPECT study

This 15-year-old patient presents with a story most concerning for a lumbosacral pars interarticularis stress fracture, or spondylolyis. Spondylolysis may develop in athletes with recurrent lumbar extension, especially if they have poor abdominal strength and control. When x-ray imaging is negative for spondlylolithesis or unilateral pars defects, and clinical suspicion remains high, a bone scan with SPECT images remains the most sensitive in identifying an acute spondylolysis. A CT scan of the lumbar spine, with thin cuts obtained through an area of concern, may be a reasonable second study to help stage a spondylolysis and can provide further details, such as fracture staging that are unavailable by bone scan. CT scan alone, however, cannot help differentiate acute from chronic lesions. While an MRI is tempting, because it does not expose the patient to radiation, it remains less sensitive than bone scan in identifying a spondylolyis, though it is of greater benefit if there is suspicion of herniated disc or other non-bony pathology. A DEXA scan is not useful in the evaluation of spondylolysis in the adolescent athlete.

1. Standaert CJ, Herring SA. Expert opinion and controversies in sports and musculoskeletal medicine: the diagnosis and treatment of spondylolysis in adolescent athletes. Arch Phys Med Rehabil 2007 Apr;88(4):537-540.

4. A 13-year-old female soccer player presents to the office with bilateral anterior knee pain. Physical examination is notable for lateral patella facet pain, ankle dorsiflexion 10 degrees, hamstring popliteal angle complement 10 degrees, and knees going into slight valgus with single-leg squat. The single most important part of physical therapy for this patient is?

   A. Strengthen VMO
   B. Strengthen gluteus medius
   C. Stretch hamstrings
   D. Stretch gastrocnemius

Correct Answer: B. Strengthen gluteus medius

This patient has patellofemoral pain syndrome (PFPS). There are several contributing factors to poor mechanics associated with PFPS. Some, such as weak hip abductors, weak quadriceps, tight hamstrings, and limited ankle dorsiflexion, are modifiable with physical therapy. Answers C and D are incorrect because the patient already has normal flexibility. The single-leg squat assesses the lower leg kinetic chain. In the vignette, the patient's knee goes into valgus with a single-leg squat. This suggests that the hip abductors are relatively weak and not firing appropriately. The correct answer is B because the gluteus medius is the major hip abductor muscle. Because no evidence is given that the quadriceps/VMO is weak, Answer A is not the correct answer for this patient.

1. Myer GD, Ford KR, Barber Foss KD, Goodman A, Ceasar A, Rauh MJ, et al. The incidence and potential pathomechanics of patellofemoral pain in female athletes. Clin Biomech (Bristol, Avon) 2010 Aug;25(7):700-707. doi: 10.1016/j.clinbiomech.2010.04.001. Epub 2010 May 14.
2. Baldon R, Serrao F, Silva R, Piva S. Effects of functional stabilization training on pain, function, and lower extremity biomechanics in women with patellofemoral pain: a randomized clinical trial. J Orthop Sports Phys Ther 2014;44(4):240-A8.
3. Myer GD, Ford KR, Di Stasi SL, Foss KD, Micheli LJ, Hewett TE. High knee abduction moments are common risk factors for patellofemoral pain (PFP) and anterior cruciate ligament (ACL) injury in girls: is PFP itself a predictor for subsequent ACL injury? Br J Sports Med 2015 Jan;49(2):118-122. doi: 10.1136/bjsports-2013-092536. Epub 2014 Mar 31.

5. A 55-year-old male presents to your office with right posterior heel pain of eight months duration. The patient notes a stabbing pain with ascending stairs as well as running, particularly uphill. Up to this point, the patient has attempted a home stretching program, as well as intermittent NSAIDs, with minimal benefit. On examination, the patient has localized pain to the Achilles insertion with palpation, single-leg raises, as well as passive ankle dorsi-flexion. In reference to the treatment of chronic insertional Achilles tendinopathy, which of the following statements is true?

   A. Full range of motion eccentric therapy programs provide greater patient satisfaction than floor-level eccentric therapy programs
   B. Low-energy shock wave therapy provides superior recovery (return to normal activity), compared to full range of motion eccentric loading therapy programs
   C. Concentric therapy programs provide superior pain relief, compared to full range of motion eccentric therapy programs
   D. Injectable therapies (including hyperosmolar dextrose and polidocanol) have been shown to be ineffective in significantly decreasing VAS pain scores

Correct Answer: B. Low-energy shock wave therapy provides superior recovery (return to normal activity), compared to full range of motion eccentric loading therapy programs

There is level 1 evidence that full-range eccentric loading showed inferior results to low-energy shock wave therapy, as applied in patients with chronic tendinopathy of the insertion of the Achilles tendon. Systematic reviews have suggested that floor-level eccentric loading provides superior pain and patient satisfaction outcomes, when compared to full-range eccentrics. The results of the systematic reviews suggest that floor-level results are comparable to low-energy shock wave therapy. These two treatment methods, however, have not been compared directly. Hyperosmolar dextrose and polidocanol injections have been shown to be effective in decreasing VAS pain scores.

1. Rompe JD, Furia J, Maffulli N. Eccentric loading compared with shock wave treatment for chronic insertional Achilles tendinopathy. A randomized, controlled trial. J Bone Joint Surg Am 2008 Jan;90(1):52-61. doi: 10.2106/JBJS.F.01494.
2. Wiegerinck JI, Kerkhoffs GM, van Sterkenburg MN, Sierevelt IN, van Dijk CN. Treatment for insertional Achilles tendinopathy: a systematic review. Knee Surg Sports Traumatol Arthrosc 2013 Jun;21(6):1345-1355. doi: 10.1007/s00167-012-2219-8. Epub 2012 Oct 6.
3. Malliaras P, Barton CJ, Reeves ND, Langberg H. Achilles and patellar tendinopathy loading programmes: a systematic review comparing clinical outcomes and identifying potential mechanisms for effectiveness. Sports Med 2013 Apr;43(4):267-286. doi: 10.1007/s40279-013-0019-z.

6. With regard to eccentric rehabilitation of hamstring strains, which of the following statements is true?

   A. Should only be performed in the shortened position to prevent re-injury
   B. Can begin as early as day two post-injury, without adversely affecting healing
   C. Has never been proven to prevent recurrent hamstring strains
   D. Can only be performed on special equipment
   E. Should have the load determined by 1RM

Correct Answer: B. Can begin as early as day two post-injury, without adversely affecting healing

Eccentric training of hamstrings has been shown to reduce the incidence of hamstring strains (both new and recurrent injury) and can be started early into rehabilitation. A number of eccentric exercises exist that have no special equipment needed (backwards lunge, "good morning" exercises, Nordic hamstrings, etc). Recent evidence shows that lengthened eccentric training may provide additional benefits and does not lead to reinjury.

1. Andrew N, Gabbe BJ, Cook J, Lloyd DG, Donnelly CJ, Nash C, et al. Could targeted exercise programmes prevent lower limb injury in community Australian football? Sports Med 2013 Aug;43(8):751-763. doi: 10.1007/s40279-013-0056-7.
2. Heiderscheit BC, Sherry MA, Silder A, Chumanov ES, Thelen DG. Hamstring strain injuries: recommendations for diagnosis, rehabilitation, and injury prevention. J Orthop Sports Phys Ther 2010;40(2):67-81.
3. Nichols AW. Does eccentric training of hamstring muscles reduce acute injuries in soccer? Clin J Sport Med 2013;23(1):85-86.
4. Sherry MA, Best TM. A comparison of 2 rehabilitation programs in the treatment of acute hamstring strains. J Orthop Sports Phys Ther 2004;34(3):116-125.

7. A 35-year-old female presents with three months of anterior knee pain, made worse with running, squatting, and using stairs. She originally presented to her primary care physician and was told she had runner's knee. She was given a referral to physical therapy, but she did not go, because of time and cost. Six months ago, she had started training for an upcoming 5 km race but had to stop due to the knee pain. She still aspires to run the race and is looking for Answers on how to return to running without knee pain. Which of the following recommendations is true with regard to patellofemoral pain?

   A. Prefabricated foot orthoses improve patellofemoral pain at three months and one year
   B. Bracing the patella has not been shown to be effective for pain reduction in the short term
   C. Taping has no role in patellofemoral pain rehabilitation
   D. A physical therapy program, consisting of quadriceps and gluteal strengthening, stretching, and patellar taping, has a moderate therapeutic effect within three months

Correct Answer: D. A physical therapy program, consisting of quadriceps and gluteal strengthening, stretching, and patellar taping, has a moderate therapeutic effect within three months

Foot orthoses do not improve outcomes at three and 12 months. Bracing the patella has level 1 evidence for reducing pain. Taping appears to give at least short-term pain relief in people with patellofemoral syndrome. Level 1 evidence shows that a multimodal physical therapy program with strengthening, stretching and taping has moderate to large therapeutic effect at three months and has at least a small therapeutic effect at 12 months.

   1. Barton CJ, Lack S, Hemmings S, Tufail S, Morrisey D. The best practice guide to conservative management of patellofemoral pain: incorporating level 1 evidence with expert clinical reasoning. Br J Sports Med 2015;49:923-934.

8. Which of the following are common sites of compression of the ulnar nerve?

   A. Cubital tunnel and Guyon's canal
   B. Cubital tunnel and pronator teres muscle
   C. Pronator teres muscle and Guyon's canal
   D. Radial tunnel and Guyon's canal

Correct Answer: A. Cubital tunnel and Guyon's canal

The ulnar nerve arises in the brachial plexus from C8 and T1 nerve roots, and closely approximates the brachial artery in the proximal arm. It then dives deeper into the posterior compartment in the midarm (arcade of Struthers). It next courses through the cubital tunnel, surrounded by fat just proximal to the ulnar groove. Ulnar nerve compression is the most common upper-extremity nerve entrapment. There are actually four areas where the ulnar nerve can be compressed at the elbow: the arcade of Struthers, medial epicondyle, cubital tunnel, and at the aponeurosis between the heads of the flexor carpi ulnaris. Distally, the ulnar nerve can be entrapped in Guyon's canal at the volar wrist—often called cyclist's palsy, from compression on the handlebars of bicycles. Pronator teres is a common site of median nerve entrapment. The radial tunnel is a common site of radial nerve entrapment.

1. Miller TT, Reinus WR. Nerve entrapment syndromes of the elbow, forearm, and wrist. AJR Am J Roentgenol 2010 Sep;195(3):585-594. doi: 10.2214/AJR.10.4817.
2. Morrey BF. Elbow and forearm. In: DeLee JC (ed). DeLee & Drez's Orthopaedic Sports Medicine. 3rd ed. Philadelphia: Saunders Elsevier, 2009:1189-1318.
3. Neal S, Fields K. Peripheral nerve entrapment and injury in the upper extremity. Am Fam Physician 2010;81(2):147-155.

Test 1 Answers, Critiques, and References

9. You are covering a high school football game when a player comes out of the game after a helmet-to-helmet tackle. When evaluating him for concussion, which of the following symptoms warrants prompt referral to the emergency department?

   A. Headache
   B. Nausea
   C. Photophobia
   D. Lethargy
   E. Retrograde amnesia

Correct Answer: D. Lethargy

Lethargy or declining level of consciousness following head injury is indicative of serious intracranial pathology and should prompt further evaluation at the nearest medical facility. Headache, nausea, photophobia, and retrograde amnesia are common in mild traumatic brain injury and do not necessarily suggest a life-threatening intracranial process. While concussions can result in a myriad of symptoms, one of the most important roles of the sideline physician is to assess and recognize catastrophic injury, so that prompt transport and evaluation can be initiated in the appropriate setting.

1. Harmon KG, Drezner J, Gammons M, Guskiewicz K, Halstead M, Herring S, et al. American Medical Society for Sports Medicine position statement: concussion in sport. Clin J Sport Med 2013;23:1-18.
2. Putakian M, Rafferty M, Guskiewicz K, Herring S, Aubry M, Cantu RC, et al. Onfield assessment of concussion in the adult athlete. Br J Sports Med 2013;47:285-288.
3. Resch JE, Kutcher JS. The acute management of sport concussion in pediatric athletes. J Child Neurol 2015 Oct;30(12):1686-1694.

10. A sophomore college football player sustains a burner during a game. Which is true regarding his neurologic examination, when determining if he is safe to return to the game?

    A. He can be cleared to return to play after experiencing bilateral numbness in both small fingers as long as his strength has returned and he is asymptomatic
    B. C6 nerve root is tested by checking the strength of the wrist extensors
    C. C7 can easily be tested by checking forearm flexion
    D. C5 innervates the triceps so it can easily be checked by forearm extension

Correct Answer: B. C6 nerve root is tested by checking the strength of the wrist extensors

By definition, a burner affects cervical nerve roots. If a patient experiences bilateral symptoms, they DO NOT have a burner and more likely have a cervical injury. Return to play would be contraindicated without further investigation. Burners may cause some stinging or numbness, and these symptoms should abate before a player is cleared. However, when examining a patient, it is the motor part of the neurologic examination that mostly determines the inability to return to the game. It is important to memorize a concise motor neurologic examination: C5—arm abduction (deltoid) and forearm flexion (bicep); C6—wrist extension (radial wrist extensor); C7—forearm extension (triceps) and wrist extension (flexor carpi radialis); C8—flexion of DIP joint of ring finger (flexor digitorum sublimis); T1—finger abduction and adduction (first dorsal interossei).

1. Kuhlman GS, McKeag DB. The "burner": a common nerve injury in contact sports. Am Fam Physician 1999 Nov 1;60(7):2035-2040, 2042.
2. Olson DE, McBroom SA, Nelson BD, Broton MS, Pulling TJ, Olson DE. Unilateral cervical nerve injuries: brachial plexopathies. Curr Sports Med Rep 2007 Jan;6(1):43-49.

11. You evaluate an 18-year-old defensive tackle for the local college football team for a preparticipation physical evaluation. He reports that in his senior season in high school, he suffered two neck injuries, both while making a tackle. The first injury involved mild neck pain, as well as burning and numbness to his left arm that lasted for 30 minutes and completely resolved. He returned to practice and play several days later. Three weeks following that injury, he experienced another hit that left him with bilateral arm and leg tingling and mild weakness lasting two days. He was hospitalized until his symptoms resolved and missed the final two games of the season. His examination today is completely normal. Regarding these two injuries, what are the most appropriate recommendations for this athlete?

   A. Clear him for full return to play, as long as he remains symptom free
   B. Clear him for full play, but refer to a neurosurgeon for further workup
   C. Disqualify him from any collision sports immediately
   D. Hold him from lifting or contact activities, obtain an MRI, and consider referral

Correct Answer: D. Hold him from lifting or contact activities, obtain an MRI, and consider referral

This athlete has suffered two different neuropraxias. The first was a brachial plexus neuropraxia (stinger), and the second was a cervical cord neuropraxia. The latter is the more concerning injury. An episode of cervical cord neuropraxia puts an athlete at increased risk for future injury, which could result in paralysis. For this reason, return-to-play decisions after these injuries are challenging. It is generally agreed upon that a multidisciplinary (sports medicine physician, neurosurgeon, athletic trainers, coaches, parents, athlete, physical therapists, etc.), collaborative effort is required in each case before considering return-to-contact activities. A single episode of cervical cord neuropraxia is not an absolute contraindication to participation; but disqualification may be the best decision for the patient until after full workup and appropriate collaboration is obtained.

1. Vaccaro AR, Klein GR, Ciccoti M, Pfaff WL, Moulton MJ, Hilibrand AJ, et al. Return to play criteria for the athlete with cervical spine injuries resulting in stinger and transient quadriplegia/paresis. Spine J 2002 Sep-Oct;2(5):351-356.
2. Cantu RV, Cantu RC. Guidelines for return to contact sports after transient quadriplegia. J Neurosurg 1994;80:592-594.
3. Watkins RG. Neck injuries in football players. Clin Sports Med 1986;5:215-246.

12. A softball pitcher continues to have precordial pain and complains of palpitations after a softball hit her in the chest. A 12-lead ECG performed by EMS at the softball park is normal. Which of the following statements is true?

   A. A normal ECG after the incident rules out a cardiac contusion
   B. A normal concentration of cardiac troponin I or T eight hours after the incident rules out cardiac damage and consequently minimizes the risk of cardiac complications
   C. Transthoracic echocardiography will detect aortic injury or isolated myocardial edema without wall motion abnormality
   D. Chronic dilated cardiac dysfunction and constrictive pericarditis can both be early complications of a cardiac contusion

Correct Answer: B. A normal concentration of cardiac troponin I or T eight hours after the incident rules out cardiac damage and consequently minimizes the risk of cardiac complications

In cardiac contusion, elevated serum cardiac troponins (both I and T) are highly sensitive and accurate for cardiac injury. Conversely, a normal concentration is a strong indicator for the absence of cardiac injury in blunt trauma. ECG changes may or may not be seen in cardiac contusion, and normal ECG alone does not rule out cardiac injury. While transthoracic echocardiography is useful, a transesophageal echo is recommended in a patient with painful chest wall injury and is also the test of choice for viewing the great vessels for detection of aortic rupture or dissection or rupture.

   1. Sybrandy KC, Cramer MJ, Burgersdijk C. Diagnosing cardiac contusion: old wisdom and new insights. Heart 2003 May;89(5):485-489.
   2. Bertinchant JP, Polge A, Mohty D, Nguyen-Ngoc-Lam R, Estorc J, Cohendy R, et al. Evaluation of incidence, clinical significance, and prognostic value of circulating cardiac troponin I and T elevation in hemodynamically stable patients with suspected myocardial contusion after blunt chest trauma. J Trauma 2000 May;48(5):924-931.

13. What items would a sports medicine physician want in the game bag to help emergently reduce a symptomatic posterior sternoclaviclar dislocation in the field?

    A. Trainer's Angel
    B. Towel roll
    C. Towel clamp
    D. Sling and swathe

Correct Answer: C. Towel clamp

Closed reduction can be attempted using traction in abduction and extension. Reduction of an acute injury usually occurs with an audible pop or snap, and the relocation can be noted visibly. However, if not successful, an assistant can grasp or push down on the clavicle in an effort to dislodge it from behind the sternum. On occasion, in a stubborn case, especially in a thick-chested person or a patient with extensive swelling, it is impossible for the assistant's fingers to obtain a secure grasp on the clavicle. The skin should then be surgically prepared, and a sterile towel clip should be used to gain purchase on the medial clavicle percutaneously. The towel clip is used to grasp completely around the shaft of the clavicle. The dense cortical bone prevents the purchase of the towel clip into the clavicle. Then, the combined traction through the arm, as well as the anterior lifting force on the towel clip, will reduce the dislocation. After the reduction, the sternoclavicular joint is stable, even with the patient's arms at the sides. However, the shoulders should be held back in a well-padded figure-of-eight clavicle strap for three to four weeks to allow for soft tissue and ligamentous healing. A Trainer's Angel is used to cut off a face mask.

1. Frank RM, Provencher MT, Fillingham Y, Romeo AA, Mazzocca AD. Injury to the acromioclavicular and sternoclavicular joints. In: Miller MD, Thompson SR (eds). DeLee & Drez's Orthopaedic Sports Medicine. 4th ed. Philadelphia: Saunders Elsevier, 2015:678-711.

14. A 15-year-old male soccer player is following up in clinic four days after being involved in a moderate-speed traffic accident. He was evaluated in the emergency department and found to have a pulmonary contusion of the right lower lobe by CT. No abnormalities were seen on chest x-ray. No other injuries were reported, and he was discharged home after a 24-hour observation in the hospital. At the present time, he states that he is a little short of breath and was sweating a lot last night while trying to sleep. Despite performing incentive spirometry as instructed, he has developed a cough. Which of the following is the next best step in the management of this patient?

   A. Repeat chest x-rays
   B. Perform a CT of the chest with IV contrast (pulmonary embolism protocol)
   C. Perform a non-contrast CT of the chest
   D. Perform a V-Q scan
   E. Start the patient on low molecular weight heparin

Correct Answer: A. Repeat chest x-rays

The most common complication from pulmonary contusion is secondary pneumonia. Repeat radiographs are the most cost effective and easily obtained study that would likely show pneumonia in this patient. The second most common complication is ARDS, hence the observation period in the hospital. A non-contrast CT of the chest would provide information on the size of the contusion, as well as any pneumonia forming. In the absence of hemodynamic instability, however, knowing the size of the contusion will not add to the treatment of the patient, making Answer C not the best choice. The remaining answers pertain to diagnosis and treatment of pulmonary embolism, which is not a common complication of pulmonary contusion, and is not likely in a low-risk patient such as the one presented.

1. Chang CJ, Dixit S. Thorax and abdominal injuries. In: Madden C, Putukian M, Young CC, McCarty EC (eds). Netter's Sports Medicine. Philadelphia: Saunders Elsevier, 2010: 379-392.
2. Caviness AC. Pulmonary contusions in children. UpToDate. Accessed October 9, 2013 at https://www.uptodate.com/contents/pulmonary-contusion-in-children.

15. A 35-year-old male aerobics instructor is seen in your clinic because he has had several months of lower abdominal and groin pain. He reports that over the past two months, the pain has increased, exacerbated by coughing or laughing. He reports no acute injury and no prior muscle strains. He stopped all physical activity for the past four weeks. An inguinal hernia is not appreciated on physical examination. X-rays, MRI, and bone scan do not show any bony abnormalities. What would be considered the best initial treatment plan for this athlete?

  A. Corticosteriod injection to the conjoined tendon sheath
  B. Reassurance and rest
  C. Non-weight-bearing and crutches for six weeks, given the patient may have occult stress fracture
  D. Conservative treatment with a comprehensive rehabilitation program to improve core strengthening and posterior abdominal wall weakness

Correct Answer: D. Conservative treatment with a comprehensive rehabilitation program to improve core strengthening and posterior abdominal wall weakness

This athlete most likely has a sports hernia, which is a disruption of the inguinal canal, characterized by a torn external oblique aponeurosis, a torn conjoined tendon, and a dehiscence between the torn conjoined tendon and inguinal ligament. A corticosteroid injection has not been shown to be an effective treatment for this problem. The patient has had symptoms for several months, including four weeks of rest without any improvement. Placing the patient on crutches is not indicated, since his radiologic studies and clinical examination do not support a bony injury requiring him to be non-weight-bearing.

  1. Morrelli V, Smith V. Groin injuries in athletes. Am Fam Physician 2001;64:1405-1414.
  2. Housner JA. Sports hernia. In: Puffer JC (ed). 20 Common Problems in Sports Medicine. New York: McGraw-Hill, 2002:148-149.

16. A 21-year-old senior female softball player presents to the clinic with left-sided abdominal pain. She says she first noticed the pain after hitting a double and sliding head-first into second base in last night's game. She was able to finish the inning, but felt like she had trouble taking a deep breath and removed herself from the game. Today, she says she is breathing okay, but still has pain with deep inspiration. She has pain with trunk rotation and bending, and bruising in the anterolateral abdomen of the left side. She has bilateral breath sounds equal in nature and is tender to palpation along her ribs and abdominal wall of the left side. A chest x-ray and vital signs are normal. Her pain has likely resulted from which of the following?

　A. Rib fracture
　B. Costochondritis
　C. Internal oblique strain
　D. Splenic hematoma

Correct Answer:　C. Internal oblique strain

The question addresses a common mechanism of tearing an abdominal wall muscle (i.e., the swinging of a bat). Rib fracture would be uncommon, even with a head-first slide. Costochondritis typically doesn't have bruising, and has a more confined area of tenderness. A splenic hematoma is possible, but would more likely present from more severe trauma, be accompanied by hemodynamic changes, or have an associated history of mono-like symptoms.

1. Connell D, Jhamb A, James T. Side strain: a tear of internal oblique musculature. AJR Am J Roentgenol 2003 Dec;181(6):1511-1517.

17. Over the past weekend, an 18-year-old male was playing tackle football with his dormitory buddies. At one point, he was running down the field for a touchdown, when another person tackled him to the ground, falling onto his chest and abdomen. He felt an immediate pain in his right upper quadrant. The pain worsened very quickly, and he was taken to the emergency room. Which of the following statements addresses the management of this patient?

A. A negative history and physical examination reliably excludes liver injury
B. Physical findings sensitive and specific for liver injury include right upper quadrant or generalized abdominal tenderness, as well as abdominal wall contusion or hematoma
C. Immediate assessment with ultrasound has replaced diagnostic peritoneal lavage and CT as the gold standard
D. Operative management (laparotomy) remains the preferred treatment in stable patients

Correct Answer: C. Immediate assessment with ultrasound has replaced diagnostic peritoneal lavage and CT as the gold standard

A history of trauma to the right upper quadrant, right rib cage, or right flank should increase the suspicion for liver injury. The patient may complain of pain in the right upper abdomen, right chest wall, or the right shoulder, due to diaphragmatic irritation. The liver is the most frequently injured organ following abdominal trauma. While abdominal tenderness and peritoneal signs are the most common findings indicative of intraabdominal injury, these are not sensitive or specific for liver injury. Physical findings associated with liver injury include right upper quadrant or generalized abdominal tenderness, abdominal wall contusion or hematoma (e.g., seat belt sign), right lower chest wall tenderness, contusion, or instability due to rib fractures. Any wounds that penetrate the right chest, abdomen, flank, or back may be related to significant liver damage. A negative history and physical examination do not reliably exclude liver injury. Other injuries are present in about 80% of patients with hepatic injury, with the mostly likely being an associated chest injury and/or injury to the spleen (the most commonly injured intraabdominal organ. Other injuries associated with a blunt mechanism include lower rib fractures, pelvic fracture, and spinal cord injury. Integration of CT in early trauma-room management and shift to non-operative management in hemodynamically stable patients resulted in improved survival and should be the gold standard management for liver trauma. Immediate assessment with ultrasound has replaced diagnostic peritoneal lavage in the resuscitation room, but computerized tomography remains the gold standard. Nonoperative management is preferred in stable patients, but laparotomy is indicated in unstable patients. Perihepatic packing, hepatotomy plus direct suture, and resectional debridement are recommended. Interventional radiological techniques are becoming more widely used, particularly in patients who are being managed nonoperatively or have been stabilized by perihepatic packing.

1. Petrowsky H, Raeder S, Zuercher L, Platz A, Simmen HP, Puhan MA, et al. A quarter century experience in liver trauma: a plea for early computed tomography and conservative management for all hemodynamically stable patients. World J Surg 2012 Feb;36(2):247-254. doi: 10.1007/s00268-011-1384-0.
2. Badger SA, Barclay R, Campbell P, Mole DJ, Diamond T. Management of liver trauma. World J Surg 2009 Dec;33(12):2522-2537. doi: 10.1007/s00268-009-0215-z.

18. A high school soccer player is struck in the abdomen with an opponent's knee while contesting a corner kick. She experiences immediate abdominal discomfort, sitting down immediately on standing. Vital signs are within normal limits on the field, but she experiences increasing discomfort and cannot return to play. Following blunt abdominal trauma in sports, which of the following is true?

   A. While rare, bowel perforation is the most frequent cause of death
   B. She can be watched at home without concern for serious injury
   C. Radiation of pain isn't helpful during assessment of need for transport
   D. Splenic rupture is the most common catastrophic injury

Correct Answer: D. Splenic rupture is the most common catastrophic injury

The spleen is the most commonly injured organ in blunt abdominal injury. Bowel perforation is much rarer in blunt trauma, compared to penetrating trauma. Organ injury is rare, but potentially catastrophic. All organs can be injured. The abdominal examination is not reported, but is absolutely necessary for initial assessment. Presence of guarding, localized tenderness, rebound, worsening symptoms, change in vital signs, nausea, and vomiting all warrant emergency evaluation, with consideration for urgent medical transport versus private car. Radiation is an ominous sign, requiring further evaluation and observation. Signs suggesting splenic injury include radiation to L shoulder, due to diaphragmatic irritation by blood (eponym Kehr's sign), and neck pain, due to intraabdominal phrenic nerve irritation by blood (eponym Seagasser's sign).

   1. Rifat SF, Gilvydis RP. Blunt abdominal trauma in sports. Curr Sports Med Rep 2003 Apr;2(2):93-97.
   2. Walter KD. Radiographic evaluation of the patient with sport-related abdominal trauma. Curr Sports Med Rep 2007 Apr;6(2):115-119.

19. You are evaluating an athlete with recurrent low back pain, with negative provocative testing for discogenic causes and negative imaging. You suspect a lumbar strain. In addition to the transversus abdominis, what muscle has been shown to have increased fatigability and a delayed onset of activity in sufferers of recurrent low back strains?

   A. Lumbar multifidus
   B. External oblique
   C. Iliocostalis
   D. Longissimus
   E. Psoas major

Correct Answer: A. Lumbar multifidus

Studies have shown that the function of the transversus abdominis and the lumbar multifidus is impaired in those patients with low back pain. A significant reduction in segmental lumbar multifidus cross-sectional area is seen in patients with acute first episode and unilateral back pain. In addition, the lumbar multifidus demonstrated greater fatigability relative to other parts of the erector spinae in patients with chronic low back pain compared with a normal population.

1. Brukner P, Khan K (eds). Clinical Sports Medicine. 4th ed. Sydney: McGraw-Hill Australia, 2011.
2. Scuderi GR, McCann PD, Bruno PJ. Sports Medicine: Principles of Primary Care. Philadelphia: Mosby, 1997.

20. A 68-year-old female, a retired nursing assistant, comes in with eight months of worsening low back pain. She denies any previous injuries or surgeries and does not recall an inciting event. X-rays of her lumbosacral spine revealed degenerative spondylolisthesis of L4-L5. What is this condition usually associated with?

   A. Peripheral neuropathy
   B. Multiple myeloma
   C. Previous scoliosis during adolescence
   D. Solitary plasmacytoma
   E. Spinal stenosis

Correct Answer: E. Spinal stenosis

Degenerative spinal spondylolisthesis may be asymptomatic, but when it is, there may be concomitant spinal stenosis. The rest of the choices listed usually are not associated with degenerative spondylolisthesis. There are several medical causes for peripheral neuropathy. Multiple myeloma and solitary plasmacytoma are plasma cell tumors. Previously diagnosed scoliosis is not known to predispose patients to degenerative spondylolisthesis in adulthood.

1. Weinstein JN, Lurie JD, Tosteson TD, Hanscom B, Tosteson AN, Blood EA, et al. Surgical versus nonsurgical treatment for lumbar degenerative spondylolisthesis. N Engl J Med 2007 May 31;356(22):2257-2270.
2. Jacobsen S, Sonne-Holm S, Rovsing H, Monrad H, Gebuhr P. Degenerative lumbar spondylolisthesis: an epidemiological perspective: the Copenhagen Osteoarthritis Study. Spine (Phila Pa 1976) 2007 Jan 1;32(1):120-125.
3. Lovell MR, Iverson GL, Collins MW, McKeag D, Maroon JC. Does loss of consciousness predict neuropsychological decrements after concussion? Clin J Sport Med 1999 Oct;9(4):193-198.

21. A 12-year-old girl tennis player and former gymnast comes to your office complaining of six months of low back pain that appears when only she serves while playing tennis. She quit gymnastics about a year ago but does not remember any issues when she was in gymnastics. Off and on, she has been taking ibuprofen as needed for pain. What is the most appropriate examination maneuver for evaluating your suspected diagnosis?

   A. Stork test
   B. Straight-leg raise test
   C. FABER test
   D. FADIR test

Correct Answer: A. Stork test

There is a clinical suspicion of spondylolysis/spondylolisthesis for this patient. A stork test is positive when pain in the area of spondylolysis with one-legged stance and hyperextension of the lumbar spine. Straight-leg test is for lumbar radiculopathy. Answers C and D are typically related to hip pathology.

1. Kim HJ, Green DW. Spondylolysis in the adolescent athlete. Curr Opin Pediatr 2011 Feb;23(1):68-72.
2. Lawrence JP, Greene HS, Grauer JN. Back pain in athletes. J Am Acad Orthop Surg 2006 Dec;14(13):726-735.
3. Standaert CJ. Low back pain in the adolescent athlete. Phys Med Rehabil Clin N Am 2008 May;19(2):287-304, ix.

22. Regarding the management of low back pain, which of the following statements is true?

A. In patients with acute low back pain, imaging results, physical examination findings, and type of injury usually correlate with chronicity or severity of symptoms
B. Acetaminophen, antidepressants, skeletal muscle relaxants, and lidocaine patches appear more effective than placebo for chronic low back pain
C. Topiramate (Topamax), select opioids, and NSAIDs appear more effective than placebo in the short-term treatment of chronic non-specific low back pain
D. Few randomized trials suggest that there is some advantage of bed rest for patients with sciatica

Correct Answer: C. Topiramate (Topamax), select opioids, and NSAIDs appear more effective than placebo in the short-term treatment of chronic non-specific low back pain

Few objective measures accurately predict progression from acute to non-specific chronic low back pain or resulting disability. Imaging results, physical examination findings, and type of injury do not correlate with chronicity or severity of symptoms. Several large case-control studies have identified non-pathology-dependent variables that are associated with back pain persistence and greater severity of symptoms. These variables include workers' compensation claim status, litigation status, comorbid mental health diagnosis, injury sustained at work versus at home, and socioeconomic factors. Acetaminophen, antidepressants (excluding duloxetine [Cymbalta]), skeletal muscle relaxants, and lidocaine patches not are more effective than placebo for chronic low back pain. Duloxetine (Cymbalta) appeared to reduce pain severity in one randomized controlled trial. For decades, bed rest was considered standard therapy for patients with acute low back pain. Multiple randomized trials have now demonstrated that recovery from pain is equally rapid and complete without bed rest. A systematic review concluded that patients advised to rest in bed may even have slightly more pain and less functional recovery than those individuals advised to remain ambulatory. Randomized trials also suggest there is no advantage to bed rest for patients with sciatica.

1. Herndon CM, Zoberi KS, Gardner BJ. Common questions about chronic low back pain. Am Fam Physician 2015 May 15;91(10):708-714.
2. Machado GC, Maher CG, Ferreira PH, Pinheiro MB, Lin CW, Day RO, et al. Efficacy and safety of paracetamol for spinal pain and osteoarthritis: systematic review and meta-analysis of randomised placebo controlled trials. BMJ 2015 Mar 31;350:h1225. doi: 10.1136/bmj.h1225.
3. Knight C, Deyo R, Staiger T, Wipf J. Treatment of acute low back pain. UpToDate. Accessed June 6, 2015 at http://www.uptodate.com/contents/treatment-of-acute-low-back-pain.

23. A 16-year-old female cheerleader presents to you with insidious onset of progressive lumbar back pain. She denies neurologic symptoms, and examination is normal, except for reproducible pain on extension. Your evaluation produces a diagnosis of unilateral spondylolysis at the L5 level. Which one of the following statements is correct?

   A. Surgery is indicated at this time, in order to keep her active in her sport
   B. She will likely never play sports again, due to risk for neurologic complications
   C. She should wear tight-fitting clothing for support under her uniform
   D. While no consensus exists to guide treatment in all cases, some period of rest is recommended, with or without bracing

Correct Answer: D. While no consensus exists to guide treatment in all cases, some period of rest is recommended, with or without bracing

Spondylolysis is one of the most, if not the most, common identifiable conditions in adolescent athletes who present with low back pain. Though no overall consensus exists, all recommendations are for a trial of conservative therapy, before surgical treatment is considered. Conservative approach includes a period of rest, with or without bracing, and with or without rehabilitation. Most athletes with mild unilateral spondylolysis who undergo treatment will have excellent results, and do not need to be given a lifetime ban from sport. While many recommend bracing, there are no studies to support tight-fitting clothing as treatment for spondylolysis.

1. McCleary MD, Congeni JA. Current concepts in the diagnosis and treatment of spondylolysis in young athletes. Curr Sports Med Rep 2007 Jan;6(1):62-66.
2. Daniels JM, Pontius G, El-Amin S, Gabriel K. Evaluation of low back pain in athletes. Sports Health 2011 Jul;3(4):336-345.

24. You suspect a patient of yours has quadrilateral space syndrome and order an electromyography (EMG) study to confirm your diagnosis. In the event that your diagnosis is correct, you would anticipate seeing neurogenic changes in which of the following muscles?

    A. Supraspinatus
    B. Infraspinatus
    C. Subscapularis
    D. Teres minor

Correct Answer: D. Teres minor

The quadrilateral space of the posterior shoulder is bound superiorly by the subscapularis and teres minor, inferiorly by the teres major, medially by the long head of triceps brachii, and laterally by the surgical neck of the humerus. This space contains the axillary nerve and posterior circumflex artery. Quadrilateral space syndrome results in injury to the axillary nerve, and, as a rule, preferentially affects the teres minor, although the deltoid may also be involved. The pathophysiology is thought to involve compression of the neurovascular bundle by fibrotic bands within the space or by hypertrophy of the muscular boundaries. On the other hand, quadrilateral space syndrome may also result from direct trauma or a ganglion, glenoid labral cyst, or paralabral cyst. The Answers A and B are incorrect, given that the supraspinatus and infraspinatus are innervated by the suprascapular nerve, although the latter muscle may also be affected by glenoid labral or paralabral cysts via compression of the nerve at the spinoglenoid notch. Answer C is incorrect, because the subscapularis is innervated by the upper and lower subscapular nerves.

1. Brown SA, Doolittle DA, Bohanon CJ, Jayaraj A, Naidu SG, Huettl EA, et al. Question quadrilateral space syndrome: the Mayo Clinic experience with a new classification system and case series. Mayo Clin Proc 2015 Mar;90(3):382-394. doi: 10.1016/j.mayocp.2014.12.012. Epub 2015 Jan 31.
2. Hoskins WT, Pollard HP, McDonald AJ. Quadrilateral space syndrome: a case study and review of the literature. Br J Sports Med 2005 Feb;39(2):e9.

25. A 25-year-old female with no past medical history presents with a one-day history of severe right-sided shoulder girdle pain. Her pain is unremitting, regardless of position, and radiates into her forearm with associated paresthesias. She does not attribute the pain to injury, although she is a front-door greeter at your hospital, and she occasionally helps patients into wheelchairs. Her pain was the most severe last night, as she was unable to sleep. Of note, she is recovering from an upper respiratory tract infection. What is the best test to help confirm the diagnosis?

    A. MRI
    B. EMG
    C. Laboratory analysis to include CMP, CBC, and an ESR
    D. X-ray of the shoulder

Correct Answer: B. EMG

The patient's symptoms are most consistent with Parsonage-Turner syndrome (PTS), also called brachial neuritis. PTS is often associated with a viral infection or as a post-surgical complication. The pain is unremitting and worse at night. The duration of pain is usually self-limiting, lasting one to two weeks. Weakness can develop as the illness progresses. An EMG is the best tool for diagnosis, due to axonal denervation involving the muscles. An MRI would be helpful to rule out other etiologies of an entrapped nerve (e.g., disc herniation, mass) or structural shoulder pathology, but it may not show changes suggesting PTS. Answer C, laboratory analysis, would help rule out infection or inflammatory conditions, but the question stem does not suggest these as the etiology. Answer D is incorrect, since x-ray films of the shoulder in PTS would appear within normal limits.

1. Feinberg JH, Radecki J. Parsonage-Turner Syndrome. HSSJ 2010 Sep;6(2):199-205.
2. Miller JD, Pruitt S, McDonald TJ. Acute brachial plexus neuritis: an uncommon cause of shoulder pain. Am Fam Physician 2000 Nov 1;62(9):2067-2072.

26. What is the most common complication found in anterior shoulder dislocations (beyond typical Hill-Sachs and Bankart lesions)?

    A. Rotator cuff tears
    B. Axillary nerve injury
    C. Greater tuberosity fractures
    D. Lesser tuberosity fracture

Correct Answer: A. Rotator cuff tears

Other than typical Bankart Lesions and Hill-Sachs lesions, rotator cuff tears are the most common injuries associated with anterior shoulder dislocations, more so than axillary nerve injuries and greater tuberosity fractures. Combined injuries are common as well, such that follow-up with ultrasound and MRI are mandatory to avoid missing a complication.

1. Atef A, El-Tantawy A, Gad H, Hefeda M. Prevalence of associated injuries after anterior shoulder dislocation: a prospective study. Int Orthop 2016 Mar;40(3):519-524. doi: 10.1007/s00264-015-2862-z.

27. A 25-year-old right-handed man has a six-month history of right shoulder pain. He denies any specific injury, but works out regularly at the gym. His pain resolves if he takes a week off. The pain is worse with weight-bearing and loading activities, such as the shoulder press and chest press. His MRI arthrogram is shown below. What is his diagnosis?

   A. Rotator cuff tear
   B. Clavicular osteolysis
   C. Labral tear
   D. Subacromial bursitis

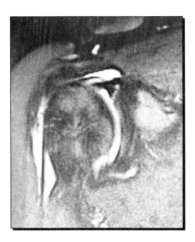
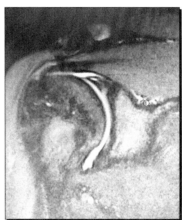

Correct Answer: C. Labral tear

The transverse oblique coronal MRI images show a superior-posterior labral tear (SLAP). The first image shows the SLAP lesion and a subtle tear of the biceps tendon, which is better delineated in the second image (contrast within the biceps tendon). These images demonstrate a type IV SLAP lesion—a bucket-handle-type tear of the labrum that extends into the bicep tendon. SLAP lesions often occur either traumatically (e.g., a FOOSH mechanism) or from repetitive overhead activity (e.g., throwing sports or weight training, as in this case). Being younger than 35, a rotator cuff tear would be very unusual without trauma. Clavicular osteolysis is common in weight lifters, but the AC joint is normal on the MRI. In addition, the MRI does not show bursitis. Labral tears commonly occur in young active people without trauma. Patients tend to feel worse with weight-bearing activities and better with rest.

1. Davis KW. Imaging pediatric sports injuries: upper extremity. Radiol Clin North Am 2010 Nov;48(6):1199-1211. doi: 10.1016/j.rcl.2010.07.020.
2. O'Kane JW, Toresdahl BG. The evidenced-based shoulder evaluation. Curr Sports Med Rep 2014 Sep-Oct;13(5):307-313. doi: 10.1249/JSR.0000000000000090.

28. A six-year-old boy is brought into the emergency room with left elbow pain and swelling, after a fall on his outstretched arm, with his elbow in extension. Despite being left-handed, he is now only using his right arm. On lateral elbow x-ray views, the anterior humeral line does not transect the capitellum. Which of the following, if also injured, could mask a developing compartment syndrome?

A. Ulnar nerve
B. Distal radius
C. Radial nerve
D. Scaphoid
E. Median nerve

Correct Answer: E. Median nerve

Knowledge of the anatomy in this area is critical to adequate evaluation and treatment of co-existing injuries associated with supracondylar fractures. This child sustained an extension-type supracondylar fracture, the most common (> 90%). With the elbow in extension, the distal fragment displaces posteriorly; it is the opposite for flexion-type supracondylar fractures. Within the area of the fracture segments are the brachial artery and the anterior interosseous nerve, both of which could be severed during the injury. A complete neurovascular examination of the distal extremity is essential and should be repeated during the evaluation. Ulnar, median, and radial sensory and motor function should be tested distally. Radial and ulnar pulses should be palpated.

If the pulse is present but decreased, other signs of perfusion, including capillary refill and the color and temperature of the hand, should be assessed. A pulse oximeter can also be used for continuous evaluation. If pulselessness is noted, an arteriography can be performed to evaluate vascular injury, although surgical exploration and concomitant correction would be more direct. Compartment syndrome is an ongoing concern, the first sign of which is pain out of proportion to the injury (e.g., requiring increasing doses of pain medication). A median nerve, typically a transient neuropraxia, could alter sensory and motor function and, therefore, mask a developing compartment syndrome in the antebrachial compartment. Distal radial fractures occur with 5% to 6% of supracondylar fractures. Scaphoid fractures are not commonly associated with supracondylar fractures. Treatment of a supracondylar fracture would involve reduction and fixation. On the other hand, if the distal extremity is pulseless and not perfused or unable to be reduced successfully, the procedure would be performed open to allow for exploration and effective reduction. Treatment of a compartment syndrome would involve fasciotomy of the involved compartment.

1. Brubacher JW, Dodds D. Pediatric supracondylar fractures of the distal humerus. Curr Rev Musculoskelet Med 2008 Dec;1(3-4):190-196.
2. Thompson JC. Netter's Concise Atlas of Orthopaedic Anatomy. Philadelphia: Saunders Elsevier, 2002.
3. Pediatric supracondylar fractures of the humerus. Wheeless' Textbook of Orthopaedics. Accessed July 27, 2014 at http://www.wheelessonline.com/ortho/pediatric_supracondylar_fractures_of_the_humerus.
4. Vascular injuries in supracondylar fracture. Wheeless' Textbook of Orthopaedics. Accessed July 27, 2014 at http://www.wheelessonline.com/ortho/vascular_injuries_in_supracondylar_frx.
5. Neurologic deficits: following supracondylar fracture. Wheeless' Textbook of Orthopaedics. Accessed July 27, 2014 at http://www.wheelessonline.com/ortho/neurologic_deficits_following_supracondylar_frx.

29. A 33-year-old female recreational golfer presents with three months of right lateral elbow pain. She has tried a counter-force elbow brace and naproxen with no improvement. On physical examination, she has tenderness in the extensor mass, 3 cm distal from the epicondyle, and pain with resisted extension of the middle finger. No sensory or motor deficits are noted on examination. What is the most common site of nerve compression associated with this patient's diagnosis?

    A. Supinator edge
    B. Arcade of Frohse
    C. ERCB edge
    D. Radial artery recurrent leash of Henry

Correct Answer: B. Arcade of Frohse

The diagnosis for this case is radial tunnel syndrome. Patients with this diagnosis often present with failed treatment for lateral epicondylitis initially. Pain will be in the proximal forearm and will be worse with resisted supination and resisted extension of the middle finger. Pain will also be more localized in the extensor mass (2 to 4 cm distal to the epicondyle) than over the lateral epicondyle. Pain stems from compression of the posterior interosseous nerve, which is a branch off the radial nerve. While the most common site of compression is the arcade of Frohse, any of the answer choices can be an area of compression. Non-operative treatment includes activity modification, temporary bracing, and NSAIDs, before considering surgical options.

1. Naam NH, Nemani S. Radial tunnel syndrome. Orthop Clin North Am 2012 Oct;43(4):529-536. doi: 10.1016/j.ocl.2012.07.022.
2. Strohl AB, Zelouf DS. Ulnar tunnel syndrome, radial tunnel syndrome, anterior interosseous nerve syndrome, and pronator syndrome. J Am Acad Orthop Surg 2017 Jan;25(1):e1-e10. doi: 10.5435/JAAOS-D-16-00010.

30. A 30-year-old elite male swimmer presents with posteromedial elbow pain, especially when the elbow reaches terminal extension during the breaststroke. He denies numbness or tingling. He has tenderness to palpation to the posteromedial elbow. He has a negative milking maneuver, with 30 to 100 degrees of flexion. There is no pain with resisted flexion of the elbow, resisted extension of the elbow, resisted pronation of the forearm, resisted wrist dorsiflexion, or resisted third-finger extension. His strength is normal in the distal extremity. Small irregular loose bodies are seen posteriorly on radiograph. What is the most likely diagnosis?

   A. Triceps tendinosis
   B. Osteochondral lesion of the radial head
   C. Medial epicondylosis
   D. Valgus extension overload

Correct Answer: D. Valgus extension overload

Valgus extension overload (VEO) is most common in throwing athletes. VEO is also seen in non-throwers, resulting from impingement of the posteromedial tip of the olecranon process on the medial wall of the olecranon fossa. The combination of posteromedial pain at the point of forceful extension and loose bodies/osteophytes in the olecranon fossa region is very suggestive of this diagnosis, particularly when combined with negative tests for other structures in the region. A provocative maneuver for VEO is a valgus stress from slight flexion moving into extension, unlike testing the ulnar collateral ligament using the milking maneuver, which is valgus stress in the arc of flexion from 30 to 100 degrees. This athlete could certainly have early posteromedial impingement, atypical ulnar neuropathy, or even a UCL injury, but given the choices, valgus extension overload is most likely.

1. Dugas JR. Valgus extension overload: diagnosis and treatment. Clin Sports Med 2010;29(4):645-654.
2. Hariri S, Safran MR. Ulnar collateral ligament injury in the overhead athlete. Clin Sports Med 2010;29(4):619-644.
3. Zellner B, May MM. Elbow injuries in the young athlete—an orthopedic perspective. Pediatr Radiol 2013;43 Suppl 1:S129-S134.

31. In the evaluation and management of ulnar collateral ligament (UCL) injury, which one of the following is correct?

   A. Point tenderness is produced at the medial epicondyle
   B. All partial tears respond well to conservative non-surgical care
   C. Varus stress is applied to the elbow in extension and shoulder abduction and external rotation
   D. MRI has 100% specificity for ulnar collateral ligament tears
   E. MR Arthrogram adds no additional benefit to the evaluation of ulnar collateral ligament tears

Correct Answer: D. MRI has 100% specificity for ulnar collateral ligament tears

UCL injury is commonly found in throwing activity. Maximum stress to the UCL is found at the late cocking and early acceleration phase of throwing. MRI has been shown to have 100% specificity for UCL tears and 57% to 79% sensitivity, which can be improved with MRA to 97%. The modified milking maneuver, with the elbow flexed to 70 degrees, is done with the shoulder in abduction and external rotation. The examiner places one thumb at medial joint line and the other hand pulls down on the patient's thumb to create a valgus stress. Low-grade partial tears have been shown to respond well to conservative care, but not high-grade partial tears.

1. Freehill MT, Safran MR. Diagnosis and management of ulnar collateral ligament injuries in throwers. Curr Sports Med Rep 2011 Sep-Oct;10(5):271-278. doi: 10.1249/JSR.0b013e31822d4000.
2. Dugas J, Chronister J, Cain EL Jr, Andrews JR. Ulnar collateral ligament in the overhead athlete: a current review. Sports Med Arthrosc Rev 2014 Sep;22(3):169-182. doi: 0.1097/JSA.0000000000000033.

32. An 18-year-old soccer player misses a potential game winning goal and punches the ground in frustration. He comes to the sideline holding his right hand and subsequently develops ecchymosis and swelling of over the dorsal aspect of his hand. There is focal tenderness over the distal fifth metacarpal, without associated lacerations or dermal injury. Plain radiographs demonstrate a fifth metacarpal neck fracture, with 20 degrees of apex dorsal angulation. (see image) What is the most appropriate next step in management?

    A. Sugar tong splint, with follow-up in 7 to 10 days
    B. Orthopedic referral for operative management
    C. Ulnar gutter splint, with follow-up in 7 to 10 days
    D. Volar splint, with follow-up in 7 to 10 days

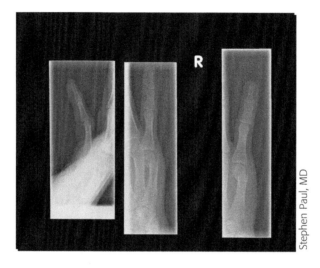

Correct Answer: C. Ulnar gutter splint, with follow-up in 7 to 10 days

An ulnar gutter splint will adequately immobilize the fourth and fifth metacarpals at the metacarpophalangeal (MCP) and carpometacarpal (CMC) joints, while still allowing for some function and motion in the second and third metacarpals. Neither a sugar tong nor a volar wrist splint provide immobilization at the MCP joint. Orthopedic referral for operative management is not necessary, since 20 degrees of angulation is within acceptable limits for this. Metacarpal neck fractures are subject to displacement, due to the action of the interosseous muscles. The interossei will cause volar displacement of the metacarpal head (dorsal angulation). Compensatory motion at the carpometacarpal (CMC) joints allows for some acceptable angulation in the fourth and fifth metacarpals. The base of the second and third metacarpals, however, is essentially fixed at the distal carpal row, which does not allow for any compensatory motion to accommodate for angulation. As a result, very little angulation is tolerated in neck fractures of the second and third metacarpals. In general, the "10-20-30-40" rule can be used to determine the acceptable limits of fracture angulation, where "10" refers to acceptable angulation in the second metacarpal and "40" refers to acceptable angulation in the fifth metacarpal (though some advocate for 30 degrees of maximum angulation in the fifth metacarpal).

1. Bloom J. Metacarpal neck fractures. UpToDate. Accessed July 7, 2015 at http://www.uptodate.com/contents/metacarpal-neck-fractures.
2. Cotterell IH, Richard MJ. Metacarpal and phalangeal fractures in athletes. Clin Sports Med 2015;34:69-98.

33. A 30-year-old female sustained a fall onto the outstretched hand (FOOSH) while snowboarding. X-rays show a non-displaced Colles' fracture. You treated her fracture appropriately and she presents to your office four weeks after her injury and complains that she cannot move her thumb towards the back of her hand. On examination, you ask her to place her hand flat onto the table, with her palm down, and she is unable to lift her thumb off of the surface. In which dorsal wrist compartment does her ruptured tendon reside?

    A. First compartment
    B. Second compartment
    C. Third compartment
    D. Fourth compartment

Correct Answer: C. Third compartment

Extensor pollicis longus (EPL) rupture is an occasional complication of non-displaced distal radius fractures. The rupture occurs most commonly at Lister's tubercle and may be due to either ischemia or attritional rupture over an osseous spike. EPL rupture most often occurs between three weeks to three months after distal radius fracture. Recent studies show that EPL rupture after distal radius fracture may not be as common as was previously thought. The tendon resides in the third dorsal compartment of the wrist as it turns around Lister's tubercle.

1. Roth KM, Blazar PE, Earp BE, Han R, Leung A. Incidence of extensor pollicis longus tendon rupture after nondisplaced distal radius fractures. J Hand Surg Am 2012 May;37(5):942-947. doi: 10.1016/j.jhsa.2012.02.006. Epub 2012 Mar 29.
2. Helal B, Chen SC, Iwegbu G. Rupture of the extensor pollicis longus tendon in undisplaced Colles' type of fracture. Hand 1982 Feb;14(1):41-47.
3. Hirasawa Y, Katsumi Y, Akiyoshi T, Tamai K, Tokioka T. Clinical and microangiographic studies on rupture of the E.P.L. tendon after distal radial fractures. J Hand Surg Br 1990 Feb;15(1):51-57.

34. A 17-year-old basketball player presents with second finger pain after "jamming" it catching a pass. Examination reveals difficulty with active extension at the DIP joint, but normal passive extension. X-ray shows no evidence of bony injury. What are the treatment components of this condition?

   A. Radial gutter cast for six weeks, followed by removable custom hand splint for six weeks
   B. Urgent referral to orthopedic hand surgeon for surgical repair
   C. Buddy tape to third finger for four to six weeks, then as needed with activity for four to six weeks
   D. Splint DIP in full extension for six to eight weeks continuously

Correct Answer: D. Splint DIP in full extension for six to eight weeks continuously

This case describes a non-bony mallet finger for which conservative therapy is recommended. This consists of splinting the DIP of the affected finger in full extension for six to eight weeks continuously. Patients should be aware that allowing the DIP to bend during this time will require the process to start over again. Answer A is incorrect, given that radial gutter casting is not necessary for a simple mallet finger and is usually used to treat a second or third metacarpal fracture. Answer B is incorrect, as surgery is not needed for a simple non-bony mallet finger. Answer C is incorrect, because buddy taping would not immobilize the DIP joint well enough and is usually used for simple, non-displaced phalanx fractures.

1. Bendre AA, Hartigan BF, Kalainov DM. Mallet finger. J Am Acad Orthop Surg 2005 Sep;13(5):336.
2. Bloom JM, Khouri JS, Hammert WC. Current concepts in the evaluation and treatment of mallet finger injury. Plast Reconstr Surg 2013 Oct;32(4):560e.
3. Borchers JR, Best TM. Common finger fractures and dislocations. Am Fam Physician 2012 Apr 15;85(8):805-810.

35. A 33-year-old male drummer presents with pain and swelling in the dorsoradial aspect of his left wrist for eight weeks. He denies any acute injury, but reports more drumming over the past four months. His symptoms, however, have impaired his ability to practice and perform, and he is very eager to return to drumming with his band. On physical examination, you note an area of soft tissue swelling, tenderness, and crepitus with active wrist movements in an area about 6 cm proximal of Lister's tubercle. You decide to include an ultrasound-guided corticosteroid injection as part of his treatment plan. Which of the following injection targets most closely approximates the locus of this patient's pathology?

   A. Between the compartment with the abductor pollicis longus and extensor pollicis brevis, and the bony surface of the distal radius
   B. Between the compartment with the extensor pollicis longus, and the bony surface of the distal radius
   C. Between the compartment with the extensor carpi radialis longus and extensor carpi radialis brevis, and the compartment with the extensor pollicis longus
   D. Between the compartment with the extensor carpi radialis longus and extensor carpi radialis brevis, and the compartment with the abductor pollicis longus and extensor pollicis brevis

Correct Answer: D. Between the compartment with the extensor carpi radialis longus and extensor carpi radialis brevis, and the compartment with the abductor pollicis longus and extensor pollicis brevis

There are a number of conditions involving tenosynovitis about the hand and wrist, including so-called "intersection syndrome." The more widely-known "proximal" intersection syndrome is characterized by tenosynovitis of the radial wrist extensors—extensor carpi radialis longus (ECRL) and extensor carpi radialis brevis (ECRB)—as well as the muscles of the extensor pollicis brevis (EPB) and the abductor pollicis longus (APL). These two groups of muscle-tendons reside in distinct extensor tendon compartments—two of six known structures: first compartment—extensor pollicis brevis (EPB) and abductor pollicis longus (APL); second compartment—extensor carpi radialis longus (ECRL) and extensor carpi radialis brevis (ECRB); third compartment—extensor pollicis longus (EPL); fourth compartment—extensor digitorum communis (EDC) and extensor digiti indicis (EDI); fifth compartment—extensor digiti minimi (EDM); and sixth compartment—extensor carpi ulnaris (ECU). The tenosynovitis and friction between the first and second compartments result in pain, swelling, and crepitus where these two compartments "intersect" in the dorsoradial distal forearm (or proximal wrist). This is typically 4 to 8 cm proximal to Lister's tubercle. Care must be taken to not confuse this syndrome with the more common De Quervain tenosynovitis, which is limited to the 1st dorsal compartment and typically presents with pain about the radial styloid. While intersection syndrome may result from direct trauma, it is more commonly associated with activities that require repetitive wrist flexion and extension. Interestingly, the literature also reports a lesser-known "distal" intersection syndrome, involving the third and second compartments over the wrist.

1. Shehab R, Mirabelli MH. Evaluation and diagnosis of wrist pain: a case-based approach. Am Fam Physician 2013 Apr 15;87(8):568-573.
2. Parellada AJ, Gopez AG, Morrison WB, Sweet S, Leinberry CF, Reiter SB, et al. Distal intersection tenosynovitis of the wrist: a lesser-known extensor tendinopathy with characteristic MR imaging features. Skeletal Radiol 2007 Mar;36(3):203-208. Epub 2006 Dec 20.
3. Browne J, Helms CA. Intersection syndrome of the forearm. Arthritis Rheum 2006 Jun;54(6):2038.

36. Which of the following strategies is helpful in counseling families of youth athletes in preventing overuse injuries from early sports specialization?

    A. Keep hourly average weekly training volumes lower than their age in years
    B. Spend less than six months participating in one sport each year
    C. Begin sports specialization after puberty
    D. Try to participate in cross-training activities during off-season training

Correct Answer: A. Keep hourly average weekly training volumes lower than their age in years

A new study by Jayanthi et al. evaluated variables related to overuse and acute injuries from sports-specialized intensive training in young athletes. The results of this investigation showed that as hourly average weekly training volumes increased, injuries increased as well. The authors suggested to keep these training volumes less than the age of the child. Answer B is incorrect, since it is recommended to take off at least three to four months per calendar year on one particular sport. Answer C is incorrect, given that sports specialization should be delayed until late adolescence, and not related to puberty. Answer D is incorrect, because cross-training during the off-season does not influence injuries from sports specialization.

1. Jayanthi NA, LaBella CR, Fischer D, Pasulka J, Dugas LR. Sports-specialized intensive training and the risk of injury in young athletes: a clinical case-control study. Am J Sports Med 2015 Apr;43(4):794-801. doi: 10.1177/0363546514567298. Epub 2015 Feb 2.
2. Feeley B, Agel J, LaPrade R. When is it too early for single sports specialization? Am J Sports Med 2016 Jan;44(1):234-241.
3. DiFiori JP, Benjamin HJ, Brenner J, Gregory A, Jayanthi N, Landry GL, et al. Overuse injuries and burnout in youth sports: a position statement from the American Medical Society for Sports Medicine. Clin J Sport Med 2014 Jan;24(1):3-20.

37. Your athletic director comes to you to schedule preparticipation evaluations for the incoming fall athletes. She would like them scheduled as close as possible to the start of school, so the athletes won't have to come to town too early. When would you recommend the physicals are optimally be done?

    A. At least one day prior to the start of the activity
    B. At least one week prior to the start of the activity
    C. At least four weeks prior to the start of the activity
    D. At least six weeks prior to the start of the activity

Correct Answer: D. At least six weeks prior to the start of the activity

In general, it is recommended that preparticipation evaluations are done at least six weeks prior to activity. This scheduling allows time for further evaluation, treatment, and rehabilitation of any problems identified in the screening process.

1. American Academy of Family Physicians, American Academy of Pediatrics, American College of Sports Medicine, American Medical Society for Sports Medicine, American Orthopaedic Society for Sports Medicine, American Osteopathic Academy of Sports Medicine. Bernhardt DT, Roberts WO (eds). Preparticipation Physical Evaluation. 4th ed. Elk Grove Village, IL: American Academy of Pediatrics, 2010.
2. Khodaee M, Madden CC, Putukian M. The preparticipation physical evaluation. In: Madden CC, Putukian M, Young CC, McCarty EC (eds). Netter's Sports Medicine. Philadelphia: Saunders Elsevier, 2010:10-23.

38. A 16-year-old high school swimmer presents for her preparticipation physical evaluation at the local high school. She denies any chest pain, syncope, pre-syncope, shortness of breath, or any significant family history of sudden cardiac death prior to the age of 50, Marfan syndrome, long QT syndrome, or hypertrophic cardiomyopathy. She denies history of asthma, seizures, or diabetes. She denies taking any medications and did not drink coffee or energy drinks today. She did not exercise or practice prior to this examination. She is not anxious and denies previous history of anxiety, hypertension, or murmurs. On examination, you find her blood pressure to be 160/110. Her examination was otherwise normal. Which three factors must you consider in order to diagnose the patient with stage 2 hypertension?

A. Age, height, weight
B. Age, weight, gender
C. Height, weight, gender
D. Age, height, gender

Correct Answer: D. Age, height, gender.

The Fourth Report on the Diagnosis, Evaluation, and Treatment of High Blood Pressure in Children and Adolescents recommended the use of standardized tables to diagnose hypertension in children. These tables were based on the age, height, and gender of children and adolescents.

1. McCambridge TM, Benjamin HJ, Brenner JS, Cappetta CT, Demorest RA, Gregory AJ, et al. Council on Sports Medicine and Fitness. Athletic participation by children and adolescents who have systemic hypertension. Pediatrics 2010 Jun;125(6):1287-1294. doi: 10.1542/peds.2010-0658.
2. National High Blood Pressure Education Program Working Group on High Blood Pressure in Children and Adolescents. The Fourth Report on the Diagnosis, Evaluation, and Treatment of High Blood Pressure in Children and Adolescents. Pediatrics 2004;114(2 suppl):555-576.
3. Khodaee M, Madden CC, Putukian M. The preparticipation physical evaluation. In: Madden CC, Putukian M, Young CC, McCarty EC (eds). Netter's Sports Medicine. Philadelphia: Saunders Elsevier, 2010:10-23.

39. After performing a preparticipation physical evaluation on an 18-year-old male with a seizure disorder, you counsel him on activity participation. Which of the following recommendations is correct?

   A. Scuba diving, skydiving, and swimming are strictly forbidden
   B. Contact sports should be avoided, since head trauma may provoke seizures
   C. Swimming is considered safe if directly supervised by trained individuals and personal flotation devices are used appropriately
   D. Exercise is detrimental, because the associated physiologic stress will often exacerbate an underlying seizure disorder
   E. Physical fitness confers no benefit to the individual with a seizure disorder

Correct Answer: C. Swimming is considered safe if directly supervised by trained individuals and personal flotation devices are used appropriately

Participation in recreational and athletic activities is important to the fitness and mental health of those individuals with seizure disorders, without causing excessive injury risk or increase in seizure activity. Numerous studies have demonstrated the positive effects of exercise in people with seizures. Though sport-specific activity recommendations should be made on a case-by-case basis, the only consistently restricted activities are scuba diving and freefall/airborne activities, such as skydiving. Safe participation in swimming may be accomplished by direct supervision from trained individuals, avoidance of open water swimming, and appropriate use of personal flotation devices. There is no evidence to suggest that contact sports pose any significant risk.

   1. Knowles BD, Pleacher MD. Athletes with seizure disorders. Curr Sports Med Rep 2012;11:16-20.
   2. Shah N. Seizures and epilepsy. In: Bracker MD (ed). The 5-Minute Sports Medicine Consult. 2nd ed. Philadelphia: Lippincott Williams & Wilkins, 2011.

40. An 18-year-old female swimmer presents to you for a preparticipation physical evaluation (PPE). In the fall, she will be attending and swimming for a NCAA Division I college, for which you are the team physician. Her history is unremarkable, except for a past medical history of Ehlers-Danlos syndrome. She has no records with her, but assures you that she has been followed by a specialist in her hometown and that she has had no issues with her illness. Other than having hypermobility, her physical examination is unremarkable. What is the next best course of action?

   A. Full clearance and participation without restriction
   B. Disqualify from competitive activity, as Ehlers-Danlos syndrome poses a significant cardiac risk
   C. Clearance deferred, pending review of medical records
   D. Cleared for participation limited to low to moderate static and dynamic activity

Correct Answer: C. Clearance deferred, pending review of medical records

Ehlers-Danlos Syndrome is a genetic disorder of connective tissue, characterized by joint hypermobility and skin extensibility. There are different forms of the Ehlers-Danlos syndrome, with one form being vascular. Patients with the vascular form of Ehlers-Danlos syndrome have increased risk of aortic rupture. According to the 36th Bethesda guidelines, these patients should not engage in any competitive athletic activity. Otherwise, if they have any other forms of the disease, the athlete has full clearance to participate. Accordingly, Answer C is correct, because of the need to confirm what type of Ehlers-Danlos syndrome she has prior to making a clearance decision.

1. American Academy of Family Physicians, American Academy of Pediatrics, American College of Sports Medicine, American Medical Society for Sports Medicine, American Orthopaedic Society for Sports Medicine, American Osteopathic Academy of Sports Medicine. Bernhardt DT, Roberts WO (eds). Preparticipation Physical Evaluation. 4th ed. Elk Grove Village, IL: American Academy of Pediatrics; 2010. Accessed August 13, 2015 at http://ebooks.aap.org/product/ppe-preparticipation-physical-evaluation.
2. Maron BJ, Ackerman MJ, Nishimura RA, Pyeritz RE, Towbin JA, Udelson JE. Task Force 4: HCM and other cardiomyopathies, mitral valve prolapse, myocarditis, and Marfan syndrome. J Am Coll Cardiol 2005 Apr 19;45(8):1340-1345.

41. A 16-year-old right-handed high school athlete presents for a preparticipation physical evaluation in order to play club sports. On physical examination, he was found to have visual acuity of 20/30 in the right eye and 20/60 in the left eye. He does not wear glasses. Which sport is not recommended for him?

   A. Gymnastics
   B. Track and field
   C. Swimming
   D. Boxing

Correct Answer: D. Boxing

A visual acuity of 20/40 or better in at least one eye is considered to provide good vision. As such, athletes with best corrected vision in one eye of less than 20/40 should be considered functionally one-eyed. The American Academy of Ophthalmology states that athletes who are functionally one-eyed must not participate in boxing, wrestling, or full-contact martial arts. Answers A and B are incorrect, given that gymnastics and track and field are considered to be eye-safe sports. Answer C is incorrect, because swimming is considered to be a low-risk sport for eye injuries.

   1. Vinger PF. A practical guide for sports eye protection. Phys Sportsmed 2000;28(6):49-69.
   2. American Academy of Family Physicians, American Academy of Pediatrics, American College of Sports Medicine, American Medical Society for Sports Medicine, American Orthopaedic Society for Sports Medicine, American Osteopathic Academy of Sports Medicine. Bernhardt DT, Roberts WO (eds). Preparticipation Physical Evaluation. 4th ed. Elk Grove Village, IL: American Academy of Pediatrics, 2010.

42. An 18-year-old male presents to clinic for a preparticipation physical evaluation so that he can be cleared to try out for his local college's football team. He has no significant past medical history, no medically related complaints, and normal vital signs. He has a normal physical examination, with the exception of an enlarged spleen palpated on his abdominal examination. What is the most appropriate next step in his management?

   A. This is an incidental finding, and he should be cleared for all sports without restrictions
   B. If the spleen is acutely enlarged, all sports should be avoided, due to risk of rupture
   C. If the spleen is chronically enlarged, no further workup is necessary
   D. He may be cleared for all noncontact activities, but all contact/collision and limited contact sports should be avoided

Correct Answer: B. If the spleen is acutely enlarged, all sports should be avoided, due to risk of rupture

While not all palpable spleens in athletes are enlarged, any time an enlarged spleen is suspected, further evaluation is necessary before clearance is given to participate in sports, due to the risk of rupture. Depending on the cause of an enlarged spleen, there is an increased risk of rupture, even with noncontact sports. It is unclear in this case whether this athlete's spleen is acutely or chronically enlarged, because he denies any significant past medical history and is asymptomatic. The differential diagnosis for an enlarged spleen is broad and includes, but is not limited to, infectious mononucleosis, hepatitis and other infectious diseases, lymphoma, immunodeficiency disorders—including HIV, autoimmune diseases, inherited diseases, and others. Enlarged spleens may also occasionally occur as a normal variant. Given the risk of splenic rupture with sports participation, further workup, including laboratory evaluation and imaging, as well as a more detailed past medical, family, and social history, should be pursued prior to clearance for sports participation.

   1. American Academy of Pediatrics Committee on Sports Medicine and Fitness. Medical conditions affecting sports participation. Pediatrics 2001;107(5):1205-1209.
   2. Kurowski K, Chandran S. The preparticipation athletic evaluation. Am Family Physician 2000;61(9):2683-2690.

Test 1 Answers, Critiques, and References

43. Which of the following is not a mental health predictor of injury and illness in student athletes?

    A. Post-traumatic stress disorder
    B. Substance abuse
    C. Reactive depression
    D. Burnout

Correct Answer: C. Reactive depression

Reactive depression is a normal response to injury in student athletes, and is different from major depression in that it does not persist or become progressive. Answer A is incorrect, because post-traumatic stress disorder has a significant correlation with post-concussive syndrome and can be a predictor of developing complications following a concussion. Answer B is incorrect, because substance abuse can cause mood changes, sleep disturbance, and disordered eating, which can all contribute to injury or illness in student athletes. Answer D is incorrect, because burnout is a predictor of overuse injury, depression, and sport dropout.

1. Brown GT (ed). Mind, Body, and Sport: Understanding and Supporting Student-Athlete Mental Wellness. Indianapolis, IN: NCAA, 2014. Accessed December 24, 2018 at https://www.naspa.org/images/uploads/events/Mind_Body_and_Sport.pdf.

44. The preparticipation physical evaluation (PPE) is utilized in several sports. Regarding each specific population, which of the following is true?

   A. 75% of patients with hypertrophic cardiomyopathy with left ventricular outflow obstruction have a murmur on physical examination
   B. Geriatric patients undergoing PPE should have a physical examination, including postural vital signs, heart murmur, femoral pulses, and screening for Marfan disease
   C. Female athletes should not be asked about their menstrual cycles, as it may lead to distrust between the physician and the athlete
   D. Athletes with intellectual disabilities do not need PPE, as they have lower reported injury rates than physically disabled and general population athletes

Correct Answer: B. Geriatric patients undergoing PPE should have a physical examination, including postural vital signs, heart murmur, femoral pulses, and screening for Marfan disease

In addition to standard physical examination, the geriatric physical examination should include postural vital signs, cardiac auscultation, femoral pulses, and Marfan screening. Answer A is incorrect, because 25% of patients with HCM and left ventricular outflow obstruction have a murmur on physical examination. Answer C is incorrect, because female athletes are at risk for the female athlete triad, which includes menstrual dysfunction, low energy availability, and decreased bone mineral density. Answer D is incorrect, because although it is true the reported injury rates are lower compared to general populations and physically disabled athletes, special needs athletes PPE should be similar to any athlete without cognitive or physical disability. Answer E is incorrect, because focusing overly on the impairment may lead to missing common medical issues.

1. Maron BJ, Araújo CG, Thompson PD, Fletcher GF, de Luna AB, Fleg JL, et al. Heart Federation; International Federation of Sports Medicine; American Heart Association Committee on Exercise, Cardiac Rehabilitation, and Prevention. Recommendations for preparticipation screening and the assessment of cardiovascular disease in masters athletes: an advisory for healthcare professionals from the working groups of the World Heart Federation, the International Federation of Sports Medicine, and the American Heart Association Committee on Exercise, Cardiac Rehabilitation, and Prevention. Circulation 2001 Jan 16;103(2):327-334.
2. Maron BJ. Hypertrophic cardiomyopathy. Lancet 1997;350(9071):127-133.
3. American Academy of Family Physicians, American Academy of Pediatrics, American College of Sports Medicine, American Medical Society for Sports Medicine, American Orthopaedic Society for Sports Medicine, American Osteopathic Academy of Sports Medicine. Bernhardt DT, Roberts WO (eds). Preparticipation Physical Evaluation. 4th ed. Elk Grove Village, IL: American Academy of Pediatrics, 2010:131-139.

45. Individuals with Down syndrome have an increased risk of atlantoaxial instability and are required to have screening neck radiographs prior to sports participation. Those identified as having atlantoaxial instability are excluded from which of the following Special Olympic sports, unless the athlete and guardian grant written consent and obtain signatures from two independent medical professionals prior to participation?

    A. Tennis
    B. Gymnastics
    C. Figure skating
    D. Athletes with atlantoaxial instability are automatically disqualified from high-risk and contact sports

Correct Answer: B. Gymnastics

Activities which pose a high risk of injury to the cervical spine include contact sports, sports at risk of uncontrolled neck flexion/extension, and any activities which involve falls from heights. In individuals with radiographic evidence of atlantoaxial instability, activities that pose a high risk of injury to the cervical spine, such as gymnastics, are restricted. Signatures from two medical providers, the athlete, and the guardian are required prior to participation in high-risk activities in the Special Olympics. Answers A and C are incorrect, because tennis and figure skating are not considered high-risk sports for neck trauma.

1. Leas DP, Banit DM, Murrey D, Darden BV. Atlantoaxial instability in Down syndrome. Medscape. Accessed July 5, 2015 at http://emedicine.medscape.com/article/1180354-overview#showall.
2. Atlantoaxial instability Down syndrome. National Down Syndrome Society. Accessed July 5, 2015 at http://www.ndss.org/Resources/Health-Care/Associated-Conditions/Atlantoaxial-Instability-Down-Syndrome.
3. Down syndrome. Pediatric Orthopedic Society of North America. Accessed July 5, 2015 at http://www.posna.org/education/StudyGuide/DownsSyndromeTrisomy21.asp.

46. When training for an endurance event, which of the following is the most critical factor to consider when planning a training regimen?

   A. Frequency
   B. Intensity
   C. Time
   D. Technique
   E. Recovery

Correct Answer: B. Intensity

The most critical factor when training for an endurance event is intensity. Intensity denotes the level of participation in the activity. If intensity is sustained at too high or too low a level, it can impact training results, as well as training frequency, time, technique, and recovery. Current recommendations for intensity levels for activity range from moderate to vigorous, estimated by $\dot{V}O_2$max testing, target heart rate calculation, or rate of perceived exertion. Frequency refers to the number of training sessions within a given time period. Although adequate frequency is important to the principle of reversibility, the anticipated frequency will depend on the intensity level of the activity, with greater frequency required for lesser intensity workouts. General physical activity recommendations for the appropriate frequency of activity range from three days a week of vigorous activity or for five or more days a week at moderate activity levels, though this may be altered for those training for an event. Time is also impacted by intensity levels. The higher the level of intensity, the less time required to participate for aerobic benefit. On the other hand, a higher level of intensity usually results in an inability to participate for an extended period of time. Recovery time is also important when training for an endurance event. As with frequency and time, the recovery time can also be dictated by the intensity of the activity, with more intense activity requiring longer recovery times.

1. American College of Sports Medicine. ACSM's Guidelines for Exercise Testing and Prescription. 10th ed. Baltimore, MD: Lippincott Williams & Wilkins, 2017.
2. Zaryski C, Kin M, Smith DJ. Training principles and issues for ultra-endurance athletes. Curr Sports Med Rep 2005 Jun;4(3):165-170.

47. Which of the following is a credible theory for why stretching may hinder athletic performance and potentially lead to injury?

   A. Increased joint stability
   B. Decreased joint-movement efficiency
   C. Increased ability of the tendon and muscle to absorb energy
   D. Decreased pain tolerance
   E. Increased strength before the recovery phase of training

Correct Answer: B. Decreased joint-movement efficiency

Although many individuals include stretching pre- or post-workout, stretching has its own risks. There are several pathophysiologic theories on why stretching may actually hinder athletic performance and potentially lead to injury. For example, stretching could increase the movement about the joint, decreasing joint-movement efficiency and joint stability, potentially leading to injury. As the muscle and tendon fibers have been stretched to capacity (due to increased stretching tolerance), their ability to absorb energy with activity decreases, which could lead to injury. Furthermore, stretching increases pain tolerance, which could allow an athlete to continue to participate when they should have stopped activity, which could not only lead to injury, but also worsen an already present condition. Stretching is also theorized to allow decreased strength before the recovery phase of training. At present, however, there is no clear data supporting pre- or post-workout stretching as a means of injury prevention.

   1. Thacker SB, Gilchrist J, Stroup DF, Kimsey CD Jr. The impact of stretching on sports injury risk: a systematic review of the literature. Med Sci Sports Exerc 2004;36(3):371-378.
   2. Guissard N, Duchateau J. Neural aspects of muscle stretching. Exerc Sport Sci Rev 2006 Oct;34(4):154-158.

48. A 10-year-old male comes into your office. He would like to start weight training for football. Which of the following statements is correct regarding weight/resistance training in pediatric athletes?

   A. Weight training will help gain size and strength
   B. Weight training may be preferable for overweight children and adolescents compared to aerobic activity
   C. Weight training should be done with standard (adult-sized) equipment
   D. Weight training is associated with growth plate injuries in skeletally immature athletes

Correct Answer: B. Weight training may be preferable for overweight children and adolescents compared to aerobic activity

Weight training in the prepubertal child is associated with strength gains. However, the strength gains are associated with improved neural activity (increased motor-unit activation and changes in motor-unit coordination, recruitment, and firing), rather than concomitant muscle hypertrophy. Answer A is incorrect, because weight training will not increase muscle size. Injury data on weight training in children has frequently implicated inappropriately sized equipment and/or poor technique as common causes of injury. Cartilage/growth plate injury is a theoretical concern with resistance training in children, but this has not been found to be a real problem in proper training programs. Multiple studies have demonstrated that weight training with appropriately sized equipment, under careful supervision with emphasis on technique, has been shown to be safe and beneficial. Finally, several studies have demonstrated improved body-composition profiles and improved glucose sensitivities for overweight children after resistance training. In addition, the dropout rates tend to be lower for resistance training programs compared to aerobic training programs in overweight youth, making resistance training a better option for overall health in those selected populations.

   1. American Academy of Pediatrics Council on Sports Medicine and Fitness, McCambridge TM, Stricker PR. Strength training by children and adolescents. Pediatrics 2008 Apr;121(4):835-840.
   2. Faigenbaum AD, Kraemer WJ, Blimkie CJ, Jeffreys I, Micheli LJ, Nitka M, et al. Youth resistance training: updated position statement paper from the National Strength and Conditioning Association. J Strength Cond Res 2009 Aug;23(5 Suppl):S60-S79.
   3. Faigenbaum AD, Myer GD. Pediatric resistance training: benefits, concerns, and program design considerations. Curr Sports Med Rep 2010 May-Jun;9(3):161-168.

49. A 45-year-old patient comes to your office interested in learning more about training for a marathon that will be run at high altitude (about 6,000 feet or 1,829 meters above sea level). He is concerned because he lives only 500 feet or 152 meters above sea level and does not travel frequently to locations considered high altitude. He is a generally healthy person and exercises regularly. Which of the following statements gives him the best opportunity to safely and effectively participate in this marathon?

   A. Endurance events are not affected as much as sprint events, therefore his training does not need to be modified
   B. Illness related to altitude (acute mountain sickness, high altitude cerebral edema) only affects those individuals who are at a high altitude longer than 72 hours
   C. Acclimatization has not been shown to improve performance for races run within three days of reaching altitude
   D. The effect of altitude on $\dot{V}O_2$max is greater on those who perform endurance events
   E. High-intensity training (i.e., hard sprints to improve speed and other interval training) is best performed at high altitude as this improves training velocity and $\dot{V}O_2$max

Correct Answer: D. The effect of altitude on $\dot{V}O_2$max is greater on those who perform endurance events

The effect of altitude is greater on endurance athletes, because they rely on high cardiac output and high pulmonary blood flow to deliver oxygen to muscles for long periods of time. The relative decrease in available oxygen at high altitude diminishes this capacity ($\dot{V}O_2$max) and can be felt at lower altitudes. The cutoff for noticeable change is often 2,000 feet or 610 meters. Sprint events are less affected, because they rely more on short bursts of energy, which do not rely on oxygen transport to produce energy. Symptoms of acute mountain sickness can present as quickly as one to two hours after arriving at high altitude, and will usually present within 24 hours. High-intensity training is best undertaken at sea level, regardless of where a competition is to be held (making Answer E incorrect). Overall, "live high, train low" is the mantra, and acclimatization is crucial in participating in endurance events at high altitude.

1. Gallagher SA, Hackett P. Acute mountain sickness and high altitude cerebral edema. UpToDate. Accessed November 3, 2014 at https://www.uptodate.com/contents/acute-mountain-sickness-and-high-altitude-cerebral-edema.
2. Levine BD, Stray-Gundersen J. High-altitude training and competition. In: Madden CC, Putukian M, Young CC, McCarty EC (eds). Netter's Sports Medicine. Philadelphia: Saunders Elsevier, 2010:158-161.
3. Hackett PH, Roach RC. High-altitude medicine. In: Auerbach PS (ed). Wilderness Medicine. 5th ed. Philadelphia: Mosby Elsevier, 2007:2-36.

50. Which type of training program provides the greatest improvement in cardiorespiratory fitness?

   A. Moderate-intensity continuous training
   B. High-intensity interval training
   C. Strength training
   D. Long aerobic workout

Correct Answer: B. High-intensity interval training

The American College of Sports Medicine recommends that adults should get at least 150 minutes of moderate-intensity per week. Exercise recommendations can be met through either 30 to 60 minutes of moderate-intensity exercise (five days per week) or 20 to 60 minutes of vigorous-intensity exercise (three days per week). Studies have shown that high-intensity interval training (HIIT) improves cardiorespiratory fitness the greatest across a broad range of populations. Patients with cardiometabolic diseases showed significantly greater increases in $\dot{V}O_2$peak following HIIT. Studies have shown the following adaptations occur significantly more with HIIT than MICT (moderate-intensity continuous training): increase in $\dot{V}O_2$peak, decrease in SBP and DBP, increase in HDL, decrease in triglycerides, decrease in fasting glucose, decrease in oxidative stress and inflammation, and increase in cardiac function.

1. Wilson M, Ellison G, Cable NT. Basic science behind the cardiovascular benefits of exercise. Heart 2015;101:758-765.
2. Nybo L, Sundstrup E, Jakobsen M, Mohr M, Hornstrup T, Simonsen L, et al. High-intensity training versus traditional exercise interventions for promoting health. Med Sci Sports Exerc 2010 Oct;42(10):1951-1958. doi: 10.1249/MSS.0b013e3181d99203.
3. Weston K, Wisloff U, Coombes J. High-intensity interval training in patients with lifestyle-induced cardiometabolic disease: a systematic review and meta-analysis. Br J Sports Med 2014 Aug;48(16):1227-1234.

51. A 33-year-old female runner returns to your clinic to follow up for patellofemoral syndrome of the left knee. As you are about to leave the room after her visit, she asks for your opinion on vitamin C supplementation in athletes to help with immune function. Which of the following is the most appropriate response?

   A. Vitamin C is an essential component to the diet, and athletes should try to consume at least 1 g per day to optimize performance
   B. Vitamin C is not an essential component to the diet, and athletes should avoid supplementation for optimal performance
   C. Vitamin C is an essential component to the diet, and athletes should try to consume approximately 200 mg per day for optimal performance
   D. Vitamin C is an essential component to the diet, and athletes should try to consume under 100 mg per day to optimize performance

Correct Answer: C. Vitamin C is an essential component to the diet, and athletes should try to consume approximately 200 mg per day for optimal performance

Antioxidant supplements are widely used by athletes to manage oxidative stress that can lead to immune dysfunction, fatigue, and muscle damage. Vitamin C, taken in doses of 200 to 1000 mg per day, can decrease oxidative stress. Current evidence suggests that Vitamin C in larger doses appears to reduce athletic performance. Smaller doses do not seem to demonstrate the same beneficial effect.

1. Braakhuis AJ. Effect of vitamin C supplements on physical performance. Curr Sports Med Rep 2012 Jul-Aug;11(4):180-184.
2. Copp SW, Ferreira LF, Herspring KF, Hirai DM, Snyder BS, Poole DC, et al. The effects of antioxidants on microvascular oxygenation and blood flow in skeletal muscle of young rats. Exp Physiol 2009 Sep;94(9):961-971. doi: 10.1113/expphysiol.2009.048223.
3. Gomez-Cabrera MC, Domenech E, Romagnoli M, Arduini A, Borras C, Pallardo FV, et al. Oral administration of vitamin C decreases muscle mitochondrial biogenesis and hampers training-induced adaptations in endurance performance. Am J Clin Nutr 2008 Jan;87(1):142-149.

52. Which one of the following is correct about vitamin D in athletes?

   A. Supplementation for an athlete with a vitamin D level below 20 ng/ml is achieved with 2000 IU of vitamin D2 daily
   B. Maximum sports health benefit is achieved at a vitamin D level of 50 ng/ml
   C. Screening athletes for vitamin D deficiency includes obtaining a serum (1,25) dihydroxyvitamin D level
   D. Dietary supplementation with vitamin D2 is more advantageous than cutaneous synthesis of vitamin D

Correct Answer: B. Maximum sports health benefit is achieved at a vitamin D level of 50 ng/ml

Peak neuromuscular benefits of vitamin D are seen at 50 ng/ml. This is well above the level of 30 ng/ml currently considered as sufficient. The sports health benefits include promotion of optimal muscle function, stress fracture prevention, and immune system effects, with a reduction of both inflammation and the incidence of colds and flu. Answer A is incorrect, because an athlete with a level below 30 ng/ml should receive supplementation. Supplementation would occur with 50,000 IU of vitamin D3 daily. Vitamin D3 supplements, which are more potent than D2, should be used for supplementation. Answer C is incorrect, because the value used for screening for vitamin D deficiency is the serum 25 hydroxyvitamin D, not the (1,25) dihydroxy level. Dietary supplementation to a level of vitamin D above 50 ng/ml can be achieved with D3, not D2. Furthermore, cutaneous synthesis of vitamin D from sunlight exposure is considered more advantageous than oral supplementation, because the process has a negative feedback loop, which prevents vitamin D accumulation and toxicity, making Answer D incorrect.

1. Shuler FD, Wingate MK, Moore GH, Giangarra C. Sports health benefits of vitamin D. Sports Health 2012 Nov;4(6):496-501. doi: 10.1177/1941738112461621.
2. Constantini NW, Arieli R, Chodick G, Dubnov-Raz G. High prevalence of vitamin D insufficiency in athletes and dancers. Clin J Sport Med 2010 Sep;20(5):368-371. doi: 10.1097/JSM.0b013e3181f207f2.

53. What is the evidence-based proportion of fat in a typical diet for natural bodybuilders?

    A. 15% to 30 %
    B. 10% to 15%
    C. 15% to 20%
    D. 30% to 40%

Correct Answer: A. 15% to 30%

In the context of natural bodybuilding contest preparation, a scientific review of the literature makes the following recommendations. Caloric intake should be set at a level that results in bodyweight losses of approximately 0.5% to 1% per week to maximize muscle retention. Within this caloric intake, most, but not all bodybuilders will respond best to consuming 2.3 to 3.1 g/kg of lean body mass per day of protein, 15% to 30% of calories from fat, and the reminder of calories from carbohydrate.

1. Helms ER, Aragon AA, Fitschen PJ. Evidence-based recommendations for natural bodybuilding contest preparation: nutrition and supplementation. J Int Soc Sports Nutr 2014 May 12;11:20. doi: 10.1186/1550-2783-11-2.0.

54. Which of the following patients would you advise further evaluation prior to initiation of an exercise program?

    A. Patient with stable CAD wanting to restart their moderate exercise regimen
    B. COPD patient with dyspnea at rest
    C. A young, well-controlled hypertensive patient without risk factors and no evidence of organ damage
    D. A well-controlled patient with epilepsy wanting to take up running for exercise

Correct Answer: B. COPD patient with dyspnea at rest

Patients with CAD may benefit from exercise-capacity testing prior to beginning an exercise program. Some patients benefit from cardiac rehabilitation programs prior to beginning a program on their own. However, COPD patients with dyspnea at rest, resting hypercapnia, or cor pulmonale should usually refrain from exercise, making Answer B the more correct choice. Well-controlled hypertensive patients with no additional cardiac risk factors or end organ damage, should be encouraged to exercise to obtain all the available cardiovascular health benefits. Patients with epilepsy who have regular seizures should avoid certain activities, including scuba diving, aviation, parachuting, archery, and auto racing, due to potential harm to self or others. Epilepsy patients who are controlled should be encouraged to exercise.

1. Pescatello LS, Franklin BA, Fagard R, Farquhar WB, Kelley GA, Ray CA, et al. American College of Sports Medicine position stand. Exercise and hypertension. Med Sci Sports Exerc 2004 Mar;36(3):533-553.
2. Fields KB, Bailey W, Barnes KP, Rainbow CR, Hudnall S. Exercise and chronic disease. In: O'Connor FG, Casa DJ, Davis BA, St. Pierre P, Sallis RE, Wilder RP (eds.) ACSM's Sports Medicine: A Comprehensive Review. Philadelphia: Lippincott Williams & Wilkins, 2013:271-275.

55. A 30-year-old male with T6 paraplegia presents to the office with a desire to begin a wheelchair exercise program. He has been gaining weight, due to a lack of activity since the injury several years ago. He wants your advice on how to safely begin an exercise program. Along with advising proper equipment, carrying water, and avoiding hot or humid days, you also advise which of the following?

   A. Wear tight leg straps to increase sympathetic tone
   B. Take 10 g of carbohydrates every 30 minutes during exercise
   C. Empty his bladder and bowels before each workout
   D. Have cervical x-rays to rule out atlantoaxial instability

Correct Answer: C. Empty his bladder and bowels before each workout

This case refers to the prevention of autonomic dysreflexia (AD), a medical emergency. AD is caused by increased sympathetic input from the splanchnic nerves, caused by noxious stimuli. The majority of cases are caused by a distended bladder (90%) or bowel (9%). Prevention includes bowel and bladder maintenance and skin care. Answer A is incorrect, given that this can induce AD (a practice known as "boosting") and is illegal in Paralympics sports. Answer B is a recommendation for a type 1 diabetic. Answer D is a recommendation for a patient with Down syndrome.

   1. Richter KJ, et al. In: Scuderi GR, McCann PD (eds). Sports Medicine: A Comprehensive Approach. 2nd ed. Philadelphia: Mosby, 2005:725-737.
   2. Klenck C, Gebke K. Practical management: common medical problems in disabled athletes. Clin J Sport Med 2007 Jan;17(1):55-60.

56. An obese patient (BMI > 30 kg/m2) without other comorbidities presents to your office. To improve compliance, one strategy for the patient's exercise prescription could include which of the following?

   A. Incorporating high-impact aerobic activities
   B. Emphasizing exercising after their morning (am) meal
   C. Strict cardiovascular prescription at 85% maximum HR for at least 30 minutes five times per week
   D. Increasing weight-bearing activities very rapidly to increase metabolism
   E. Start with non-weight-bearing activities, such as swimming and recumbent bike

Correct Answer: E. Start with non-weight-bearing activities, such as swimming and recumbent bike

In 2015-2016, the prevalence of obesity was 39.8% among adults and 18.5% among youth in the United States. As such, exercise prescription remains extremely important for both the sports medicine specialist and the primary care provider for these patients. Guidelines are specific for a generalized exercise prescription. Cardiovascular exercise should take place at least five days per week, with the patient maintaining 85% of their maximum predicted HR for at least 20 minutes. In addition, progressive resistance training should be performed two to three days per week. Subsequent data also exists for patients with comorbidities. This specific case deals with an obese patient without other comorbidities. A provider should prescribe non-weight-bearing activities at first to avoid increased stress on the lower extremities. The compliance rate alone for obese patients is very poor secondary to either pain or discouragement. Thus, the patient should perform as much exercise as they can (not the firm 20 minutes as previously stated) to increase compliance. In addition, the patient should exercise prior to the morning meal to help with digestion. The lower the impact of the exercise prescription, the higher the compliance.

   1. American College of Sports Medicine. ACSM's Guidelines for Exercise Testing and Prescription. 10th ed. Philadelphia: Lippincott Williams & Wilkins, 2017.
   2. Hales CM, Carroll MD, Fryar CD, Ogden CL. Prevalence of obesity among adults and youth: United States, 2015-2016. NCHS data brief, no. 288. Hyattsville, MD: National Center for Health Statistics, 2017. Accessed March 4, 2019 at https://www.cdc.gov/nchs/data/databriefs/db288.pdf.

57. Which of the following is true regarding exercise among patients with type 2 diabetes?

   A. Muscular contractions stimulate blood glucose transport via an additive mechanism not impaired by insulin resistance or type 2 diabetes
   B. Blood glucose remains stable during physical activity, due to an increased reliance on fat to fuel muscular activity as intensity increases
   C. There is little risk of hypoglycemia with moderate aerobic exercise, even in patients using exogenous insulin or insulin secretagogues
   D. Persons with type 2 diabetes should undertake no more than 120 minutes per week of moderate to vigorous aerobic exercise, spread out during at least three days during the week

Correct Answer: A. Muscular contractions stimulate blood glucose transport via an additive mechanism not impaired by insulin resistance or type 2 diabetes

It is well established that physical activity improves blood glucose control. While insulin-stimulated blood glucose uptake into skeletal muscle predominates at rest and is impaired in type 2 diabetes, muscular contractions stimulate blood glucose transport via a separate additive mechanism not impaired by insulin resistance or type 2 diabetes. Physical activity causes increased glucose uptake into active muscles balanced by hepatic glucose production, with a greater reliance on carbohydrates to fuel muscular activity as intensity increases. There is little risk for hypoglycemia with moderate aerobic exercise in those patients not using exogenous insulin or insulin secretagogues. Those patients who are using these medications may need to adjust their dose as they undergo physical activity. Current physical activity recommendations for patients with type 2 diabetes are to undertake at least 150 minutes per week of moderate to vigorous aerobic exercise spread out during at least three days during the week. In addition to aerobic training, persons with type 2 diabetes should undertake moderate to vigorous resistance training at least two to three days per week.

1. Colberg SR, Sigal RJ, Fernhall B, Regensteiner JG, Blissmer BJ, Rubin RR, et al. Exercise and type 2 diabetes: the American College of Sports Medicine and the American Diabetes Association: joint position statement. Diabetes Care 2010 Dec;33(12):e147-e167. doi: 10.2337/dc10-9990.
2. Madden KM. Evidence for the benefit of exercise therapy in patients with type 2 diabetes. Diabetes Metab Syndr Obes 2013;6:233-239.
3. American Diabetes Association. Standards of medical care in diabetes—2014. Diabetes Care 2014 Jan;37 Suppl 1:S14-S80. doi: 10.2337/dc14-S014.

58. A pregnant woman wants to learn more about what activities she can participate in during pregnancy. Which of the following activities should be avoided during pregnancy?

   A. Swimming
   B. Elliptical machine
   C. Cycling
   D. Light exercise, including weight training

Correct Answer: C. Cycling

Healthy pregnant women with uncomplicated singleton pregnancies are at low risk of adverse maternal or fetal exercise-related events when participating in moderate-intensity activities. Pregnant women are advised to participate in activities that minimize the risk of balance loss and joint and ligament trauma to the body, as well as to avoid activities that could cause trauma to the fetus. Exercise recommendations for pregnant women include 150 minutes per week of moderate-intensity activity. Bicycle riding, especially during the second and third trimesters, should be avoided because of changes in balance and the risk of falling. Exposure to the extremes of air pressure, such as in scuba diving and high-altitude exercise in non-acclimatized women, should also be avoided.

1. Bredin SS, Foulds HJ, Burr JF, Charlesworth SA. Risk assessment for physical activity and exercise clearance: in pregnant women without contraindications. Can Fam Physician 2013 May;59(5):515-517.
2. Exercise during pregnancy. ACSM Current Comment. Accessed May 1, 2015 at https://www.acsm.org/access-public-information/brochures-fact-sheets/fact-sheets.

59. Which of the following is true of exercise in patients with osteoporosis?

   A. In postmenopausal women, impact exercises can increase BMD in the hip and spine
   B. Weight-bearing exercises are more beneficial than non-weight-bearing, high-force exercises in preventing bone loss and fractures in post-menopausal women
   C. Swimming can improve BMD in postmenopausal women
   D. Smoking cessation will improve overall health but will not reduce risk of osteoporosis

Correct Answer: A. In postmenopausal women, impact exercises can increase BMD in the hip and spine

Answer B is incorrect, given that non-weight-bearing, high-force exercises are more beneficial than weight-bearing exercises in preventing bone loss and fractures in post-menopausal women. Answer C is incorrect, because swimming does not improve BMD in post-menopausal women. Answer D is incorrect, as smoking cessation can reduce the risk of osteoporosis.

1. Howe TE, Shea B, Dawson LJ, Downie F, Murray A, Ross C, et al. Exercise for preventing and treating osteoporosis in postmenopausal women. Cochrane Database Syst Rev 2011 Jul 6;(7):CD000333. doi: 10.1002/14651858.CD000333.pub2.
2. Bethel M. Osteoporosis treatment and management. Medscape. Accessed June 25, 2015 at http://emedicine.medscape.com/article/330598-treatment#d12.

60. Which of the following statements is true regarding athletic equipment and the prevention of injury?

    A. Ankle bracing is better than taping in prevention of recurrent ankle sprains
    B. Mouthpieces help prevent concussion
    C. Soccer headgear helps prevent concussion
    D. Knee bracing helps prevent ACL injury

Correct Answer: A. Ankle bracing is better than taping in prevention of recurrent ankle sprains

Good evidence exists that ankle bracing reduces incidence of recurrent ankle sprains. Most evidence supports ankle bracing over ankle taping in primary and secondary injury. The evidence is stronger for bracing over taping in prevention. Mouthpieces reduce orofacial injuries, but no conclusive evidence exists on prevention of concussion. The current evidence is not conclusive for the use of soccer headgear in the prevention of concussion. Knee braces have not been conclusively demonstrated in the literature to prevent ACL tears and would not be the most correct answer.

1. Trojian TH, Mohamed N. Demystifying preventive equipment in the competitive athlete. Curr Sports Med Rep 2012 Nov-Dec;11(6):304-308. doi: 10.1249/JSR.0b013e31827558c8.
2. Cohen RS, Balcom TA. Current treatment options for ankle injuries: lateral ankle sprain, Achilles tendonitis, and Achilles rupture. Curr Sports Med Rep 2003 Oct;2(5):251-254.

61. You are the medical director for a marathon race, and you review the epidemiologic data on the common causes of mortality among marathon runners. What is the most common cause of death during a marathon in the United States?

    A. Coronary artery disease (CAD)
    B. Hypertrophic cardiomyopathy
    C. Exercise-associated hyponatremia (EAH)
    D. Cardiac arrhythmias

Correct Answer: A. Coronary artery disease (CAD)

In the United State, the death rate for marathon running over the past decade was found to be at 0.75 per 100,000 finishers. CAD is the main cause of cardiac arrest and mortality during marathons. Most cardiac arrest and death happen at or close to the finish line. EAH is serious problem among marathon runners, but rarely is fatal.

1. Mathews SC, Narotsky DL, Bernholt DL, Vogt M, Hsieh YH, Pronovost PJ, et al. Mortality among marathon runners in the United States, 2000-2009. Am J Sports Med 2012 Jul;40(7):1495-1500. doi: 10.1177/0363546512444555. Epub 2012 May 4.
2. Kim JH, Malhotra R, Chiampas G, d'Hemecourt P, Troyanos C, Cianca J, et al. Race Associated Cardiac Arrest Event Registry (RACER) Study Group. Cardiac arrest during long-distance running races. N Engl J Med 2012 Jan 12;366(2):130-140.
3. Webner D, DuPrey KM, Drezner JA, Cronholm P, Roberts WO. Sudden cardiac arrest and death in United States marathons. Med Sci Sports Exerc 2012 Oct;44(10):1843-1845.

62. In the planning and preparation for a large mass participation international sporting event, there are many factors that should be considered. One environmental consideration is that of severe inclement weather. Which of the following should be part of the planning for such an occurrence?

    A. Appropriate number of medical supplies should be monitored
    B. Lead medical physicians should have good communication with local weather reporters
    C. A safe area must be designated for athletes and spectator protection, in the event evacuation is required due to inclement weather
    D. Environmental planning should be managed by local authorities, not the medical personnel

Correct Answer: C. A safe area must be designated for athletes and spectator protection, in the event evacuation is required due to inclement weather

In the event of severe inclement weather, the medical team must be aware of potential local weather conditions. The medical and event plan should include a safe place for both athletes and spectators, in the event that an evacuation is deemed necessary in order to provide safety. Although adequate medical supplies are part of event management, if severe inclement weather creates a hazard, this must take priority. Mass casualty, such as an active shooter or bomb threat, would be escalated to local authorities.

1. Rubin AL. Safety, security, and preparing for disaster at sporting events. Curr Sports Med Rep 2004 Jun;3(3):141-145.
2. Vasquez MS, Fong MK, Patel LJ, Kurose B, Tierney J, Gardner I, et al. Medical planning for very large events: Special Olympics World Games Los Angeles 2015. Curr Sports Med Rep 2015 May-Jun;14(3):161-164.
3. Franc-Law JM. A community-based model for medical management of a large scale sporting event. Clin J Sport Med 2006 Sep;16(5):406-411.

63. You are responding as part of the medical team to athletes and spectators who have been victims of a mass casualty in a sports arena due to an active shooter. Local authorities have cleared the area to begin medical treatment. There are multiple victims with extremity, as well as chest, wounds. Which of the following is the best course of action?

    A. Begin CPR on any patient without a pulse
    B. Apply tourniquets to all extremity wounds high and tight and label the time, and move on to the next patient
    C. Apply pressure to chest wounds in sight only
    D. Begin CPR on any patients without a pulse and look for an AED

Correct Answer: B. Apply tourniquets to all extremity wounds high and tight and label the time, and move on to the next patient

In cases of mass casualty as the scenario at hand, the goal is to help as many of the victims as possible in an efficient manner. All victims with open wounds on the extremities should have tourniquets placed high and tight. The time should be labeled, so when the victim is further cared for, members of the team in the emergency room have this information readily available. Chest wounds should be evaluated to ensure an entrance and exit wound. A chest seal should be applied directly to the skin. CPR in this setting, as well as AED, would not be the priority, because time would be inefficiently used.

1. Franc-Law JM. A community-based model for medical management of a large scale sporting event. Clin J Sport Med 2006 Sep;16(5):406-411.
2. Rubin AL. Safety, security, and preparing for disaster at sporting events. Curr Sports Med Rep 2004 Jun;3(3):141-145.
3. Vasquez MS, Fong MK, Patel LJ, Kurose B, Tierney J, Gardner I, et al. Medical planning for very large events: Special Olympics World Games Los Angeles 2015. Curr Sports Med Rep 2015 May-Jun;14(3):161-164.

64. Which of the following is true regarding children and sports activity?

   A. Preteen athletes most commonly injure lower limbs, whereas teenagers injure upper limbs
   B. Salter-Harris II fractures generally require surgical intervention
   C. Joint dislocations and ligamentous injuries are more common than buckle and other types of fractures
   D. Physes close on average at 14.5 years of age in girls and 16.5 years of age in boys
   E. Non-union of fractures are common in the immature skeleton

Correct Answer: D. Physes close on average at 14.5 years of age in girls and 16.5 years of age in boys

After physeal closing, injury patterns are similar to those in adults, but physes close at about 15 years of age in girls and 17 years of age in boys. Preteens have injuries in the upper limbs, including contusions, strains, and simple fractures. Teenagers more commonly injure the lower limbs, knee injury being the most common. Salter-Harris II fractures are the most common type of physeal fracture at the transphyseal location, with extension into the epiphysis and extending into the joint. These do not often require surgical intervention. Because open epiphyses are three to five times weaker than the surrounding capsular and ligamentous tissues, fractures are more common than dislocations and ligamentous injuries. Non-union is rare, because the immature skeleton forms callous early and heals quickly. Non-unions are more common in adults than children.

1. Madden CC, Putukian M, Young CC, McCarty EC (eds). Netter's Sports Medicine. Philadelphia: Saunders Elsevier, 2010.
2. Carson S, Woolridge DP, Colletti J, Kilgore K. Pediatric upper extremity injuries. Pediatr Clin N Am 2006 Feb;53(1):41-67.
3. Arora R, Fichadia U, Hartwig E, Kannikeswaran N. Pediatric upper-extremity fractures. Pediatr Annals 2014;43(5):196-204.

65. The parents of a young female soccer player solicit your advice regarding general injury prevention strategies during an office visit. In providing recommendations, which of the following injury prevention methods has been proven effective?

    A. Neck strengthening programs for concussion
    B. Mouthguards for concussion
    C. Bracing for anterior cruciate ligament injury
    D. Neuromuscular training programs for anterior cruciate ligament injury
    E. Stretching programs for groin injury

Correct Answer: D. Neuromuscular training programs for anterior cruciate ligament injury

Neuromuscular training programs can effectively reduce the risk of anterior cruciate ligament (ACL) injury in certain athletes. However, evidence for prophylactic bracing to reduce ACL injury risk is lacking. There is no conclusive evidence to suggest that the use of mouthguards or increasing neck strength reduces concussion risk. A significant reduction in the incidence of sport-related groin injuries following completion of a groin injury prevention program has not been demonstrated.

1. Benson BW, McIntosh AS, Maddocks D, Herring SA, Raftery M, Dvorak J. What are the most effective risk-reduction strategies in sport concussion? Br J Sports Med 2013 Apr;47(5):321-326.
2. Esteve E, Rathleff MS, Bagur-Calafat C, Urrutia G, Thorborg K. Prevention of groin injuries in sports: a systematic review with meta-analysis of randomised controlled trials. Br J Sports Med 2015 Jun;49(12):785-791.
3. Labella CR, Hennrikus W, Hewett TE, Council on Sports Medicine and Fitness, Section on Orthopaedics. Anterior cruciate ligament injuries: diagnosis, treatment, and prevention. Pediatrics 2014 May;133(5):e1437-e1450.

66. Which of the following is true regarding sports participation in the athlete with a solitary kidney?

   A. Before clearing an athlete with a solitary kidney for sports, testing should be undertaken to ensure normal kidney function
   B. Kidney injuries are a common occurrence in sports
   C. Traumatic kidney injuries in sports usually warrant urgent surgery and have high potential to be catastrophic
   D. Athletes with one kidney should be discouraged from participation in contact or collision sports
   E. Specialized padding has been proven to be beneficial in protecting a solitary kidney from injury

Correct Answer: A. Before clearing an athlete with a solitary kidney for sports, testing should be undertaken to ensure normal kidney function

Athletes with a solitary kidney should be qualified for all sports, and there should be a thorough discussion of potential risks and benefits with the athlete and their family. Imaging should be undertaken to ensure normal position and anatomy. Normal kidney function should be ensured as well. Kidney injuries in sports are extremely rare. They seldom require surgical intervention or have been shown to be catastrophic. Specialized padding may provide some extra protection, but this has not been proven.

1. Grinsell MM, Butz K, Gurka MJ, Gurka KK, Norwood V. Sport-related kidney injury among high school athletes. Pediatrics 2012 Jul;130(1):e40-e45.
2. Brophy RH, Gamradt SC, Barnes RP, Powell JW, Delpizzo JJ, Rodeo SA, et al. Kidney injuries in professional American football: implications for management of an athlete with one functioning kidney. Am J Sports Med 2008 Jan;36(1):85-90.
3. Grinsell MM, Showalter S, Gordon K, Norwood V. Single kidney and sports participation: perception versus reality. Pediatrics 2006 Sep;118(3):1019-1027.

Test 1 Answers, Critiques, and References

67. You are performing a preparticipation physical evaluation (PPE) on the new college quarterback. It is noted in his history that he has cystic fibrosis. Prior to matriculating at the school, he played a full four years of high school football without a problem. Which of the following recommendations would you make as team physician?

    A. The athlete is not cleared because he has cystic fibrosis
    B. The athlete is cleared for full participation without further testing
    C. The athlete is required to have pulmonary function testing prior to clearance to evaluate lung capacity
    D. The athlete is required to have an exercise treadmill test prior to clearance to evaluate oxygen saturation during exercise
    E. The athlete is required to have an induced sputum culture to see if he needs prophylactic antibiotics during play

Correct Answer: D. The athlete is required to have an exercise treadmill test prior to clearance to evaluate oxygen saturation during exercise

A high number of athletes with the diagnosis of cystic fibrosis are participating in competitive sports across the United States and around the world. For the sports medicine physician, it is important to identify athletes with cystic fibrosis in order to avoid crisis or flares early on. One of the most important occurrences with CF patients would be heat illness. Patients with cystic fibrosis need acclimatization and good hydration to reduce the risk of heat illness. In addition, an athlete needs an individual assessment at the PPE. Generally, all sports may be played if oxygenation remains satisfactory during a graded exercise test. Answer A is incorrect, given that many athletes participate in sports. Answer B is incorrect, because further testing is required. Answer C is incorrect, because PFTs will not change the management when an athlete is exercising. Although it would provide helpful information, it would not necessarily change therapy or preclude clearance. Answer E is incorrect, as many CF patients are on prophylactic antibiotics. On the other hand, the sputum culture would not change athletic management.

1. Rice SG, American Academy of Pediatrics Council on Sports Medicine and Fitness. Medical conditions affecting sports participation. Pediatrics 2008 Apr;121(4):841-848.
2. Moorcroft AJ, Dodd ME, Morris J, Webb AK. Individualised unsupervised exercise training in adults with cystic fibrosis: a 1 year randomised controlled trial. Thorax 2004 Dec;59(12):1074-1080.
3. Copley J. Stretching techniques: static, passive, active, dynamic, ballistic, and isometric stretches. Suite101.com Media Inc. Accessed June 20, 2010 at http://fitness.suite101.com/article.cfm/stretching_techniques?sms_ss=email.

68. Which of the following statements regarding participation in competitive sports is most accurate in a patient with aortic stenosis (AS)?

   A. Patients with mild AS may participate in all sports and require no follow-up after initial testing
   B. Patients with moderate AS are allowed to participate in moderate-intensity static sports if an exercise tolerance test demonstrates satisfactory exercise capacity without symptoms or ECG changes, and the patient has a normal blood pressure response to exercise
   C. Patients with asymptomatic severe AS may participate in low-static- and low-dynamic-intensity competitive sports
   D. Patients with symptomatic moderate AS may participate in low-static- and low-dynamic-intensity sports with serial evaluations of AS severity on at least an annual basis
   E. Patients with severe AS should not engage in a low-intensity recreational walking program after being excluded from competitive sports, due to increased risk for syncope

Correct Answer: B. Patients with moderate AS are allowed to participate in moderate-intensity static sports if an exercise tolerance test demonstrates satisfactory exercise capacity without symptoms or ECG changes, and the patient has a normal blood pressure response to exercise

In patients with AS, the risk of sudden cardiac death increases with increasing severity of the disease. This is particularly true as the patient becomes symptomatic (dyspnea, syncope, angina pectoris). The 36th Bethesda conference eligibility recommendations for competitive athletes with cardiovascular abnormalities discusses patients with aortic stenosis. While patients with mild AS can participate in all sports, they require at least annual evaluation of the severity of the disease. Patients with asymptomatic, moderate AS may participate in low-static and low-dynamic sports. Participation in moderate-static and moderate-dynamic sports may be allowed if the patient undergoes an exercise tolerance test and demonstrates satisfactory exercise capacity without symptoms or ECG changes, and has a normal blood pressure response to exercise. This makes Answer B more accurate than Answer A. Patients with symptomatic moderate AS and severe AS should not engage in any competitive sports. This makes Answers C and D incorrect. The guidelines only address participation in competitive sports. Patients with AS of any severity may participate in non-competitive activities. This makes Answer E incorrect.

   1. Maron BJ, Zipes DP. Introduction: eligibility recommendations for competitive athletes with cardiovascular abnormalities-general considerations. J Am Coll Cardiol 2005 Apr 19;45(8):1318-1321.

69. A 25-year-old male Italian soccer player presents to you for his preparticipation physical evaluation. He complains of some shortness of breath with exercise. His family history is significant for an older brother who died from a heart-related issue while training in the military. Physical examination was within normal limits. Because of his family history, you decide to order a 12-lead ECG. The ECG shows T wave inversion in leads V1 to V3. A terminal notch in the QRS complex is noted (see image). You refer your patient to the cardiologist, where he undergoes a two-dimensional echocardiogram, which shows an enlarged, hypokinetic right ventricle, with a thin RV free wall. Your patient undergoes a cardiac biopsy, and several days later, you get a pathology report which reads "fibro-fatty infiltration of right ventricular free wall." What is your diagnosis based on the above?

    A. Hypertrophic cardiomyopathy
    B. Arrythmogenic right ventricular dysplasia
    C. Anomalous coronary artery
    D. Prolonged QT syndrome

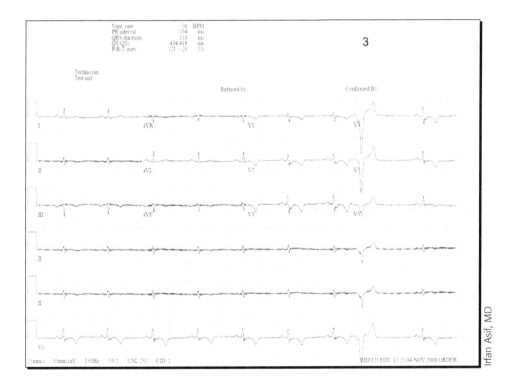

Correct Answer: B. Arrythmogenic right ventricular dysplasia

Arrhythmogenic right ventricular dysplasia is usually inherited in an autosomal dominant pattern, with variable expression. Up to 80% of individuals with ARVD present with syncope or sudden cardiac death. The pathogenesis of ARVD is largely unknown. Normal right ventricular muscle tissue is replaced with fatty or fibro/fatty tissue. Arrhythmias due to ARVD typically arise from the right ventricle.

The type of arrhythmia ranges from frequent premature ventricular complexes to ventricular tachycardia to ventricular fibrillation. There is a long asymptomatic lead-time in individuals with ARVD. Individuals in their teens may not have any characteristics of ARVD on screening tests. Many individuals have symptoms associated with ventricular tachycardia, such as palpitations, light-headedness, or syncope. Others may have symptoms and signs related to right ventricular failure, such as lower extremity edema and liver congestion, with elevated hepatic enzymes. Unfortunately, sudden death may be the first manifestation of disease.

ARVD is a progressive disease. Over time, the right ventricle becomes more involved, leading to right ventricular failure. The right ventricle will fail before there is left ventricular dysfunction. However, by the time the individual has signs of overt right ventricular failure, there will be histological involvement of the left ventricle. Eventually, the left ventricle will also become involved, leading to biventricular failure.

Hypertrophic cardiomyopathy is a disease of the myocardium in which a portion of the myocardium is hypertrophied without any obvious cause. It is perhaps most well-known as a leading cause of sudden cardiac death in young athletes. The occurrence of hypertrophic cardiomyopathy is a significant cause of sudden unexpected cardiac death in any age group, as well as a cause of disabling cardiac symptoms. Some abnormalities seen are due to LVH and include voltage abnormalities, ST segment and T wave abnormalities, prominent Q waves, and signs of LA enlargement. The ECG in a patient with an anomalous coronary artery is usually negative and patients are usually asymptomatic. Prolonged Q-T syndrome would be suspected if the QT intervals corrected for heart rate (QTc) is longer than 0.44 seconds. However, a normal QTc can be more prolonged in females (up to 0.46 sec).

1. Corrado D, Pelliccia A, Bjørnstad HH, Vanhees L, Biffi A, Borjesson M, et al. Cardiovascular pre-participation screening of young competitive athletes for prevention of sudden death: proposal for a common European protocol. Consensus Statement of the Study Group of Sport Cardiology of the Working Group of Cardiac Rehabilitation and Exercise Physiology and the Working Group of Myocardial and Pericardial Diseases of the European Society of Cardiology. Eur Heart J 2005 Mar;26(5):516-524.
2. Wren C. Screening for potentially fatal heart disease in children and teenagers. Heart 2009 Dec;95(24):2040-2046. doi: 10.1136/hrt.2009.172858.

70. As part of a preparticipation physical evaluation, a 20-year-old previously healthy, asymptomatic African-American male college long distance runner has an ECG performed. Which of the following ECG findings is abnormal in athletes and warrants additional testing?

    A. Sinus arrhythmia
    B. Incomplete right bundle branch block
    C. Mobitz type II second degree AV block
    D. QRS voltage criteria for LVH

Correct Answer: C. Mobitz type II second degree AV block

Mobitz type II second degree AV block (see image below) can be indicative of underlying structural disease. It is characterized by sudden loss of p-wave conduction, with prior PR prolongation. In the ECG shown below, note the P waves with a loss of conduction and no QRS complex (arrows). There is no PR prolongation in the beats prior, and there is no PR shortening in the beats following (Mobitz type I). Mobitz type II second degree AV block in an athlete is not due to increased vagal tone, and should prompt evaluation for underlying conduction disease. Mobitz type II should be differentiated from Mobitz type I (Wenckebach), which can be attributed to a functional block from increased vagal tone. Heart rate can vary with inspiration and expiration. Up to 55% of well-trained athletes have sinus arrhythmia. Up to 40% of well-trained athletes have IRBBB, especially endurance athletes. This condition is believed to occur because of RV remodeling and increased RV cavity size, which causes an increase in conduction time rather than a delay in the His-Purkinje system. An increase in vagal tone can create a Mobitz type I pattern. It should correct to a 1:1 conduction pattern with exercise. A well-trained athlete can have a physiologic increase in chamber size or wall thickness. This is more commonly true in Black/African athletes. If there is non-voltage criteria for LVH, further investigation is needed.

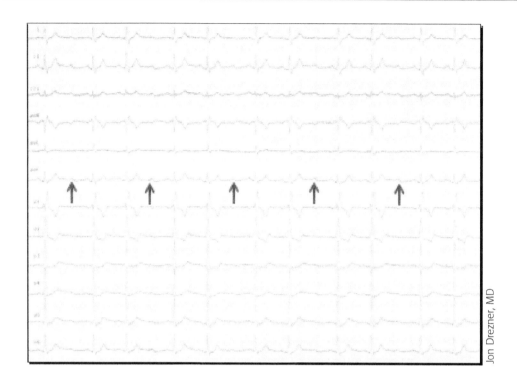

1. Drezner JA, Ackerman MJ, Cannon BC, Corrado D, Heidbuchel H, Prutkin JM, et al. Abnormal electrocardiographic findings in athletes: recognising changes suggestive of primary electrical disease. Br J Sports Med 2013 Feb;47(3):153-167. doi: 10.1136/bjsports-2012-092070.
2. Drezner JA, Fischbach P, Froelicher V, Marek J, Pelliccia A, Prutkin JM, et al. Normal electrocardiographic findings: recognising physiological adaptations in athletes. Br J Sports Med 2013 Feb;47(3):125-136. doi: 10.1136/bjsports-2012-092068.

71. During the athletic preparticipation physical evaluation, which of the following findings would be concerning for hypertrophic cardiomyopathy?

    A. Normal auscultation findings
    B. Widening of second heart sound
    C. Midsystolic murmur that gets louder with standing or Valsalva maneuver
    D. Systolic ejection murmur at the upper right sternal border

Correct Answer: C. Midsystolic murmur that gets louder with standing or Valsalva maneuver

Patients with hypertrophic cardiomyopathy may present with normal auscultatory findings. A harsh midsystolic murmur that gets louder or longer with standing or Valsalva maneuver should, however, raise clinical concern. Patients may have a positive family history of hypertrophic cardiomyopathy, premature sudden cardiac death, or recurrent syncopal episodes, and personal history of exertional chest pain or syncope. Widening of the second heart sound (physiological split) is considered normal. A harsh systolic ejection murmur at the upper right sternal border is seen in patients with aortic stenosis.

1. Giese EA, O'Connor FG, Depenbrock PJ, Oriscello RG. The athletic preparticipation evaluation: cardiovascular assessment. Am Fam Physician 2007 Apr;75(7):1008-1014.
2. Kurowski K, Chandran S. The preparticipation athletic evaluation. Am Fam Physician 2000 May 1;61(9):2683-2690.

72. During the preparticipation physical evaluation for athletes, you should look for non-cardiac signs of cardiovascular disease. Which of the following is a physical finding of Marfan syndrome?

    A. Thumb sign
    B. Elbow hyperextension
    C. Fibrillin-1 mutation
    D. Pes cavus

Correct Answer: A. Thumb sign

To detect thumb sign, ask the patient to wrap the fingers of one hand around their other wrist. If the thumb and 5th digit overlap, that is a positive thumb sign. Limited elbow extension may be present in patients with Marfan, but is not a specific sign for it.

1. Mirabelli MH, Devine MJ, Singh J, Mendoza M. The preparticipation sports evaluation. Am Fam Physician 2015 Sep 1;92(5):371-376.
2. Glorioso J Jr, Reeves M. Marfan syndrome: screening for sudden death in athletes. Curr Sports Med Rep 2002 Apr;1(2):67-74.

Test 1 Answers, Critiques, and References

73. While evaluating a child for a preparticipation physical evaluation, you auscultate a murmur at the upper left sternal border. It is a crescendo-decrescendo murmur, and you are debating between a pathological murmur and an innocent murmur. Which of the following is true?

   A. An atrial septal defect (ASD) would have a murmur that has a normal S2 split and moves with respiration
   B. Pulmonic stenosis would present as a quiet murmur that can also be confused with an innocent murmur
   C. Patients with an ASD may also have a diastolic murmur that sounds like a rumble across the tricuspid valve area
   D. This murmur may be the initial finding in a patient with aortic stenosis
   E. If this murmur decreases in intensity when the patient stands, it could be a finding of hypertrophic cardiomyopathy

Correct Answer: C. Patients with an ASD may also have a diastolic murmur that sounds like a rumble across the tricuspid valve area

ASDs are often confused with innocent murmurs on evaluation, and special care needs to be used in evaluating the pediatric patient. A patient with an ASD may have a diastolic and systolic murmur, but the diastolic murmur is not always heard. An innocent murmur would have a normal S2 split and move with respiration. An atrial septal defect would present with a murmur that is widely split and fixed, i.e., does not move with respiration. Pulmonic stenosis would present with a loud murmur and is not often confused with an innocent murmur. Aortic stenosis would be a murmur found at the upper right sternal border. When evaluating a patient for hypertrophic cardiomyopathy, the murmur would increase in intensity when changing positions from sitting to standing.

   1. McConnell ME, Adkins SB, Hannon DW. Heart murmurs in pediatric patients: when do you refer? Am Fam Physician 1999 Aug;60(2):558-565.
   2. American Academy of Family Physicians, American Academy of Pediatrics, American College of Sports Medicine, American Medical Society for Sports Medicine, American Orthopaedic Society for Sports Medicine, American Osteopathic Academy of Sports Medicine. Bernhardt DT, Roberts WO (eds). Preparticipation Physical Evaluation. 4th ed. Elk Grove Village, IL: American Academy of Pediatrics, 2010.

74. A 13-year-old male middle school soccer player presents for a preparticipation physical evaluation (PPE). He is asymptomatic, has a normal physical examination, and his family history is negative for cardiovascular disease. His PPE should include?

    A. An electrocardiogram, because he is male
    B. An electrocardiogram, because he plays soccer
    C. An electrocardiogram, because he is 13 years old
    D. An electrocardiogram is not routinely indicated

Correct Answer: D. An electrocardiogram is not routinely indicated

Experts agree that screening for sudden cardiac death in young athletes is indicated prior to competitive athletics. At a minimum, a history and physical examination should be completed. There is debate, however, whether to include an electrocardiogram (ECG) into the screening process. If it is included, the ECG must be interpreted with modern, athlete-specific standards, and the appropriate infrastructure must be in place. In addition, in this age group, there may be juvenile T wave inversion patterns that may be present. Hence, if an ECG is included, it may be best to do so in high-school-aged athletes and older.

1. Maron BJ, Friedman RA, Kligfield P, Levine BD, Viskin S, Chaitman BR, et al. Assessment of the 12-lead ECG as a screening test for detection of cardiovascular disease in healthy general populations of young people (12-25 years of age): a scientific statement from the American Heart Association and the American College of Cardiology. Circulation 2014 Oct 7;130(15):1303-1334.
2. Roberts WO, Asplund CA, O'Connor FG, Stovitz SD. Cardiac preparticipation screening for the young athlete: why the routine use of ECG is not necessary. J Electrocardiol 2015 May-Jun;48(3):311-315. doi: 10.1016/j.jelectrocard.2015.01.010. Epub 2015 Jan 28.

75. Which of the following statements regarding endurance and fluid replacement exercise is true?

    A. Older athletes have increased thirst sensitivity when dehydrated
    B. Prehydration has not been proven to help prevent dehydration during exercise
    C. Hydration plans should have a goal of preventing > 2% weight loss from water deficit
    D. Body size and speed should be disregarded when developing hydration plans

Correct Answer: C. Hydration plans should have a goal of preventing > 2% weight loss from water deficit

Older athletes have decreased thirst sensitivity when dehydrated. Prehydration with fluids and electrolytes is part of proper planning before endurance events, especially those greater than one hour in duration. Answer D is incorrect. In endurance events, a person's age, sex, body size, and running speed all affect the sweat rate and, therefore, the fluid and electrolyte loss. Rehydration plans should be customized to those factors. Hydration plans have a primary goal of trying to prevent a > 2% water weight loss in endurance events, as well as maintain electrolyte balance. Urine specific gravity or pre- and post-weight measurements during training are acceptable tools to assist in this goal.

1. American College of Sports Medicine, Sawka MN, Burke LM, Eichner ER, Maughan RJ, Montain SJ, et al. American College of Sports Medicine position stand. Exercise and fluid replacement. Med Sci Sports Exerc 2007 Feb;39(2):377-390.

76. A 15-year-old female soccer player complains of right hip pain. Her pain began one week ago, after running sprints at soccer practice. Lifting her leg, flexing her hip, and running make the pain worse. On exam, she is focally tender over the anterior superior iliac spine (ASIS). Pelvic x-rays reveal that she is skeletally immature. You diagnose her with ASIS apophysitis. Which muscle originates at the location of her injury?

    A. Sartorius
    B. Rectus femoris
    C. Biceps femoris, long head
    D. Gracilis

Correct Answer: A. Sartorius

The sartorius originates at the anterior superior iliac spine and inserts at the proximal medial tibia, as part of the pes anserinus (along with gracillis and semitendinosis). Actions of the sartorius include hip and knee flexion, hip abduction, external rotation of the hip, and internal rotation of the tibia. The rectus femoris originates at the anterior inferior iliac spine (AIIS). The long head of biceps femoris originates at the ischial tuberosity; its short head originates at the linea aspera on the femur. The gracilis originates near the pubic symphysis.

1. Thompson JC. Netter's Concise Orthopaedic Anatomy. 2nd ed. Philadelphia: Saunders Elsevier, 2010.
2. Longo UG, Ciuffreda M, Locher J, Maffulli N, Denaro V. Apophyseal injuries in children's and youth sports. Br Med Bull 2016 Dec;120(1):139-159. Epub 2016 Nov 23.
3. Singer G, Eberl R, Wegmann H, Marterer R, Kraus T, Sorantin E. Diagnosis and treatment of apophyseal injuries of the pelvis in adolescents. Semin Musculoskelet Radiol 2014;18(5):498-504.

77. Which of the following statements is true of congenital coronary artery anomalies?

   A. Diagnosis is based on abnormalities on 12-lead electrocardiogram
   B. Coronary artery anomalies are the most common cause of sudden cardiac death in athletes
   C. The most common anomaly is a single right coronary artery, with an absent left coronary artery
   D. All athletes with anomalous coronary arteries will experience symptoms (e.g., chest pain, syncope) at some point in time
   E. Blood flow may be compromised during exertion, resulting in ischemia and fatal arrhythmia

Correct Answer: E. Blood flow may be compromised during exertion, resulting in ischemia and fatal arrhythmia

Anomalous coronary arteries are the second leading cause of sudden cardiac death in young athletes in the United States behind hypertrophic cardiomyopathy. While a single right coronary artery (RCA), with an absent left coronary artery (LCA), has been described, the anomalous artery is usually an LCA originating from the right sinus of Valsalva or an RCA originating from the left sinus of Valsalva. Because the anomalous artery courses between the aorta and pulmonary trunk, it is thought that the vessel is compressed, and blood flow is compromised during exertion. This can result in ischemia and fatal arrhythmia. Clinical presentation includes chest pain, dizziness, syncope, and palpitations. On the other hand, many athletes remain asymptomatic prior to sudden cardiac death. A high index of suspicion is essential in making the diagnosis, since the 12-lead electrocardiogram is often interpreted as normal. While echocardiography and coronary angiography have traditionally been used in making the diagnosis, coronary CT has now become a useful diagnostic modality as well.

   1. Basilico FC. Cardiovascular disease in athletes. Am J Sports Med 1999;27(1):108-121.
   2. Rommel M, Griffin R, Harrison EE. Coronary anomalies: cardiac CT evaluation of the symptomatic adult athlete. Curr Sports Med Rep 2007;6(2):85-92.

78. Which of the following is true of hypertrophic cardiomyopathy (HCM)?

    A. HCM is a genetic disorder with an autosomal recessive pattern of inheritance
    B. HCM is characterized by right ventricular wall thickness of > 5 mm
    C. The murmur associated with HCM is exacerbated by the Valsalva maneuver
    D. Most patients have detectible signs of HCM before sudden death
    E. Gold standard for diagnosis is cardiac CT

Correct Answer: C. The murmur associated with HCM is exacerbated by the Valsalva maneuver

HCM, which is autosomal dominant in familial inheritance, is characterized by right ventricular wall thickness of 15 mm. The upper limit of normal wall thickness is 12 mm, and the gray zone is 13 to 14 mm. Valsalva maneuvers and position changes to standing will increase the murmur. On occasion, no murmur is present. Because most patients have no presenting signs or symptoms before sudden death, a thorough family history is critical for a physician to obtain for optimal screening. Echocardiography is the gold standard test, and ECG is the first diagnostic test for suspicion of HCM.

1. Elliot PM, McKenna WJ. Clinical manifestations of hypertrophic cardiomyopathy. UpToDate. Accessed December 1, 2014 at https://www.uptodate.com/contents/hypertrophic-cardiomyopathy-clinical-manifestations-diagnosis-and-evaluation.
2. Maron BJ, Maron MS. Hypertrophic cardiomyopathy. Lancet 2013 Jan 19;381(9862):242-255. doi: 10.1016/S0140-6736(12)60397-3. Epub 2012 Aug 6.

79. A 15-year-old male comes to you for his preparticipation physical evaluation. He has a positive family history of Marfan syndrome in an older sibling, who has been restricted from collision sports. By history, this young man denies any ocular, cardiovascular, or pulmonary concerns. On examination, he is found to have positive wrist and thumb signs, pes planus, minor pectus carinatum, joint hypermobility, and a high arched palate. You find no skin or cardiopulmonary abnormalities on examination. Which statement is correct for further assessment of this child?

   A. Although he has positive family history and skeletal findings, there is no evidence for involvement of a third system, therefore no additional workup is needed
   B. Send for ophthalmology evaluation and transesophageal echocardiogram
   C. Get a one-time normal radiograph of the lumbar spine and both hips to rule out protrusio acetabulae and scoliosis and, if normal, no additional workup is needed
   D. No additional workup is needed; simply ban the child from contact or collision sports, as a precaution

Correct Answer: C. Get a one-time normal radiograph of the lumbar spine and both hips to rule out protrusio acetabulae and scoliosis and, if normal, no additional workup is needed

Marfan syndrome has a reported incidence of two to three in 10,000 and is the most common inherited connective tissue disorder. The diagnosis of Marfan syndrome is based on the Ghent nosology. Clinical features in the skeletal, ocular, cardiovascular, pulmonary, and integumentary systems are used to define major criteria or partial involvement. Two additional systems include the dura and genetic findings.

The diagnosis requires a minimum of major criteria in two systems and the involvement of a third. In this case, the child has positive family history and fits criteria for at least involvement of the skeletal system. Additional skeletal measurements and radiographs could be done to further evaluate for scoliosis, protrusio acetabula, and upper to lower body segment ratio. Radiographs of the lumbar spine and hips would further clarify the skeletal criteria, but these findings are age-related and will change over time.

With the knowledge of positive family history and the involvement of the skeletal system, the ocular and cardiovascular systems need to be evaluated as well. Referral for transesophageal echocardiogram and ophthalmology evaluation is advised. If this child's ocular and echocardiogram evaluations were normal, a pelvic MRI to detect dural ectasia may be indicated, if a positive finding would make the diagnosis. Furthermore, in younger athletes with suspected Marfan syndrome who do not fulfill the Ghent diagnostic criteria, repeat clinical evaluations should be offered.

Sports participation in those with Marfan syndrome depends on which organ systems are involved and to what extend they are affected. Generally, participation in moderate-static/low-dynamic sports can be allowed if normal aortic root, normal to mild mitral valve abnormalities, and no family history of sudden death exist. These athletes are advised to have repeat cardiovascular evaluations every six months. Collision sports may not be advisable, due to cardiovascular and ocular risks. Depending on the extent of the organ system involvement, some Marfan syndrome athletes will be limited to only low-intensity sports.

1. Glorioso J Jr, Reeves M. Marfan syndrome: screening for sudden death in athletes. Curr Sports Med Rep 2002 Apr;1(2):67-74.
2. Dean J. Management of Marfan syndrome. Heart 2002 Jul;88(1);97-103.
3. Maron BJ, Ackerman MJ, Nishimura RA, Pyeritz RE, Towbin JA, Udelson JE. Task Force 4: HCM and other cardiomyopathies, mitral valve prolapse, myocarditis, and Marfan syndrome. J Am Coll Cardiol 2005 Apr 19;45(8):1340-1345.

80. A 19-year-old male college lacrosse player complains of a "racing and pounding" heart beat intermittently during lacrosse practice for the past two weeks. It lasts for a few minutes and then resolves. He denies any chest pain, syncope, radiation, nausea, or difficulty breathing. He is otherwise healthy and has no family history of cardiac disease or unexplained sudden death. You obtain an ECG (see image), which shows normal sinus rhythm, with a delta wave and a shortened PR interval. To determine if the patient has the antidromic or orthodromic form of this condition, what would you do next to test for this?

A. Signal averaged ECG
B. Transesophageal echocardiogram
C. Cardiac MRI
D. Electrophysiology study
E. 12 lead ECG treadmill stress test

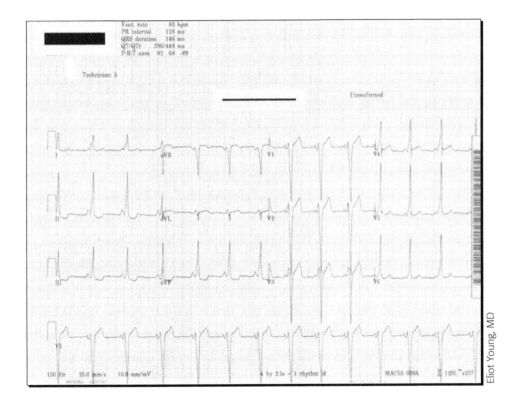

Correct Answer: D. Electrophysiology study

This patient's ECG is consistent with Wolff-Parkinson-White (WPW), a preexcitation syndrome. In WPW, an accessory pathway exists between the atria and ventricles, which can lead to an arrhythmia, due to electrical flow through this aberrant pathway. Though a low risk, WPW can be a cause of sudden cardiac death; the risk of sudden death in patients with WPW is estimated to be one in every 1000 patient-years of follow-up. An electrophysiology (EP) study can help determine if the conduction through the aberrant pathway is orthodromic (from the ventricles back to the atria) or antidromic (from the atria to the ventricles). The antidromic conduction may place the patient at higher risk for ventricular fibrillation. The other studies will not be able to determine whether this patient has the orthodromic or antidromic form of WPW.

1. Sarubbi B. The Wolff-Parkinson-White electrocardiogram pattern in athletes: how and when to evaluate the risk for dangerous arrhythmias. The opinion of the paediatric cardiologist. J Cardiovasc Med (Hagerstown) 2006 Apr;7(4):271-278.
2. Rao AL, Salerno JC, Asif IM, Drezner JA. Evaluation and management of Wolff-Parkinson-White in athletes. Sports Health 2014 Jul;6(4):326-332.
3. Colucci RA, Silver MJ, Shubrook J. Common types of supraventricular tachycardia: diagnosis and management. Am Fam Physician 2010 Oct 15;82(8):942-952.

81. Which of the following is correct?

   A. Congenital sensorineural deafness is associated with long QT syndrome
   B. Albuterol should be encouraged in patients with suspected congenital prolonged QT interval
   C. Taking ciprofloxacin does not prolong the QT interval
   D. Athletes with known prolonged QT can be cleared to run the 110 meter hurdles, but not to run the 1500 meters in track and field

Correct Answer: A. Congenital sensorineural deafness is associated with long QT syndrome

Sudden cardiac death in young athletes is rare. Long QT syndrome is not the most common cause of sudden cardiac death, but there are important clinical issues related to long QT. Most deaf children and adults do not have long QT syndrome. There is an association with deafness, however. This is an inherited genetic association. Many common medications, including some stimulants, prolong the QT interval. This is particularly important for patients with a borderline QT interval or those currently using other medications, where an altered QT interval is a potential side effect. Drug-drug interactions can affect the QT enough to lead to disaster. Albuterol has been shown to prolong the QT interval, in addition to causing hypokalemia. Cardiac clearance for sprinters and hurdlers is essentially the same as cardiac clearance for middle distance runners. Sprinters may run many miles during a workout, and distance runners will sprint during their training and races. Ciprofloxacin and other floroquinolones have been linked to injury to soft tissues, including tendon rupture, and to prolongation of the QT interval.

1. Gomez AT, Prutkin JM, Rao AL. Evaluation and management of athletes with long QT syndrome. Sports Health 2016 Nov/Dec;8(6):527-535. doi: 10.1177/1941738116660294. Epub 2016 Aug 6.
2. Kapetanopoulos A, Kluger J, Maron BJ, Thompson PD. The congenital long QT syndrome and implications for young athletes. Med Sci Sports Exerc 2006 May;38(5):816-825.
3. Maron BJ, Zipes DP. Introduction: eligibility recommendations for competitive athletes with cardiovascular abnormalities-general considerations. J Am Coll Cardiol 2005 Apr 19;45(8):1318-1321.

82. Which of the following test results is considered the most sensitive test for diagnosing exercise-induced bronchospasm in athletes?

   A. A decrease of FEV1 by 10% in a field-exercise challenge test
   B. A drop of FEV1 of 10% from baseline in an eucapnic voluntary hyperventilation test
   C. A decrease of 20% of FEV1 from baseline on a methacholine challenge test
   D. An elevation of exhaled nitric oxide greater than 15 ppb
   E. All of the above

Correct Answer: E. All of the above

There are several acceptable methods used to diagnose exercise-induced bronchospasm (EIB) in athletes, including a challenge with exercise, inhaled mannitol, or eucapneic voluntary hyperventilation (EVH), followed by spirometry. The International Olympic Committee has adopted the EVH test as the preferred method, due to its relative ease of completion and excellent sensitivity. In a field-exercise challenge test, a fall from baseline of 15% is considered a positive test, but a fall of 10% is considered abnormal and indicative of airway hyperreactivity, but not definitive for EIB. A positive test with the methacholine challenge test is a drop of 20% of FEV1 from baseline, but it has not been shown to be as sensitive as EVH. An elevated exhaled nitric oxide indicates possible airway inflammation, but it has not been shown to reliably diagnose EIB.

1. Millward D, Paul S, Brown M, Porter D, Stilson M, Cohen R, et al. The diagnosis of asthma and exercise-induced bronchospasm in Division 1 athletes. Clin J Sport Med 2009;19(6):482-486.
2. Holzer K, Brukner P. Screening of athletes for exercise-induced bronchoconstriction. Clin J Sport Med 2004 May;14(3):134-138.
3. MacCallum DS, Comeau D. Exercise-induced bronchoconstriction. Curr Sports Med Rep 2016 May-Jun;15(3):128-129.

83. A 25-year-old very competitive female track athlete notes that she develops throat tightness, dyspnea, and an audible inspiratory stridor while running during competition. Her symptoms seem to resolve within five minutes of stopping her event. The symptoms seem to be very mild or be absent during her routine training and practice. What is her most likely diagnosis?

    A. Asthma
    B. Exercise-induced bronchospasm
    C. Vocal cord dysfunction
    D. Malingering

Correct Answer: C. Vocal cord dysfunction

Vocal cord dysfunction (VCD) is often misdiagnosed as exercise-induced bronchospasm (EIB). A careful history, focusing on the key differences between these two disorders, will allow differentiation in most cases. VCD often begins during exercise and resolves within five minutes of exercise cessation. The episodes typically begin and end abruptly with symptoms of throat tightness/choking. The individual responds poorly to prophylactic beta-2 agonists. The hallmark symptom is dyspnea that occurs in conjunction with an audible inspiratory stridor. The patient with EIB characteristically has symptoms beginning three to five minutes following exercise termination and peaking within 15 minutes of the end of the exercise. The abnormal breathing sensation is commonly localized to the chest and includes the following symptoms: shortness of breath, difficulty breathing, expiratory wheezing, cough (locker room cough), chest pain or tightness, decreased exercise endurance, and/or the lack of interest in or avoidance of physical activities. Prophylactic beta-2 agonists are effective. Unlike vocal cord dysfunction, in EIB, arterial blood gases and spirometry are usually abnormal. Broncho-provocation challenges are the gold standard for diagnosis for EIB.

1. Pope JS, Koenig SM. Pulmonary disorders in the training room. Clin Sports Med 2005 Jul;24(3):541-564, viii.
2. Rundell KW, Spiering BA. Inspiratory stridor in elite athletes. Chest 2003;123(2):468-474.
3. Fallon KE. Upper airway obstruction masquerading as exercise induced bronchospasm in an elite road cyclist. Br J Sports Med 2004;38(4):E9.

84. A 30-year-old male presents with worsening hip pain over the past six months. He points to the area of the groin as the area of maximal pain and demonstrates a "C sign." He recalls stepping funny in a pothole a few years ago while running, but no other trauma or injury. He reports pain is worst with internal rotation of the hip in yoga. He reports catching without locking. You suspect a labral tear, with possible femoral acetabular impingement (FAI). Which of the following clinical tests will be most helpful to confirm your suspected diagnosis?

   A. FABER (flexion abduction external rotation) test
   B. Impingement test (internal rotation of the hip while flexed to 90 degrees)
   C. Thomas test (flexion of the unaffected hip causing concomitant flexion of the affected hip)
   D. Ober's test

Correct Answer: B. Impingement test (internal rotation of the hip while flexed to 90 degrees)

The most common presentation of femoral acetabular impingement is groin pain that is worsened by prolonged sitting (i.e., prolonged hip flexion) and/or activity. Patients sometimes inadvertently perform the C sign to describe their pain by gripping the lateral hip, just above the greater trochanter, between the abducted thumb and index finger. On physical examination, terminal hip motion may be limited, especially with internal rotation. Pain is often elicited by the impingement sign when the hip is flexed to 90 degrees and internally rotated. The impingement sign has been shown to be present in more than 90% of patients who later have the diagnosis of FAI confirmed on x-ray or during surgery. FABER test has been used as a provocative maneuver for sacroiliac joint pathology, but can also be positive with lumbar spine pathology. The Thomas test evaluates for hip flexion contracture, while the Ober's test evaluates for tightness of the iliotibial band.

1. Ito K, Leunig M, Ganz R. Histopathologic features of the acetabular labrum in femoroacetabular impingement. Clin Orthop Relat Res 2004 Dec;(429):262-271.
2. Peters CL, Erickson JA. Treatment of femoro-acetabular impingement with surgical dislocation and debridement in young adults. J Bone Joint Surg 2006 Aug;88(8):1735-1741.
3. Murphy S, Tannast M, Kim YJ, Buly R, Millis MB. Debridement of the adult hip for femoroacetabular impingement: indication and preliminary clinical results. Clin Orthop Relat Res 2004 Dec;(429):178-181.

85. While working as the team physician for a local high school football team, you are approached by the parents of one of the junior linebackers. Recently, after his second episode of transient quadriparesis, the player had an MRI showing severe cervical spinal stenosis and cord compression. He was advised by the neurosurgical specialist to no longer play football or other contact sports. He now exhibits no neurologic signs or symptoms. Both the player and his parents voice understanding of the risk of catastrophic injury, yet desire for him to continue playing, so that he can "hopefully get a college scholarship and possibly play professionally one day." What is the best course of action to protect yourself legally if the player were to resume playing football?

   A. Have the player complete an "exculpatory waiver" or "risk release," releasing the physician and the activity sponsor from any liability
   B. Have the player and his parents complete an "exculpatory waiver" or "risk release," releasing the physician and the activity sponsor from any liability
   C. Have the player and his parents hand-write and sign a letter indicating their understanding of the risks of continued participation
   D. Complete a standard waiver indicating the risks of continued participation and have it signed by the player and his parents, and then allow the athlete to return, since both the player and the parents voiced understanding of the risks

Correct Answer: C. Have the player and his parents hand-write and sign a letter indicating their understanding of the risks of continued participation

Secondary to the goal of safety for the athlete is the goal of limiting legal risk for the physician. In situations where the athlete (and parent(s) or guardian) desires to return-to-play against medical recommendations, some legal experts recommend that the physician have the parents or guardians and the athlete write, in their own words, and in their own handwriting, a signed letter indicating their understanding of the risks of continued participation. A video recording of the parents and the athlete stating that they clearly understand both the condition and the associated risks is an alternative. Either of these options would help prove to a jury that the parents and the athlete had proper understanding of the risks that might occur with continued participation.

An "exculpatory waiver" is a "risk release" that indicates that the signer is fully informed of the inherent risk of participation against medical advice and that they assume said risk. This also serves as a promise not to sue the physician or the activity sponsor in the event of a catastrophic outcome. Unfortunately, courts have often invalidated contracts releasing physicians from liability.

Because the player in this scenario is a minor, he has limited legal capacity. Any decision made, or contract signed, would require the support of his parents or legal guardians. A signed standard waiver should be avoided, because it may use language that the athlete and his parents would not normally use, and they may not fully understand the risks involved. Voiced understanding would not be sufficient to limit legal risk for the physician in this situation.

1. American Academy of Family Physicians, American Academy of Pediatrics, American College of Sports Medicine, American Medical Society for Sports Medicine, American Orthopaedic Society for Sports Medicine, American Osteopathic Academy of Sports Medicine. Bernhardt DT, Roberts WO (eds). Preparticipation Physical Evaluation. 4th ed. Elk Grove Village, IL: American Academy of Pediatrics, 2010:23-25.
2. Mitten MJ. Team physicians and competitive athletes: allocating legal responsibility for athletic injuries. Univ Pittsbg Law Rev 1993;55(1):129-169.

86. A 35-year-old female long distance runner who is training for a marathon by running 50-70 miles per week presents with a one-month history of right anterior hip and groin pain. The pain develops after two miles of running and is alleviated by stopping. Her examination demonstrates right anterior groin tenderness to palpation over the pubic ramus, as well as pain with hopping on the affected leg. Which of the following statements is correct with regard to the diagnosis of a pubic ramus stress fracture?

   A. Men are more susceptible to pubic rami stress fractures than women
   B. A positive radionuclide bone scan definitively confirms the diagnosis of a pubic ramus stress fracture
   C. A small avulsion fracture off the inferior pubic ramus is pathognemonic of a pubic ramus stress fracture
   D. Pubic rami stress fractures are caused by the adductor and gracilus muscles pulling on the lateral aspect of the pubic ramus

Correct Answer: D. Pubic rami stress fractures are caused by the adductor and gracilus muscles pulling on the lateral aspect of the pubic ramus

Pubic rami stress fractures are relatively rare, involving only 1.25% of all stress fractures. They are more commonly seen in military recruits and female runners. An increase in the incidence of pubic rami stress fractures corresponds to the increase in female participation in marathon running. Women are more susceptible to pubic rami stress fractures than men for unknown reasons, but may be related to the different anatomical configuration of the female pelvis or differences in gait.

Although highly sensitive in the detection of stress fractures, radionuclide bone scintigraphy lacks specificity and provides poor anatomical detail. It has been reported to be falsely positive in as high as 32% of patients presenting with hip or groin pain. This is presumably due to high osteoblastic activity in the area because of high stress loads and constant remodeling. Periosteitis, adductor tendonitis, and avulsion fractures are other causes of a positive bones scan.

An MRI has both sensitivity and specificity for detecting pubic rami stress fractures, as well as those arising from the femoral neck, acetabulum, and sacrum. A fatigue fracture of traumatic etiology involving the bony attachment of the gracilis muscle to the pubic ramus is termed the gracilis syndrome. This results in an avulsion fracture of the tendinous insertion of the gracilis muscle at the anterior edge of the inferior pubic ramus. Pubic rami stress fractures differ from other sites as being caused by a response to tensile forces, rather than compressive forces. The tensile forces are produced by muscular forces of the adductor and gracilis muscles pulling on the lateral aspect of the pubic ramus during hip extension.

Radiographic evaluation with plain films has shown limited usefulness in the diagnosis of pelvic and femoral neck stress fractures. Bony changes typically lag behind onset of symptoms by two to four weeks, and 50% of patients who have stress fractures never exhibit changes on plain films. Flamingo-view plain films are useful in diagnosing osteitis pubis. These views are performed anteroposteriorly with alternating unilateral lower extremity weight-bearing. Instability of the pubic symphysis, which is characteristic of osteitis pubis, is suggested when the symphysis is widened more than 7 mm or when the top surfaces of the superior pubic rami move more than 2 mm.

1. Nelson EN, Kassarjian A, Palmer WE. MR imaging of sports-related groin pain. Magn Reson Imaging Clin N Am 2005 Nov;13(4):727-742.
2. Morelli V, Espinoza L. Groin injuries and groin pain in athletes: part 2. Prim Care 2005 Mar;32(1):185-200.
3. Wiley JJ. Traumatic osteitis pubis: the gracilis syndrome. Am J Sports Med 1983 Sep-Oct;11(5):360-363.

87. Which of the following is considered a significant risk for hamstring strain injury?

    A. Previous hamstring strain
    B. Young age (adolescent)
    C. Female gender
    D. Hamstring to quadriceps ratio of 0.6

Correct Answer: A. Previous hamstring strain

The cause of hamstring strain injury is multifactorial. In an evidence-based systematic review, several significant risk factors for hamstring strain injury were identified, including a previous history of hamstring strain injury (the most commonly reported significant risk for recurrence). In that regard, previously injured athletes were two to six times more likely to suffer subsequent strains. Increasing age is also a factor (athletes between 23 to 25 years were between 1.3 and 3.9 times more likely to suffer strains, and in increasing age groups, the risk was shown to increase by 30% annually). In addition, race can be a consideration (Black athletes were significantly more likely to suffer hamstring strains). Participation at higher levels of competition can also affect the level of risk (hamstring strain was infrequently reported in amateur sport, but prevalence was significantly greater [$p < .01$] in higher levels of competition). Female gender has not been shown to be a risk factor for hamstring strain. The hamstring-to-quadriceps ratio is used as a measure for return to play, with the goal being 0.5 to 0.6.

1. Prior M, Guerin M, Grimmer K. An evidence-based approach to hamstring strain injury: a systematic review of the literature. Sports Health 2009 Mar;1(2):154-164.
2. Mann G, Shabat S, Friedman A, Morgenstern D, Constantini N, Lowe J, et al. Hamstring injuries. Orthopedics 2007 Jul;30(7):536-540; quiz 541-542.
3. Clanton TO, Coupe KJ. Hamstring strains in athletes: diagnosis and treatment. J Am Acad Orthop Surg 1998 Jul-Aug;6(4):237-248.

88. You move to a rural area, where you are the only sports physician in town. You want to set up a relationship with the local high school to become their team physician. This high school, however, only has one athletic trainer and has never had a team physician before. They ask you what your role will be. Which of the following is a role of the team physician?

   A. Provide for appropriate education and counseling regarding nutrition, strength and conditioning, ergogenic aids, substance abuse, and other medical problems that could affect the athlete
   B. Provide medical advice for the teachers and the custodian
   C. Ask the high school athletic director to establish a chain of command for injury and illness management
   D. Dismiss the need for proper documentation and medical record keeping

Correct Answer: A. Provide for appropriate education and counseling regarding nutrition, strength and conditioning, ergogenic aids, substance abuse, and other medical problems that could affect the athlete

The role of a team physician includes providing appropriate education and counseling regarding nutrition, strength and conditioning, ergogenic aids, substance abuse, and other medical conditions that could affect the athlete. Answer B is incorrect, because it is not the role of the team physician to provide medical advice for the teachers and other school staff. Answer C is incorrect, because it is the role of the team physician and not that of the athletic director to establish a chain of command for injury and illness management. Answer D is incorrect, because it is the role of the team physician to establish proper documentation and medical recordkeeping.

1. Herring SA, Kibler WB, Putukian M. Team Physician Consensus Statement: 2013 update. Med Sci Sports Exerc 2013 Aug;45(8):1618-1622.

89. A 16-year-old cross country skier presents with her mother for management of her exercise-induced bronchospasm. She has not been diagnosed with asthma, and has been managed with an inhaled beta-2 agonist prior to exercise, along with a proper warm-up. Unfortunately, she is still experiencing chest tightness and wheezing when racing, which is affecting her participation. Her mother wants to know what else can be done. Which of the following is the next best step in management?

   A. Add an inhaled corticosteroid 15 minutes prior to exercise
   B. Add a diet high in omega-3 fatty acids
   C. Add an oral beta-2 agonist, along with methylxanthines, 15 minutes prior to exercise
   D. Add inhaled cromolyn sodium 15 minutes prior to exercise

Correct Answer: D. Add inhaled cromolyn sodium 15 minutes prior to exercise

The combination of inhaled cromolyn and a beta-2 agonist has been shown to be effective for the treatment of exercise induced bronchospasm (EIB). There is conflicting evidence about omega-3 fatty acids in the treatment of EIB. It would not be the next step in management once beta-2 agonists alone fail. Oral beta-2 agonists and methylxanthines are not effective for treatment. Inhaled corticosteroids can be helpful in managing underlying asthma if present, but should not be used as a short-acting prophylactic agent.

1. National Asthma Education and Prevention Program. Expert Panel Report 3 (EPR-3): Guidelines for the Diagnosis and Management of Asthma-Summary Report 2007. J Allergy Clin Immunol 2007 Nov;120(5 Suppl):S94-S138.
2. Parsons JP, Hallstrand TS, Mastronarde JG, Kaminsky DA, Rundell KW, Hull JH, et al. An official American Thoracic Society clinical practice guideline: exercise-induced bronchoconstriction. Am J Respir Crit Care Med 2013 May 1;187(9):1016-1027.
3. Storms WW. Asthma associated with exercise. Immunol Allergy Clin North Am 2005;25(1):31.

90. A 32-year-old female has been training for a marathon for four months. She complains of right lateral knee pain, exacerbated with running, climbing stairs, and riding a bicycle. The pain is reproducible to palpation along the lateral knee, 2 cm superior to joint line. Range of motion is pain-free and normal. There is no joint effusion. She has decreased her mileage over the last two weeks and has tried local ice application and oral anti-inflammatory medications, which have provided temporary improvement. What should be the next consideration in treatment?

A. Stop training
B. Physical therapy
C. Corticosteroid injection
D. Referral to orthopaedic surgeon

Correct Answer: B. Physical therapy

Iliotibial band syndrome is a common cause of knee pain. Repetitive knee flexion and extension results in excess friction and local inflammation of the distal iliotibial band, as it slides over lateral femoral condyle. Diagnosis is made by history and physical examination. Initial goal of treatment is reduction of inflammation using ice, anti-inflammatory medication, and activity modification. Once the acute inflammation improves, treatment should begin with a stretching program targeting the iliotibial band and hip and plantar flexors, with progression to a strengthening program focusing on the gluteus medius. This can be achieved through physical therapy. If symptoms persist, a local corticosteroid injection can be considered. For refractory cases that fail conservative treatment, referral to an orthopaedic sports surgeon for surgical release of the iliotibial band is occasionally indicated.

1. Khaund R, Flynn SH. Iliotibial band syndrome: a common source of knee pain. Am Fam Physician 2005 Apr 15;71(8):1545-1550.
2. Calmbach WL, Hutchens M. Evaluation of patients presenting with knee pain: part II. Differential diagnosis. Am Fam Physician 2003 Sep 1;68(5):917-922.

91. A fit 58-year-old male with bright red rectal bleeding and known hemorrhoids presents to your office following a rowing marathon. Which one of the following is appropriate?

    A. Treat his hemorrhoids conservatively, avoid constipation, and watch for further bleeding
    B. Ask to see him in the office for a rectal examination and guaiac assessment, and follow his case clinically if the guaiac test is negative
    C. Ask him to call the office if the bleeding recurs, otherwise, no other assessment is needed
    D. A colonoscopy should be recommended

Correct Answer: D. A colonoscopy should be recommended

The athlete has experienced rectal bleeding. A negative guaiac at this point does not change the history of rectal bleeding in this adult. Rectal bleeding in adults may indicate cancer, especially in his age group. Hemorrhoids are common. Sports can commonly exacerbate hemorrhoids. Given his age, it is important to carry a high index of suspicion for GI malignancy when evaluating GI bleeding. With a colonoscopy, you are able to either diagnose an important GI condition contributing to bleeding or allow the athlete to be reassured that he may continue his endurance activities. Exercise-induced intestinal ischemia may also produce lower gastrointestinal bleeding. Endoscopy within one to two days is required to diagnose ischemia in these cases, otherwise the visible mucosal changes diagnostic for this condition may resolve.

 1. Pfenninger JL, Zainea GG. Common anorectal conditions: part I. Symptoms and complaints. Am Fam Physician 2001 Jun 15;63(12):2391-2398.
 2. Feinman M, Haut ER. Lower gastrointestinal bleeding. Surg Clin North Am 2014 Feb;94(1):55-63. doi: 10.1016/j.suc.2013.10.005.

92. Regarding strength training in children and adolescents, which of the following is true?

   A. There is no minimal age requirement for participation in strength training, but each participant should have the maturity to accept and follow directions
   B. Strength training does not improve performance or reduce the risk of injury in children and adolescents
   C. Strength training does not increase strength in children, because they do not have enough testosterone
   D. Strength training is unsafe and stunts growth

Correct Answer: A. There is no minimal age requirement for participation in strength training, but each participant should have the maturity to accept and follow directions

There is no minimal age requirement for participation in strength training, but each participant should have the maturity to accept and follow directions (usually around seven or eight years of age). If a child is capable of participating in an organized youth sport, they are capable of participating in some form of program designed to condition the body to meet the physical demands imposed by the sport. Answer B is incorrect. Greater transfer of strength and power to motor performance can be achieved by using resistance exercises that closely simulate the actions of the specific sport. Participation in an overall conditioning program may indirectly reduce the risk or lessen the severity of sports-related injuries. Physical conditioning, including strength training, may reduce the risk of injury during normal daily physical activities. An overall conditioning program that includes strength training may help prepare unconditioned youth for the demands of sports practice and competition.

The difference between the response to strength training in children and adolescents may be related to differences in circulating androgen levels, but other factors appear to contribute. The ability of strength training to increase strength in adolescents is well established. Increases in strength in adolescents are due to the combined effects of neural adaptations and increases in muscle mass (hypertrophy). The training-induced strength gains observed in children are due to neural adaptations, rather than hypertrophy. Answer D is incorrect. With appropriate supervision, strength training may have a favorable influence on bone growth and development during childhood and adolescence. Evidence that strength training in a controlled environment affects the growth of young participants is lacking.

1. Faigenbaum AD, Myer GD. Resistance training among young athletes: safety, efficacy and injury prevention effects. Br J Sports Med 2010 Jan;44(1):56-63.
2. Myer GD, Quatman CE, Khoury J, Wall EJ, Hewett TE. Youth versus adult "weightlifting" injuries presenting to United States emergency rooms: accidental versus nonaccidental injury mechanisms. J Strength Cond Res 2009 Oct;23(7):2054-2060.
3. Vehrs PR. Physical activity and strength training in children and adolescents: an overview. UpToDate. Accessed May 28, 2015 at http://www.uptodate.com/contents/physical-activity-and-strength-training-in-children-and-adolescents-an-overview.

93. A 10-year-old male soccer player comes to the office complaining of two weeks of right knee pain. He reports the pain began after he struck the ball really hard when trying to shoot the ball. Since then, he has had persistent pain with running and kicking the ball. The pain is located at the inferior aspect of his patella. He denies any popping, swelling, or locking. His parents report that he usually will begin to limp after 30 minutes of playing soccer. He reports pain associated with running around playing in the backyard, as well as while using stairs. On examination, he has full active range of motion of both knees, with no extension lag. He is tender at the inferior pole of the patella on the right, and no effusion is present. He has pain with resisted knee extension test on the affected side. He has a mildly antalgic gait. You obtain the x-ray shown below. What is the diagnosis?

A. Patellar sleeve fracture
B. Osgood-Schlatter disease
C. Tibial tubercle avulsion fracture
D. Sinding-Larsen-Johannson syndrome
E. Patellar tendonitis

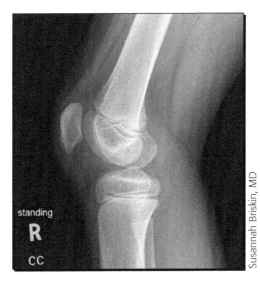

Correct Answer: D. Sinding-Larsen-Johannson syndrome

This patient falls into the classic age range for Sinding-Larsen-Johannson (SLJ), an osteochondrosis of the inferior pole of the patella. It occurs in 8- to 12-year-olds, and is more common in males than females. Typically, symptoms may occur after a single traumatic incident, or as a result of overuse. SLJ is treated conservatively with stretching, icing, and restricting painful activity if the athlete is limping. Bracing may be used occasionally, as well as formal physical therapy.

In this patient, the pain localizes to the inferior aspect of the patella, and on x-ray there is splintering in this location. Traction enthesophytes can sometimes be seen as well. He complains of overuse type pain with any activity (running, kicking, stairs) that requires him to activate the quad, and hence pull on the inferior pole of the patella. A patellar sleeve fracture can happen at this age. On the other hand, it is typically an acute injury that results in an extension lag on examination and weakness with resisted knee extension. Classic x-ray findings include a patella alta.

Osgood-Schlatter (OS) occurs in a slightly older age range, usually 11- to 15-year-olds, when rapid growth spurt is happening. OS pain localizes to the tibial tubercle apophysis. On this x-ray, the tibial tubercle apophysis has not begun to fuse yet. A tibial tubercle avulsion fracture is usually an acute injury that occurs around 15 years of age. As a rule, a sudden quad contraction (going up for a layup) induces the injury. A sudden pull or pop is felt, and the patient is unable to continue playing. An extension lag will be present on examination. X-rays should reveal the avulsion fracture. This patient is too young for patellar tendonitis. The tibial tubercle physis should be closed or nearly closed before patellar tendon pain begins at the inferior pole of the patella.

1. Stein CJ, Micheli LJ. Overuse injuries in youth sports. Phys Sportsmed 2010;38(2):102-108.
2. Atanda A Jr, Shah SA, O'Brien K. Osteochondrosis: common causes of pain in growing bones. Am Fam Physician 2011 Feb 1;83(3):285-291.
3. Valentino M, Quiligotti C, Ruggirello M. Sinding-Larsen-Johansson syndrome: a case report. J Ultrasound 2012 Jun;15(2):127-129.

Test 1 Answers, Critiques, and References

94. An 18-year-old female recreational athlete reports insidious onset of left-sided knee pain. The pain is pressure-like, behind the patella and worse with prolonged sitting. She denies any injury, swelling, locking, or instability. You find a tight lateral retinaculum on examination. Which of the examination findings suggest a tight retinaculum that can be seen with this condition?

   A. Decreased patella glide
   B. Positive single-leg squat
   C. Positive patella compression
   D. Positive patella apprehension

Correct Answer: A. Decreased patella glide

A tight lateral retinaculum decreases patellar glide, since it restricts medial motion. The patella, which can be divided into four quadrants, should glide symmetrically. Answer B is incorrect, since it relates to weak core/pillar muscles. While core weakness is associated with an increased risk of anterior knee pain, it is not diagnostic for a tight lateral retinaculum. Answer C is incorrect, since compression of the patellofemoral joint can elicit pain, due to chondral injury to the inferior patellar cartilage (chondromalacia patellae), but does not address patellar stability. Answer D is incorrect, since patellar apprehension is related to lateral patellar instability in the setting of patellar subluxation or dislocation. This test does not address the laxity or tightness of the lateral retinaculum. Conversely, it does address the integrity of the medial patellar stabilizers (medial retinaculum/medial patellofemoral ligament).

1. Hiemstra LA, Kerslakea S, Irving C. Anterior knee pain in the athlete. Clin Sports Med 2014 Jul;33(3):437-459.
2. Servi JT. Patellofemoral joint syndromes. Medscape. Accessed December 1, 2014 at http://emedicine.medscape.com/article/90286-overview.

95. A 17-year-old football player complains of a six-month chronic history of vague knee pain in the anteromedial aspect of the knee. The pain is worsened with activities such as squatting, lunging, and going up and down stairs. It is relieved with icing and ibuprofen. There is no history of trauma. His knee examination is unremarkable, with the exception of a tender cord-like structure on the anteromedial aspect of the knee that reproduces a popping sensation and pain with extension from a flexed position. A diagnosis of plica syndrome is made. Which of the following is the mainstay of treatment for this condition?

   A. Activity modification, ice, scheduled anti-inflammatories, and physical therapy
   B. Immobilization with a straight leg brace for four weeks
   C. Orthopedic surgical referral for removal
   D. Medial heel wedges and a corticosteroid injection

Correct Answer: A. Activity modification, ice, scheduled anti-inflammatories, and physical therapy

Plica syndrome is a painful condition of the knee, commonly seen in runners and other athletes. A normal plica is a thin, vascular structure that is easily deformable, often appearing as a thin, narrow veil of tissue arthroscopically. An abnormal plica is an intra-articular band of thick, fibrotic tissue which can cause pain and a popping sensation by rubbing across either the medial femoral condyle or undersurface of the patella. It is typically a diagnosis of exclusion, when other causes of anterior knee pain have been ruled out. Plica syndrome is more common in people who have some degree of genu valgum. The mainstay of treatment is activity modification, ice, anti-inflammatories, and physical therapy to address the biomechanical factors that play a role in its pathophysiology. Immobilization can be attempted after a course of the aforementioned treatment, but is not a first choice. Surgical removal can be curative, but should be considered only after other conservative measures have failed. Medial heel wedges can help in patients with genu valgum, but will not solve the issue alone. There is little evidence to support the routine use of a corticosteroid injection in a painful plica.

1. Bellary SS, Lynch G, Housman B, Esmaeili E, Gielecki J, Tubbs RS, et al. Medial plica syndrome: a review of the literature. Clin Anat 2012 May;25(4):423-428. doi: 10.1002/ca.21278.
2. Kent M, Khanduja V. Synovial plicae around the knee. Knee 2010 Mar;17(2):97-102.

96. Which of the following drugs is a risk factor for exertional rhabdomyolysis?

   A. Ibuprofen
   B. Sertraline
   C. Fexofenadine
   D. Lisinopril
   E. Methylphenidate

Correct Answer: A. Ibuprofen

NSAIDs, in general, are a risk factor for exertional rhabdomyolysis. This may be due to their direct effects on the kidney. NSAID use may also be associated with concomitant conditions, such as infection. Other drugs that are risk factors include analgesics, colchicine, statins, macrolides, anticholinergics, and recreational drugs. Fexofenadine is a non-sedating antihistamine without anticholinergic side effects. Anticholinergic antihistamines, such as diphenhydramine, would pose a risk. Lisinopril and sertraline have not been found to be risk factors. Other risk factors include sickle cell trait, eccentric exercise, heat stress, trauma, infection, and myopathy.

1. Clarkson PM. Exertional rhabdomyolysis and acute renal failure in marathon runners. Sports Med 2007;37(4-5):361-363.
2. Moeckel-Cole SA, Clarkson PM. Rhabdomyolysis in a collegiate football player. J Strength Condition Res 2009;23(4):1055-1059.
3. George M, Delgaudio A, Salhanick S. Exertional rhabdomyolysis—when should we start worrying? Case reports and literature review. Pediatr Emerg Care 2010 Nov;26(11):864-866.

97. A football player is seeing you for a knee injury sustained in a recent game. Following the game, he noticed his left knee did not feel right. He played the entire game, but the left knee felt like it was going to give out when he was running and planting. As you examine the player, you are concerned that he may have suffered an injury to his posterior cruciate ligament. Which of the following is true regarding injury to the posterior cruciate ligament (PCL) in sport?

    A. Injury to the PCL in sport is common and accounts for the majority of knee-ligament injuries in sport
    B. The pivot shift test is the most sensitive and specific physical examination test for PCL injury
    C. A common mechanism for injury to the PCL in sport is a fall onto a flexed knee
    D. Most PCL injuries require surgery in order to allow athletes to return to sport

Correct Answer: C. A common mechanism for injury to the PCL in sport is a fall onto a flexed knee

Injury to the posterior cruciate ligament in sport is relatively uncommon, making up 3% of all ligamentous knee injuries. These injuries are often subtle, and athletes may not remember a specific mechanism of injury. The most common mechanism in sport for injury to the PCL is a fall onto a flexed knee with a plantarflexed foot. The most sensitive and specific physical examination test is the posterior drawer test. Most PCL injuries are treated nonoperatively with rehabilitation, and most athletes recover well and return to sport within six weeks following treatment.

1. Margheritini F, Rihn J, Musahl V, Mariani PP, Harner C. Posterior cruciate ligament injuries in the athlete: an anatomical, biomechanical and clinical review. Sports Med 2002;32(6):393-408.
2. McCallister DR, Petrigliano FA. Diagnosis and treatment of posterior cruciate ligament injuries. Curr Sports Med Rep 2007;6(5):293-299.

98. Avulsion of the iliotibial band off of Gerdy's tubercle, biceps femoris avulsion off of the fibular head, and popliteus avulsion are most like associated with which of the following knee injuries?

    A. Posterolateral complex injury
    B. Patellar dislocation
    C. Medial collateral ligament sprain
    D. Lateral meniscal tear

Correct Answer: A. Posterolateral complex injury

Mechanical forces of hyperextension and varus stress that are associated with posterior lateral complex injuries can cause avulsion injuries involving ilitotiibial band, biceps femoris, and popliteus, along with injuries to the cruciate ligaments. The injury forces associated with patellar dislocation, medial collateral ligament sprain, and lateral mensical tear are not associated with these avulsion injuries.

   1. Vinson E, Major N, Helms C. The posterolateral corner of the knee. AJR Am J Roentgenol 2008 Feb;190(2):449-458.

99. An athlete you see in clinic had 3+ proteinuria on a routine dipstick a week ago on his checkup. As per protocol, 48 hours later, abstaining from heavy exercise, you obtain a morning urinalysis (UA) in which the protein persists at 2+. There is no personal or family history of renal disease, anemia, hypertension, or medication usage (e.g., protein powder supplements, NSAIDs, antibiotics) that would suggest organic disease. What is the best next step in your workup of proteinuria?

   A. Referral for kidney biopsy
   B. Order a CBC, renal function, including full metabolic panel, fasting blood glucose
   C. 24-hour urine collection test
   D. Refer to nephrologist
   E. CT scan with thin cuts through renal, ureter and bladder

Correct Answer: C. 24-hour urine collection test

Proteinuria is present in up to 70% of athletes after exertion and in 5% to 85% of all screening UAs. Exertional proteinuria usually ranges from 2+ to 3+ by dipstick measurement. It is caused by alterations in renal hemodynamics with vigorous exercise. These changes include an acute decrease in renal blood flow with maintenance of glomerular filtration rate, along with elevations in renin, angiotensin II, and ADH. In this case, the proteinuria has persisted, despite testing after a period of rest. The next step would be to collect a 24-hour urine specimen and quantitatively measure the amount of protein excreted. Persons younger than 30 years who excrete less than 2 gm of protein per day and have a normal creatinine clearance should be tested for orthostatic or postural proteinuria. It is characterized by increased protein excretion in the upright position, but normal protein excretion when the patient is supine.

To diagnose orthostatic proteinuria, split urine specimens are obtained for comparison. The first morning void is discarded. A 16-hour daytime specimen is obtained, with the patient performing normal activities and finishing the collection by voiding just before bedtime. An eight-hour overnight specimen is then collected. The daytime specimen typically has an increased concentration of protein, with the nighttime specimen having a normal concentration. Patients with true glomerular disease have reduced protein excretion in the supine position, but it will not return to normal (less than 50 mg per eight hours), as it will with orthostatic proteinuria. Answer A is incorrect, because a kidney biopsy would not be indicated at this time. Answer B is incorrect, given that the labs listed will not rule out orthostatic proteinuria. Answer D is incorrect, since referral to a nephrologist may be needed once benign orthostatic proteinuria could be ruled out. Answer E is incorrect, as there is no role for CT imaging at this point.

1. Burroughs KE. Renal and genitourinary problems. In: Madden CC, Putukian M, Young CC, McCarty EC (eds). Netter's Sports Medicine. Philadephia: Saunders Elsevier, 2010:215.
2. Carroll MF, Temte JL. Proteinuria in adults: a diagnostic approach. Am Fam Physician 2000 Sep 15;62(6):1333-1340.

100. A 35-year-old male long distance recreational cyclist presents to your office with acute perineal pain and numbness. He is riding his bicycle several days per week. His genitourinary and neurologic examination is normal, and you offer a diagnosis of pudendal neuropathy. What is the most appropriate initial step in management?

   A. Medical management with gabapentin
   B. Physical therapy to address pelvic stabilization
   C. Ultrasound-guided nerve block
   D. Attention to bicycle fit and saddle adjustment
   E. Permanent cessation of bicycling

Correct Answer: D. Attention to bicycle fit and saddle adjustment

Perineal and genital pain and numbness are common complaints of recreational cyclists, typically resulting from pudendal neuropathy or entrapment. Diagnosis is primarily clinical after other lumbosacral and urogenital conditions have been excluded. Short-term cessation of bicycle riding is often recommended initially. However, symptoms may recur upon resumption of cycling if bicycle fit, saddle position, and saddle type are not addressed, which is the mainstay of treatment. Neither physical therapy nor medications play a significant role in the management of pudendal neuropathy. Selective anesthetic nerve block may be attempted, but only after conservative measures have failed.

1. Martinez JM. Bicycle seat neuropathy. Medscape. Accessed July 20, 2012 at http://emedicine.medscape.com/article/91896.
2. Asplund C, Barkdull T, Weiss BD. Genitourinary problems in bicyclists. Curr Sports Med Rep 2007 Oct;6(5):333-339.

101. You are at the finish line medical aid station of a 161 km (100 miles) ultramarathon race in Arizona in April. You see a runner with fatigue and mild dizziness, who has completed the race in 25 hours. Otherwise, he is able to drink fluids. He has been urinating regularly and provides you his urine sample, which is bright yellow. His dizziness improves significantly after drinking some fluids. You decide to check him with a blood analyzer, and you note his creatinine (Cr) is 1.4 mg/dL (reference range 0.6 to 1.3 mg/dL) and his creatine kinase (CK) is 1,400 U/L (reference range 30 to 223 U/L). What would you do next?

   A. Advise him to keep drinking fluid and follow up only if he develops worsening of symptoms or his urine turns to dark color
   B. Give a bolus of 1 l of intravenous (IV) normal saline and recheck his creatinine and creatine kinase
   C. Treat his rhabdomyolysis with acidification of urine
   D. Refer him to a nearby hospital

Correct Answer: A. Advise him to keep drinking fluid and follow up only if he develops worsening of symptoms or his urine turns to dark color

Reference range for CK does not apply for athletic population after strenuous and long exercise. Significant elevation of CK level and mild elevation of Cr occur as a result of running ultramarathons. The majority of athletes with significantly elevated CK levels and mild elevation in Cr (possible mild acute kidney injury based on current criteria) are asymptomatic and require no major medical attention. Therefore, in clinical settings, asymptomatic athletes with elevated CK levels and mild Cr elevation (possible mild AKI) can be managed with oral rehydration and monitored with clinical symptoms. IV fluid is only indicated if there is a diagnosis of exertional rhabdomyolysis with the presence of myoglobinuria (sometimes presents with dark urine) and AKI or inability to adequately rehydrate the athlete with oral rehydration.

1. Magrini D, Khodaee M, San-Millán I, Hew-Butler T, Provance AJ. Serum creatine kinase elevations in ultramarathon runners at high altitude. Phys Sportsmed 2017 May;45(2):129-133.
2. Hoffman MD, Ingwerson JL, Rogers IR, Hew-Butler T, Stuempfle KJ. Increasing creatine kinase concentrations at the 161-km Western States Endurance Run. Wilderness Environ Med 2012 Mar;23(1):56-60.
3. Khodaee M, Changstrom BG, Hoffman MD. Commercialised portable intravenous fluids in sports: placing vulnerable athletes at risk. Br J Sports Med 2018 Nov 9. pii: bjsports-2018-099855. doi: 10.1136/bjsports-2018-099855. Epub ahead of print.

102. A 37-year-old female triathlete presents with left lower extremity pain. She has been training for a marathon and has been increasing the intensity of her workout over the past month. On her examination, she has point tenderness over her mid-tibia and has a positive tuning fork sign. X-ray is negative for a fracture, but you order a bone scan that reveals a posterior mid-shaft tibial stress fracture. She is adamant about being able to compete in her marathon next month. What is the best option in this situation?

    A. Instruct her to continue her training and complete her race
    B. Refer her to physical therapy
    C. Put her in a pneumatic brace, with activity modification
    D. Refer her to orthopedic surgery for immediate surgery

Correct Answer: C. Put her in a pneumatic brace, with activity modification

This patient has a posterior tibial stress fracture and may have several dynamic variables that increase her risk of these stress fractures, including increases in instantaneous and average vertical loading rates and peak tibial shock. Since these fractures are located on the compression side, most heal uneventfully with conservative treatment and have an average recovery time of approximately 12 weeks with rehabilitation and graded return to activity. While not ideal, activity modification and a pneumatic brace may allow her to complete her race in a month. She should be instructed to use pain as her guide, however, as worsening pain may require greater rest. Vitamin D could be of benefit, but a serum level should be checked prior to initiating therapy. A high-risk tibial stress fracture would be in the anterior tibia, where there could be delayed union or non-union. These stress fractures, also known as the "dreaded back line," can be career-ending for athletic professionals. Some anterior tibial stress fractures may be managed conservatively, but consultation with an orthopedic surgeon is warranted, as early fixation with an intramedullary nail may result in an expedited return to activity.

1. Black W, Hosey RG, Johnson JR, Evans-Rankin K, Rankin WM. Common upper and lower extremity fractures. In: South-Paul JE, Matheny SC, Lewis EL (eds). Current Diagnosis & Treatment: Family Medicine. 4th ed. New York: McGraw-Hill, 2015.
2. DiFiori JP, Benjamin HJ, Brenner J, Gregory A, Jayanthi N, Landry GL, et al. Overuse injuries and burnout in youth sports: a position statement from the American Medical Society for Sports Medicine. Clin J Sport Med 2014 Jan;24(1):3-20.
3. Gollotto K, Rosero E, Connor C, Hezel J. Sports rehabilitation. In: Maitin IB, Cruz E (eds). Current Diagnosis & Treatment: Physical Medicine & Rehabilitation. New York: McGraw-Hill, 2015.

103. Which of the following is the correct relationship of the median nerve of the wrist?

    A. Radial side of the palmaris longus tendon
    B. Ulnar side of the palmaris longus tendon
    C. Anterior to the palmaris longus tendon
    D. Posterior to the flexor pollicis longus tendon

Correct Answer: A. Radial side of the palmaris longus tendon

The median nerve lies radial and posterior to the palmaris longus tendon, and anterior to the flexor pollicis longus tendon. The palmaris longus tendon is an important landmark when performing an injection of the carpal tunnel/median nerve.

1. McDonagh C, Alexander M, Kane D. The role of ultrasound in the diagnosis and management of carpal tunnel syndrome: a new paradigm. Rheumatology (Oxford) 2015 Jan;54(1):9-19. doi: 10.1093/rheumatology/keu275. Epub 2014 Aug 12.
2. Wilson D, Allen GM. Imaging of the carpal tunnel. Musculoskelet Radiol 2012 Apr;16(2):137-145. doi: 10.1055/s-0032-1311765. Epub 2012 May 30.

104. Which of the following statements is true regarding nail disorders in athletes?

   A. The risk of ingrown toenails can be minimized by having the athlete wear shoes that are snug and minimize the sliding of the foot inside the shoe
   B. Trimming the toenails in a curved arc just distal to the free edge will minimize the risk of ingrown toenails
   C. Any collections of dark fluid beneath the nail bed should be immediately drained with a red-hot paper clip
   D. The persistence of a linear black band or streak running the length of the nail warrants further evaluation
   E. The treatment of choice for onychomycosis is a topical antifungal

Correct Answer: D. The persistence of a linear black band or streak running the length of the nail warrants further evaluation

The persistence of a linear black band or streak running the length of the nail may represent a melanocytic nevus or malignant melanoma of the nail matrix and warrants further evaluation. The risk of recurring ingrown toenails and subungual hematoma can minimized by having the athlete wear shoes that are at least 2 cm longer than the longest toe. Cutting the toenail straight across and with enough length to clear the nail bed minimizes the risk of ingrown toenails. While subungual hematomas may be drained by pressing a red hot paper clip end (as well as drilling with an 18-gauge needle or the use of an electrocautery unit), there is no need to do so, unless the patient is having symptoms. Asymptomatic onychomycosis does not need to be treated. However, if treatment is chosen, oral antifungals are the treatment of choice.

   1. Batts KB. Dermatology. In: O'Connor FG, Sallis RE, Wilder RP, St. Pierre P (eds). Sports Medicine: Just the Facts. New York: McGraw-Hill, 2005:149-157.

105. You see a high school football player in the training room for an injury which occurred yesterday morning. He says his dog bit him on the arm. On examination, there is a 4-cm long laceration. The wound is fairly deep, but you see no injury to bone, muscle, or tendon. There is minimal erythema or swelling. He believes he had a tetanus shot within the last five years. What is the best initial management to prevent infection?

   A. Suture the wound
   B. Use a cyanoacrylate tissue adhesive to close the wound
   C. Irrigate and debride
   D. Give a Td booster

Correct Answer: C. Irrigate and debride

The best initial management of bite wounds or lacerations is to irrigate and debride with a minimum of 200 ml of normal saline. Wound closure can be considered for lacerations that have been open less than 12 hours, but not in this case, since it has been a full day. Contraindications to laceration repair are wounds more than 12 hours old, animal bites (except on face), and puncture wounds. Tissue adhesives may be used to close certain lacerations but are also contraindicated for animal bites, puncture wounds and contaminated wounds. A tetanus booster should also be considered if this patient has had less than three doses lifetime or the last dose was over five years ago. Antibiotic treatment with amoxicillin/clavulanate should also be considered for dog and cat bites to prevent infection of Pasteurella multocida, but does not replace irrigation as the best initial management.

1. Pfenninger JL, Fowler GC. Procedures for Primary Care. 2nd ed. St. Louis, MO: Mosby, 2003:158-160.
2. Hollander JE, Singer AJ. Laceration management. Ann Emerg Med 1999 Sep;34(3):356-367.
3. Bruns TB, Worthington JM. Using tissue adhesive for wound repair: a practical guide to dermabond. Am Fam Physician 2000 Mar 1;61(5):1383-1388.

106. A 13-year-old male presents at your clinic after sustaining an injury during skiing. His lower left leg was cut by his ski blade (see image below). His past medical and social histories are unremarkable. What would be the best management option after irrigating the wound?

   A. A referral to an orthopedic surgeon
   B. Wound closure with tissue adhesives (e.g., Dermabond)
   C. Wound closure with 4/0 silk
   D. Wound closure with 4/0 monofilament nylon
   E. Wound closure with 4/0 polyglycolic acid sutures (e.g., Vicryl)

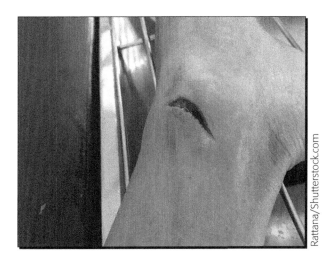

Correct Answer: D. Wound closure with 4/0 monofilament nylon

This laceration should be closed with non-absorbable sutures, such as monofilament nylon suture. Due to poor tensile strength, silk sutures should not be used. This laceration is too wide and too deep for tissue adhesives to work. There is no need to refer this patient to orthopedic surgery.

   1. Forsch RT. Essentials of skin laceration repair. Am Fam Physician 2008 Oct 15;78(8):945-951.
   2. Aukerman DF, Sebastianelli WJ, Nashelsky J. Clinical inquiries. How does tissue adhesive compare with suturing for superficial lacerations? J Fam Pract 2005 Apr;54(4):378.
   3. Brown DJ, Jaffe JE, Henson JK. Advanced laceration management. Emerg Med Clin North Am 2007 Feb;25(1):83-99.

107. In relation to exercise and its effects on the immune system, which of the following is correct?

    A. Exercising while acutely ill leads to enhancement of the immune system called the open window
    B. Moderate, short bouts of exercise can increase circulating IgA levels, leading to a decreased risk of infection
    C. High-intensity exercise stimulates T-cell proliferation, leading to a decreased risk of a viral infection
    D. Endurance running for longer than 60 minutes leads to a decreased rate of infection

Correct Answer: B. Moderate, short bouts of exercise can increase circulating IgA levels, leading to a decreased risk of infection

Regular, mild to moderate exercise in brief increments seems to enhance the immune system by increasing circulating neutrophils, lymphocytes, and salivary IgA levels. Upper respiratory tract infections were decreased 20% to 30% in moderate exercisers compared to sedentary individuals. Conversely, prolonged high-intensity exercise appears to depress the immune system. Answer A is incorrect, because exercising while acutely ill has been shown to cause temporary depressions in the immune system, leading to what is referred to as the "open window." Answer C is incorrect, because high-intensity exercise decreases T-cell proliferation, potentially leading to an increase in viral infections. Answer D is incorrect, because endurance running has been shown to increase the rate of infection. One study showed that 68% of ultramarathon runners contracted an upper respiratory tract infection after a race.

1. Dick NA, Diehl JJ. Febrile illness in the athlete. Sports Health 2014 May;6(3):225-231.

108. A 25-year-old soccer athlete presents to your office for further evaluation of bilateral lower extremity pain associated with numbness of the first web space of the foot. The onset of symptoms typically begins after running for 10 minutes and ceases immediately after rest. Which of the following describes the pathophysiology?

   A. An abnormal increase in muscle compartment pressure interferes with tissue circulation, causing temporary ischemia and neurological deficits
   B. During exercise, muscles are perfused, but neurologic structures are compressed
   C. Compartment pressures increase, due to hyperperfusion
   D. Improved muscle blood flow during exercise results in ischemic pain and impaired muscle function

Correct Answer: A. An abnormal increase in muscle compartment pressure interferes with tissue circulation, causing temporary ischemia and neurological deficits

The case describes clinical symptoms of chronic exertional compartment syndrome (CECS). Pathophysiologic changes cause an abnormal increase in muscle compartment pressure, which interferes with tissue circulation, causing ischemia and neurological deficits. These generally reverse once the athlete ceases activity. Patients with CECS generally have poor muscle perfusion in a confined and often non-compliant compartment that will, in turn, compress neurovascular structures. Compression is temporary and resolves once activity is discontinued. Compartment pressures increase, but there is usually a decrease in perfusion. Poor blood flow during exercise contributes to ischemic pain and impaired muscle function.

1. Aweid O, Del Buono A, Malliaras P, Iqbal H, Morrissey D, Maffulli N, et al. Systematic review and recommendations for intracompartmental pressure monitoring in diagnosing chronic exertional compartment syndrome of the leg. Clin J Sport Med 2012 Jul;22(4):356-370.
2. Blackman PG. A review of chronic exertional compartment syndrome in the lower leg. Med Sci Sports Exerc 2000 Mar;32(3 Suppl):S4-S10.
3. Pedowitz RA, Hargens AR, Mubarak SJ, Gershuni DH. Modified criteria for the objective diagnosis of chronic compartment syndrome of the leg. Am J Sports Med 1990 Jan-Feb;18(1):35-40.

109. A 43-year-old female runner presents to clinic with medial ankle and foot pain. She states the pain has been present for three months and is gradually getting worse. She reports no specific injury or trauma. She has taken ibuprofen, rested, and used ice, with some improvement. However, the pain recurs when she resumes running. Her examination is remarkable for tenderness and mild swelling posterior and inferior to the medial malleolus. Subtle weakness is appreciated with resisted plantarflexion and inversion of the foot compared to the opposite side. With weight-bearing inspection, a mild pes deformity is present. What is the most appropriate treatment option?

    A. Tenosynovectomy with tendon debridement
    B. Orthotic with rehabilitation exercises
    C. Corticosteroid injection within the posterior tibialis tendon sheath
    D. Rigid foot-ankle brace with activity

Correct Answer: B. Orthotic with rehabilitation exercises

The clinical vignette describes a patient with posterior tibialis tendon dysfunction (PTTD). Symptoms of PTTD are commonly present for months or years before patients decide to seek help. The history usually involves an insidious onset of pain and swelling along the course of the tendon in the medial ankle and foot. As the condition worsens, a gradual collapse of the medial longitudinal arch occurs and a hind foot valgus deformity develops. The posterior tibialis tendon can be palpated through its course along the medial side of the ankle to assess for its integrity and for the presence of any tenosynovitis, which may manifest as tenderness or swelling. The strength of the posterior tibialis tendon can be evaluated by placing the foot in slight plantarflexion and eversion. The patient is then asked to invert and further plantarflex the foot against resistance while the examiner palpates for the posterior tibialis tendon to determine its integrity and the site of maximum tenderness.

The treatment of PTTD is based on the severity and stage of the dysfunction and includes both non-operative and operative options. Most patients can be treated conservatively. Initially, a period of rest and avoidance of activities that worsen pain should be advised. Patients may switch to a lower-impact activity, such as cycling or swimming. Patients should be encouraged to use ice and can take acetaminophen or non-steroidal anti-inflammatory medication, as tolerated. Reducing flatfoot deformity, while allowing ankle movement, may minimize the progression of PTTD. For patients with associated mild pes planus, an over-the-counter orthotic may prove adequate in relieving pain related to the posterior tibialis tendon. The remaining options are incorrect, because they are utilized for more moderate to severe pathology than what is described in the question stem.

In patients with associated moderate-to-severe pes planus, a custom-fitted orthotic may be necessary. Semi-rigid, rigid, and articulated foot-ankle braces have been used in the treatment of PTTD. These can help maintain the heel in neutral alignment and support the medial longitudinal arch of the foot, reducing the stress on the posterior tibialis tendon. Operative management of PTTD is normally reserved for patients in whom a trial of at least six months of conservative therapy has failed or who have progressive symptoms and deformity.

1. Erol K, Karahan AY, Kerimoğlu Ü, Ordahan B, Tekin L, Şahin M, et al. An important cause of pes planus: the posterior tibial tendon dysfunction. Clin Pract 2015 Feb 5;5(1):699.
2. Yao K, Yang TX, Yew WP. Posterior tibialis tendon dysfunction: overview of evaluation and management. Orthopedics 2015 Jun;38(6):385-391.

110. A wrestler comes in during his preseason training with concerns of localized hair loss of his posterior scalp. This is associated with about six weeks of pruritis and an occasional burning sensation. On examination, you observe mild erythema over a well-demarcated patch of alopecia, with small black dots noted flush to the surface of the skin. He has a single, moderately tender, enlarged occipital lymph node, but otherwise his dermatological and remaining examination is negative. Which of the following is true regarding this condition?

   A. Precautions for avoiding sharing of hats and combs is not necessary
   B. Monitoring liver function is recommended, with medicines required for treatment
   C. This condition responds well to topical medication
   D. A minimum of 72 hours of treatment is required by NCAA prior to return to competition

Correct Answer: B. Monitoring liver function is recommended, with medicines required for treatment

The condition described is tinea capitis, specifically black dot tinea capitis (BDTC). Treatment for this condition needs to be systemic, given that the hair follicles are affected. Possible antifungal options include terbinafine, itraconazole, ketoconazole, or griseofulvin. With each of these, hepatotoxicity or hepatic failure is a rare but potential side effect. Thus, it is recommended to obtain baseline and repeat liver function tests every four to six weeks during treatment to monitor his condition. Answer A is incorrect, as the fungal fomites may be spread by the sharing of items, such as combs, brushes, hats, or barrettes. Answer C is incorrect, because topical antifungal medications do not penetrate the follicles well and are ineffective for treatment. Answer D is incorrect, given that the NCAA states that a minimum of two weeks of systemic therapy is required for tinea capitis (for tinea corporis, the antifungal treatment may be topical and only 72 hours of treatment is required).

1. Wilson EK, Deweber K, Berry JW, Wilckens JH. Cutaneous infections in wrestlers. Sports Health 2013 Sep;5(5):423-437.
2. Bannerman E, Stevenson JH. Dermatology issues in sports. Curr Sports Med Rep 2017 Jul-Aug;16(4):219-220.

111. While in the athletic training room on a Tuesday, you are asked to see a 17-year-old high school wrestler with a rash on his arm. On examination, there are two raised, scaly, ring-shaped lesions, with irregular erythematous borders on the volar aspect of his left arm (see image). He asks if he can wrestle in the upcoming regional championships the coming Saturday. In addition to recommending an appropriate occlusive covering on the affected site, what would you advise him?

    A. May compete without further restriction
    B. May compete if he has a minimum of 72 hours of treatment with an oral antiviral
    C. May compete if he has a minimum of 120 hours of treatment with an oral antifungal
    D. May compete if he has a minimum of 72 hours of treatment with a topical or oral antifungal

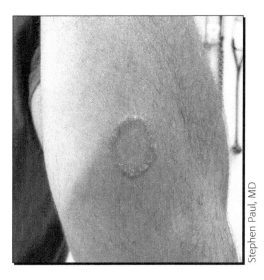

Correct Answer: D. May compete if he has a minimum of 72 hours of treatment with a topical or oral antifungal

Tinea corporis (ringworm) presents as a circular or ring-shaped, scaly, raised plaque, with irregular erythematous borders, often with central clearing. It commonly occurs in athletes secondary to direct contact transmission, and is spread via fomites in the athletic environment. The head, neck, and upper extremities are most commonly affected. Treatment with antifungal medications may be topical or oral, and continuation of treatment has been recommended for one week after clinical resolution. Extensive or multiple superficial lesions respond best to oral therapy. Suppression and prophylaxis doses that have been successful include fluconazole (100 to 200 mg once weekly) or itraconazole (400 mg every other week) for recurrent infections. Return to play guidelines for athletes with tinea corporis outline a minimum of 72 hours of topical or oral antifungal treatment, as well as appropriate occlusive covering of the affected site either until resolution or until the athlete is disqualified from participation.

1. Likness LP. Common dermatologic infections in athletes and return-to-play guidelines. J Am Osteopath Assoc 2011 Jun;111(6):373-379.
2. Bannerman E, Stevenson JH. Dermatology issues in sports. Curr Sports Med Rep 2017 Jul-Aug;16(4):219-220.
3. Zinder SM, Basler RSW, Foley J, Scarlata C, Vasily DB. National Athletic Trainers' Association position statement: skin diseases. J Athl Train 2010 Jul-Aug;45(4):411-428.

112. A 15-year-old male lacrosse player presents with a three-month history of left shin pain. He was diagnosed with a stress fracture and has been wearing a fracture boot for six weeks without improvement. The pain, which is worse at night, is relieved by ibuprofen. His imaging is below. What is the most appropriate next step?

   A. Strict non-weight-bearing
   B. Continue the fracture boot for six weeks
   C. Radiofrequency ablation
   D. Bone scan

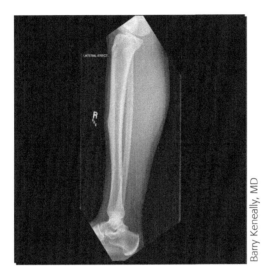

Correct Answer: C. Radiofrequency ablation

This patient has an osteoid osteoma. This is a benign tumor, which typically causes pain in teenagers and young adults that is worse at night and is often relieved by NSAIDs. The imaging shown is typical with a central nidus surrounded by sclerosis and edema. Treatment of choice is radiofrequency ablation, which is curative.

1. Athwal P, Stock H. Osteoid osteoma, a pictorial review. Conn Med 2014 Apr;78(4):233-235.
2. Boscainos PJ, Cousins GR, Kulshreshtha R, Oliver TB, Papagelopoulos PJ. Osteoid osteoma. Orthopedics 2013 Oct 1;36(10):792-800.

113. During knee flexion, the primary restraints to medial and lateral translation of the patella change. When the knee is in 30 to 60 degrees of flexion, what is the primary restraint?

   A. Vastus medialis oblique (VMO)
   B. Medial patellofemoral ligament (MPFL)
   C. Femoral trochlear groove
   D. Lateral retinaculum

Correct Answer: C. Femoral trochlear groove

From 0 to 30 degrees of flexion, the primary restraint is the MPFL. This ligament attaches from the medial patella to the medial femoral condyle. Secondary restraints are VMO and lateral retinaculum. From 30 to 90 degrees of flexion, the patella has entered the trochlear groove, which is the primary restraint. Contact from the patella moves from inferior to superior poles of the patella. At 90 degrees, the patellar tendon contacts the trochlear groove and begins to absorb some of the compressive forces.

1. Sherman SL, Plackis AC, Nuelle CW. Patellofemoral anatomy and biomechanics. Clin Sports Med 2014 Jul;33(3):389-401.
2. Koh JL, Stewart C. Patellar instability. Clin Sports Med 2014 Jul;33(3):461-476. doi: 10.1016/j.csm.2014.03.011. Epub 2014 May 29.

114. Which of the following nerves innervates the skin of the first dorsal web space of the foot?

    A. Sural nerve
    B. Saphenous nerve
    C. Lateral plantar nerve
    D. Deep peroneal nerve

Correct Answer: D. Deep peroneal nerve

The saphenous nerve supplies skin on medial side pf the foot, and the sural nerve supplies the lateral foot. The continuation of superficial peroneal nerve supplies the dorsum of the foot, except for the first dorsal web space, which is innervated by the deep peroneal nerve on the plantar surface. The lateral plantar nerve supplies the lateral one-fourth, and the medial plantar nerve supplies the medial three-fourths.

1. Crafts RC (ed). A Textbook of Human Anatomy. 2nd ed. New York: John Wiley & Sons, 1979:407.

115. A 17-year-old high school wrestler with a prior history of herpes skin outbreaks presents to you with a "typical outbreak" for him—a vesicular rash, with some surrounding erythema to his left anterior chest. There is no evidence of drainage or axillary lymphadenopathy. His examination is otherwise normal. He is hoping to compete tomorrow. Which is the most appropriate choice for treatment and return-to-play recommendations?

A. Begin acyclovir, hold him from wrestling or other contact sports, and reevaluate in five days
B. Cover the area with a sterile dressing, and allow the patient to participate tomorrow
C. Begin acyclovir, hold from wrestling for two days
D. Begin acyclovir, cover the area, and allow the patient to participate tomorrow

Correct Answer: A. Begin acyclovir, hold him from wrestling or other contact sports, and reevaluate in five days

Herpes simplex virus (HSV) is a common communicable condition in athletes, especially wrestlers. Current guidelines for return to play for recurrent HSV outbreaks are: (1) treatment with antiviral for 120 hours prior to participation, (2) blisters must be dry, with a firm adherent crust at the time of competition, and (3) no areas of active infection should be covered to allow participation. The guidelines are similar for initial outbreaks with the addition of: (4) no new blisters or vesicles for 72 hours prior to participation, and (5) no systemic symptoms (fever, malaise, etc.). Answers B, C, and D are incorrect due to the aforementioned guidelines. Reevaluation after 120 hours of treatment to assess for new or active lesions is indicated prior to allowing the athlete to return to wrestling.

1. Klossner D. 2012-13 NCAA Sports Medicine Handbook. 23rd ed. Indianapolis, IN: NCAA, 2012:60-64.
2. Zinder SM, Basler RS, Foley J, Scarlata C, Vasily DB. National Athletic Trainers' Association position statement: skin diseases. J Athl Train 2010 Jul-Aug;45(4):411-428.
3. Adams B. New strategies for the diagnosis, treatment, and prevention of herpes simplex in contact sports. Curr Sports Med Rep 2004 Oct;3(5):277-283.

116. A Division I wrestler comes in for evaluation of a non-itchy skin breakout on his trunk. He states that he is feeling well, without fever, malaise, or other systemic symptoms. Within a 1 cm region, there are three small, firm, shiny, dome-shaped papules, each approximately 3 mm in size. On closer examination, these lesions have a shallow indentation and sit on a non-erythematous base (see image). He has a tournament in six days and wants to compete. According to NCAA regulations, which option for management will give him the best chance for participating?

   A. Acyclovir 800 mg orally twice daily for five days, and no new lesions for 72 hours prior to competition
   B. Mupirocin 2% ointment applied three times daily, without new lesions for 48 hours prior to competition
   C. Terbinafine 250 mg orally daily for at least 72 hours prior to competition
   D. Curettage and cover the area with a gas-permeable membrane with tape

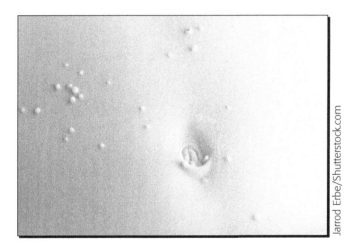

Correct Answer: D. Curettage and cover the area with a gas-permeable membrane with tape

The skin lesion described is molluscum contagiosum, a member of the poxvirus family. This virus is spread by direct skin-to-skin contact. The infection is characterized by firm, dome-shaped papules on the skin, often 2 to 5 mm in diameter. The surface is shiny and pink, with a central umbilication. Treatment methods vary including curettage, cryotherapy, podophyllotoxin, cantharidin, imiquimod, potassium hydroxide, salicylic acid, and topical retinoids. Strong evidence is lacking for any single method. NCAA regulations state that the lesions, if localized, can be covered with a gas-permeable membrane with tape, otherwise, the lesions must be curetted or removed. Answer A is incorrect, because this regimen of acyclovir is the treatment for recurrent herpes gladiatorum. Answer B is incorrect, given that topical Mupirocin 2% is the treatment of choice for areas of limited impetigo. Answer C is incorrect, because this terbinafine regimen is for treatment of tinea capitis.

1. Wilson EK, Deweber K, Berry JW, Wilckens JH. Cutaneous infections in wrestlers. Sports Health 2013 Sep;5(5):423-437.
2. Parsons JT. 2014-15 NCAA Sports Medicine Handbook. 25th ed. Indianapolis, IN: NCAA, 2014. Accessed June 29, 2015 at https://www.ncaapublications.com/p-4374-2014-15-ncaa-sports-medicine-handbook.aspx.
3. Isaacs SN. Molluscum contagiosum. UpToDate. Accessed June 29, 2015 at http://www.uptodate.com/contents/molluscum-contagiosum?.

117. A 38-year-old female presents to your clinic with foot pain that began six weeks ago. She is an avid runner, but states that she has not made any changes to her training program or changed her shoes or running surface recently. She describes the pain as a burning sensation that radiates to her toes. What is the most common location for the lesion causing her pain?

   A. Between the second and third metatarsals
   B. Between the third and fourth metatarsals
   C. Between the fourth and fifth metatarsals
   D. Between the first and second metatarsals

Correct Answer: B. Between the third and fourth metatarsals

This clinical vignette describes a Morton's neuroma, a non-neoplastic, perineural, fibrous proliferation involving a plantar digital nerve. These lesions are most commonly found between the third and fourth metatarsals, followed by the second and third metatarsal space. These lesions can be seen on MRI and ultrasound. The presence of a lesion should be correlated with clinical findings because lesions smaller than 5 mm may not be clinically relevant.

   1. Thomson CE, Gibson JN, Martin D. Interventions for the treatment of Morton's neuroma. Cochrane Database Syst Rev 2004;(3):CD003118.
   2. Richardson DR, Dean EM. The recurrent Morton neuroma: what now? Foot Ankle Clin 2014 Sep;19(3):437-449.

118. You are providing skin checks at your high school's wrestling tournament. Upon close inspection, you notice that one wrestler has a scabbed-over lesion, with a small amount of discharge (see image below). He appears surprised, stating that he did not notice the lesion until just now. What would be your recommendations?

   A. He is allowed to participate today, as long as the lesion remains covered
   B. He is not allowed to participate until the lesion is dry, he has no new skin lesions for 48 hours, and he has completed 48 hours of directed antibiotics
   C. He is not allowed to participate until the lesion is dry, he has no new skin lesions for 24 hours, and he has completed 24 hours of directed antibiotics
   D. He is not allowed to participate until the lesion is dry, he has no new skin lesions for 48 hours, and he has completed 72 hours of directed antibiotics

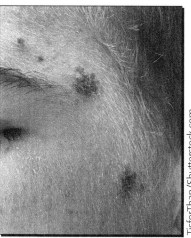

Correct Answer: D. He is not allowed to participate until the lesion is dry, he has no new skin lesions for 48 hours, and he has completed 72 hours of directed antibiotics

This wrestler likely has a bacterial skin infection. Given the skin-to-skin contact required in his sport, specific guidelines must be used to allow this athlete to return to sport. Requirements for his return include: all lesions must be scabbed over with no oozing or discharge, no new skin lesions for at least 48 hours, and completion of 72 hours of directed antibiotics. If new lesions continue to develop or drain after 72 hours, you should consider MRSA, and you must then have 10 days of treatment. Active infections may not be covered for competition. Answers A, B, and C are incorrect, because only Answer D meets these requirements.

1. Zinder SM, Basler RSW, Foley J, Scarlata C, Vasily DB. National Athletic Trainers' Association position statement: skin diseases. J Athl Train 2010 Jul-Aug;45(4):411-428.
2. Likness LP. Common dermatologic infections in athletes and return-to-play guidelines. J Am Osteopath Assoc 2011;111(6):373-379.

119. Which of following is a true statement with respect to adolescent idiopathic scoliosis?

   A. The less ossification there is at the iliac apophysis, the greater the potential for curve progression
   B. Tanner-Whitehouse methods of assessment use the epiphyses of the small bones in the foot to stage skeletal maturity
   C. The Risser grade is a measure of vertebral apophyseal fusion
   D. The majority of idiopathic scoliosis cases have a curvature that is convex to the left side

Correct Answer: A. The less ossification there is at the iliac apophysis, the greater the potential for curve progression

The lower the Risser score, the more potential for progression of curvature and for growth. The Risser score reflects the amount of fusion at the iliac apophysis. The Tanner-Whitehouse methods of calculating the digital skeletal age utilize the distal radius and ulna, as well as the small bones of the wrist. Most adolescent idiopathic scoliosis (AIS) cases (85% to 90%) are convex to the right. If the convexity is to the left, there is increased association with other pathology.

1. Horne JP, Flannery R, Usman S. Adolescent idiopathic scoliosis: diagnosis and management. Am Fam Phys 2014 Feb 1;89(3):193-198.
2. Sanders JO, Khoury JG, Kishan S, Browne RH, Mooney JF 3rd, Arnold KD, et al. Predicting scoliosis progression from skeletal maturity: a simplified classification during adolescence. J Bone Joint Surg Am 2008 Mar;90(3):540-553. doi: 10.2106/JBJS.G.00004.

120. You have been treating a 36-year-old male runner for chronic recalcitrant right plantar fasciitis for several months. His pain has been consistently located at the plantar aspect of the calcaneus around the medial calcaneal tuberosity, without other bony tenderness, and worsens from the morning throughout the day while walking for his job. He denies numbness or paresthesias and has 5/5 strength in his foot, although he notes occasional discomfort when flexing or abducting his toes. He has had only limited response to treatments, including rest, night splinting, direct and indirect fascial massage and flexibility, oral medications, and a trial of booting and orthotics. Ultrasound imaging two months prior demonstrated a calcaneal osteophyte at the insertion of the plantar fascia and a mild thickening of the fascia itself, without evidence of degeneration. Due to his pain, limitations, and the chronicity of the problem, you decide to obtain an MRI. What would you expect to find on the MRI?

    A. Rupture of the plantar fascia
    B. Edema within the abductor digiti minimi
    C. Calcaneal stress fracture
    D. Tenosynovitis of the flexor digitorum longus

Correct Answer: B. Edema within the abductor digiti minimi

This patient has a history, examination, and imaging findings that are suggestive of plantar fasciitis. However, he has lacked significant improvement, despite a prolonged period of multiple appropriate conservative measures. As such, consideration of an expanded differential is needed. Baxter's (inferior calcaneal) neuropathy, which may be responsible for up to 20% of cases of heel pain, either can be almost indistinguishable from plantar fasciitis, or can exist concomitantly with it. There are some additional indications in this instance that suggest this as the diagnosis: progressive pain throughout the day, whereas plantar fasciitis is usually worse in the mornings and evenings; discomfort with toe flexion/abduction (Baxter's nerve innervates the abductor digiti minimi and variably innervates the flexor digitorum brevis and quadratus plantae); and the presence of an enthesophyte, which may increase the risk of entrapment. There is nothing in the history or examination to suggest rupture in the interval since the ultrasound was performed. Accordingly, Answer A is incorrect. Because calcaneal stress fractures typically result in more severe and diffuse pain throughout the calcaneus, rather than focal pain at the medial tuberosity, Answer C is unlikely. While pain from an injury to the flexor digitorum longus may be provoked by toe flexion, pain is typically located at the medial malleolus. Furthermore, injury to this tendon is relatively uncommon.

1. Porter DA, Schon LC. Baxter's The Foot and Ankle in Sport. 2nd ed. Philadelphia: Mosby Elsevier, 2008:226-240.

121. A 20-year-old college football player sustained an ankle injury in the first quarter of a game while being tackled. You evaluate him at halftime. He is able to partially bear weight on his injured ankle. He recalls his ankle being in a dorsiflexed position while sustaining an eversion injury. Which of the following would most likely suggest a syndesmotic ankle injury?

   A. Pain to palpation over the anterior talofibular ligament
   B. Pain along the anterior ankle when an external rotation force is placed on the ankle with the proximal leg stabilized and the ankle dorsiflexed
   C. Pain along the mid-calf level, with compression of the proximal fibula and tibia
   D. Decreased range of motion with plantarflexion

Correct Answer: B. Pain along the anterior ankle when an external rotation force is placed on the ankle with the proximal leg stabilized and the ankle dorsiflexed

Answer B describes a positive external rotation test (see image below) The ankle mortice is loaded and externally rotated, with an abnormal causing higher ankle pain. Although there is limited evidence-based literature regarding diagnostic accuracy and reliability of this test, a systematic review showed the external rotation test to have the highest inter-rater reliability. Answer A is incorrect, because it describes an inversion lateral ankle sprain. Answer C is incorrect, because it describes a negative squeeze test. A positive squeeze test causes pain at the syndesmosis. Answer D is incorrect, because limited plantarflexion is a very nonspecific sign and can be caused by many conditions.

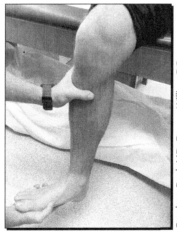

Stephen Paul, MD, Darren Willius, DO, Arie DeGrio, MD

1. Kellett JJ. The clinical features of ankle syndesmosis injuries: a general review. Clin J Sport Med 2011 Nov;21(6):524-529.
2. Sman AD, Hiller CE, Refshauge KM. Diagnostic accuracy of clinical tests for diagnosis of ankle syndesmosis injury: a systematic review. Br J Sports Med 2013 Jul;47(10):620-628.
3. Williams GN, Jones MH, Amendola A. Syndesmotic ankle sprains in athletes. Am J Sports Med 2007 Jul;35(7):1197-1207.

122. Which of the following is true concerning iron deficiency anemia?
    A. Males are more commonly affected than females
    B. Risk factors include chronic illness, heavy menstrual blood loss, and obesity
    C. Athletic performance is never affected by iron deficiency anemia
    D. Ferritin levels remain normal until the late stages of iron deficiency anemia

Correct Answer: B. Risk factors include chronic illness, heavy menstrual blood loss, and obesity

Iron deficiency anemia is the most common true anemia in athletes. Females are more commonly affected than males. Adolescent risk factors include chronic illness, heavy menstrual blood loss, obesity, and malnourishment. Athletic performance, as well as cognitive function, can be impaired in adolescents with iron deficiency anemia. Ferritin levels are abnormal in the early stages of the disease.

1. Dewoolkar A, Patel ND. Iron deficiency and iron deficiency anemia in adolescent athletes: a systematic review. Int J Child Health Hum Dev 2014;7(1):11-19.
2. Camaschella C. Iron-deficiency anemia. N Engl J Med 2015 May 7;372(19):1832-1843.

123. Which is the most common associated findings in athletic pseudo-anemia due to exercise?

   A. Normal hemoglobin; low MCV; low ferritin
   B. Low hemoglobin; normal MCV; normal/low ferritin
   C. Low hemoglobin; low MCV; elevated/normal ferritin
   D. Low hemoglobin; high MCV; normal/low ferritin

Correct Answer: B. Low hemoglobin; normal MCV; normal/low ferritin

Answer A describes iron-deficient anemia, with a normal (or low) hemoglobin, low MCV and MCHC (mean corpuscular hemoglobin concentration), and low ferritin (hypochromic, microcytic anemia). Answer C describes a mild Thalassemia pattern of low hemoglobin, low MCV, and elevated (or normal) ferritin. Answer D describes a pattern commonly seen with foot-strike hemolysis, which presents with low hemoglobin, high MCV, and normal (or low) ferritin.

Athletic pseudo (dilutional) anemia describes a pattern often seen in high-performing athletes, in whom the exercise ultimately is a reversible plasma-builder. With exercise, there is initially a hemoconcentration and up to 10% to 20% decrease in plasma volume, due to sweat, increased mean arterial pressure, and osmotic pressure, due to lactic acid, which in net moves fluid from blood to tissue. The body response is to kick in the renin/aldosterone/vasopressin system, which increases salt, albumin, and water to the blood, causing plasma increase. This plasma increase actually increases cardiac output and oxygen delivery. One of the results is "anemia," due to diluted values of hemoglobin and possibly low amounts of ferritin in the plasma, without affecting red blood cell mass.

1. Eichner ER. Anemia in athletes, news on iron therapy, and community care during marathons. Curr Sports Med Rep 2018;17(1):2-3.
2. Eichner ER. Sports anemia, iron supplements and blood doping. Med Sci Sports Exerc 1992;24(9 Suppl):S315-S318.
3. Mairbaurl H. Red blood cells in sports: effects of exercise and training on oxygen supply by red blood cells. Front Physiol 2013 Nov 12;4:332.
4. Kong WN, Gao G, Chang YZ. Hepcidin and sports anemia. Cell Biosci 2014;4(19):1-11.

124. A 14-year-old soccer player kicked the soccer ball during an abrupt pass and felt intense pain in the anterior groin. She was unable to return to play. Which of the following supports the diagnosis of a pelvic avulsion fracture at the origin of the rectus femoris?

   A. Pain at the pubic tubercle
   B. Pain at the anterior margin of the iliac crest
   C. Pain at the anterior superior iliac spine
   D. Pain at the anterior inferior iliac spine

Correct Answer: D. Pain at the anterior inferior iliac spine

The rectus femoris originates from the anterior inferior iliac spine. Apophyseal avulsion fractures are usually acute, and the displaced fragment may be bony or cartilaginous. The mechanism of injury is typically from a violent muscle contraction that occurs across an open apophysis. Sudden onset of pain, swelling, and weakness are the usual symptoms of an apophyseal avulsion fracture. Answer A is incorrect, because pain at the pubic tubercle is more likely from an injury to the adductor muscle group. Answer B is incorrect, because iliac crest avulsion fractures usually occur with the sudden contraction of the abdominal muscles that are opposed by simultaneous contraction of the gluteus medius and tensor fascia latae. This may result from activities such as excessive arm swing and trunk rotation while running, or a sudden change in direction. Answer C is incorrect, because anterior superior iliac spine avulsion (ASIS) occurs during sudden contraction of the sartorius when the hip is extended with the knee flexed.

1. Jawetz ST, Shah PH, Potter HG. Imaging of physeal injury: overuse. Sports Health 2015 Mar;7(2):142-153.
2. Kjellin I, Stadnick ME, Awh MH. Orthopaedic magnetic resonance imaging challenge: apophyseal avulsions at the pelvis. Sports Health 2010 May;2(3):247-251.
3. Moore D. Rectus femoris. Ortho Bullets. Accessed July 6, 2015 at http://www.orthobullets.com/anatomy/10057/rectus-femoris.

125. A 15-year-old female swimmer presents to your office with a complaint of mild neck stiffness for the last week. She has a past medical history significant for polyarticular juvenile idiopathic arthritis (JIA), which she has had since she was eight years old. It primarily involves the joints in her hands. She has been stable on her disease-modifying antirheumatic drugs prescribed by her rheumatologist. On examination, she is noted to have mild decreased extension of her cervical spine, but no tenderness, however. Given her past medical history, x-rays of her cervical spine are ordered. What is the most likely finding to be seen on these x-rays?

   A. Cervical spine fusion
   B. Normal x-rays
   C. Spinal stenosis
   D. Spondylolysis

Correct Answer: A. Cervical spine fusion

Cervical spine fusion is common in children with JIA and usually appears after the disease has been present for months to years. This complication is not an uncommon finding in children who had disease onset in their first decade of life. Targeted and earlier treatment has led to a decrease in this complication. However, decreased neck extension, even if asymptomatic, is usually a sign that they have arthritis. This can lead to subluxation of C2 on C3. Cervical spine fusion may also occur. Spinal stenosis is a narrowing of the spinal canal which may lead to neurological symptoms and deficits. Spondylolysis refers to a defect in the pars interarticulars of the lumbar spine (or very rarely thoracic spine), due to either a stress fracture or degenerative changes.

1. Kimura Y. Systemic juvenile idiopathic arthritis: clinical manifestations and diagnosis. UpToDate. Accessed June 20, 2015 at www.uptodate.com.
2. DeWitt EM, Kimura Y, Beukelman T, Nigrovic PA, Onel K, Prahalad S, et al. Consensus treatment plans for new-onset systemic juvenile idiopathic arthritis. Arthritis Care Res (Hoboken) 2012 Jul;64(7):1001-1010. doi: 10.1002/acr.21625.
3. Sherry D. Juvenile idiopathic arthritis. Medscape. Accessed June 20, 2015 at http://emedicine.medscape.com/article/1007276-clinical#b6.

126. A 12-year-old male baseball pitcher presents to the office with four months of experiencing mild intermittent right groin pain. Pain is an intermittent dull ache. It does not prevent him from playing. He reports running normally in his baseball games with no pain. He is the star pitcher on his all-star team, and is looking forward to playing this weekend. On physical examination, he has mild pain with right hip internal rotation, but full ROM compared to the left. Bilateral hip strength is normal. Gait is normal. Hamstrings and iliopsoas hip flexors are tight (the popliteal angle is 45 degrees bilaterally), a positive Thomas test. X-rays of the pelvis are shown below. What is the next best step in management?

   A. Follow up with orthopedic surgeon next week, do not play in baseball game this weekend
   B. Okay to play in baseball game, follow up if the pain increases
   C. Immediate transport to the emergency department for urgent orthopedic evaluation
   D. Referral to physical therapy to stretch hamstrings and hip flexors and follow up in four weeks

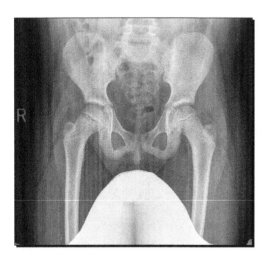
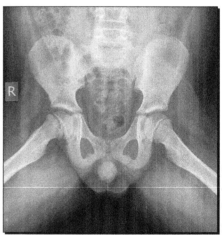

Correct Answer: C. Immediate transport to the emergency department for urgent orthopedic evaluation

X-rays demonstrate a mild right slipped capital femoral epiphysis. The Klein's line, drawn along the superior femoral neck does not intersect with the epiphysis. While apparently stable in the office, this condition is an orthopedic emergency. A slide into the base, or a minor fall, could cause further slip. The blood supply to the epiphysis is tenuous, and further injury could lead to avascular necrosis of the epiphysis. If this happens, there are no good treatment options, and long-term outcomes are uniformly poor. As such, he needs to be transported to the emergency department immediately. Treatment includes non-weight-bearing (wheelchair) and surgical pinning of the epiphysis within 24 hours. Waiting to see the orthopedic surgeon the following week is not appropriate. Physical therapy, while appropriate to address his muscle inflexibility, does not address the slip.

1. Novais EN, Millis MB. Slipped capital femoral epiphysis: prevalence, pathogenesis, and natural history. Clin Orthop Relat Res 2012 Dec;470(12):3432-3438.
2. Peck DM, Voss LM, Voss TT. Slipped capital femoral epiphysis: diagnosis and management. Am Fam Physician 2017 Jun 15;95(12):779-784.
3. Millis MB, Novais EN. In situ fixation for slipped capital femoral epiphysis: perspectives in 2011. J Bone Joint Surg Am 2011 May;93 Suppl 2:46-51.

127. A 20-year-old male collegiate wrestler sustained a severe injury to his right shoulder during the beginning of the wrestling season. He required surgery, which precluded him from participating for the remainder of the season. He is in his junior year, and during his sophomore year, achieved multiple All-Conference honors, and was anticipated to be an All-American this year. His surgery and initial post-operative rehabilitation with his athletic trainer were unremarkable, and he was progressing on schedule. About six weeks post-op, he began having more trouble with rehabilitation. He described severe pain, became very angry, and stopped reporting for therapy, stating that it was painful and a waste of his time. A thorough evaluation by his surgeon did not reveal any structural reason for the setback. His friends disclose that he has been more withdrawn and angry, and he also recently broke up with his long-time girlfriend. Which is the best approach in the continuing treatment of this athlete?

   A. Modify the rehabilitation protocol to allow for more recovery time and a less strenuous schedule
   B. Prescribe pain medications to be taken prior to rehabilitation, as the pain response is most likely responsible for his set-back
   C. Report to the coaches that he is now non-compliant with his treatment
   D. Discuss and implement techniques for coping with stress and other psychological factors involved in injury recovery of a high-level athlete
   E. Recommend transfer of care to a physical therapist instead of the athletic trainer currently overseeing the rehabilitation process

Correct Answer: D. Discuss and implement techniques for coping with stress and other psychological factors involved in injury recovery of a high-level athlete

Dealing with an injured athlete can present unique challenges during the recovery process. While ruling out reinjury or another organic cause of the pain is absolutely necessary, when none is found, it is important to consider the psychological aspects of recovery. Due to high levels of stress, pressure to return quickly, and a possibility of never returning to sport, athletes can exhibit a wide spectrum of responses. While not all athletes display negative responses, many will exhibit denial, anxiety, depression, anger, resentment, frustration, hopelessness, loneliness, worthlessness, impatience, and overall negativity. There are several variables that may help predict a negative response, and the aforementioned athlete has several of them: he is male, participates at a very high level, had a very serious injury requiring surgery, and the injury occurred during the season, requiring him to miss time. Studies have shown that implementing healthy coping mechanisms, including becoming more informed and involved about the injury and recovery process, have helped to increase treatment adherence rates and reduce stress. The other options in the question either serve to mask the problem or add more stress to the situation.

1. Bauman J. Returning to play: the mind does matter. Clin J Sport Med 2005 Nov;15(6):432-435.
2. Herring SA, Kibler WB, Putukian M. The team physician and the return-to-play decision: a consensus statement-2012 update. Med Sci Sports Exerc 2012 Dec;44(12):2446-2448.

128. A 13-year-old male presents with medial anterior knee pain. No knee effusion is present. X-rays and subsequent MRI show an osteochondritis dissecans lesion in the medial femoral condyle. The articular cartilage surface is intact; the physis is open. What is the next most appropriate step in management?

   A. Physical therapy
   B. Activity modification
   C. Surgery
   D. Observation

Correct Answer: B. Activity modification

The aforementioned vignette describes a stable, newly diagnosed osteochondritis dissecans (OCD) lesion in a skeletally immature individual. The primary initial treatment of a stable OCD lesion in a skeletally immature athlete is non-operative. Consensus therapeutic modalities include protected weight-bearing with crutches, locked hinged knee-bracing, unloader bracing, and simple activity modification—the avoidance of sports and impact activities. Answer B is correct, because it is the only treatment that reduces loading of the affected area. In the vignette, the lesion by MRI criteria is stable, so surgery in not initially indicated. Surgery in a skeletally immature individual is only indicated for unstable or detached lesions or lesions that have failed conservative therapy. Since initial therapy should be something that decreases knee-loading forces, Answers A and D are not appropriate.

1. Yang JS, Bogunovic L, Wright RW. Nonoperative treatment of osteochondritis dissecans of the knee. Clin Sports Med 2014 Apr;33(2):295-304.
2. Wall EJ, Vourazeris J, Myer GD, Emery KH, Divine JG, Nick TG, et al. The healing potential of stable juvenile osteochondritis dissecans knee lesions. J Bone Joint Surg Am 2008 Dec; 90(12):2655-2664.
3. Chambers HG, Shea KG, Anderson AF, Jojo Brunelle TJ, Carey JL, Ganley TJ, et al. American Academy of Orthopaedic Surgeons clinical practice guideline on: the diagnosis and treatment of osteochondritis dissecans. J Bone Joint Surg Am 2012 Jul 18;94(14):1322-1324.

129. Although exercise is one form of treatment for a patient with depression, patients seen in a sports medicine setting are not immune to depression. Second-generation antidepressants, most commonly selective serotonin reuptake inhibitors (SSRIs), have been shown to be an effective pharmacological treatment for depression. How soon should a patient be seen after initiating pharmacological treatment for depression?

    A. Within one month
    B. Within two weeks
    C. Within two months
    D. In six months

Correct Answer: B. Within two weeks

Patients with depression are at increased risk for suicide (up to 20 times normal), and starting an antidepressant does not decrease this risk. In fact, there is evidence of an increase in suicidal thoughts and behavior after starting antidepressant medication in some populations. This increased risk for suicide attempts is greater in the first one to two months of medication treatment. Therefore, as described in a recent clinical guidelines statement from the American College of Physicians and given a "strong recommendation" with "moderate quality evidence," patient monitoring should begin one to two weeks after medication is initiated.

1. Adams SM, Miller KE, Zylstra RG. Pharmacologic management of adult depression. Am Fam Physician 2008 Mar 15;77(6):785-792.
2. Qaseem A, Snow V, Denberg TD, Forciea MA, Owens DK, Clinical Efficacy Assessment Subcommittee of American College of Physicians. Using second-generation antidepressants to treat depressive disorders: a clinical practice guideline from the American College of Physicians. Ann Intern Med 2008 Nov 18;149(10):725-733.

130. A 10-year-old right-handed baseball catcher presents to your clinic with one month of right shoulder pain. He denies any acute injury to the shoulder, but states that his pain has progressively worsened over time. When the pain first started, he was pitching and decided to switch to catcher to give his arm a rest. Despite this switch, his pain has persisted. He has noticed that his accuracy and velocity have significantly decreased in the last week. Your examination is unhelpful, since the patient has diffuse tenderness to palpation, and most of your special tests are positive. You are suspicious the patient has Little League shoulder, so you order shoulder x-rays. You review the films with the patient and his father. Given that the x-rays look within normal limits, the father insists that he continues to play baseball and take ibuprofen for pain before his games. What is your next best step?

    A. Provide the family reassurance and encourage them to monitor their son for any worsening pain
    B. Consider obtaining an x-ray of the contralateral shoulder to compare with his opposite shoulder
    C. Allow the patient to continue to play catcher, but not pitch, while you start him in physical therapy
    D. Order an MRI to help definitively diagnose the etiology of the patient's pain

Correct Answer: B. Consider obtaining an x-ray of the contralateral shoulder to compare with his opposite shoulder

Despite his normal appearing x-rays, with this history, the clinician must maintain a high index of suspicion for proximal humeral epiphysiolysis (Little League shoulder). This condition is caused by the repetitive loading of the humerus due to the torque and distraction forces required during throwing. This can cause microtrauma to the proximal humeral physis, which is substantially weaker than the surrounding bone. Despite going from pitcher to catcher, this position will likely also require a large quantity of high velocity throws. It has been shown that increased shoulder pain is associated with throwing more than 800 pitches per season, with the cumulative effect, rather than the acute effect, being the most important factor.

The diagnosis of proximal humeral epiphysiolysis is made by radiograph. Widening of the proximal humeral physis is seen best on plain radiograph, using an anteroposterior view of the shoulder, with the arm in external rotation. Because this widening may be found in asymptomatic pitchers, clinical correlation with symptoms is important. Widening may be subtle, and comparative radiographs of the opposite shoulder should be performed to help confirm the diagnosis. Answer A is incorrect: since you suspect a stress injury, you should not allow him to continue to throw. Answer C is incorrect, because the initial treatment for this injury is rest, followed by physical therapy to address biomechanical flaws and a throwing progression prior to return to sport. Answer D is incorrect, because this diagnosis typically does not require an MRI.

1. Sciascia A, Kibler BLW. The pediatric overhead athlete: what is the real problem? Clin J Sport Med 2006;16(6):471-477.

131. The following question refers to noninstitutionalized or community-dwelling asymptomatic adults without a history of fractures (defined as not residing in an assisted living facility, nursing home, or other institutional care setting). Which of the following statements is true regarding vitamin D supplementation and the prevention of fractures in adults without a history of osteoporosis or vitamin D deficiency?

   A. In community-dwelling, postmenopausal women, daily supplementation with ≤ 400 IU of vitamin D3 and ≤ 1,000 mg of calcium has no net benefit for the primary prevention of fractures
   B. There is clear evidence regarding the benefit of daily vitamin D and calcium supplementation for the primary prevention of fractures
   C. There are no risks to supplementation with 400 IU or less of vitamin D3 and 1,000 mg or less of calcium
   D. The USPSTF recommends against vitamin D supplementation to prevent falls in community-dwelling adults 65 years or older who are at increased risk of falls because of a history of recent falls or vitamin D deficiency

Correct Answer: A. In community-dwelling, postmenopausal women, daily supplementation with ≤ 400 IU of vitamin D3 and ≤ 1,000 mg of calcium has no net benefit for the primary prevention of fractures

The USPSTF concludes that in postmenopausal women, there is adequate evidence that daily supplementation with 400 IU of vitamin D3, combined with 1,000 mg of calcium, has no effect on the incidence of fractures. However, there is inadequate evidence about the effect of higher doses of combined vitamin D and calcium supplementation on fracture incidence in noninstitutionalized postmenopausal women. Answer B is incorrect. In premenopausal women and in men, there is inadequate evidence to determine the effect of combined vitamin D and calcium supplementation on the incidence of fractures. Answer C is incorrect. Although the magnitude of harm has been assessed as small, evidence indicates that supplementation with 400 IU or less of vitamin D3 and 1,000 mg or less of calcium increases the incidence of renal stones. In the Women's Health Initiative, a statistically increased incidence of renal stones occurred in women taking supplemental vitamin D and calcium. One woman was diagnosed with a urinary tract stone for every 273 women who received supplementation over a seven-year follow-up period. Answer D is incorrect. The USPSTF recommends vitamin D supplementation (the median dose of vitamin D in available studies was 800 IU) to prevent falls in community-dwelling adults 65 years or older who are at increased risk of falls because of a history of recent falls or vitamin D deficiency (B recommendation).

1. U.S. Preventive Services Task Force. Vitamin D and calcium supplementation to prevent fractures in adults: recommendation statement. Am Fam Physician 2014 Jun 1;89(11):896C-896E.
2. Bordelon P, Ghetu MV, Langan RC. Recognition and management of vitamin D deficiency. Am Fam Physician 2009 Oct 15;80(8):841-846.

132. A high school freshman who normally throws the shotput comes into the office with severe hip pain that started yesterday after he ran the relay the last day of track practice. He was sprinting around the track and felt a pop. He fell and could not continue running. He was helped off the field and given crutches by his athletic trainer. On examination, he is tender to palpation over the anterior hip and cannot flex the hip more than a few degrees without significant pain. An x-ray in the office confirms your diagnosis of minimally displaced avulsion of the anterior superior iliac spine. Which of the following is true?

   A. The ASIS avulsion is due to a forceful contraction of the rectus femoris during sprinting
   B. You call your orthopedic partner to get the patient on the schedule for ORIF
   C. This type of injury may be misdiagnosed as an acute muscle strain
   D. CT scan is never helpful if this is a possible diagnosis on your differential

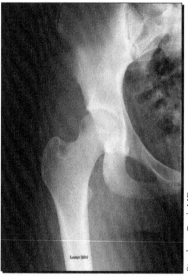

Correct Answer: C. This type of injury may be misdiagnosed as an acute muscle strain

ASIS avulsion fractures cause hip flexor weakness and may be confused with a hip flexor strain. ASIS avulsion fracture are common in athletes with open physes. The avulsion usually occurs with forceful contraction of the sartorius and tensor fascia lata. The rectus femoris originates on the anterior inferior iliac spine, not the anterior superior iliac spine. Conservative treatment with rest and protected weight-bearing is usually successful. Only for large displacements greater than 3 cm is surgery needed. CT can be helpful if the avulsed fragment is very small and not seen on x-ray.

   1. Moeller JL. Pelvic and hip apophyseal avulsion injuries in young athletes. Curr Sports Med Rep 2003 Apr;2(2):110-115.

133. What is the medication class that is least likely to cause hypoglycemia during exercise?

   A. Insulin
   B. Sulfonylurea
   C. Biguanide
   D. Meglitinides

Correct Answer: C. Biguanide

Biguanides decrease hepatic gluconeogenesis and increase glucose utilization in peripheral tissues. It is not associated with exercise-associated hypoglycemia. Individuals with type 2 diabetes are likely to develop hypoglycemia during exercise when using insulin or insulin secretagogues because of inappropriately high levels of insulin in relationship to the athlete's blood sugar. Meglitinides and sulfonylureas are insulin secretagogues which stimulate pancreatic beta cell insulin production. The ADA recommends supplementing with 15 g of carbohydrate prior to exercise if the measured blood sugar is less than or equal to 100 mg/dL.

1. Colberg SR, Sigal RJ, Fernhall B, Regensteiner JG, Blissmer BJ, Rubin RR, et al. Exercise and type 2 diabetes: the American College of Sports Medicine and the American Diabetes Association: joint position statement executive summary. Diabetes Care 2010 Dec;33(12):2692-2696.
2. Harris GD, White RD. Diabetes in the competitive athlete. Curr Sports Med Rep 2012 Nov-Dec;11(6):309-315.
3. Shugart C, Jackson J, Fields KB. Diabetes in sports. Sports Health 2010;2(1):29-38.

134. A thin 26-year-old male runner presents to your office with complaints of intermittent numbness and tingling over the distal anterolateral right lower leg and the dorsum of the right foot, sparing the web space of the first two toes. Upon further questioning, he reveals that this only occurs when he sits with his right leg crossed over his left leg, with the lateral aspect of his right lower leg approximately 8 cm proximal to the lateral malleolus resting on his contralateral knee. It will resolve quickly over a period of about 15 seconds after uncrossing the leg. The patient obliges to demonstrate his seated position. You examine him after he is able to recreate his symptoms and note normal vascular status on examination. You advise the patient to stop sitting in this fashion. Compressing of what structure is likely leading to his complaints?

   A. Deep peroneal nerve
   B. Popliteal artery
   C. Superficial peroneal nerve
   D. Lateral tibialis nerve
   E. L5 nerve root

Correct Answer: C. Superficial peroneal nerve

The superficial peroneal nerve provides motor innervation of the lateral compartment of the lower leg, including the peroneus brevis and peroneus longus. More pertinent to the question, it provides sensory innervation to the anterolateral distal one third of the leg and the dorsum of the foot, with the exception of the web space of the first and second toe, which is innervated by the deep peroneal nerve. The nerve, as its name suggests, becomes very superficial, existing in the subcutaneous tissue after piercing the fascia on average 10 to 12 cm proximal to the lateral malleolus. The patient, when sitting in this fashion, is able to compress his superficial peroneal nerve after it pierces the fascia, resulting in his symptoms. The deep peroneal nerve is incorrect, as it provides sensory to the webspace between the 1st and 2nd toes. Answer B is incorrect, as there is no evidence of diminished pulses on examination or any other evidence of popliteal artery entrapment. Answer D is incorrect, because the lateral tibialis nerve does not exist. Answer E, the L5 nerve root, is also incorrect, because while the dermatomal innervation does include part of the dorsum of the foot and anterolateral lower leg, the great toe and lesser toe are both innervated by different nerve roots.

   1. Harrast MA, Finnoff JT. Sports Medicine: Study Guide and Review for Boards. New York: Demos Medical Publishing, 2012.
   2. Madden CC, Putukian M, Young CC, McCarty EC (eds). Netter's Sports Medicine. Philadelphia: Saunders Elsevier, 2010.

135. A 20-year-old athlete comes into your office for counseling on a recent diagnosis of HIV. The athlete wants to know if they can exercise and take part in their sport. What advice do you give the athlete?

   A. Per NCAA regulations, an athlete with HIV cannot participate in an NCAA sport
   B. It is detrimental to the health of an HIV positive patient to participate in exercise
   C. Research has shown a high risk of HIV transmission in athletics
   D. HIV transmission risk is rare in athletics, although the risk is higher in some contact sports

Correct Answer: D. HIV transmission risk is rare in athletics, although the risk is higher in some contact sports

The risk of transmission is rare in athletics. Sports such as mixed martial arts, boxing, and professional wrestling have high risks, due to the amount of blood during the event. Answer A is incorrect. The NCAA does not limit participate based on HIV status. Answer B is incorrect. Research shows that there is no detrimental effect on the health of a person with HIV. Research is still being conducted to see if it has a positive effect. Answer C is incorrect. There has not been a documented case of HIV transmission in athletics. There was a question of transmission during a soccer collision, but sexual contacts could not be ruled out.

1. Clem KL, Borchers JR. HIV and the athlete. Clin Sports Med 2007 Jul;26(3):413-424.
2. Klossner D. Blood-borne pathogens and intercollegiate athletics. In: 2010-11 NCAA Sports Medicine Handbook. 21st ed. Indianapolis, IN: NCAA, 2010;66-71.
3. Luke A, d'Hemecourt P. Prevention of infectious diseases in athletes. Clin Sports Med 2007 Jul;26(3):321-344.

136. A seven-year-old male presents to your clinic with a limp of recent onset. He has difficulty localizing his pain, but states that he did fall off his skateboard onto his knee several weeks ago, before his limp started. He has no other medical problems or significant past medical history. He denies any recent illnesses or fevers. He plays soccer and baseball. His parents have noticed the limp has gotten worse, but it has not kept him from playing his sports. What is your next course of action?

    A. Full knee examination with four view knee x-rays, and if negative, prescribe RICE and close observation
    B. AP and frog-leg lateral hip x-rays to rule-out slipped capital femoral epiphysis
    C. Complete examination of bilateral lower extremities with x-rays, and if negative, consider advanced imaging of the hip
    D. Provide parental reassurance, given that this is likely benign growing pains that should respond to rest, ice, and NSAIDs

Correct Answer: C. Complete examination of bilateral lower extremities with x-rays, and if negative, consider advanced imaging of the hip

Given this patient's age and presentation, the clinician should have a high index of suspicion for Legg-Calve-Perthes disease (LCP). It is very important to know that initial radiographs can often be normal, such that serial examinations and/or a bone scan or MRI may be required to make the diagnosis. LCP is a syndrome of idiopathic osteonecrosis (avascular necrosis) of the hip. While it can present as isolated hip pain, the presentation will commonly include a limp as well. This can be either acute or insidious in onset. The normal age range is between 3 and 12 years, with peak incidence at five to seven years of age. LCP can be bilateral in 10% to 20% of patients. The male-to-female ratio is 4:1 or greater, and African-Americans are rarely affected. Answer A is incorrect, because even though it is important to examine the knee given his history, this is a distractor, and the clinician should not forget to consider hip pathology if nothing is found on knee examination. Answer B is incorrect, because slipped capital femoral epiphysis is unlikely in this age group and is seen more commonly in an obese, African-American adolescent. Answer D is incorrect, because growing pains should not cause a child to have a progressively worsening limp.

1. Nigrovic PA. Overview of hip pain in childhood. UpToDate. Accessed June 30, 2015 at http://www.uptodate.com/contents/overview-of-hip-pain-in-childhood?source=machine Learning&search=legg+calve+perthes+disease+children&selectedTitle=1%7E21§ionRank=1&anchor=H14#H14.
2. Clark MC. Overview of the causes of limp in children. UpToDate. Accessed June 30, 2015 at http://www.uptodate.com/contents/overview-of-the-causes-of-limp-in-children?source=search_result&search=leg+calve+perthes&selectedTitle=2%7E150.
3. Waite BL, Krabak BJ. Examination and treatment of pediatric injuries of the hip and pelvis. Phys Med Rehabil Clin N Am 2008 May;19(2):305-318.

137. A 42-year-old female runner presents to your office with a history of multiple joint pain that started after her return from a sprint distance triathlon in Michigan last week. Her diet, menses, and weight are unchanged. She runs about 15 to 20 miles a week, swims three miles per week and bikes 50 miles a week. She denies a fever but does feel flushed at times. No history of autoimmune condition exists in her family. Her vitals are normal and afebrile. She has a normal musculoskeletal examination outside of subjective joint soreness. Her skin examination shows the following lesion on her abdomen. The test you would most likely order FIRST is?

   A. CBC
   B. Lyme titre
   C. ANA
   D. Rheumatoid factor
   E. Thyroid stimulating hormone

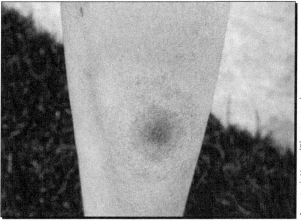

Correct Answer: B. Lyme titre

Image is of erythema chronicum migrans, which is pathognomonic for Lyme's disease. In addition, the patient traveled to a Lyme-endemic area.

1. Meyerhoff JO, Steele RW, Zaidman GW. Lyme disease. Emedicine. Accessed July 13, 2014 at http://www.emedicine.com/MED/topic1346.htm.
2. DuPrey KM. Lyme disease in athletes. Curr Sports Med Rep 2015 Jan;14(1):51-55.

138. A 20-year-old military recruit comes into your office, concerned because he has been unable to run more than three or four miles at a time, due to right-leg cramping and weakness. Eventually, the pain forces him to stop running. He has been following a training plan without major increases in distance or time. His past medical history includes a left wrist fracture from a fall as a teenager. On examination, his pelvis is symmetrical without rashes. Palpation reveals moderate tightness of both lower extremities, right more than left. His distal pulses are 2+, with normal capillary refill. Reflex testing reveals 2+ patellar and Achilles reflexes. Proprioception is normal, although you find diminished sensation on the plantar surface of his right foot. With strength testing, he is weak with toe flexion and foot inversion. Compartment syndrome is highest on your differential, but which compartment is most likely affected?

   A. Anterior compartment
   B. Deep posterior compartment
   C. Lateral compartment
   D. Superficial posterior compartment

Correct Answer: B. Deep posterior compartment

This is a case of exertional compartment syndrome of the lower leg. In this condition, the fascia is noncompliant to the expansion of muscle volume from exercise, resulting in a reversible ischemic environment that causes pain and weakness in the affected limb. An understanding of the anatomy of the leg helps to narrow in on the compartment involved. There are four compartments of the lower leg: anterior, lateral, superficial posterior, and deep posterior. The deep posterior compartment includes the tibialis posterior muscle, the long toe flexors, the peroneal artery, and the tibial nerve. When pressures are increased, toe flexion and foot inversion can be affected, and there is numbness on the plantar aspect of the foot.

Answer A is incorrect, because the anterior compartment contains the tibialis anterior muscle, the deep peroneal nerve, and the long toe extensors. Increased pressures would cause loss of sensation to the first web space and weakness with foot dorsiflexion. Answer C is incorrect, given that the lateral compartment contains the peroneus longus and brevis muscles and the superficial peroneal nerve. If affected, this would result in decreased strength of foot eversion and diminished sensation to the dorsal foot. Answer D is incorrect, as the superficial posterior compartment is comprised of the gastrocnemius and soleus muscles, as well as the distal segment of the sural nerve. If pressures were increased in this compartment, examination would reveal numbness of the lateral foot and distal calf.

1. Glorioso JE Jr, Wilckens JH. Compartment syndrome testing. In: Wilder RP, O'Connor FG, Magrum EM (eds). Running Medicine. 2nd ed. Monterey, CA: Healthy Learning, 2014:213-220.
2. Roscoe D, Roberts AJ, Hulse D. Intramuscular compartment pressure measurement in chronic exertional compartment syndrome: new and improved diagnostic criteria. Am J Sports Med 2015 Feb;43(2):392-398.
3. Tucker AK. Chronic exertional compartment syndrome of the leg. Curr Rev Musculoskelet Med 2010 Oct;3(1-4):32-37.

139. A six-year-old male presents to his primary care physician, complaining of a one-month history of progressive heel pain that worsens with increased activity. The pain initially started when he began kindergarten, which his parents attributed to him being more active. They have now noticed that he will intermittently limp and is complaining of pain on a daily basis. They have not tried any interventions up to this point in time. His mom feels that he limits his daytime activities to minimize pain. On examination, he is tender to palpation overlying the calcaneus primarily on the plantar and medial and lateral aspects. He has full range of motion of ankles, knees, and hips, without effusion. There is no swelling, and he is not limping in clinic today. He hops on his toes on the involved side to minimize pain. What do you do next?

   A. Recommend conservative treatment for Sever's disease
   B. Obtain radiographs of the patient's foot to evaluate for the appearance of the calcaneal apophysis
   C. Provide mom with reassurance that this is most likely related to his growth and will spontaneously resolve
   D. Recommend further evaluation with a CBC, ESR, CRP, and rheumatologic panel

Correct Answer: B. Obtain radiographs of the patient's foot to evaluate for the appearance of the calcaneal apophysis

Although this child's history sounds like Sever's disease, he is on the younger end of the spectrum for this diagnosis. Sever's disease can generally be treated conservatively with ice, anti-inflammatory medications, stretching, heel cups, and activity modification. Most children presenting with heel pain from Sever's disease are 9 to 11 years of age. Some children as young as five or six may have started to ossify their calcaneal apophysis and may have heel pain from Sever's syndrome, but radiographs should be obtained in younger children to determine if there is presence of the apophysis. If there is no apophysis seen on radiographs, further evaluation should be performed, generally starting with laboratory workup for alternative causes of heel pain in young children such as rheumatologic conditions, infection, and malignancies (tumor/leukemia). This more invasive workup can be avoided if there is evidence of ossification of the calcaneal apophysis on radiographs.

Growing pains, also known as nocturnal pains of childhood are a diagnosis of exclusion. There are several features in this child's history that make this diagnosis less likely, including his complaints of pain during the day, his intermittent limp, and the modification of his activities. The typical presentation of growing pains is pain that only occurs in the evening and at night, which can wake children from sleep. It does not interfere with daily activities, and it is worse on days that children are more active. Furthermore, it responds to anti-inflammatory medications, massage, and heat, and typically occurs in long bones and is non-focal. The focal nature of this child's pain also rules against growing pains.

1. Sawyer JR, Kapoor M. The limping child: a systematic approach to diagnosis. Am Fam Physician 2009 Feb;79(3):215-224.
2. Heel pain and Sever's disease. HealthyChildren.org. Accessed July 3, 2014 at http://www.healthychildren.org/English/health-issues/injuries-emergencies/sports-injuries/Pages/Heel-Pain-and-Severs-Disease.aspx.

140. What are the four structures that form the boundaries of the quadrilateral space?

   A. Teres major, teres minor, humeral neck, long head of triceps
   B. Infraspinatus, teres minor, humeral neck, long head of triceps
   C. Infraspinatus, teres minor, deltoid, long head of the triceps
   D. Teres major, teres minor, deltoid, humeral neck

Correct Answer: A. Teres major, teres minor, humeral neck, long head of triceps

The four structures composing the borders of the quadrilateral (quadrangular) space are the teres major, teres minor, humeral neck, and long head of the triceps. Answers B-D all contain anatomical structures that do not help form borders for the quadrilateral space.

1. Neal SL, Fields KB. Peripheral nerve entrapment and injury in the upper extremity. Am Fam Physician 2010;81(2):147.
2. Hoskins WT, Pollard HP, McDonald AJ. Quadrilateral space syndrome: a case study and review of the literature. Br J Sports Med 2005;39(2):e9.

141. A 16-year-old female basketball player presents with five days of sore throat, fever, and fatigue. On examination, she has an exudative pharyngitis and posterior cervical lymphadenopathy. She has a playoff game scheduled for the weekend and wants to know if she can play. Which of the following tests is the most sensitive and could assist with the decision to allow the athlete to play?

   A. Heterophile antibody-latex agglutination (Monospot)
   B. Viral capsid antigen IgM
   C. Viral capsid antigen IgG
   D. Complete blood count

Correct Answer: B. Viral capsid antigen IgM

This athlete has the classic presentation for mononucleosis. Hoagland's criteria for the diagnosis of mononucleosis includes fever, pharyngitis, lymphadenopathy, and positive serologic markers. Mononucleosis commonly has a lymphocytosis of 50% or more and atypical lymphocytes of 10% or more. The CBC is less sensitive than either the heterophile or viral capsid antigen antibody tests. Up to 25% of heterophile antibody tests ordered in the first week of symptoms will be negative. By the second week, the false negative rate decreases to 5% to 10%, and by the third week of illness, it is down to 5%. If a more sensitive diagnostic test is needed, then a viral capsid antigen IgM can be ordered. It has a sensitivity of 97% (95% to 99%) and a specificity of 94% (89% to 99%). Antibodies to viral capsid antigen are produced slightly earlier than the heterophile antibody and are more specific for EBV infection. The viral capsid IgG antibody persists past the stage of acute infection and signals the development of immunity.

1. Ebell MH. Epstein-Barr virus infectious mononucleosis. Am Fam Physician 2004 Oct 1;70(7):1279-1287.
2. Lennon P, Crotty M, Fenton JE. Infectious mononucleosis. BMJ 2015 Apr 21;350:h1825. doi: 10.1136/bmj.h1825.

142. A 16-year-old male competitive soccer player competes year-round on his high school team, as well as on a club team. He has displayed declining performance, despite intense training. His grades have been worsening at school over the past six months, and he has recently lost weight, due to decreased appetite. He reports achy calf muscles. What is the best diagnosis?

   A. Iron deficiency
   B. Overtraining
   C. Mononucleosis
   D. Somatization

Correct Answer: B. Overtraining

Overtraining syndrome is a decline in performance, despite aggressive training. It is believed to be due to a multitude of factors, such as constant high levels of physiologic or emotional stress, fatigue, immune system failure, and insufficient recovery time. Athletes who experience burnout may go through a variety of psychological, physiological, or hormonal changes. Iron deficiency and mononucleosis typically do not cause decline in academic performance. Somatization is characterized by a multitude of physical complaints that last for years.

1. Brenner JS, American Academy of Pediatrics Council on Sports Medicine and Fitness. Overuse injuries, overtraining, and burnout in child and adolescent athletes. Pediatrics 2007 Jun;119(6):1242-1245.
2. Cardoos N. Overtraining syndrome. Curr Sports Med Rep 2015 May-Jun;14(3):157-158. doi: 10.1249/JSR.0000000000000145.

143. Which of the following muscle fiber types is most often associated with early fatigue and predominately anaerobic activity?

A. Type I
B. Type Iα
C. Type IIA
D. Type IIB

Correct Answer: D. Type IIB

Type I fibers are slow-twitch, oxidative (aerobic), high mitochondria content and blood supply, and slow to fatigue. Type Iα is not a muscle fiber type. Type IIA fibers are fast-twitch, oxidative-glycolytic (aerobic/anaerobic), with high mitochondrial content and blood supply—not as slow to fatigue as type I, but more resistant than type IIB. This is the muscle fiber type most commonly associated with hypertrophy in resistance training. Type IIB fibers are fast-twitch, glycolytic (anaerobic), with fewer mitochondria and blood supply. They are faster to fatigue, but can produce highest force and tension.

1. Hart JM, Ingersoll CD, Kuenze CM. Weightlifting. In: O'Connor FG, Casa DJ, Davis BA, St. Pierre P, Sallis RE, Wilder RP (eds.) ACSM's Sports Medicine: A Comprehensive Review. Philadelphia: Lippincott Williams & Wilkins, 2013:741.
2. Zierath JR, Hawley JA. Skeletal muscle fiber type: influence on contractile and metabolic properties. PLoS Biol 2004 Oct;2(10):e348.

144. A 10-year-old gymnast reports acute onset right buttock pain after doing the splits. Examination reveals tenderness to palpation over the right ischium. She has difficulty actively extending the hip and increased pain with passive hip flexion. Based on the history and physical examination, what would you recommend?

    A. X-rays to evaluate for apophyseal avulsion fracture
    B. Rest for treatment of a hamstring strain
    C. Rehabilitation for treatment of piriformis syndrome
    D. Oral steroid course for treatment of a lumbar radiculopathy

Correct Answer: A. X-rays to evaluate for apophyseal avulsion fracture

This is a classic case of an ischial tuberosity apophyseal avulsion fracture. Pelvic avulsion fractures occur at the site of the apophyses, given that the apophyses are the weakest link. Apophyses are secondary ossification centers. Apophyseal avulsion fractures occur while apophyses are open and before the center is fused, primarily in children/adolescents 11 to 17 years old (though pelvic aphophyses can stay open even into the young twenties). The greatest weakness occurs at the time the apophyses appear.

There are seven main apophyses around the hip and pelvis. The apophyses are the sites of attachments for the large muscles. The apophyses and their corresponding muscle attachment are all listed as follows: 1) ischial tuberosity (hamstrings)—the most common site of avulsion; 2) anterior superior iliac spine (sartorius; tensor fasciae latae); 3) anterior inferior iliac spine (rectus femoris); 4) iliac crest (abdominal musculature); 5) lesser trochanter (iliopsoas); 6) greater trochanter (gluteus muscles); and 7) symphysis pubis (adductor longus).

In adolescents, avulsion injuries should be considered in all patients with apparent muscle strains, because underlying associated apophyseal avulsion fractures can be missed if no radiographic evaluation is done. Apophyseal avulsion fractures can occur acutely or chronically. When acute, the mechanism of avulsion is either a sudden violent forceful muscle contraction (e.g., kicking, running, jumping) or excessive passive lengthening (e.g., gymnasts/cheerleaders performing the splits). Presentation is sudden shooting pain referred to the involved apophysis, with decreased strength/loss of involved muscular function. Chronic cases occur due to traction from repetitive trauma, with ultimate displacement of the apophysis. These patients may present with more indolent symptoms and often do not recall an acute trauma, but a gradual increase in pain with activity and after activity. The physical examination clues to diagnosis of the chronic apophyseal avulsion are tenderness to palpation over the affected apophysis and increased pain, with resisted activation of the attached muscle group. When considering pelvic apophyseal avulsion, x-rays (AP and frog-leg laterals) are the primary workup modality. Bilateral films are often helpful for comparison to be certain that the finding is a true avulsion fracture and not a normal adolescent variant.

1. Paletta GA Jr, Andrish JT. Injuries about the hip and pelvis in the young athlete. Clin Sports Med 1995 Jul;14(3):591-628.

145. A 16-year-old male presents to your office for a preparticipation physical evaluation. He is a competitive high-school wrestler, and has previously missed several competitions due to herpes simplex infections. Upon further questioning, he admits to six episodes during the last year, with no episodes prior to that. His father, who is also his wrestling coach, would like to have him started on suppression therapy during the season. He is asymptomatic today. What would you recommend?

   A. No medication, until you can verify active lesions
   B. Acyclovir 400 mg five times daily during wrestling season
   C. HSV serology testing to confirm the diagnosis, and valacyclovir 1 g daily during wrestling season
   D. Griseofulvin 500 mg daily during wrestling season

Correct Answer: C. HSV serology testing to confirm the diagnosis, and valacyclovir 1 g daily during wrestling season

This athlete likely has recurrent herpes simplex infections. Prior to initiating suppression therapy, evidence indicates that HSV serology testing should be performed. Once confirmed, 1 gram daily of valacyclovir is an appropriate dose for an individual with 10 episodes per year. Answer A is an option, but may cause the athlete to miss further competitions. Because the recommended dosage of acyclovir for chronic daily suppression is 400 mg twice daily, not five times daily, Answer B in incorrect. Answer D is a treatment option for fungal skin infections, not herpes simplex.

1. Likness LP. Common dermatologic infections in athletes and return-to-play guidelines. J Am Osteopath Assoc 2011 Jun;111(6):373-379.
2. Zinder SM, Basler RSW, Foley J, Scarlata C, Vasily DB. National Athletic Trainers' Association position statement: skin diseases. J Athl Train 2010 Jul-Aug;45(4):411-428.

146. You are the physician covering a mid-summer track and field meet, conducted at a local college for middle school athletes. It is already 90 degrees Fahrenheit (32.2 degrees Celsius) at 9 o'clock in the morning, and local weather forecasts are predicting record highs with 80% humidity. You are extremely concerned for heat illness in the athletes. Which of the following is true regarding pediatric athletes?

   A. Children have a smaller body-surface-to-body-mass ratio than adults, making children more likely to gain heat from the environment
   B. Children have decreased heat production per kilogram of body mass when compared to adults, leading to slower increases in body temperature in warm weather
   C. The sweating rate in children is lower than in adults, making it harder for children to dissipate heat through sweat evaporation
   D. When dehydrated, the body temperature in children rises slower than in an adult

Correct Answer: C. The sweating rate in children is lower than in adults, making it harder for children to dissipate heat through sweat evaporation

The sweat rate in children is lower than that in adults, increasing the risk for heat illness in children, as there is decreased heat dissipation from sweat evaporation. Answer A is incorrect, because children have a larger body-surface-area-to-body-mass ratio than adults. Answer B is incorrect, because children have increased heat production per kilogram of body mass, which leads to faster increases in body temperature in warm environments. Answer D is incorrect, because the body temperature in children increases faster when dehydrated compared to adults.

1. Smolander J, Bar-Or O, Korhonen O, Ilmarinen J. Thermoregulation during rest and exercise in the cold in pre- and early pubescent boys and in young men. J Appl Physiol (1985) 1992 Apr;72(4):1589-1594.
2. Falk B. Effects of thermal stress during rest and exercise in the paediatric population. Sports Med 1998 Apr;25(4):221-240.

147. A 12-year-old male baseball pitcher presents to the office with medial elbow pain that began gradually. On examination, he is Tanner stage 2, with pain over the medial epicondyle area, mild pain with valgus stress, negative Tinel's over medial elbow. He has normal elbow and wrist strength. What is his most likely diagnosis?

    A. Medial epicondylitis
    B. Ulnar collateral ligament strain
    C. Medial epicondyle apophysitis
    D. Medial epicondyle avulsion fracture

Correct Answer: C. Medial epicondyle apophysitis

In this vignette, the patient still has an open medial epicondyle apophysis, given his age. Since the apophysis is structurally weaker than the surrounding ligaments, repetitive valgus stress from throwing will result in irritation of the apophysis, rather than causing a primary injury of the surrounding soft tissue. While avulsion fractures of the medial epicondyle occur in skeletally immature athletes, the history is usually specific for an acute event, usually with a pop felt, rather than gradual onset.

1. Wilk KE, Marina LC, Cain EL, Dugas JR, Andrews JR. Rehabilitation of the overhead athlete's elbow. Sports Health 2012 Sep;4(5):404-414.
2. Congeni J. Elbow. In: Harris SS, Anderson SJ (eds). Care of the Young Athlete. 2nd ed. Itasca, IL: American Academy of Pediatrics, 2010:343-353.

148. In a patient diagnosed with a C6 cervical radiculopathy on the right-hand side, what would you expect to find?

   A. Pain radiating from the neck to the lateral arm and the right thumb, weak biceps and wrist extensors, decreased sensation along the lateral forearm and thumb, and an altered brachioradialis reflex compared to the contralateral side
   B. Pain radiating into the shoulder and right lateral arm, decreased sensation along the right lateral arm, and an altered biceps reflex on the right side
   C. Pain in the lower neck and trapezius region, as well as a sensory deficit in a cape distribution
   D. Pain in the ulnar region of the right forearm, weakness in the right intrinsic finger muscles, and a decreased sensation on the right ulnar aspect of the forearm

Correct Answer: A. Pain radiating from the neck to the lateral arm and the right thumb, weak biceps and wrist extensors, decreased sensation along the lateral forearm and thumb, and an altered brachioradialis reflex compared to the contralateral side

A C6 nerve root radiculopathy on the right typically presents with any or all of the following: pain radiating from the neck to the lateral arm and the right thumb, a weak biceps and wrist extensors, decreased sensation along the lateral forearm and thumb, and an altered brachioradialis reflex compared to the contralateral side. Pain radiating into the shoulder and right lateral arm, decreased sensation along the right lateral arm, and an altered biceps reflex on the right side describes a C5 nerve root radiculopathy. Pain in the lower neck and trapezius region, as well as a sensory deficit in a cape distribution, describes a C4 nerve root radiculopathy. Pain in the ulnar region of the right forearm, weakness in the right intrinsic finger muscles, and a decreased sensation on the right ulnar aspect of the forearm describes a T1 nerve root radiculopathy.

1. Rhee JM, Yoon T, Riew KD. Cervical radiculopathy. J Am Acad Orthop Surg 2007;15(8):486-494.
2. Polston DW. Cervical radiculopathy. Neurol Clin 2007;25(2):373-385.

149. You are evaluating a 27-year-old recreational tennis player. She felt some searing chest wall pain on her dominant side while extending for a forehand shot three days ago. On her examination today, you notice substantial bruising along the anterior chest wall, suggesting some soft-tissue injury. You begin by palpating the pectoralis major muscle. Of the following points, which one is least helpful when trying to palpate the pectoralis major?

A. Sternum
B. Clavicle
C. Second to sixth ribs
D. Humerus
E. Coracoid process

Correct Answer: E. Coracoid process

Answers A and C are the origins of the sternal head of the pectoralis major: sternum and ribs two to six. Answer B, specifically, the medial clavicle is the origin of the clavicular head. The humerus, Answer D, is the insertion of the muscle on the intertubercular groove (outer lip). Answer E refers to the insertion of the pectoralis minor, which has its origin on the third to fifth ribs, and also inserts on the scapula.

1. Williams PL, Warwick R, Dyson M, Bannister LH (eds). Gray's Anatomy. 37th ed. Edinburgh: Churchill Livingstone, 1989;610-611.
2. Knipe H, Pacifici S. Pectoralis major. Radiopaedia. Accessed January 10, 2015 at http://radiopaedia.org/articles/pectoralis-major-1.
3. Pectoralis minor. University of Washington Department of Radiology. Accessed January 10, 2015 at http://www.rad.washington.edu/academics/academic-sections/msk/muscle-atlas/upper-body/pectoralis-minor.

150. Which of the following statements is true concerning the respiratory system during pregnancy?

    A. Tidal volume decreases
    B. Vital capacity is unchanged
    C. Minute ventilation is unchanged
    D. Reserve volumes increase

Correct Answer: B. Vital capacity is unchanged

During pregnancy, both tidal volume and minute ventilation increase, while reserve volumes decrease. As a result, the vital capacity remains unchanged.

1. Ireland ML, Nattiv A (eds). The Female Athlete. New York: Saunders, 2002:186.
2. Emans SJ, Grace E, Hoffer FA, Gundberg C, Ravnikar V, Woods ER. Estrogen deficiency in adolescents and young adults: impact on bone mineral content and effects of estrogen replacement therapy. Obstet Gynecol 1990 Oct;76(4):585-592.
3. Drinkwater BL, Nilson K, Chesnut CH 3rd, Bremner WJ, Shainholtz S, Southworth MB. Bone mineral content of amenorrheic and eumenorrheic athletes. N Engl J Med 1984 Aug 2;311(5):277-281.

151. A 21-year-old male presents to your clinic with lower back pain that began suddenly after performing a squatting exercise at the campus recreation center four weeks ago. He has been resting and taking ibuprofen, but the pain is not improving. Which examination findings support the diagnosis of an L3/L4 disc herniation?

    A. Numbness along the lateral aspect of the foot
    B. An absent patellar reflex
    C. Weakness with plantarflexion of the foot
    D. Weakness with extension of the great toe

Correct Answer: B. An absent patellar reflex

Sensory loss over the medial malleolus and weakness with ankle dorsiflexion would also indicate nerve impingement at the level of L3/L4. Answers A and C are incorrect, given that numbness in this region of the foot and weakness with plantarflexion of the ankle would indicate neurologic compromise at L5/S1. Answer D is incorrect, because weakness of the extensor hallucis longus would correspond with a herniation at L4/L5. Sensory loss would be found over the third metatarsal phalangeal joint if the L5 nerve was affected.

1. Gregory DS, Seto CK, Wortley GC, Shugart CM. Acute lumbar disk pain: navigating evaluation and treatment choices. Am Fam Physician 2008 Oct 1;78(7):835-842.
2. Lauerman W, Russo M. Thoracolumbar spine disorders in the adult. In: Miller MD, Thompson SR (eds). DeLee & Drez's Orthopaedic Sports Medicine. 4th ed. Philadelphia: Saunders Elsevier, 2015.

152. A 25-year-old male who is preparing to travel to high altitude requests a prescription for acetazolamide. He denies prior altitude illness. He has no underlying chronic disease. Which statement is true of this medication?

   A. Masks the symptoms of acute mountain sickness
   B. Causes decreased urination
   C. Will cause a dry cough and increasing dyspnea at increasing altitude
   D. Could cause paresthesias of hands, feet, and periorbital region

Correct Answer: D. Could cause paresthesias of hands, feet, and periorbital region

Acetazolamide is well accepted as a means for speeding acclimatization. It is reported to reduce the incidence and severity of acute mountain sickness, but it does not mask symptoms of acute mountain sickness. The usual recommended dose is acetazolamide 500 mg per day, starting at least one day before ascent and continued until descent has begun. Lower doses of acetazolamide, 125 mg twice daily, have been shown to be as effective as higher doses, with reportedly fewer and less severe side effects. Side effects include paresthesias of the periorbital region, hands, and feet, as well as diuresis. Another side effect is the report that fizzy drinks seem to taste flat. Acetazolamide may also improve general performance through aiding a restful night's sleep. A cough and dyspnea at high altitude are not caused by acetazolamide, but these symptoms could be related to high altitude pulmonary edema. As a result, these symptoms should not be ignored. It is important to remember that the use of acetazolamide is NOT a substitute for good knowledge of acute mountain sickness and a sensible plan for assent.

1. Luks AM, McIntosh SE, Grissom CK, Auerbach PS, Rodway GW, Schoene RB, et al. Wilderness Medical Society practice guidelines for the prevention and treatment of acute altitude illness: 2014 update. Wilderness Environ Med 2014 Dec;25(4 Suppl):S4-S14. doi: 10.1016/j.wem.2014.06.017.
2. Imray C, Wright A, Subudhi A, Roach R. Acute mountain sickness: pathophysiology, prevention, and treatment. Prog Cardiovasc Dis 2010 May-Jun;52(6):467-484. doi: 10.1016/j.pcad.2010.02.003.
3. Plant T, Aref-Adib G. Travelling to new heights: practical high altitude medicine. Br J Hosp Med (Lond) 2008 Jun;69(6):348-352.

153. A 24-year-old female patient presents to your office with right ear pain and decreased hearing. It started three days ago while she was ascending from scuba diving. She denies recent illness. She denies any discharge from the ear. Her examination shows a bloody infiltrate in the middle ear. How should this be treated?

   A. Symptomatic relief
   B. Tympanotomy
   C. Typmanostomy tube
   D. Antibiotics

Correct Answer: A. Symptomatic relief

Middle ear barotrauma will most likely resolve on its own. The patient may try symptomatic relief with medications, but will likely not have any relief with decongestants or other medications. Answers B and C are incorrect, because the blood from the middle ear will be absorbed by the body. It does not need to be drained. Answer D is incorrect, since antibiotics should only be used when the tympanic membrane has ruptured and the contents have been contaminated.

1. Azizi MH. Ear disorders in scuba divers. Int J Occup Environ Med 2011 Jan;2(1):20-26.
2. Lee Y, Ye BJ. Underwater and hyperbaric medicine as a branch of occupational and environmental medicine. Ann Occup Environ Med 2013 Dec 19;25(1):39. doi: 10.1186/2052-4374-25-39.
3. Vernick DM. Ear barotrauma. UpToDate. Accessed June 17, 2015 at http://www.uptodate.com/contents/ear-barotrauma?source=machineLearning&search=barotrauma&selectedTitle=1%7E94§ionRank=1&anchor=H6#H6.

154. Which of the following statements is true regarding innervation of the hamstring?

    A. The hamstring musculotendinous unit is solely innervated by the tibial branch of the sciatic nerve
    B. The hamstring musculotendinous unit is solely innervated by the peroneal branch of the sciatic nerve
    C. The biceps femoris is innervated by both the peroneal branch and the tibial branch of the sciatic nerve
    D. The semimembranosus is innervated by both the peroneal branch and the tibial branch of the sciatic nerve

Correct Answer: C. The biceps femoris is innervated by both the peroneal branch and the tibial branch of the sciatic nerve

The hamstring is commonly a victim of strain injury. One factor that makes the hamstring more susceptible to injury is its dual innervation. The hamstring makes forceful, but sometimes uncoordinated, contractions due to this dual innervation. The short head of the biceps femoris is innervated by the peroneal branch of the sciatic nerve. All other hamstring muscles, including the long head of the biceps femoris, are innervated by the tibial branch of the sciatic nerve.

1. Cox KD. Hamstring strain. In: Bracker MD (ed). The 5-Minute Sports Medicine Consult. 2nd ed. Philadelphia: Lippincott Williams & Wilkins, 2011:288-289.
2. Opar DA, Williams MD, Shield AJ. Hamstring strain injuries: factors that lead to injury and re-injury. Sports Med 2012 Mar 1;42(3):209-226. doi: 10.2165/11594800-000000000-00000.

155. A 15-year-old female who plays soccer presents to your clinic with a two-month history of anteromedial knee pain. She denies any injury, and her pain comes and goes. The pain is worse with the knee in flexion, and she complains of some painful popping as well. Her examination shows tenderness to palpation just medial to the patellofemoral joint, with palpation of a rope-like structure and some localized swelling to the same area. There is no joint effusion. Ligaments are intact on examination. McMurray's and Thessaly's tests are negative. What is your suspected diagnosis and what imaging would you order to confirm your diagnosis?

    A. Medial plica syndrome; MRI
    B. Medial meniscal tear; MRI
    C. Medial plica syndrome; no imaging
    D. Pes anserine bursitis; ultrasound

Correct Answer: C. Medial plica syndrome; no imaging

Medial meniscal tear is unlikely in a 15-year-old without an injury, no tenderness to palpation over the affected joint line, and negative special testing. An MRI is the appropriate test to confirm a suspected meniscal tear. Pes anserine bursitis is incorrect, due to the location of the tenderness to palpation. Furthermore, no rope-like structure is typically palpable with bursitis either. No imaging is necessary to confirm a bursitis. Medial plica syndrome is the correct diagnosis, due to location of pain, tenderness to palpation, and palpation of a rope-like structure. Painful popping and pseudo-locking can also be present. No imaging is needed to confirm or diagnose a plica syndrome.

    1. Gregory AJ. Plica syndrome. UpToDate. Accessed July 6, 2015 at https://www.uptodate.com/contents/plica-syndrome.
    2. Biedert RM, Sanchis-Alfonso V. Sources of anterior knee pain. Clin Sports Med 2002 Jul;21(3):335-347, vii.

156. A 12-year-old female soccer player presents to your sports medicine clinic with a right wrist injury. She was playing soccer yesterday, when she fell onto her right arm. After developing pain and swelling, she was taken to a local emergency room, where x-rays revealed a Salter-Harris type II fracture of the right distal radius. Which one of the following statements regarding Salter-Harris type II fracture is correct?

   A. The most common type of Salter-Harris fracture
   B. A fracture through the physis and epiphysis
   C. An intra-articular fracture at risk for chronic disability
   D. Best visualized with diagnostic ultrasound

Correct Answer: A. The most common type of Salter-Harris fracture

The Salter-Harris classification system is used to describe growth plate fractures in skeletally immature patients. A Salter-Harris type II fracture is the most common form and involves a fracture through the physis and metaphysis of a long bone. Salter-Harris type II fractures rarely cause growth disturbance and typically do not cause chronic functional disability. By definition, Salter-Harris type II fractures do not involve the joint space. If x-rays do not reveal adequate detail for treatment planning of the fracture, Salter-Harris fractures are best visualized with computed tomography (CT) or magnetic resonance imaging (MRI).

1. Moore W. Salter-Harris fracture imaging. Medscape. Accessed December 2, 2015 at http://emedicine.medscape.com/article/412956-overview.

157. What is the best treatment for an athlete with a tarsal navicular stress fracture?

    A. Minimum of four weeks of non-weight-bearing cast immobilization
    B. Minimum of six weeks of non-weight-bearing cast immobilization
    C. Weight-bearing-boot immobilization for four to six weeks, followed by rehabilitation and progression based on symptoms
    D. Surgical intervention to return the athlete to sport sooner

Correct Answer: B. Minimum of six weeks of non-weight-bearing cast immobilization

Treatment with at least six weeks of non-weight-bearing (NWB) cast immobilization, followed by gradual weight-bearing in a boot for four to six weeks, until pain free, for the treatment of navicular stress fractures will provide at least as good of a result, if not slightly better, than surgery for this injury. This specific regimen of conservative treatment can provide a 96% successful outcome, compared to 82% with surgical intervention. Answer A is incorrect as described above. This shortened period of NWB cast immobilization produced a success rate of only 77%. Answer C is incorrect, given that this regimen demonstrated the poorest outcome of the aforementioned choices, showing a success rate of 47%, with an average return to play, for those who could, of 5.7 months. Answer D is incorrect, based on the aforementioned discussion.

1. Torg JS, Moyer J, Gaughan JP, Boden BP. Management of tarsal navicular stress fractures: conservative versus surgical treatment: a meta-analysis. Am J Sports Med 2010 May;38(5):1048-1053.
2. Jones MH, Amendola AS. Navicular stress fractures. Clin Sports Med 2006 Jan;25(1):151-158.
3. Shindle MK, Endo Y, Warren RF, Lane JM, Helfet DL, Schwartz EN, et al. Stress fractures about the tibia, foot, and ankle. J Am Acad Orthop Surg 2012 Mar;20(3):167-176.

158. A collegiate distance runner has been seeing you for chronic exertional lower leg pain for over six months. She has tried a period of rest, medication, and physical therapy. Testing to date has been normal, including plain radiographs, bone scan, intra-compartmental pressure measurement, and EMG/NCS. You decide to proceed with yet another study to evaluate this young runner's leg pain. What is an important consideration in ordering your next imaging study or test?

   A. Perform the study with the foot in neutral, passive dorsiflexion, and maximum active plantarflexion
   B. Add contrast to the study for better visualization
   C. Have the patient rest for several weeks, before performing the next study
   D. Ensure the patient is fasting after midnight the day before

Correct Answer: A. Perform the study with the foot in neutral, passive dorsiflexion, and maximum active plantarflexion

A runner with chronic exertional leg pain can be difficult to diagnose. Often the initial differential includes periostitis, stress injuries/fractures, and maybe chronic exertional compartment syndrome. In this patient, you are told that she failed conservative care and had normal testing to rule out the usual differential. Additional considerations in the athlete should be nerve or arterial entrapment. Diagnosis of popliteal artery entrapment can be done through ultrasound, ankle brachial indices (ABI), or MRI/MRA, but in neutral position, these studies may be normal. Therefore, you need to remember to ask for the same images to be done with the patient in dorsiflexion and plantarflexion. In addition, having the patient as symptomatic as possible is helpful, so have her remain active. Contrast or fasting has no effect on this diagnosis.

1. Getzin A, Veigel J. Compartment syndrome, anterior. In: Bracker MD (ed). The 5-Minute Sports Medicine Consult. 2nd ed. Philadelphia: Lippincott Williams & Wilkins, 2011:88-89.
2. Sarwark JF (ed). Overuse syndromes. Essentials of Musculoskeletal Care. 4th ed. Rosemont, IL: AAOS, 2010:158-164.
3. Madden CC, Putukian M, Young CC, McCarty EC (eds). Netter's Sports Medicine. Philadelphia: Saunders Elsevier, 2010:429-437.

159. A 45-year-old ultramarathon runner presents to your office two days after his most recent ultramarathon complaining of anterior ankle pain. He reports no pain during the race, but significant anterior ankle pain starting the morning after the race. He is able to bear weight on the ankle, but has pain with walking and has not yet attempted running. There is mild swelling and no ecchymosis. On examination, there is crepitus as you palpate over a tendon closer to the medial aspect of the anterior ankle. He has pain with resisted dorsiflexion and inversion, and he has no pain with resisted great toe extension. Which muscle tendon is the source of his symptoms?

    A. Extensor hallucis longus
    B. Extensor digitorum longus
    C. Fibularis (peroneus) tertius
    D. Tibialis anterior

Correct Answer: D. Tibialis anterior

The tibialis anterior tendon passes over the medial aspect of the anterior ankle and contributes significantly to dorsiflexion and inversion. The extensor hallucis longus is incorrect, because, while it contributes to dorsiflexion and less so to inversion, the patient has no pain with resisted great toe extension (which is its greatest function). The extensor digitorum longus is incorrect, because it is located more centrally on the anterior ankle and contributes to dorsiflexion, but not inversion. The fibularis (peroneus) tertius is incorrect, because, while it contributes to dorsiflexion, it assists in eversion, not inversion.

1. Clemente CD. Anatomy: A Regional Atlas of the Human Body. Baltimore, MD: Lippincott Williams & Wilkins, 1997.
2. Hreljac A. Etiology, prevention, and early intervention of overuse injuries in runners: a biomechanical perspective. Phys Med Rehabil Clin N Am 2005 Aug;16(3):651-667, vi.

160. The most accurate test for a posterior cruciate ligament (PCL) injury is which of the following?

    A. Posterior sag test
    B. Quadriceps active test
    C. Posterior drawer test
    D. Reverse pivot-shift test
    E. Pivot-shift test

Correct Answer: C. Posterior drawer test

The PCL runs from the lateral border of the medial femoral condyle to the indentation between the posterior medial and lateral tibial plateaus. Common mechanisms of injury include a direct injury to the anterior tibia with the knee flexed and the foot plantarflexed (resulting in posterior displacement) and rapid/forced knee hyperextension or hyperflexion. Acutely, if isolated, symptoms of a PCL tear (e.g., stiffness, mild swelling, posterior knee pain) may be mild and go relatively unnoticed by the athlete. The examination of the athlete with a lower extremity injury should begin with an assessment of the athlete's alignment and gait. With a PCL disruption, mild varus and external rotation may be noted. The most accurate test for PCL integrity is the posterior drawer test, performed with the knee in 90 degrees of flexion, the foot planted in neutral position, and the hip flexed at 45 degrees. After being pulled anteriorly, the proximal tibia is pushed posteriorly, and the examiner assesses the degree of displacement, ranging from grade I to grade III. Grade I displacement ranges from 0 to 5 mm, grade II ranges from 5 to 10 mm, and grade III is greater than 10 mm. A grade III PCL tear is likely associated with other ligamentous injuries.

With the posterior sag test, performed with the patient supine and the knees and hips in 90 degrees of flexion, the PCL-deficient tibia will sag below the level of the normal side. The quadriceps active test is performed with the knee in 90 degrees of flexion, the foot planted in neutral, and the hip flexed at 45 degrees. The athlete is instructed to slide the foot down the examination table, requiring quadriceps contraction. In the PCL-deficient leg, that contraction will result in anterior movement of the tibia. Greater than 2 mm of movement is considered positive. The reverse pivot-shift test is used to evaluate a combined PCL and posterolateral corner (PLC) injury. It is performed with the knee in 90 degrees of flexion, the foot planted in neutral, and the hip flexed at 45 degrees. The examiner externally rotates the tibia, while extending the knee. At 20 to 30 degrees of flexion, the iliotibial band pulls on the tibia, causing an anterior shift in the PCL- and PLC-deficient knee. The pivot-shift test, with a high positive predictive value, evaluates for the presence of an anterior cruciate ligament (ACL) injury.

1. Grover M. Evaluating acutely injured patients for internal derangement of the knee. Am Fam Physician 2012;85(3):247-252.
2. McAllister DR, Petrigliano FA. Diagnosis and treatment of posterior cruciate ligament injuries. Curr Sports Med Rep 2007 Oct;6(5):293-299.

161. A 40-year-old male runner presents to your clinic with right lateral knee pain. This has been going on for the past six months and worsened with running or walking downhill. On palpation, the pain is localized to the lateral femoral condyle. Ober's test and Noble's test are equivocal. McMurray's test is normal, and hyperflexion of his knee does not reproduce his pain. Varus stress test of the knee is normal. The pain is reproduced with resisted active internal rotation of the tibia with the patient lying prone and his knee flexed to 30 degrees. X-rays of the knee are normal. The patient has been in physical therapy for the past four months, without any improvement of his pain. What is your diagnosis?

   A. Iliotibial band syndrome
   B. Lateral meniscus tear
   C. Lateral collateral ligament sprain
   D. Popliteus tendinopathy

Correct Answer: D. Popliteus tendinopathy

The popliteus muscle has three origins: lateral femoral condyle anterior and inferior to the lateral collateral ligament origin, posterior horn of the lateral meniscus, and the fibular head. The strongest origin is the one on the lateral femoral condyle. The tendon travels from its origin posteromedially through the popliteal hiatus to insert onto the posterior tibia proximally above the soleal line. Injuries to the popliteus tendon may be due to acute trauma or chronic overuse. Chronic injuries often occur with excessive downhill running, walking, or backpacking. Pain to palpation is best appreciated by placing the affected leg in a figure-of-four position and palpating the origin just anterior to the lateral femoral condyle. It may be difficult to localize the pain on physical examination, due to the proximity of the iliotibial band, popliteus tendon, and the lateral collateral ligament. The pain from popliteus may be reproduced with the patient prone, the knee flexed to 30 degrees, and resistance applied to active internal rotation of the tibia. Answer A is incorrect, because, while iliotibial band syndrome may mimic the symptoms of popliteus tendinopathy, there should not be pain with resisted active internal rotation of the tibia with the patient prone and the knee flexed to 30 degrees. Answer B is incorrect, because lateral meniscus tears should be associated with joint line tenderness, a positive McMurray's test, and pain with hyperflexion of the knee. Answer C is incorrect, because lateral collateral ligament injuries are usually associated with acute trauma, as well as with a positive varus stress test.

1. Tria AJ, Johnson CD, Zawadsky JD. The popliteus tendon. J Bone Joint Surg Am 1989;71(5):714-716.
2. Blake SM, Treble NJ. Popliteus tendon tenosynovitis. Br J Sports Med 2005 Dec;39(12):e42; discussion e42.
3. Petsche TS, Selesnick SH. Popliteus tendinitis: tips for diagnosis and management. Phys Sportsmed 2002;30(8):27-31.

162. A 16-year-old male pitcher is pitching in the high school playoffs. Being a sports medicine physician, you are interested in watching his biomechanics. Which of the following events in the pitching motion best describes the late cocking phase?

   A. Starting with initial movement of the contralateral lower extremity and ending with the elevation of the lead leg to its highest point and the ball being removed from the glove
   B. Starting when the lead leg reaches its maximum height and the ball is removed from the glove and ending when the lead foot contacts the pitching mound
   C. Starting with lead foot contact and ending with the point of maximal external rotation of the throwing shoulder
   D. Starting with maximal external rotation of the throwing shoulder and ending with ball release
   E. Starting with ball release and ending with maximal humeral internal rotation and elbow extension

Correct Answer: C. Starting with lead foot contact and ending with the point of maximal external rotation of the throwing shoulder

The pitching motion is a coordinated series of movements aimed at transferring energy to throw the ball, often at a high velocity. Breakdowns in this movement may predispose the athlete to injury. Thus, it is important to identify the movements in the pitching motion in order to identify these breakdowns. The late cocking phase occurs between lead foot contact and the point of maximal external rotation of the throwing shoulder. Maximum valgus torque occurs at the end of the late cocking phase. Answer A describes the windup phase. Answer B describes the early cocking phase. Answer D describes the acceleration phase. Answer E describes the deceleration phase.

1. Seroyer ST, Nho SJ, Bach BR, Bush-Joseph CA, Nicholson GP, Romeo AA. The kinetic chain in overhand pitching: its potential role for performance enhancement and injury prevention. Sports Health 2010;2(2):135-146.
2. Edmonds EW, Dengerink DD. Common conditions in the overhead athlete. Am Fam Physician 2014;89(7):537-541.

163. Tibial plateau fractures are uncommon, occurring in less than 1% of all fractures. What are the indications for surgery for tibial plateau fracture?

   A. Athletes wishing for faster return to play
   B. Osteoporosis, age over 65 years, or other co-morbidities
   C. Lateral margin location
   D. Displaced fracture, compartment syndrome, neurovascular compromise, or knee laxity or instability

Correct Answer: D. Displaced fracture, compartment syndrome, neurovascular compromise, or knee laxity or instability

With additional indication for surgical intervention, if there is an open fracture. Return-to-play time is not enhanced by surgical intervention in fractures that do not otherwise require surgery. This type of fracture is much more common in the elderly, osteoporotic, or otherwise compromised patient. These findings are indications for attempted non-operative treatment, rather than operative treatment. The majority of all tibial plateau fractures are located at the lateral margin. This fact, by itself, is in no way an indication for surgery.

   1. O'Connor FG, Sallis RE, Wilder RP, St. Pierre P (eds). Sports Medicine: Just the Facts. New York: McGraw-Hill, 2005.

164. While performing an examination on a patient who presented to your clinic for hand weakness, you notice that she is unable to hold her fingers in abduction against resistance on the right, but is able to on the left. Sensation is intact over both upper extremities, as is her strength in extension and flexion of the wrist and fingers. Her Hoffman's sign is negative bilaterally. Which of the following would most likely explain these physical examination findings?

   A. A spinal cord lesion causing myelopathy at the level of C5
   B. A disc bulge at C4 causing central cord compression
   C. Compression of the deep branch of the ulnar nerve at the wrist
   D. Compression of the superficial branch of the ulnar nerve at the wrist
   E. Compression of the inferior trunk of the brachial plexus

Correct Answer: C. Compression of the deep branch of the ulnar nerve at the wrist

The physical examination findings on this patient are strictly motor in origin and are seen in lesions of the ulnar nerve. The ulnar nerve branches after passing through Guyon's canal into a deep and superficial branch. The deep branch is a motor branch to the interosseous muscles of the hand, while the superficial branch has a sensory component responsible for sensation of the ring and little finger. The lack of sensory symptoms makes Answer D incorrect. Myelopathy typically presents with upper motor neuron signs, such as a positive Hoffman's test. Answer A is incorrect, given that her Hoffman's test is negative, and a C5 myelopathy would not manifest in this manner. A central cord compression most commonly produces bilateral symptoms, making Answer B incorrect. Compression of the inferior trunk of the brachial plexus would produce symptoms in the distribution of the median nerve as well, making Answer E incorrect.

   1. Thompson JC. Netter's Concise Orthopaedic Anatomy. 2nd ed. Philadelphia: Saunders Elsevier, 2010.
   2. Stoller DW. The wrist and hand. Stoller's Atlas of Orthopaedics and Sports Medicine. Philadelphia: Lippincott Williams & Wilkins, 2008:811-906.

165. You saw a 32-year-old male in your office seven days ago, and you diagnosed him with lumbar radiculopathy. As part of the treatment plan, you place him on a two-week course of naproxen 500mg twice daily. He returns to your office today complaining of epigastric pain. You diagnose him with NSAID-induced gastritis. The patient questions you on other possible adverse reactions to taking NSAIDs. Which of the following is true regarding adverse reactions to NSAIDs?

   A. NSAID-induced gastritis is due to a lack of gastric mucosa, protective leukotriene production inhibited by NSAIDs
   B. Interstitial nephritis is a prostaglandin mediated kidney injury seen in patients taking NSAIDs
   C. Celecoxib, a COX-2 inhibitor, has an increased incidence of clotting dysfunction compared to nonselective NSAIDs, because of inhibition of COX-2's synthesis of thromboxane
   D. Side effects of NSAIDs are due to the pharmacologic action of the drug itself or an Ig-E mediated drug hypersensitivity reaction
   E. NSAIDs irreversibly bind to platelets, leading to increases in bleeding time

Correct Answer: D. Side effects of NSAIDs are due to the pharmacologic action of the drug itself or an Ig-E mediated drug hypersensitivity reaction

Side effects of NSAIDs are related to the direct pharmacologic action of the medication, such as inhibition of gastro-protective prostaglandins, leading to gastritis, or they are related to an IgE mediated allergic hypersensitivity reaction, such as interstitial nephritis or urticaria. Answer A is incorrect, because NSAIDs do not block leukotriene synthesis, and prostaglandins are responsible for the protection of the gastric mucosa. Answer C is incorrect, because thromboxane is produced through COX-1, and thromboxane is not synthesized by COX-2. Answer B is incorrect. Interstitial nephritis is not prostaglandin mediated, but rather an IgE mediated hypersensitivity reaction. Renal azotemia may be caused by decreased prostaglandin mediated arteriole vasodilation, but interstitial nephritis is a hypersensitivity reaction. Answer E is incorrect, because aspirin is the only NSAID that irreversibly binds platelets, where other NSAIDs are competitive, reversible inhibitors of platelets.

1. Kowalski ML, Stevenson DD. Classification of reactions to nonsteroidal antiinflammatory drugs. Immunol Allergy Clin North Am 2013 May;33(2):135-145.
2. Feucht CL, Patel DR. Analgesics and anti-inflammatory medications in sports: use and abuse. Pediatr Clin North Am 2010 Jun;57(3):751-774.

166. Creatine enhances athletic performance by which mechanism?

    A. Decreasing lactate threshold
    B. Increasing muscle phosphocreatine concentration
    C. Decreasing calcium uptake in sarcoplasmic reticulum
    D. Earlier muscle glycogen use

Correct Answer: C. Decreasing calcium uptake in sarcoplasmic reticulum

Phosphocreatine is a readily available source of energy to regenerate ATP from ADP in the absence of oxygen that does not generate lactate. Phosphocreatine decreases lactate production and increases the lactate threshold. It also increases the calcium uptake in the sarcoplasmic reticulum resulting in a more rapid and forceful muscle contraction. Some research suggests enhanced glycogen stores when creatine is combined with glycogen-depleting exercise.

1. Cooper R, Naclerio F, Allgrove J, Jimenez A. Creatine supplementation with specific view to exercise/sports performance: an update. Int J of Int Soc Sports Nutr 2012;9(1):33-44.
2. Liddle DG, Conner DJ. Nutritional supplements and ergogenic aids. Prim Care 2013 Jun;40(2):487-505.

167. Which of the following diagnostic tests is most likely to help confirm the diagnosis of piriformis syndrome?

   A. Straight leg raise
   B. Freiburg sign
   C. X-ray pelvis
   D. MRI pelvis
   E. EMG

Correct Answer: B. Freiburg sign

The piriformis muscle lies within the gluteal triangle. It originates about the anterior aspect of the sacrum, travels through the greater sciatic foramen, and inserts on the upper medial greater trochanter. Of note, the sciatic nerve generally runs deep to the piriformis and exits the greater sciatic foramen inferior to the piriformis and superior to the gemellus. The piriformis function depends, in part, on the hip position. With the hip in flexion, the piriformis serves as a hip abductor; with the hip in extension, it serves as a hip external rotator. Piriformis syndrome is believed to be caused by gluteal trauma, post-traumatic scarring, and/or functional sciatic entrapment. Examination of a patient with sciatic symptoms and a concern for piriformis syndrome should include palpation of the area (aim for the sciatic notch), during which 94% of sufferers will have pain. It is important to note that many patients with lumbar spine referred pain will also have pain in this location with palpation.

Patients will also likely have a positive Freiburg or straight-leg raise sign. Freiburg testing involves putting the hip in extension and internal rotation, and having the patient externally rotate the hip against resistance. A test resulting in pain or sciatica symptoms is positive in 63% of sufferers of piriformis syndrome. Straight-leg raise results in sciatica symptoms from piriformis syndrome in one-third of sufferers. A straight-leg raise, however, is positive in many sufferers of sciatica and commonly indicates a lumbar spine etiology with a herniated disc. Diagnostic studies are not particularly helpful in confirming the diagnosis of piriformis syndrome. X-ray and MRI, however, might be used to identify other hip and spinal causes of sciatica symptoms. It is important to first rule out a lumbar spine etiology for any patient complaining of radiating leg symptoms. EMG has not conclusively demonstrated altered neuromuscular electrical activity, though a delayed H reflex with the limb in a provocative position has been proposed as one way to evaluate for piriformis syndrome.

1. Cass SP. Piriformis syndrome: a cause of nondiscogenic sciatica. Curr Sports Med Rep 2015 Jan;14(1):41-44. doi: 10.1249/JSR.0000000000000110.
2. Franklyn-Miller A, Falvey E, McCrory P. The gluteal triangle: a clinical patho-anatomical approach to the diagnosis of gluteal pain in athletes. Br J Sports Med 2009 Jun;43(6):460-466. doi: 10.1136/bjsm.2007.042317. Epub 2008 Nov 19.

168. Physiologic and performance effects of human growth hormone (hGH) include which of the following?

    A. Increases muscle strength
    B. Decreases heart rate
    C. Increases lean body mass
    D. Increases workload capacity

Correct Answer: C. Increases lean body mass

Scientific evidence has failed to show an ergogenic effect with hGH. They have shown increases in lean body mass, basal metabolic rate, and heart rate. There is no benefit in muscle strength, power, or workload capacity. Adverse effects include soft tissue edema, fatigue, hyperlipidemia, erectile dysfunction, arthralgias, and irreversible facial, jaw, and skull bone growth.

1. Momaya A, Fawal M, Estes R. Performance-enhancing substances in sports: a review of the literature. Sports Med 2015 Apr;45(4):517-531.
2. Liddle DG, Conner DJ. Nutritional supplements and ergogenic aids. Prim Care 2013 Jun;40(2):487-505.
3. Birzniece V. Doping in sport: effects, harm and misconceptions. Intern Med J 2015 Mar;45(3):239-248. doi: 10.1111/imj.12629.

169. A 73-year-old female presents to your office because she heard that flexibility exercises are important for older individuals. Her goal is to be able to maintain her activities of daily living, like dressing and walking. She wants to know how often and when to stretch. Which of the following best summarizes the current recommendations regarding stretching?

   A. Flexibility exercises should be performed at least twice a week for at least 10 minutes and be done when the body is warmed up
   B. Flexibility exercises should be performed daily, but held for 10 seconds or less due to age-related tendinopathy
   C. Flexibility exercises should be performed at least twice a week for 10 minutes at the beginning of the workout
   D. Flexibility exercises should not be performed after age 65

Correct Answer: A. Flexibility exercises should be performed at least twice a week for at least 10 minutes and be done when the body is warmed up

Answer A is correct based on the American College of Sports Medicine position statement on Exercise and Physical Activity in Older Adults. Answer B is incorrect, because it is best to slowly stretch into the desired position and hold for 10 to 30 seconds. Answer C is incorrect, given that current recommendations indicate that the body should be warmed up prior to stretching for maximum benefit. Answer D is incorrect, as stretching can be performed at any age.

   1. Morey M. Physical activity and exercise in older adults. UpToDate. Accessed June 1, 2014 at https://www.uptodate.com/contents/physical-activity-and-exercise-in-older-adults.
   2. American College of Sports Medicine, Chodzko-Zajko WJ, Proctor DN, Fiatarone Singh MA, Minson CT, Nigg CR, et al. American College of Sports Medicine position stand. Exercise and physical activity for older adults. Med Sci Sports Exerc 2009 Jul;41(7):1510-1530. doi: 10.1249/MSS.0b013e3181a0c95c.
   3. Takeshima N, Rogers NL, Rogers ME, Islam MM, Koizumi D, Lee S. Functional fitness gain varies in older adults depending on exercise mode. Med Sci Sports Exerc 2007 Nov;39(11):2036-2043.

170. A 33-year-old white female presents with a 14-month history of pelvic pain following the birth of her son. She has abnormal x-rays of the pelvis. She had improved with rest, but experienced aggravation of her pain with return to running. Diagnosis of osteitis pubis was confirmed by examination and MRI of pelvis. She was successfully treated with injection of the pubic symphysis with steroid, sacroiliac stabilization belt, and physical therapy. Which of the following is a true statement about osteitis pubis?

    A. Osteitis pubis is generally a surgical problem
    B. Osteitis pubis is generally treatable with rest and rehabilitation
    C. Osteitis pubis is rarely seen in running athletes
    D. Osteitis pubis is best imaged by radiograph of the pelvis

Correct Answer: B. Osteitis pubis is generally treatable with rest and rehabilitation

Osteitis pubis is generally a non-surgical problem, which can be managed with rest and rehabilitation through physical therapy. Often, anti-inflammatory medications, such as oral or injected steroids, are helpful to manage the pain. Surgery is rarely needed, but can be useful in some refractory cases. Osteitis pubis is most often seen in running sports, specifically distance running and soccer, and in ice hockey as well. MRI is the best way to confirm osteitis pubis, although it can be seen on plain radiographs. Widening can also be seen with ultrasound and is one way to track the condition in pregnant patients. It is important to note that many women who have previously carried a pregnancy may have asymptomatic abnormalities on imaging.

1. McKim KR, Taunto JE, Kirchner GD. The effectiveness of a compression short in the treatment of athletes with osteitis pubis. Clin J Sport Med 1999 Apr;9(2):112.
2. Lovell G, Galloway H, Hopkins W, Harvey A. Osteitis pubis and assessment of bone marrow edema at the pubic symphysis with MRI in an elite junior male soccer squad. Clin J Sport Med 2006 Mar;16(2):117-122.

171. Which of the following is a physiologic adaptation to ascent to high altitude?

   A. A decrease in cardiac output
   B. An increase in pulmonary artery pressure
   C. Worsening ventilation-perfusion matching
   D. A decrease in alveolar ventilation

Correct Answer: B. An increase in pulmonary artery pressure

On ascent to high altitude, several physiologic mechanisms occur to accommodate to the low partial pressure of oxygen. Cardiac output increases (Answer A), pulmonary artery pressure increases (Answer B), and ventilation and perfusion matching is improved (Answer C). Alveolar ventilation is increased (Answer D), stimulated by the carotid body. Each of these adaptations are aimed to improved oxygen uptake from the atmosphere and delivery to the peripheral tissues.

1. Schoene RB. Illnesses at high altitude. Chest 2008;134(2):402-416.
2. Luks AM, McIntosh SE, Grissom CK, Auerbach PS, Rodway GW, Schoene RB, et al. Wilderness Medical Society practice guidelines for the prevention and treatment of acute altitude illness: 2014 update. Wilderness Environ Med 2014 Dec;25(4 Suppl):S4-S14. doi: 10.1016/j.wem.2014.06.017.

172. What is the maximal lactate steady state (MLSS) during exercise testing?

   A. Refers to the exercise intensity at which blood lactate removal is surpassed by lactate production, and lactate begins to accumulate above baseline levels
   B. Refers to the highest exercise intensity at which no significant rise in blood lactate occurs with continued exercise over time
   C. Refers to when blood lactate concentration rises by 1 mmol/L above exercise baseline
   D. Occurs during exercise at a respiratory exchange ratio (RER or R) of 0.85

Correct Answer: B. Refers to the highest exercise intensity at which no significant rise in blood lactate occurs with continued exercise over time

The main energy systems for exercising muscles are the immediate (phosphagen; ATP-creatine phosphate), the short-term (glycolytic; pyruvate-lactic acid), and the long-term (oxidative) systems. The immediate system fuels maximal power for less than 10 seconds. The short-term system allows for high-intensity activity for less than three minutes. The long-term system allows for moderate-low-intensity muscle activity for an unlimited amount of time, theoretically. This requires oxygen, and is therefore an aerobic system. The immediate and short-term systems are anaerobic. In order for the short-term system to continue, pyruvate is converted to lactate, which moves into the circulation as blood lactate, indicating anaerobic glycolytic activity. During an exercise test, blood lactate is initially at a baseline steady state. The long-term system predominates, and lactate removal mechanisms match the lactate being produced by glycolytic processes. With increases in exercise intensity, more energy is required by the exercising muscles. If this requirement is met by the long-term system, the lactate will remain in a steady state.

With further increases in exercise intensity, however, this ability to provide enough energy will eventually be strained, and the short-term system becomes more active to help meet the energy requirement, producing more lactate. Once lactate production exceeds lactate removal, lactate levels begin to rise. The exercise intensity at which blood lactate rises by 1 mM above exercise baseline is called the lactate threshold. With continued exercise testing, a second lactate steady state is reached, representing equilibrium between up-regulated lactate removal and lactate-producing processes. However, with continued increases in exercise intensity, the lactate removal mechanisms are again overwhelmed, and lactate begins to rise again. The point just before this rise, the highest exercise intensity at which no significant rise in blood lactate occurs with continued exercise, is the maximal lactate steady state. During exercise, where the oxidative system predominates, the respiratory exchange ratio (RER; $\dot{V}CO_2/\dot{V}O_2$), will lie between 0.7 and 1.0. So, an RER of 0.85 would still represent aerobic system predominance and baseline lactate levels. Once the RER exceeds 1.0, bicarbonate is being consumed to buffer increases in blood lactate and more CO_2 is being expired, signifying an increase in short-term system activity.

1. McArdle WD, Katch FI, Katch VL. Exercise Physiology: Energy, Nutrition, and Human Performance. 5th ed. Baltimore, MD: Lippincott Williams & Wilkins, 2001:161-162.
2. Gaesser GA, Poole DC. The slow component of oxygen uptake kinetics in humans. Exerc Sport Sci Rev 1996;24:35-71.
3. Beaver WL, Wasserman K, Whipp BJ. Bicarbonate buffering of lactic acid generated during exercise. J Appl Physiol (1985) 1986 Feb;60(2):472-478.

173. What is the correct physiological adaptation of the respiratory system to exercise?
    A. Mean arterial PCO_2 decreases, due to increased ventilatory rate
    B. Ventilation to perfusion ratios (V/Q) become more uneven throughout the lung tissues
    C. Increase in arterial pH, due to rapid renal buffering
    D. Increase in pulmonary blood flow as a percentage of cardiac output

Correct Answer: D. Increase in pulmonary blood flow as a percentage of cardiac output

During respiratory adaptation to exercise, O_2 consumption, as well as CO_2 production, is increased, which matches increased ventilation rate. Mean values for arterial PO_2 and arterial PCO_2 do not change. V/Q ratios are more evenly distributed throughout the lungs during exercise when compared to rest. Arterial pH is not changed, except under conditions of very strenuous exercise, when it may decrease.

1. Costanzo LS. Board Review Series: Physiology. 2nd ed. Baltimore, MD: Lippincott Williams & Wilkins, 2001.
2. McArdle WD, Katch FI, Katch VL. Exercise Physiology: Energy, Nutrition, and Human Performance. Philadelphia: Lippincott Williams & Wilkins, 2009:253-269.

174. A 16-year-old male volleyball player presented to your office six weeks ago with the complaint of vague posterior right shoulder pain and no history of trauma. He was referred to physical therapy for rotator cuff and periscapular strengthening, with little success. Unfortunately, his symptoms have continued, and he is unable to play volleyball, secondary to pain and weakness. He denies any numbness or tingling. On examination, he demonstrates supraspinatus and infraspinatus weakness. X-rays of the right shoulder are unremarkable. An MRI of the right shoulder demonstrates supraspinatous and infraspinatous muscle edema, but no evidence of bursitis, tendinopathy, or a tearing of the rotator cuff. You suspect a neuropathy. Given the information about this patient, what is the most likely diagnosis?

    A. Compression of the seventh cervical nerve root
    B. Suprascapular neuropathy, with compression at the transverse scapular ligament
    C. Suprascapular neuropathy, with compression at the spinoglenoid ligament
    D. Axillary nerve injury

Correct Answer: B. Suprascapular neuropathy, with compression at the transverse scapular ligament

Answer A is incorrect, given that the symptoms listed would not occur with isolated C7 nerve root compression. Answer B is correct, because weakness of the supraspinatous and infraspinatus is caused by suprascapular nerve compression at the level of the suprascapular notch, which is where the transverse scapular ligament is located. Answer C is incorrect, because suprascapular neuropathy with compression at the spinoglenoid ligament would cause only infraspinatus weakness. Answer D is incorrect, given that axillary nerve injury does not result in rotator cuff weakness and often presents with numbness and tingling in the lateral shoulder following anterior dislocation.

1. Trojian T. Suprascapular neuropathy. Medscape. Accessed May 30, 2015 at http://emedicine.medscape.com/article/92672-overview.
2. Safran MR. Nerve injury about the shoulder in athletes, part 1: suprascapular nerve and axillary nerve. Am J Sports Med 2004 Apr-May;32(3):803-819.

175. Which of the following is associated with barefoot running?

A. Rearfoot landing
B. Increased stride length
C. Increased cadence
D. Increased foot eversion moment
E. Decreased proprioception

Correct Answer: C. Increased cadence

Due to increased ground reaction forces with a rearfoot landing, barefoot runners tend to land on their midfoot or forefoot. To accomplish that feat, they shorten their stride length. To maintain their running speed, they then increase their cadence. Barefoot running affects the motion of all the lower extremity joints, including decreased foot eversion moments, due to decreased total heel width while barefoot. As shoes decrease proprioception, barefoot running is associated with increased proprioceptive capability, resulting in better stability and lighter ground impacts, which may modulate the risk of certain injuries.

1. Altman AR, Davis IS. Barefoot running: biomechanics and implications for running injuries. Curr Sports Med Rep 2012 Sep-Oct;11(5):244-250. doi: 10.1249/JSR.0b013e31826c9bb9.
2. Kindred J, Trubey C, Simons S. Foot injuries in runners. Curr Sports Med Rep 2011;10(5):249-254.
3. Lieberman DE. What we can learn about running from barefoot running: an evolutionary medical perspective. Exerc Sport Sci Rev 2012;40(2);63-72.

176. Which of the following best describes the anatomy and/or function of the posterolateral corner structures of the knee?

    A. The fibular collateral ligament is the primary dynamic restraint to varus stress
    B. The popliteus tendon is a static stabilizer against varus stress
    C. The popliteofibular ligament is an important stabilizer of tibial external rotation
    D. The anterior cruciate ligament is a major restraint to tibial internal and external rotation
    E. The posterior cruciate ligament is the primary static restraint to varus stress

Correct Answer: C. The popliteofibular ligament is an important stabilizer of tibial external rotation

The posterolateral corner (PLC) of the knee is anatomically complex and composed of several structures, providing both static and dynamic restraint. Amongst these structures, the popliteofibular ligament is an important stabilizer of external rotation. The fibular collateral ligament serves as a static restraint to varus stress. The popliteus tendon is a static and dynamic stabilizer of posterolateral rotation of the knee. The anterior cruciate ligament helps to restrain the knee against rotatory loads, but is not considered part of the PLC. The fibular collateral ligament, rather than the posterior cruciate ligament, is the primary static restraint to varus stress.

1. Levy BA, Stuart MJ, Whelan DB. Posterolateral instability of the knee: evaluation, treatment, results. Sports Med Arthrosc Rev 2010 Dec;18(4):254-262.
2. Voos JE, Mauro CS, Wente T, Warren RF, Wickiewicz TL. Posterior cruciate ligament: anatomy, biomechanics, and outcomes. Am J Sports Med 2012 Jan;40(1):222-231.

177. In the clinical evaluation of anterior hip and groin pain, which of the following pain generators is most correctly paired with its correlating finding on physical examination?

   A. Tensor fascia lata tendon—tenderness to palpation between femoral pulse and the pubic symphysis
   B. Adductor longus muscle—tenderness to palpation between femoral pulse and the anterior superior iliac spine
   C. Pectineus muscle—tenderness to palpation over femoral pulse
   D. Rectus femoris tendon—tenderness to palpation over the anterior superior iliac spine

Correct Answer: C. Pectineus muscle—tenderness to palpation over femoral pulse

In the clinical evaluation of many musculoskeletal conditions, tenderness to palpation of a structure is an important clue in determining the pain generator, and may be critical in the successful amelioration of the patient's symptoms. Without assistive technology and imaging guidance, the astute physician must rely on surface landmarks, visuospatial knowledge of anatomy, and manual dexterity to accomplish this aim. Several structures are often reliably palpable on physical examination and serve as dependable surface landmarks, including the anterior superior iliac spine (ASIS), anterior inferior iliac spine (AIIS), the femoral pulse (approximating the femoral neurovascular bundle), pubic tubercle, and pubic symphysis. It is also important to know where each soft tissue structure lies in relation to these landmarks to accurately correlate tenderness to the correct structure. The tensor fascia lata takes its origin from the anterior iliac crest, just lateral to the ASIS. The rectus femoris tendon takes its origin from the AIIS and superior roof of the acetabulum, both located inferior to the ASIS. The pectineus muscle belly lies deep, slightly medial to the femoral nerve, artery, and vein. Deep palpation at the femoral pulse would also result in palpation of the pectineus muscle. The adductor longus tendon and muscle lie medial to the pectineus, between the femoral pulse and the pubic symphysis.

   1. Thompson JC. Pelvis. Netter's Concise Orthopaedic Anatomy. 2nd ed. Philadelphia: Saunders Elsevier, 2010:219-248.
   2. Stoller DW. The hip: anatomy and pathology. Stoller's Atlas of Orthopaedics and Sports Medicine. Philadelphia: Lippincott Williams & Wilkins, 2008:161-259.

178. Which of the following best describes the relationship of the structures implicated in intersection syndrome?

   A. The abductor pollicis longus (APL) and extensor pollicis brevis (EPB) cross over extensor carpi radialis longus (ECRL) and extensor carpi radialis brevis (ECRB)
   B. The abductor pollicis longus (APL) and abductor pollicis brevis (APB) cross over extensor carpi radialis longus (ECRL) and extensor carpi radialis brevis (ECRB)
   C. The extensor carpi radialis longus (ECRL) and extensor carpi radialis brevis (ECRB) cross over abductor pollicis longus (APL) and extensor pollicis brevis (EPB)
   D. The extensor carpi radialis longus (ECRL) and extensor carpi radialis brevis (ECRB) cross over abductor pollicis brevis (APB) and extensor pollicis longus (EPL)

Correct Answer: A. The abductor pollicis longus (APL) and extensor pollicis brevis (EPB) cross over extensor carpi radialis longus (ECRL) and extensor carpi radialis brevis (ECRB)

Intersection syndrome identifies an overuse tenosynovitis of the forearm that occurs at the "intersection" of the first extensor compartment (abductor pollicis longus and extensor pollicis brevis), which lies dorsal to the second extensor compartment (extensor carpi radialis longus and extensor carpi radialis brevis). Answer B is incorrect, because it does not describe the first extensor compartment correctly. Answer C is incorrect, because it does not describe the correct anatomic relationship of the extensor compartments. Answer D is incorrect, because it describes the second and third extensor compartments. Intersection syndrome occurs in patients who perform motions requiring repetitive wrist extension, such as rowers, weight lifters, drummers, and hedge trimmers. Clinical symptoms occur a few centimeters proximal to the wrist on the dorsal aspect of the forearm.

1. Boggess BR. Evaluation of the adult with subacute or chronic wrist pain. UpToDate. Accessed July 7, 2015 at http://www.uptodate.com/contents/evaluation-of-the-adult-with-subacute-or-chronic-wrist-pain.
2. Montechiarello S, Miozzi F, D'Ambrosio I, Giovagnorio F. The intersection syndrome: ultrasound findings and their diagnostic value. J Ultrasound 2010 Jun;13(2):70-73.
3. Kaneko S, Takasaki H. Forearm pain, diagnosed as intersection syndrome, managed by taping: a case series. J Orthop Sports Phys Ther 2011 Jul;41(7):514-519.

179. Atlantoaxial instability can be an acquired or existing condition that places a young athlete at risk for spinal cord injury. Which ligament is the primary stabilizer of the atlantoaxial joint?

    A. The transverse atlantal ligament
    B. The alar ligament
    C. The posterior longitudinal ligament
    D. The anterior longitudinal ligament

Correct Answer: A. The transverse atlantal ligament

The primary static stabilizer of the upper c-spine is the transverse atlantal ligament, which lies posterior to the dens, supporting the articulation of the dens with the anterior arc of C1. It is disruption of this ligament that causes the vast majority of atlantoaxial instability. This makes A correct. The alar ligament attaches C1 and C2 to the occiput and is typically not involved in atlantoaxial instability. The anterior and posterior longitudinal ligaments are the primary stabilizers of the lower cervical spine. They lie in front and behind the vertebral bodies, respectively. They are typically not involved with instability of the upper cervical spine.

1. Netter FH. Atlas of Human Anatomy. 2nd ed. Philadelphia: Elsevier Science, 1997:22-30.
2. Miller M, Sekiya JK. Basic anatomy of the spinal column. In: Miller M, Sekiya JK (eds). Sports Medicine: Core Knowledge in Orthopaedics. Philadelphia: Mosby, 2006:419-422.
3. Snyder RL. Neck injuries. In: Madden CC, Putukian M, Young CC, McCarty EC (eds). Netter's Sports Medicine. Philadelphia: Saunders Elsevier, 2010:326-331.

180. As the head team physician for a Division I college, you have been caring for the starting center for the football team. You have seen him weekly in the training room for the last three weeks. His blood pressure, on these three separate training room visits, has been determined to be in the stage 2 hypertension range. A thorough workup has been performed, without identifying any secondary causes for the elevated blood pressure or evidence of end organ damage. In addition to lifestyle modifications that have failed to this point, you determine that the athlete will need to be treated with medication to control the blood pressure. The patient has no known medication allergies. Which would be the best medication to initiate treatment?

A. Hydrochlorothiazide
B. Metoprolol XL
C. Diltiazem
D. Lisinopril

Correct Answer: D. Lisinopril

Vasodilators, including angiotensin-converting enzyme (ACE) inhibitors or angiotensin receptor blockers (ARBs) tend to be the best tolerated. These agents have no major adverse effects on energy metabolism and do not impair maximum oxygen uptake. ARBs produce similar blood pressure lowering and hemodynamic patterns as ACE inhibitors, but have fewer side effects, such as cough and angioedema. Long-acting dihydropyridine calcium channel blockers may be an option in athletes as well, but a major side effect can be lower extremity edema, making this a less desirable choice in young athletes when compared to ACE inhibitors and ARBs. Care should be taken when using ACE inhibitors and ARBs in young females, due to the concern for fetal injury if used during pregnancy. The standard of care is not to avoid using these medications in women of childbearing potential, but rather to counsel them regarding pregnancy avoidance and in contraception use.

Answer A is the wrong answer, because hydrochlorothiazide can affect electrolyte concentrations due to urinary loss of magnesium and potassium, which can contribute to muscle cramping and cardiac arrhythmias. This effect can be especially pronounced in warmer weather, with increased sweating potential and risk for heat illness. In addition, all classes of diuretics are banned, because they can mask the presence of anabolic steroids, making their use void in any athlete undergoing drug testing. Answer B is the incorrect answer, because the beta-blocker class of anti-hypertensives may adversely affect athletic performance, due to a decrease in VO_2max and cardiac output and alterations in fuel use, thermoregulation, and skeletal muscle recruitment patterns. These medications may also exacerbate underlying asthma. If this class of medication is used, then a selective beta-blocker is a better choice. As with diuretics, this class of medication is banned in specific precision sports, such as shooting, archery, diving, and figure skating, due to their beneficial effects on anxiety and tremor. Answer C is the wrong answer, because diltiazem is in the class of nondihydropyridine calcium channel blockers. This class of medication is not as effective as the dihydropyridine class of calcium channel blockers for blood pressure control. Nondihydropyridine calcium channel blockers (verapamil, diltiazem) are more commonly given for rate control in patients with atrial fibrillation or for control of angina.

1. Leddy JJ, Izzo J. Hypertension in athletes. J Clin Hypertens 2009 Apr;11(4):226-233.
2. Ciocca M, Stafford H, Laney R. The athlete's pharmacy. Clin Sports Med 2011 Jul;30(3):629-639.

181. When performing a palpation landmark-guided injection of the carpal tunnel, which of the following observations indicate that the needle tip is in an acceptable position for introducing the injectant?

   A. Resistance is encountered when initially depressing the plunger
   B. The patient reports numbness, tingling, and burning upon placing the needle bevel at the target
   C. A small amount of blood enters the barrel upon initially drawing the plunger
   D. The needle shaft does not move with voluntary finger movements

Correct Answer: D. The needle shaft does not move with voluntary finger movements

Percutaneous injections of solutions, using a sterile hypodermic needle and syringe, have long been an important mainstay in the treatment of musculoskeletal ailments. It is important to be familiar with the components of the modern hypodermic needle and syringe. From distal to proximal, the needle has a tip (includes a point and a bevel), lumen (bore), shaft (cannula), hilt, and hub. There are also frequently caps and other safety devices associated with the needle. Most syringes will have two main components: a barrel and a plunger. The most distal part of the barrel includes an adapter tip, in order to interface with the needle and other devices (e.g., Luer-Lock tip). The barrel often features calibrated scale markings and finger flanges. The most distal part of the plunger is the plunger head and seal (traditionally made of rubber), followed by the plunger stem and thumb rest.

Depending on the injectant introduced, the resulting outcome of injection procedures add therapeutic, ameliorative, and diagnostic value in the management of these patients. In general, accuracy and precision in the placement of the needle tip is important, not only for the efficacy of the injection, but for the safety of the procedure. For example, a popular injectant solution includes a corticosteroid and local anesthetic. Avoidance of injecting these solutions intravascularly is essential in order to avoid cardiac complications. By drawing back on the plunger, the clinician would be able to visualize any blood from a cannulated blood vessel, and withhold injecting the solution accordingly. Resistance to plunger depression would suggest that the needle tip has been placed in a tendon or ligament structure, and may be an indication to withhold proceeding with the injection. After introducing the needle into the wrist, should voluntary finger movements cause the needle to move or sweep, the needle tip may have been placed into a tendon and should be redirected. Numbness, tingling, and burning before injecting suggests that the needle tip or shaft have been placed in a nerve or near enough to risk intraneural injection. In general, the goal of the landmark-guided carpal tunnel injection is to inject the solution into the carpal tunnel by cannulating the space in an extravascular, extra-neural, and extra-tendinous manner.

1. Ball C. The early development of intravenous apparatus. Anaesth Intensive Care 2006 Jun;34 Suppl 1:22-26.
2. Kotwal A. Innovation, diffusion and safety of a medical technology: a review of the literature on injection practices. Soc Sci Med 2005 Mar;60(5):1133-1147.
3. Denkler K. Helpful hints for injections of wrist and hand region. Am Fam Physician 2003;68(10):1912.

182. With proper skin cleansing and the use of aseptic technique, the risk of introducing infection into a sterile joint via knee aspiration can be reduced. What is this reduced risk?

    A. 1:100
    B. 1:1,000
    C. 1:10,000
    D. 1:100,000

Correct Answer: C. 1:10,000

With proper skin cleansing and the use of aseptic technique, the risk of introducing infection into a sterile joint via knee aspiration can be less than 1:10,000.

1. Gill S. Knee arthrocentesis. Medscape. Accessed June 27, 2015 at http://emedicine.medscape.com/article/79994-overview.

Test 1 Answers, Critiques, and References

183. You are moonlighting in an urgent care clinic when a 23-year-old male presents with a right shoulder injury he sustained while playing football with some friends. After thoroughly examining the patient, you obtain shoulder x-rays that confirm an anterior shoulder dislocation (see image). As soon as you touch the patient to attempt your reduction, he screams in pain and demands you give him pain medication. What is your best next step?

   A. Provide the patient intravenous sedation and reattempt your reduction using an external rotation technique
   B. Continue with your reduction, despite his requests to avoid muscle spasm
   C. Inject a small amount of intra-articular lidocaine using a posterior glenohumeral approach, and then re-attempt your reduction using a scapular manipulation technique
   D. Provide the pain medication he prefers and reattempt your reduction, starting with the Milch technique

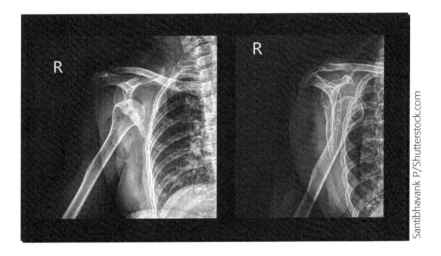

Correct Answer: C. Inject a small amount of intra-articular lidocaine using a posterior glenohumeral approach, and then re-attempt your reduction using a scapular manipulation technique

While the best time to reduce an anterior shoulder dislocation is acutely on the playing field, in most clinical scenarios like this one, you will find the patient requires some form of medication prior to reduction. Answer A is incorrect, because you are in the urgent care setting, with limited resources, and intravenous sedation would likely not be available. Also, it has been shown in one study that reductions of acute anterior shoulder dislocations can be achieved equally well in patients who receive an intra-articular injection compared to those who receive intravenous sedation. These reductions were found to be no more painful, less costly and required shorter recovery time. Answer B is incorrect, because muscle spasm is likely unavoidable at this point, and you do not want to put the patient through a painful procedure. With regard to the reduction technique utilized, there are several approaches that can be used and there is no one best technique. Acceptable techniques include scapular manipulation, the external rotation technique, the Rockwood technique, and the Stimson maneuver. If reduction is not achieved with the external rotation approach, the Milch technique can be added. To perform this technique, abduct the externally rotated arm into an overhead position. Reduction is achieved by applying gentle traction in line with the humerus and direct pressure over the humeral head, with the clinician's thumb in the axilla. Answer D is incorrect, because you would not want to perform the Milch technique prior to attempting one of the other aforementioned techniques.

1. Sherman SC. Shoulder dislocation and reduction. UpToDate. Accessed June 30, 2015 at http://www.uptodate.com/contents/shoulder-dislocation-and-reduction?.
2. McCormack RG. Intra-articular lidocaine or intravenous sedation for reduction of shoulder dislocations? Clin J Sport Med 2004;14(4):252-253.

184. A 37-year-old, right-hand-dominant female who is an avid golfer complains of right dorsal forearm pain with activity for three months. She does not recall any trauma. On physical examination, there is tenderness over the radial head with minimal wrist extensor weakness and pain, with resisted supination of an extended forearm with wrist flexion. Radiographs are negative. She has tried icing, an elbow sleeve, oral NSAIDs, and occupational therapy for lateral epicondylitis, without significant improvement. What other diagnosis should be considered at this time?

   A. Radial tunnel syndrome
   B. Cubital tunnel syndrome
   C. Lateral epicondylitis
   D. Medial epicondylitis

Correct Answer: A. Radial tunnel syndrome

Radial tunnel syndrome is characterized by compression of the superficial branch of the radial nerve at the radial tunnel. Because this is a sensory nerve branch only, no motor weakness should be present. Pain radiates into the dorsal forearm and increases with repetitive supination and especially with pronation. Radial tunnel syndrome is often mistaken for lateral epicondylitis (tennis elbow). One distinction between lateral epicondylitis and radial tunnel syndrome is the location of palpable pain: over the radial neck anteriorly (radial tunnel), over the extensor carpi radialis brevis (lateral epicondylitis). The radial nerve dives deep at the elbow to become the posterior interosseous nerve.

In lateral epicondylitis, pain is at the extensor carpi radialis brevis and increases with resisted wrist dorsiflexion with the elbow in extension. In medial epicondylitis (golfer's elbow), pain is localized at the medial epicondyle to the pronator teres and flexor carpi radialis muscles. Cubital tunnel syndrome involves entrapment of the ulnar nerve at the elbow, causing potential medial elbow pain associated with paresthesias along the distal forearm and fourth and fifth digits.

1. Neal S, Fields KB. Peripheral nerve entrapment and injury in the upper extremity. Am Fam Physician 2010 Jan 15;81(2):147-155.
2. Moradi A, Ebrahimzadeh MH, Jupiter JB. Radial tunnel syndrome, diagnostic and treatment dilemma. Arch Bone Jt Surg 2015 Jul;3(3):156-162.

185. A 16-year-old male presents to your clinic for follow-up from the emergency department. He was seen three days ago for a fracture. On review of his discharge paperwork, you notice he was diagnosed with a non-displaced, bicortical distal radial metaphysis fracture. There was no reduction performed in the emergency department. He has pain with pronation and supination and is tender to palpation over the fracture site. You repeat radiographs in the clinic and confirm that the fracture has not moved since initial presentation. You decide to treat this fracture with an appropriately molded cast and not refer for surgery. Which is the most correct application of the cast for the treatment of this fracture?

   A. Placement of a short-arm cast with the wrist in flexion and ulnar deviation
   B. Placement of a long-arm cast with the wrist in flexion and ulnar deviation, the forearm in neutral position, and the elbow flexed at 90 degrees
   C. Placement of a long-arm cast with the wrist in mild extension and ulnar deviation, the forearm in neutral position, and the elbow flexed at 90 degrees
   D. Placement of a long-arm cast with the wrist in mild extension and ulnar deviation, the forearm in supination, and the elbow flexed at 90 degrees
   E. Placement of a long-arm cast with the wrist in mild extension and ulnar deviation, the forearm in pronation, and the elbow flexed at 90 degrees

Correct Answer: C. Placement of a long-arm cast with the wrist in mild extension and ulnar deviation, the forearm in supination, and the elbow flexed at 90 degrees

While there is some controversy as to whether a short or long-arm cast is preferred in the treatment of non-displaced fractures, the aforementioned short-arm option is incorrectly molded. In cases of non-displaced metaphyseal fractures, the forearm should be neutral in respect to pronation and supination, and the wrist should be in functional position (which is slightly in extension and slightly in ulnar deviation), in order to prevent unnecessary stiffness. This makes all answers except for C incorrect. The long-arm cast does not allow for pronation and supination once hardened, which provides pain relief in the early stages of healing. The cast should be changed to a short-arm cast in two to three weeks to allow the patient to move the elbow to avoid stiffness, which in children can happen very quickly. Care should be taken to monitor the fracture with periodic x-rays to evaluate any potential drift of the radius due to the effects of the supinator and pronator teres muscles.

   1. Schweich P. Closed reduction and casting of distal forearm fractures in children. UpToDate. Accessed September 2, 2014 at https://www.uptodate.com/contents/closed-reduction-and-casting-of-distal-forearm-fractures-in-children.
   2. Waters PM, Bae DS. Fractures of the distal radius and ulna. In: Beaty JH, Kasser JR (eds). Rockwood and Wilkins' Fractures in Children. 7th ed. Philadelphia: Lippincott Williams & Wilkins, 2010:292-346.
   3. Diaz-Garcia RJ, Chung KC. Common myths and evidence in the management of distal radius fractures. Hand Clin 2012 May;28(2):127-133.

186. You are seeing a 16-year-old soccer player with the eye injury noted in the picture. Which of the following statements is true?

   A. This injury, which is often caused by sneezing, should be treated with topical antibiotics and followed up in your office within 24 to 48 hours
   B. This is an uncommon injury in sports, as it is mostly seen in motor vehicle trauma
   C. This injury can be associated with sickle cell disease, hemophilia, and Von Willebrand's disease
   D. This is usually an isolated injury to the posterior chamber of the eye

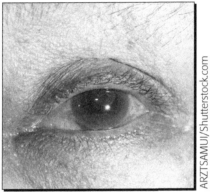

Correct Answer: C. This injury can be associated with sickle cell disease, hemophilia, and Von Willebrand's disease

This is a hyphema, which represents blood in the anterior chamber of the eye. While trauma is the most common cause, patients with underlying RBC or bleeding disorders are also at higher risk. As a rule, larger hyphemas will be obvious during general inspection of the eye, but smaller ones may only be noted by shining a light source tangentially across the eye or during a fundoscopic or slit-light eye examination. Answer A is incorrect for many reasons. As opposed to many corneal injuries, topical antibiotics are not the mainstay of treatment for this problem. Sneezing is usually associated with subconjunctival hemorrhages, which are usually a benign problem. Hyphemas are potentially serious eye injuries, indicating another possible underlying structural eye injury that can raise intraocular pressure. Therefore, the workup for a hyphema mandates a visual acuity test, pupillary response, intraocular pressure measurement, and slit-lamp examination, mandating that athletes with this problem be seen by an ophthalmologist or in the emergency department. Answer B is incorrect, since 50% of traumatic hyphemas are attributed to sports trauma. Answer D is incorrect, as hyphemas involve the anterior chamber of the eye.

1. Weber TS. Training room management of eye conditions. Clin Sports Med 2005 Jul;24(3):681-693.
2. Pokhrel PK, Loftus SA. Ocular emergencies. Am Fam Physician 2007 Sep 15;76(6):829-836.
3. Wipperman JL, Dorsch JN. Evaluation and management of corneal abrasions. Am Fam Physician 2013 Jan 15;87(2):114-120.

Test 1 Answers, Critiques, and References

187. What is an important physical finding in head trauma?

   A. Battle's sign
   B. Castell's sign
   C. Kehr's sign
   D. Tactile fremitus

Correct Answer: A. Battle's sign

Battle's sign is ecchymosis over the mastoid, which can be indicative of a skull fracture. Castell's sign is a percussion test for splenomegaly. Kehr's sign is shoulder pain caused by splenic rupture. Tactile fremitus is a test for pneumothorax.

1. Kutcher JS, Giza CC. Sports concussion diagnosis and management. Continuum (Minneap Minn) 2014 Dec;20(6 Sports Neurology):1552-1569. doi: 10.1212/01.CON.0000458974.78766.58.

188. Your last patient of the day is a 17-year-old male soccer player complaining of progressive left-sided scrotal pain over the past eight hours. He reports a kick to the scrotum and groin during a collision with another player in a game earlier this morning. He has developed nausea and vomiting in the past hour. On physical examination, his left testicle is elevated and oriented transversely compared to the right testicle. What is the next step in management of this athlete?

A. Manual detorsion, followed by ice pack and compression to the scrotum
B. Referral to the emergency department for an emergent evaluation by urology
C. Schedule for urgent ultrasound within 24 to 48 hours
D. Urinalysis and CBC with differential

Correct Answer: B. Referral to the emergency department for an emergent evaluation by urology

The patient is exhibiting classic signs of testicular torsion, which is a medical emergency. Delays in diagnosis and definitive treatment can result in decreased fertility or loss of a testis. Immediate referral to a urologist for surgical exploration is critical. Although the likelihood of testicular salvage decreases if the patient has been symptomatic more than six to eight hours, all highly suspicious cases of testicular torsion should be referred emergently to urology. A high index of suspicion should be maintained for all patients who have two or more of the following: pain less than 24 hours, elevated testicle, transverse lie of the testicle, nausea or vomiting, and abnormal cremasteric reflex. Answer A is incorrect, because manual detorsion is typically unsuccessful in patients with symptoms greater than six hours and does not replace the need for surgical exploration. Answer C is incorrect, because obtaining advanced imaging should not delay the immediate referral to urology for emergent surgical consultation. Answer D is incorrect, because laboratory tests are typically negative in cases of testicular torsion.

1. Ogunyemi O, Abel E, Weiker M, Kim E. Testicular torsion. Medscape. Accessed July 10, 2015 at http://emedicine.medscape.com/article/2036003.
2. Sharp VJ, Kieran K, Arlen AM. Testicular torsion: diagnosis, evaluation, and management. Am Fam Physician 2013 Dec 15;88(12):835-840.
3. Galejs L, Kass E. Diagnosis and treatment of the acute scrotum. Am Fam Physician 1999 Feb 15;59(4):817-824.

189. You are the physician at the finish line tent of a large marathon when a 44-year-old female runner collapses 100 meters before the finish line. The athlete is confused, sweating profusely, and cannot walk. A rectal temperature is obtained, revealing a temperature of 103 degrees Fahrenheit (39.4 degrees Celsius). Which of the following methods is the most effective treatment?

    A. Help the athlete walk it off
    B. Continuous spraying of cool water
    C. Apply ice to the neck, axilla, and groin
    D. Ice water immersion

Correct Answer: D. Ice water immersion

The athlete has heat stroke, despite only having a temperature of 103 degrees Fahrenheit (39.4 degrees Celsius). Since the athlete has mental confusion, this demonstrates there is end organ damage, and she needs to be cooled rapidly. Ice water is the preferred method of cooling a heat stroke patient. It can cool at a rate of 0.25 degrees Fahrenheit (-17.6 degrees Celsius) per minute. While the other answers will provide cooling, these other methods do not provide rapid enough cooling.

1. Gaffing SL. Cooling methods for heatstroke victims. Ann Intern Med 2000 Apr 18;132(8):678.
2. American College of Sports Medicine, Armstrong LE, Casa DJ, Millard-Stafford M, Moran DS, Pyne SW, et al. American College of Sports Medicine position stand. Exertional heat illness during training and competition. Med Sci Sports Exerc 2007 Mar;39(3):556-572.

190. Which of the following statements is correct regarding an epidural and subdural hematoma?

  A. Only subdural hematomas can be monitored by CT scan and managed non-operatively
  B. Subdural hematomas more commonly exhibit a higher Glasgow Coma Score (GCS) on admission to the emergency department
  C. An epidural hematoma is normally due to a bleeding middle meningeal artery, caused by a temporal skull fracture
  D. A subdural hematoma on CT scan demonstrates localized bleeding between the dura and skull
  E. If treated early, prognosis for subdural hematoma is better than that for epidural hematoma

Correct Answer: C. An epidural hematoma is normally due to a bleeding middle meningeal artery, caused by a temporal skull fracture.

Epidural hematoma (EDH) and subdural hematoma (SDH) are neurosurgical emergencies that should be identified quickly and triaged to a nearby trauma center. EDH can often occur with a concomitant skull fracture overlying the temporal bone. EDH is due to laceration of the middle meningeal artery, with the bleeding found between the dura and the skull. SDH is usually due to a brain parenchymal laceration, with bleeding within the dura. An EDH may be seen more commonly in sports, while SDH is seen in high-impact trauma (e.g., motor vehicle accidents, falls, and assaults). The hallmark of an EDH is a brief loss of consciousness after a head injury, followed by a "lucid" interval. The patient is temporarily neurologically intact during the lucent period, but may deteriorate rapidly. With SDH, most patients present with loss of consciousness after a severe head injury (a lower Glasgow Coma Scale and therefore poorer prognosis). SDH less frequently presents with a lucid interval. CT scan is the test of choice in diagnosing both of these conditions. Non-operative management may be indicated in patients who are neurologically stable after an EDH, but those with a SDH often require emergent evacuation of the hemorrhage, unless it is small and stable.

1. McBride W. Intracranial epidural hematoma in adults. UpToDate. Accessed December 21, 2018 at https://www.uptodate.com/contents/intracranial-epidural-hematoma-in-adults.
2. McBride W. Subdural hematoma in adults: etiology, clinical features, and diagnosis. UpToDate. Accessed December 21, 2018 at https://www.uptodate.com/contents/subdural-hematoma-in-adults-etiology-clinical-features-and-diagnosis.
3. Morris SA, Jones WH, Proctor MR, Day AL. Emergent treatment of athletes with brain injury. Neurosurgery 2014 Oct;75 Suppl 4:S96-S105.
4. Davis G, Marion DW, Le Roux P, Laws ER, McCrory P. Clinics in neurology and neurosurgery—extradural and subdural haematoma. Br J Sports Med 2010 Dec;44(16):1139-1143.

191. A 22-year-old male soccer player is stung by a bee on the practice field. He approaches you on the sideline and is quickly noted to have pronounced wheezing. You run for your medical bag and when you return moments later his wheeze is less audible but he is still in respiratory distress. You notice that his lips are beginning to swell, and he is increasingly panicked. After telling the athletic trainer at your side to call 911, what is your first action?

   A. Establish intravenous access
   B. Administer 0.5 mL of Epinephrine (1:1,000) intramuscularly
   C. Administer 0.3 mL of Epinephrine (1:100,000) subcutaneously
   D. Give the patient 50 mg of diphenhydramine, monitor closely, and repeat every four hours as needed

Correct Answer: B. Administer 0.5 mL of epinephrine (1:1,000) intramuscularly

This patient is experiencing anaphylaxis. This hypersensitivity reaction can occur within minutes of an insect sting and can progress quickly from mild urticaria to respiratory distress, collapse, and death. The treatment is immediate administration of epinephrine. The 0.5 mL dose of 1:1,000 concentration is recommended to be given intramuscularly, as this has been found to absorb more quickly than subcutaneous injections. Diphenhydramine may be given in response to an allergic reaction, but it is not first-line therapy for anaphylaxis. Albuterol may be given to asthmatic patients who present with exacerbation, but it is not helpful in response to anaphylaxis. IV access should be obtained, if feasible, but this should occur after epinephrine administration.

   1. Mustafa SS. Anaphylaxis. Medscape. Accessed July 15, 2011 at http://emedicine.medscape.com/article/135065-overview.
   2. Tang AW. A practical guide to anaphylaxis. Am Fam Physician 2003 Oct 1;68(7):1325-1333.

192. What sign helps to differentiate a simple pneumothorax from a tension pneumothorax?

    A. Tracheal deviation away from the affected side
    B. Unilateral chest pain
    C. Dyspnea
    D. Open wound to the chest

Correct Answer: A. Tracheal deviation away from the affected side

A simple pneumothorax may be spontaneous or traumatic. Spontaneous pneumothorax is more likely to occur in sports that involve a change in intrathoracic pressure, such as weight lifting and scuba diving. Traumatic pneumothorax is more likely to occur secondary to rib fracture. A tension pneumothorax will occur when a pneumothorax is accompanied by progressive accumulation of air in the pleural space, with the resultant increase in intrathoracic pressure causing a shift of the mediastinal structures away from the pneumothorax, as well as a decrease in venous return and cardiac output. An open pneumothorax is a pneumothorax accompanied by open wound to the chest (sucking chest wound). The other choices can be seen in all three types of pneumothorax, simple, tension, or open. Tracheal deviation away from the affected side will only be seen in a tension pneumothorax. Tracheal deviation away from the affected side will be accompanied by jugular venous distension and hypotension.

1. Hull JH, Ansley L, Robson-Ansley P, Parsons JP. Managing respiratory problems in athletes. Clin Med 2012 Aug;12(4):351-356.
2. Partridge RA, Coley A, Bowie R, Woolard RH. Sports-related pneumothorax. Ann Emerg Med 1997 Oct;30(4):539-541.

Test 1 Answers, Critiques, and References

193. A 32-year-old male soccer player suffered a contusion of his left lower leg against the goal post while playing. He developed swelling and tenderness over his left tibia. He is taken to the emergency room after the game finished. X-rays showed a non-displaced tibial shaft fracture (see images). He is immobilized with a cast and sent home. Five hours later, he comes back to the hospital, complaining of terrible pain that is worsening and does not respond to prescribed narcotics. On arrival, he starts complaining of tingling of the left lower extremity that he did not have when he came to the emergency room before. He has normal sensation and normal peripheral pulses of lower extremities. He is given IV narcotics, but pain is not going away. What is the most appropriate next step in the management of this case?

    A. Admit him to the hospital for observation, keep his leg in the cast with constant elevation, and consult orthopedics the next day
    B. Remove the cast and place a splint instead, discharge him from the hospital, and tell him to keep ice and elevation at all times when resting and to follow up with orthopedics as an outpatient
    C. Consult the neurologist on call immediately
    D. Remove the cast and immediately consult the foot and ankle orthopedist on call

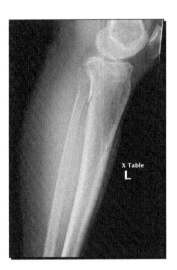
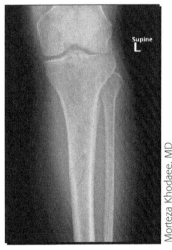

Morteza Khodaee, MD

Correct Answer: D. Remove the cast and immediately consult the foot and ankle orthopedist on call

This athlete most likely has acute compartment syndrome (ACS) at the left lower leg level. Diagnosis depends on a high clinical suspicion and an understanding of risk factors, pathophysiology, and subtle physical examination findings. The typical high-risk scenario for ACS is a male patient younger than 35 years of age, involved in a high energy sport or a roadway collision, resulting in a tibial shaft fracture. He will go on to develop acute compartment syndrome of the leg in less than 10 hours and require emergent fasciotomy. Diagnosis of ACS in this patient is primarily a clinical one, but can be confirmed with invasive intra-compartmental pressure monitoring or non-invasive near infrared spectroscopy (NIRS). Therefore, consulting a specialist who can perform emergent compartment testing and emergent fasciotomy is the right Answer. ACS occurs as a result of two factors occurring in isolation or simultaneously: an increase in the contents of an enclosed space (e.g., bleeding) and/or a decrease in the volume of a space (e.g., tight cast). In this case, leaving the patient in a cast will be contraindicated. Also, as previously mentioned, he will likely need emergent fasciotomy. This patient cannot be sent home. He will likely need emergent fasciotomy. Consulting a neurologist is not indicated. The management of ACS is surgical.

1. Mabvuure NT, Malahias M, Hindocha S, Khan W, Juma A. Acute compartment syndrome of the limbs: current concepts and management. Open Orthop J 2012;6:535-543.
2. Taylor RM, Sullivan MP, Mehta S. Acute compartment syndrome: obtaining diagnosis, providing treatment, and minimizing medicolegal risk. Curr Rev Musculoskelet Med 2012 Sep;5(3):206-213.
3. Erdoss J, Dlaska C, Szatmary P, Humenberger M, Vecsei V, Hajdu S. Acute compartment syndrome in children: a case series in 24 patients and review of the literature. Int Orthop 2011 Apr;35(4):569-575.

194. A 44-year-old male travels from Florida to a ski resort in Colorado at an altitude of 9,600 feet (2,926 m) in one day for a ski vacation. He has been there before and had no problems during that trip. One day after arriving, he began complaining of a headache and some minor nausea, with trouble sleeping. His mental status was normal. Which of the following is true?

    A. This patient has early HACE, as a result of the altitude change in one day
    B. This patient would likely benefit from acetazolamide
    C. This patient would likely benefit from sildenafil
    D. This patient would likely benefit from using over-the-counter Ginkgo biloba

Correct Answer: B. This patient would likely benefit from acetazolamide

This patient has traveled above 2,800 m in one day and has the symptoms of acute mountain sickness (AMS), including headache, nausea, and difficulty sleeping. This is considered mild AMS. Treatments include descent or oxygen, as well as acetazolamide, and in some cases, dexamethasone. Sildenafil and Ginkgo Biloba are not recommended for treatment of mild AMS, but may have a role in prevention.

1. Luks AM, McIntosh SE, Grissom CK, Auerbach PS, Rodway GW, Schoene RB, et al. Wilderness Medical Society practice guidelines for the prevention and treatment of acute altitude illness: 2014 update. Wilderness Environ Med 2014 Dec;25(4 Suppl):S4-S14. doi: 10.1016/j.wem.2014.06.017.

195. According to the most recent AMSSM position stand on concussion management (based on 2012 statement), which of the following is correct in the immediate assessment of a suspected concussion injury?

   A. Standard sideline tests are reliable across age, ethnic, and sports groups
   B. Neuroimaging should be ordered for all athletes
   C. There should be no same-day return to play for any athlete diagnosed with a concussion
   D. Only physicians should be allowed to make the diagnosis of a concussion injury
   E. Balance disturbance is both a sensitive and specific indicator of concussion injury

Correct Answer: C. There should be no same-day return to play for any athlete diagnosed with a concussion

There are no studies validating consistency in any of the recognized standard sideline assessments when comparing age groups, ethnicity of athletes, or sports type. It is also unclear if these tests are more useful if a pre-injury baseline test was completed. Neuroimaging should only be obtained when there is concern for intra-cerebral bleeding. The majority of these injuries are not associated with visible brain trauma on conventional CT and MRI brain imaging protocols. Any licensed healthcare provider who has requisite training and competency in the diagnosis and management of concussion may make the diagnosis and remove the athlete from play. Balance impairment is very specific, but not very sensitive. Sideline balance assessment must take into account fatigue, lower extremity injury, field and weather conditions, shoe or cleat type, and any assistive bracing or taping of the lower extremity. It is clear now that athletes suspected of concussion injury should not be allowed to return to play in the same game, given the risk of compounded or worsened injury.

   1. Harmon KG, Drezner J, Gammons M, Guskiewicz K, Halstead M, Herring S, et al. American Medical Society for Sports Medicine position statement: concussion in sport. Clin J Sport Med 2013 Jan;23(1):1-18.

196. An 18-year-old male rugby player is involved in a high-velocity collision during a match. He falls to the ground, clutching his left knee, saying he felt a "big pop." Your on-field examination shows marked laxity, with varus and valgus stress of the knee in full extension and a positive Lachman's maneuver. Palpation of the dorsalis pedis and posterior tibialis pulses are diminished in left leg. What is the next appropriate step for management?

    A. Reassure the athlete that he has suffered a sprain
    B. Arrange for an MRI for suspected anterior cruciate ligament (ACL) tear
    C. Emergent transportation to a local ED for an angiogram to evaluate for popliteal artery injury
    D. Keep the athlete on the sideline and check serial ankle brachial indexes (ABI), watching for worsening signs of ischemia

Correct Answer: C. Emergent transportation to a local ED for an angiogram to evaluate for popliteal artery injury

True knee dislocations, defined as a loss of tibiofemoral articulation and multiple ligament injuries, need to be treated as potential orthopedic emergencies. The recognized mechanism is typically a high-velocity impact, but case reports have shown non-contact knee dislocations may occur as well. Popliteal artery injuries occur in up to 40% of these injuries, and a delay in recognition by eight hours can lead to irreversible limb ischemia, requiring above-the-knee amputation. Patients suspected of having multiple ligaments disrupted or marked laxity should be emergently referred to a local ED that is equipped to handle vascular emergencies. The knee joint should be reduced if still grossly dislocated or pulses are absent. It is important to keep in mind that a knee dislocation with spontaneous relocation could harbor a vascular injury as well. If any hard signs of vascular injury are present (e.g., expanding hematoma, absent pulses, bruit, or hemorrhage), the patient should receive an immediate intraoperative popliteal angiogram by a vascular surgeon. Any patient with an ABI > 0.90 and present distal pulses may be admitted and observed with serial examinations, plus ABIs for at least 24 hours, because a vascular injury may mature from an initial discreet, intimal tear. Prior to surgical ligament reconstruction, a duplex ultrasound is needed to confirm the integrity of the popliteal artery, evaluate normal flow, and rule out intimal tears that could present post-operatively.

1. Nicandri GT, Chamberlain AM, Wahl CJ. Practical management of knee dislocations: a selective angiography protocol to detect limb-threatening vascular injuries. Clin J Sport Med 2009 Mar;19(2):125-129.
2. Goga IE, Gongal P. Severe soccer injuries in amateurs. Br J Sports Med 2003 Dec;37(6):498-501.
3. Putukian M, McKeag DB, Nogle S. Noncontact knee dislocation in a female basketball player: a case report. Clin J Sport Med 1995 Oct;5(4):258-261.

197. Which of the following is true regarding commotio cordis?

    A. Little League Baseball now requires the batter to wear chest protectors for prevention in children under 12 years of age
    B. The apparent mechanism for death is ventricular fibrillation, induced by an abrupt blunt precordial blow during a specific time in the cardiac cycle
    C. Baseballs thrown at 20 mph, a blow in the left area of the heart, and blunt impacts are associated with more deadly outcomes in commotio cordis
    D. With rapid defibrillation, cardiac support, and AED maneuvers, greater than 25% of individuals may survive commotio cordis
    E. Impact must occur within the QRS of the cardiac cycle in order for ventricular fibrillation to occur and cause commotio cordis

Correct Answer: B. The apparent mechanism for death is ventricular fibrillation, induced by an abrupt blunt precordial blow during a specific time in the cardiac cycle

Ventricular fibrillation is the mechanism of death for commotio cordis and is induced by the blunt precordial blow that occurs in the upslope of the T wave and causes sudden death in athletes. Little League Baseball has discussed chest protectors and has reviewed comfort, fit and effectiveness, but no requirements are currently in place. Baseballs thrown at more than 40 mph and blows in the center of the chest and precordial area are associated with more deadly outcomes. Despite rapid defibrillation and AED maneuvers, less than 10% of patients with commotio cordis survive.

1. Link MS. Pathophysiology, prevention, and treatment of commotio cordis. Curr Cardiol Rep 2014;16(6):495. doi: 10.1007/s11886-014-0495-2.
2. Walker J, Calkins H, Nazarian S. Evaluation of cardiac arrhythmia among athletes. Am J Med 2010 Dec;123(12):1075-1081.

198. A 26-year-old male triathlete presents to your clinic with a right shoulder injury after a crash during the bike stage of a race three days prior. He reports that he was 10 miles into the stage when he felt slightly dizzy for a split second. The next thing he remembered was that he was on the ground. He was taken to the emergency department, where shoulder x-rays were negative. He also had a normal ECG and normal head CT. He denies any symptoms other than mild pain to his right shoulder. His examination is normal except for abrasion (road rash) to his right upper arm. He is hoping for clearance to participate in an event next weekend. What is the best management plan for this patient?

    A. Provide wound care instructions, and clear the patient to participate as tolerated
    B. Obtain a repeat ECG and an echocardiogram. If both tests are normal, clear him to participate
    C. Refer him to cardiology and only clear him for running (not cycling or swimming) until further assessment
    D. Hold him from any athletic participation and refer him to cardiology

Correct Answer: D. Hold him from any athletic participation and refer him to cardiology

This athlete suffered a syncopal episode during exertion, which increases his risk significantly for ominous cardiac abnormalities. He will require a full cardiac workup before clearance for any athletic participation can be considered. While a repeat ECG and echocardiogram are reasonable tests to obtain, it is general consensus that these athletes should be worked up and cleared by, or in conjunction with, a cardiologist, given that additional testing (such as event monitor or stress testing) may be indicated.

1. O'Connor FG, Levine BD, Childress MA, Asplundh CA, Oriscello RG. Practical management: a systematic approach to the evaluation of exercise-related syncope in athletes. Clin J Sport Med 2009 Sep;19(5):429-434.
2. Colivicchi F, Ammirati F, Santini M. Epidemiology and prognostic implications of syncope in young competing athletes. Eur Heart J 2004 Oct;25(19):1749-1753.
3. Natarajan B, Nikore V. Syncope and near syncope in competitive athletes. Curr Sports Med Rep 2006 Dec;5(6):300-306.

199. You are covering a high school football game when one of the players goes in for a tackle with his head down and does not immediately get up off the field. You suspect an acute cervical spine injury. Which of the following pieces of equipment should be removed while you maintain in-line cervical stabilization and await emergency transport?

   A. Facemask
   B. Helmet
   C. Shoulder pads
   D. Remove no equipment

Correct Answer: A. Facemask

The facemask should be removed to allow for airway management in the event of airway collapse, especially in the case of a high cervical injury. The helmet should never be removed alone. When removing football equipment, it is an "all or none" approach (i.e., helmet and shoulder pads always come off together). The helmet and shoulder pads should be left in place, however, until the athlete has been transported to the hospital. Generally, initial radiographs are taken with equipment on, while the athlete is still on the spine board. Even in cases where the athlete appears stable, it is prudent to remove the facemask before transport. Facemask removal is best done by a person with experience, and two methods of removal should always be available (screwdriver and trainer's angels, for example).

1. Waninger KN. Management of the helmeted athlete with suspected cervical spine injury. Am J Sports Med 2004 Jul-Aug;32(5):1331-1350.
2. Jacobson B, Cendoma M, Gdovin J, Cooney K, Bruening DJ. Cervical spine motion during football equipment-removal protocols: a challenge to the all-or-nothing endeavor. Athl Train 2014 Jan-Feb;49(1):42-48.

200. A 45-year-old female with type 2 diabetes mellitus on oral medications and insulin has recently started an exercise program after speaking with you for recommendations. She often finds herself unable to complete the one-hour exercise class, as she is diaphoretic and weak. She reports mild dizziness and increased thirst, as well as a fast pulse. A trainer finds her blood sugar to be 45 mg/dL. What recommendation is true regarding her situation?

   A. She should try to exercise in the evening, because hypoglycemia is more likely in the morning than the evening due to diurnal variation in growth hormone and cortisol
   B. She has exercise-induced hypoglycemia and should always check her blood sugar 30 minutes before exercise, with goals in the range of 150 to 200 mg/dL
   C. If her blood sugar is higher than 250 mg/dL, she is safe to exercise, as hyperglycemic numbers are safer than hypoglycemic numbers during exercise
   D. In order to prevent these episodes, she should exercise before meals, instead of afterwards, and keep her pre-meal insulin and medications the same
   E. Since her class is only one hour long, she needs adequate hydration, rather than extra carbohydrate snacks to avoid hypoglycemia

Correct Answer: B. She has exercise-induced hypoglycemia and should always check her blood sugar 30 minutes before exercise, with goals in the range of 150 to 200 mg/dL

Checking her blood sugar 30 minutes before exercise and after exercise is optimal. She should keep pre-exercise blood sugars in the range of 150 to 200 mg/dL. Hypoglycemia is least likely when exercising in the morning and most likely when exercising in the evening, due to diurnal variation in growth hormone and cortisol. If blood sugars before exercise are starting at 250 to 300 mg/dL, her blood sugar may actually rise, rather than fall, during exercise. Exercising while hyperglycemic can be just as dangerous as hypoglycemic. She should decrease pre-meal insulin, and exercise about 30 to 60 minutes after a meal, in order to keep her blood sugars adequate during and after exercise. If exercising longer than 45 minutes, she will need to consume food containing carbohydrates equal to one or two exchanges, with fluid every 30 minutes during the exercise in order avoid hypoglycemia. Post-exercise hypoglycemia may also occur several hours to a full day after intense or prolonged exercise, because of increased insulin sensitivity and depletion of muscle and liver glycogen stores. In order to prevent this, she needs to reduce pre-exercise insulin, increase pre-, intra-, and post-exercise carbohydrate intake, and monitor post-exercise blood sugars frequently, even at night, considering snacks as necessary.

1. Barclay L. New recommendations regarding exercise and type 2 diabetes issued. Medscape. Accessed October 1, 2012 at https://www.medscape.org/viewarticle/533929.
2. Colberg SR, Sigal RJ, Fernhall B, Regensteiner JG, Blissmer BJ, Rubin RR, et al. The American College of Sports Medicine and the American Diabetes Association: joint position statement executive summary. Diabetes Care 2010 Dec;33(12):2692-2696.
3. American College of Sports Medicine and American Diabetes Association joint position statement. Diabetes mellitus and exercise. Med Sci Sports Exerc 1997 Dec;29(12):i-vi.

4

Test 2 Answers, Critiques, and References

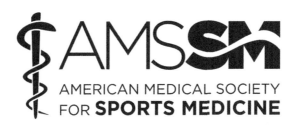

1. A 20-year-old collegiate soccer player presents to the training room with a complaint of groin pain that radiates to the testicle, a situation that has been going on for about four months. He cannot identify an acute injury as a cause. The pain is worse after practices or games, and has been increasing in intensity. He has not lost any weight, and there has been no recent increase in his level of training. He does not complain of any lumps in the groin. On exam, the testicle is normal in size, and no masses are present. No hernia, provocation, or bulge is palpated, even with Valsalva maneuvers. You elicit pain with resisted hip flexion, and with palpation of the posterior inguinal wall and pubic tubercle. The single-leg hop test does not elicit pain. What is the most likely diagnosis?

    A. Acute adductor strain
    B. Sports hernia
    C. Femoral neck stress fracture
    D. Inguinal hernia

Correct Answer: B. Sports hernia

A sports hernia is a syndrome of chronic pain due to injury and or weakness of the complex of the posterior inguinal canal, conjoined tendon, and the common adductor origin. It is most common in cutting sports, such as football, basketball, soccer, and hockey. Rehabilitation includes balancing shear forces/strength across the pelvis, relative rest, and occasionally surgery. The history does not suggest an acute injury to the adductors. Femoral neck stress fracture is less likely, because the patient is able to tolerate a single-leg hop, and he has not had a recent increase in physical activity or weight loss. There are no palpable findings of an inguinal hernia noted on exam, even with Valsalva.

1. Caudill PH, Nyland JA, Smith CE, Yerasimides J, Lach J. Sports hernias: a systematic literature review. Br J Sports Med 2008 Dec;42(12):954-964. doi: 10.1136/bjsm.2008.047373. Review.
2. Johnson JD, Briner WW. Primary care of the sports hernia: recognizing an often-overlooked cause of pain. Phys Sportsmed 2005 Feb;33(2):35-39. doi: 10.3810/psm.2005.02.50.
3. Lee AD, Briner WW. Sports hernias. In: Bracker MD (ed). The 5-Minute Sports Medicine Consult. 2nd ed. Philadelphia: Lippincott Williams & Wilkins, 2011:552-553.

2. A 20-year-old ballet dancer presents with sudden proximal posterior thigh pain after practice yesterday. He had been practicing for a performance, when he felt a pop during his grande jeté. Which of the following would limit his return to participation?

   A. Full concentric strength
   B. Injury involving the proximal free tendon
   C. Active straight leg raise deficit
   D. Pain-free range of motion

Correct Answer: B. Injury involving the proximal free tendon

This athlete has sustained a type II hamstring injury, which involves the proximal free hamstring tendon of the semimembranosus, near the ischial tuberosity. These types of injuries typically are common in dancers and occur due to excessive stretch of the hamstrings, and can take quite some time to heal and allow return to full function and activity. Longer recovery and return-to-play considerations include the presence of pain over the injury site, the site location (longer time to return for injuries at the proximal free tendon), and the presence of a passive straight-leg raise deficit. Recovery protocols should include eccentric strength training (after full concentric strength obtained), shockwave therapy, soft tissue mobilization, and a graduated return to play. Return to play can occur when pain has resolved, strength is returned, and motion is full. Lack of complete healing is a leading risk factor of reinjury. In contrast to type II injuries, type I hamstring injuries are eccentric injuries, occurring when the muscle contracts at the terminal swing phase in running. The long head of the biceps femoris is typically injured at the proximal muscle-tendon junction, a common site of injury for strains. Concentric, and then eccentric, strength training, with pain-free motion, are components of recovery for type I injuries as well.

1. Drezner JA. Practical management: hamstring muscle injuries. Clin J Sport Med 2003 Jan;13(1):48-52.
2. Chu SK, Rho ME. Hamstring injuries in the athlete: diagnosis, treatment, and return to play. CSMR 2016 May-Jun;15(3):184-190. doi: 10.1249/JSR.0000000000000264.

3. Which of the following has a significant association with the risk of future ankle sprains?

    A. Current ankle taping
    B. Previous contralateral ankle injury
    C. Positive single-leg balance test
    D. Current ankle bracing

Correct Answer: C. Positive single-leg balance test

The association between a positive single-leg balance test (SLB) and future ankle sprains is significant. Controlling for confounding variables, the relative risk for an ankle sprain with a positive SLB test was 2.54 (95% confidence interval, 1.02 to 6.03) in a recent study. Athletes with a positive SLB test who did not tape their ankles had an increased likelihood of developing ankle sprains. The relative risk for ankle sprain for a positive SLB test and negative taping was 8.82 (1.07 to 72.70). A history of previous ankle injury was not associated with future ankle sprains in this study, though ipsilateral injury has been shown to be a risk factor previously.

1. Trojian TH, McKeag DB. Single leg balance test to identify risk of ankle sprains. Br J Sports Med 2006 Jul;40(7):610-613. doi: 10.1136/bjsm.2005.024356.
2. Janssen KW, Kamper SJ. Ankle taping and bracing for proprioception. Br J Sports Med 2013 May;47(8):527-528. doi: 10.1136/bjsports-2012-091836. Epub 2012 Oct 26.

4. Which of the following has evidence-based support for use in the rehabilitation of acute ankle sprains?

   A. Electrical stimulation
   B. External ankle supports
   C. Acupuncture
   D. Therapeutic ultrasound

Correct Answer: B. External ankle supports

External ankle supports, such as walking boots and functional ankle braces, are evidence-based options for use in the treatment and rehabilitation of ankle sprains, both in the acute phase and for prevention of recurrent ankle injury. Although commonly used in many different clinical settings, electrical stimulation, acupuncture, and therapeutic ultrasound lack similar evidence-based support for use with this injury.

1. van den Bekerom MP, van der Windt DA, Ter Riet G, van der Heijden GJ, Bouter LM. Therapeutic ultrasound for acute ankle sprains. Cochrane Database Syst Rev 2011 Jun 15;(6):CD001250. doi: 10.1002/14651858.CD001250.pub2.
2. Feger MA, Goetschius J, Love H, Saliba SA, Hertel J. Electrical stimulation as a treatment intervention to improve function, edema or pain following acute lateral ankle sprains: a systematic review. Phys Ther Sport 2015 Nov;16(4):361-369. doi: 10.1016/j.ptsp.2015.01.001. Epub 2015 Jan 26.
3. Kim TH, Lee MS, Kim KH, Kang JW, Choi TY, Ernst E. Acupuncture for treating acute ankle sprains in adults. Cochrane Database Syst Rev 2014 Jun 23;(6):CD009065. doi: 10.1002/14651858.CD009065.pub2.

5. The men's soccer athletic trainer at the university you cover asks for your opinion on an athlete. One of the starting players was home in Ecuador for the summer and tore his Achilles tendon. He had surgery, and the coach wants to know the fastest way for him to get back to playing. Following an acute Achilles tendon rupture and subsequent surgical repair, which of the following postoperative rehabilitation protocols is safe, and associated with earlier return to function and significantly higher subjective patient outcomes (patient satisfaction)?

   A. Non-weight-bearing in a rigid cast for at least six weeks
   B. Early, dynamic postoperative ankle motion and weight-bearing in a brace
   C. Early loading with eccentric exercises using heavy weights
   D. Stair-climbing protocol, with multiple, prolonged sessions per week
   E. Isometric stretching using a fixed weight

Correct Answer: B. Early, dynamic postoperative ankle motion and weight-bearing in a brace

A recent meta-analysis of randomized controlled trials and a review of literature regarding time to return to play, complications, and subjective patient outcomes following an acute Achilles tendon rupture and subsequent surgical repair supports the use of early, dynamic postoperative ankle motion and weight-bearing using a brace. Non-weight-bearing status in a rigid cast (Answer A) is a postoperative method used following surgical repair, and while safe, it does not lead to early return to function and patient satisfaction scores as significantly as does the early, dynamic postoperative ankle motion and weight-bearing in a brace. Answers C, D, and E are not appropriate in the acute postoperative period.

1. McCormack R, Bovard J. Early functional rehabilitation or cast immobilization for the postoperative management of acute Achilles tendon rupture? A systematic review and meta-analysis of randomized controlled trials. Br J Sports Med 2015 Oct;49(20):1329-1335. doi: 10.1136/bjsports-2015-094935. Epub 2015 Aug 17.
2. Phan K, Campbell RJ, Kamper SJ. Early weight-bearing and rehabilitation versus immobilization following surgical Achilles tendon repair (PEDro synthesis). Br J Sports Med 2016 Dec;50(24):1550-1551. doi: 10.1136/bjsports-2016-096310. Epub 2016 May 18.

6. A 42-year-old male baseball pitcher player presents to your office with a history of shoulder impingement and corresponding signs on physical exam. Which of the following conditions has the most relevance for successful rehabilitation of this problem?

   A. Scapulothoracic dyskinesis
   B. Prominence of the lateral border of the scapula
   C. Increased internal, compared to external, range of motion of the shoulder
   D. Mild pain and limited weakness of the rotator cuff immediately after pitching

Correct Answer: A. Scapulothoracic dyskinesis

Scapulothoracic dyskinesis is an abnormal set of motions and positions affecting the relative position of the scapula and the proximal humerus. Etiologies include nerve or muscle injury, muscle inhibition, and glenohumeral stiffness or laxity. Mechanical dysfunction may result in impingement and insufficient translation of energy from the lower body. Prominence of the medial, as opposed to the lateral, border of the scapula is often seen with scapulothoracic dyskinesis. Glenohumeral internal range of motion deficit (GIRD) is often seen in throwing athletes with shoulder pain and can be treated with sleeper stretch, among other rehabilitation approaches. Mild weakness of the rotator cuff can be seen even in asymptomatic pitchers if tested immediately after pitching, likely from fatigue and/or pain. More significant weakness would be a cause for concern, however.

1. Young C. Throwing injuries of the upper extremity: clinical presentation and diagnostic approach. UpToDate. Accessed December 1, 2018 at https://www.uptodate.com/contents/throwing-injuries-of-the-upper-extremity-clinical-presentation-and-diagnostic-approach.
2. Kibler WB, Ludewig PM, McClure PW, Michener LA, Bak K, Sciascia AD. Clinical implications of scapular dyskinesis in shoulder injury: the 2013 consensus statement from the "Scapular Summit." Br J Sports Med 2013 Sep;47(14):877-885. doi: 10.1136/bjsports-2013-092425. Epub 2013 Apr 11.

7. A 14-year-old female soccer player presents to the office with a two-week history of right anterior knee pain, without a preceding injury. Physical examination shows full range of motion, no effusion, and intact ligaments. She has pain over the lateral patella facet. Hamstring and iliotibial band flexibility are normal. Her knee goes into valgus with one-leg squat. X-rays are normal. What is the most appropriate initial management of this condition?

   A. MRI knee
   B. Physical therapy, with an emphasis on hip strengthening
   C. Patella-stabilizing brace
   D. Physical therapy, with an emphasis on vastus medialis strengthening

Correct Answer: B. Physical therapy, with an emphasis on hip strengthening

In this case, her history and physical examination are most consistent with the patellofemoral pain syndrome. Recent meta-analyses from 2016 have concluded that physical therapy, with an emphasis on both knee and hip function, has both short-term and long-term benefits, and is the preferred therapy for patellofemoral pain syndrome. Since she has evidence of weak functional hip abductors (i.e., her knee goes into valgus with a single-leg squat), physical therapy should target hip girdle strength, rather than her vastus medialis. Those same meta-analyses did not find any definitive evidence for taping or bracing, making a patella-stabilizing brace an incorrect choice. MRI is not indicated, because her history and her physical exam do not suggest internal derangement.

1. Crossley KM, Stefanik JJ, Selfe J, Collins NJ, Davis IS, Powers CM. 2016 patellofemoral pain consensus statement from the 4th International Patellofemoral Pain Research Retreat, Manchester. Part 1: terminology, definitions, clinical examination, natural history, patellofemoral osteoarthritis and patient-reported outcome measures. Br J Sports Med 2016 Jul;50(14):839-843. doi: 10.1136/bjsports-2016-096384. Epub 2016 Jun 24.
2. Crossley KM, van Middelkoop M, Callaghan MJ, Collins NJ, Rathleff MS, Barton CJ. 2016 patellofemoral pain consensus statement from the 4th International Patellofemoral Pain Research Retreat, Manchester. Part 2: recommended physical interventions (exercise, taping, bracing, foot orthoses and combined interventions). Br J Sports Med 2016 Jul;50(14):844-852. doi: 10.1136/bjsports-2016-096268. Epub 2016 May 31.

8. A 19-year-old female soccer goalie receives a direct blow to the face from blocking a shot on goal. She develops pain and blurred vision in the right eye, and is removed from the field. On exam, you see a collection of blood in the anterior chamber of the right eye and diagnose her with a hyphema. Appropriate management includes which of the following?

   A. Since the hyphema collection covers less than 25% of anterior chamber, she may continue playing with the use of protective eyewear
   B. Advise patient to rest, safely apply ice, take anti-inflammatory as needed for pain, and follow up with her ophthalmologist within the next one to two days
   C. Start antibiotic ointment immediately, as there is a high likelihood of developing associated bacterial infection
   D. Refer to ophthalmologist for prompt evaluation

Correct Answer: D. Refer to ophthalmologist for prompt evaluation

A hyphema is an accumulation of blood in the anterior chamber of the eye. It is most often caused by blunt trauma to the eye, leading to microvascular injury to the ciliary mechanism. Symptoms may include pain, swelling, blurred vision, photophobia, and pupillary constriction or dilatation. This requires prompt evaluation by an ophthalmologist. Treatment includes a rigid, nonocclusive shield, a period of limited activity or bed rest, head elevation, discontinuation of aspirin and NSAIDs, and close follow-up. Potential long-term effects and complications include glaucoma, particulate accumulation in the anterior chamber, and rebleeding. The patient should be monitored closely during the first few days after injury, as this is the highest-risk time frame for rebleeding.

1. Schaefer MP. Head, ears, eyes, nose, and throat injuries and conditions. In: Harrast MA, Finnoff JT (eds). Sports Medicine Study Guide and Review for Boards. New York: Demos Medical Publishing, 2012:336-337.
2. Oldham GW. Hyphema. American Academy of Ophthalmology. EyeWiki. Accessed December 2, 2018 at https://eyewiki.aao.org/Hyphema.

9. A 15-year-old lacrosse player presents for concussion assessment from an injury suffered the previous day. His parents say he was hit from behind and think the opponent's stick or elbow hit the back of his skull. The player and his parents are concerned about his headache, dizziness, and bruising to the right mastoid area. He reports ongoing symptoms that have not improved, including headache, sleep disturbance, dizziness, and neck pain. On exam, the patient has moderate tenderness along his occiput, his temporal bones, and ecchymoses superficial to his mastoid area. You remember reading about "Battle's sign" describing ecchymoses along the mastoid area. This exam finding is suspicious for?

   A. Vestibular problem
   B. Cervical spine injury
   C. Skull fracture
   D. Tumor

Correct Answer: C. Skull fracture.

A mastoid ecchymosis after trauma is suspicious for a skull fracture that may have been missed or inadequately imaged. While CT scans are not helpful in most concussions, they are indicated when Battle's sign is present to assess for skull fracture and intracranial hemorrhage. While he is experiencing vestibular symptoms, his mastoid ecchymosis in the setting of trauma is more concerning for a missed skull fracture, and not indicative of an injury to the vestibular nucleus or semicircular canal. A cervical spine injury could be present, but Battle's sign is not specifically associated with neck injuries. A tumor is unlikely to be associated with this finding.

1. Tubbs RS, Shoja MM, Loukas M, Oakes WJ, Cohen-Gadol A. William Henry Battle and Battle's sign: mastoid ecchymosis as an indicator of basilar skull fracture. J Neurosurg 2010 Jan;112(1):186-188. doi: 10.3171/2008.8.JNS08241.
2. Collins JM, Krishnamoorthy AK, Kubal WS, Johnson MH, Poon CS. Multidetector CT of temporal bone fractures. Semin Ultrasound CT MR 2012 Oct;33(5):418-431. doi: 10.1053/j.sult.2012.06.006.

10. When it comes to concussions, which of the following has less evidence to support it as a risk factor for an athlete to suffer a concussion?

    A. Prior concussion
    B. Participation in collision sports
    C. Female gender
    D. Participation in women's lacrosse

Correct Answer: D. Participation in women's lacrosse

High-quality evidence for risk modifiers in concussion remains sparse. Prior concussion, collision sports, female sex, and (for females) participation in women's soccer are the strongest known risk factors. Evidence for most other factors is inconclusive.

1. Matuszak JM, McVige J, McPherson J, Willer B, Leddy J. A practical concussion physical examination toolbox: evidence-based physical examination for concussion. Sports Health 2016 May-Jun;8(3):260-269. doi: 10.1177/1941738116641394.
2. Scopaz KA, Hatzenbuehler JR. Risk modifiers for concussion and prolonged recovery. Sports Health 2013 Nov;5(6):537-541. doi: 10.1177/1941738112473059.

11. During a karate tournament, an eight-year-old male has a primary tooth knocked out. After a thorough examination, it was found to be a complete avulsion, with no fracture. No swelling of his gum line is noted, and there are no concerns for airway obstruction. What do you do with the tooth?

   A. Stop the bleeding and do nothing with the tooth
   B. Place the tooth in Hank's Balanced Salt Solution
   C. Place the tooth in normal saline solution
   D. Place the tooth in his mouth next to his buccal mucosa
   E. Place the tooth in room-temperature tap water

Correct Answer: A. Stop the bleeding and do nothing with the tooth

A primary tooth should never be replanted. Ideally, replantation of an avulsed permanent tooth should occur within 5 to 10 minutes. The success of replantation is much less likely after 20 minutes. Answers B, C, and D are all viable solutions if the tooth is unable to be replanted prior to seeing a dentist. While long-term storage (> 20 minutes) in water (Answer E) has an adverse effect on periodontal ligament healing, sit is a better choice than dry storage.

1. Young EJ, Macias CR, Stephens L. Common dental injury management in athletes. Sports Health 2015 May;7(3):250-255. doi: 10.1177/1941738113486077.
2. American Academy on Pediatric Dentistry Council on Clinical Affairs. Guideline on management of acute dental trauma. Pediatr Dent 2008-2009;30(7 Suppl):175-183.

12. A 20-year-old elite rower presents to your office complaining of worsening pain over her right chest wall for the past few weeks. Recently, she has developed point tenderness over the sixth rib. After examining her, you are concerned about a possible stress fracture. Which of the following is true regarding stress fractures of the ribs?

   A. Stress fractures tend to have acute onset and are often associated with obvious deformity at the fracture site
   B. Chronic stress of upper body muscles, which attach to the ribs, can result in stress fractures of the ribs
   C. Increased shortness of breath, pain, cyanosis, and subcutaneous emphysema are commonly seen with stress fractures of the ribs
   D. Serial rib series radiographs would be used in this athlete to diagnose her stress fracture and to monitor healing

Correct Answer: B. Chronic stress of upper body muscles, which attach to the ribs, can result in stress fractures of the ribs

Because there are multiple muscle attachments of the rib to the neck and upper extremities, chronic stress can lead to stress fractures. Stress fractures of the ribs are more likely to occur in sports with increased upper body demands, such as golf, rowing, baseball, tennis, racquet sports, and weight lifting. Overuse and poor technique can contribute to rib stress fractures. Stress fractures of the rib present with gradual onset of rib pain, with or without deformity. Symptoms such as increasing shortness of breath, pain, cyanosis, and subcutaneous emphysema may indicate serious life-threatening conditions requiring emergent attention. Serial rib series radiographs are not necessary for isolated fractures of ribs 5-9. Rib series radiographs are indicated if ribs 1-2 or ribs 9-12 are involved. Furthermore, stress fractures typically are not visible on plain films of the chest until very late in their healing, when they develop a visible callus. Often a bone scan of the chest wall is the preferred instrument to diagnose rib stress fractures early in the pathologic process.

1. Davis BA, Finnoff JT. Diagnosis and management of thoracic and rib pain in rowers. Curr Sports Med Rep 2003 Oct;2(5):281-287.
2. Baker R. Fracture, rib. In: Bracker MD (ed). The 5-Minute Sports Medicine Consult. 2nd ed. Philadelphia: Lippincott Williams & Wilkins, 2011:246-247.
3. Karlson K, French A. Initial evaluation and management of rib fractures. UpToDate. Accessed December 2, 2018 at www.uptodate.com/contents/initial-evaluation-and-management-of-rib-fractures.

13. A 19-year-old female presents to the campus health service with anterior shin pain, ongoing now for three weeks. She denies any trauma, disordered eating, or infrequent menstrual periods. She is on the Ultimate Frisbee team and they are a month into the season. Her pain now starts with practice, and on long practice days or game days her shins stay sore afterwards. She noted recently it hurts to walk—but resting does not relieve the pain; it is residual. Also, she reports the area of pain on the shin is much more localized than before. There is no numbness or tingling. What is the most likely diagnosis?

    A. Chronic exertional compartment syndrome (CECS)
    B. Shin splints (medial stress syndrome)
    C. Common peroneal nerve entrapment
    D. Stress reaction to the tibia
    E. Popliteal artery entrapment

Correct Answer: D. Stress reaction to the tibia

This scenario has some of the distinguishing characteristics of a stress reaction: no obvious trauma, increasing pain over time with increasing stress or load, no noticeable relief from a brief rest, and no numbness or tingling. The correct answer is stress reaction. Note, early on, radiographs may be difficult to demonstrate a clear periosteal reaction or later stress fracture. Stress reactions often are the result of too much microdamage to the bone (a normal response to stress/load) that cannot keep up with remodeling. Exam will reveal a local, small area of focal/point tenderness along the medial tibia. The mechanism causing bone breakdown is often an increase in the load and/or stress and a decrease in the surface area where the applied stress/load is applied. Risk factors include female athlete triad, increase in load/stress (intensity, duration, training surface), leg length discrepancy, and muscle weakness.

CECS will classically have symptoms with onset of activity (often predictable), and a pause or rest in the activity will result in abatement of symptoms and recurrence with resumption of activity. Shin splints (medial stress syndrome) are very similar, but often the symptoms do not linger after an activity. Also of note, on exam the palpable tenderness along the medial tibia is extensive (8 to 12 cm). Common peroneal nerve entrapment is noted for burning pain or numbness on the lateral aspect of the lower leg, below the knee. Patients may have inability to dorsiflex the foot. Popliteal artery entrapment syndrome is noted for increasing pain, with or without swelling, and cramping sensation in the lower extremity. Numbness is often present. It is more common in males than females. Exam demonstrates decreased pulses with active plantarflexion or passive dorsiflexion. MRI/MRA and arteriography are diagnostic.

1. Haddad SF. Stress fractures. Medscape. Accessed March 4, 2019 at https://emedicine.medscape.com/article/1270244-overview#showall.

14. Which of the following is true regarding adolescent idiopathic scoliosis management?

    A. Scoliosis screening is recommended by the United States Preventive Services Task Force (USPSTF)
    B. Initial evaluation includes MRI of the thoracolumbar spine to measure the Cobb angle
    C. Individuals with adolescent idiopathic scoliosis often need more than observation alone
    D. Apex right curves (dextroscoliosis) are most common in patients with idiopathic scoliosis. Back pain and left curves (levoscoliosis) should prompt concern for other spinal disease, such as tumor
    E. Indications for surgery are largely functional and should use the Cobb angle as the sole criteria for intervention

Correct Answer: D. Apex right curves are most common in patients with idiopathic scoliosis. Back pain and left curves should prompt concern for other spinal disease, such as tumor

Levoscolisosis is much less common than dextroscoliosis in adolescent idiopathic scoliosis, and may instead indicate another disorder. These individuals will require more thorough workup, often including MRI. Screening for scoliosis is NOT recommended by the United States Preventive Services Task Force (USPSTF). Initial evaluation includes radiography (not MRI) to measure the Cobb angle. Individuals with adolescent idiopathic scoliosis generally do well with observation alone, which is why screening is not warranted. Indications for surgery are complex and should not use the Cobb angle as the sole criteria.

1. Dolan LA, Weinstein SL. Surgical rates after observation and bracing for adolescent idiopathic scoliosis: an evidence-based review. Spine (Phila Pa 1976) 2007 Sep 1;32(19 Suppl):S91-S100.
2. Weiss HR, Goodall D. The treatment of adolescent idiopathic scoliosis (AIS) according to present evidence. A systematic review. Eur J Phys Rehabil Med 2008 Jun;44(2):177-193.

15. Which of the following statements is true regarding proximal humeral epiphysiolysis (Little League shoulder)?

    A. It typically occurs in pitchers aged 8 to 10 years old
    B. A widened proximal humeral physis on plain radiograph clinches the diagnosis
    C. The athlete is usually pain-free until the acute onset of pain
    D. It is caused by repetitive loading of the shoulder with both torque and distraction forces

Correct Answer: D. It is caused by repetitive loading of the shoulder with both torque and distraction forces

Proximal humeral epiphysiolysis is caused by repetitive loading of the humerus with the torque and distraction forces of throwing that cause microtrauma and irritation of the proximal humeral physis, which is substantially weaker than the surrounding bone. It typically presents in pitchers who are 11 to 16 years old. Asymptomatic pitchers often have widened proximal humeral physis on plain radiograph. The athlete usually complains of progressively worsening, non-focal shoulder pain with throwing.

1. Murachovsky J, Ikemoto RY, Nascimento LG, Serpone Bueno R, Strose E, Almeida LH. Does the presence of proximal humerus growth plate changes in young baseball pitchers happen only in symptomatic athletes? An x-ray evaluation of 21 young baseball pitchers. Br J Sports Med 2010 Feb;44(2):90-94. doi: 10.1136/bjsm.2007.044503. Epub 2008 Feb 28.
2. Osbahr DC, Kim HJ, Dugas JR. Little League shoulder. Curr Opin Pediatr 2010 Feb;22(1):35-40. doi: 10.1097/MOP.0b013e328334584c.
3. Young C. Throwing injuries of the upper extremity: clinical presentation and diagnostic approach. UpToDate. Accessed December 2, 2018 at https://www.uptodate.com/contents/throwing-injuries-of-the-upper-extremity-clinical-presentation-and-diagnostic-approach.

16. A 21-year-old, right-hand-dominant collegiate starting pitcher has been struggling with progressive, intermittent soreness in his right shoulder that is relieved with rest and worsens with continued pitching. Despite normal x-rays, rotator cuff sports ultrasound, and appropriate physical therapy, he continues to struggle and is moved to the bullpen to decrease his workload. Over the weekend, he goes rope-swinging at the local river with his teammates, and accidentally falls hard onto the lateral right shoulder. He has immediate severe pain, but the x-rays at the local ER are normal. A CT scan shows a one-part anatomical neck fracture of the proximal humerus. What is the best treatment option for this patient at this time?

   A. Routine icing with a shoulder sling and swathe, and allow the fracture to heal non-operatively over the next six to eight weeks
   B. Let him know his pitching career is in jeopardy and treat the fracture conservatively over the next six to eight weeks with early functional rehabilitation
   C. Refer to the orthopedic surgeon for ORIF, due to potential disruption of the blood supply and risk of avascular necrosis of the humeral head
   D. Obtain an MRI to evaluate the rotator cuff tendon for a potential supraspinatus tear that occurred with the fracture in order to expedite a recovery program

Correct Answer: C. Refer to the orthopedic surgeon for ORIF, due to potential disruption of the blood supply and risk of avascular necrosis of the humeral head

The anterolateral branch, or arcuate artery, of the anterior humeral circumflex artery provides the entire blood supply to the humeral head and is at risk of being disrupted with an anatomical neck fracture, resulting in an increased risk of avascular necrosis. Accordingly, Answer C is correct. Answers A and B are incorrect, because they emphasize conservative treatment over surgical fixation. A stable one-part fracture of the surgical neck (most common) could be treated non-operatively, but this situation states that the fracture is at the anatomical neck. Answer D is incorrect, because, although there is concern for a supraspinatus tear given his past history, it is not the best treatment option at the present time.

1. Gerber C, Schneeberger AG, Vinh TS. The arterial vascularization of the humeral head. An anatomical study. J Bone Joint Surg Am 1990 Dec;72(10):1486-1494.
2. Hettrich CM, Boraiah S, Dyke JP, Neviaser A, Helfet DL, Lorich DG. Quantitative assessment of the vascularity of the proximal part of the humerus. J Bone Joint Surg Am 2010 Apr;92(4):943-948. doi: 10.2106/JBJS.H.01144.
3. Proximal humerus fractures. Orthobullets. Accessed December 4, 2018 at https://www.orthobullets.com/trauma/1015/proximal-humerus-fractures.

17. You are asked by a colleague for assistance in interpreting a right-shoulder MRI arthrogram following injury. You make note of a tear of the posteroinferior labrum and an impaction fracture of the antero-medial humeral head. Which of the following most accurately describes the mechanism of injury?

    A. Acute strike to the right shoulder from a posteroinferior direction
    B. Repetitive overuse
    C. Trauma sustained during a tonic-clonic seizure
    D. Trauma sustained from improper technique tackling in football

Correct Answer: C. Trauma sustained during a tonic-clonic seizure

The aforementioned findings are consistent with a posterior shoulder dislocation (reverse Bankart, reverse Hill-Sachs). While rare in general, this is more commonly seen with seizures or electrocutions. Answer A is incorrect, given that this describes an injury pattern for a typical anterior shoulder dislocation. Answer B is incorrect, because this describes some form of rotator cuff injury. Answer D is incorrect, as this is a common mechanism of injury for a cervical spine injury.

1. Misamore GW, Sallay PI, Didelot W. A longitudinal study of patients with multidirectional instability of the shoulder with seven- to ten-year follow-up. J Shoulder Elbow Surg 2005 Sep-Oct;14(5):466-470.
2. Radiographs for posterior shoulder dislocation. Wheeless' Textbook of Orthopaedics. Accessed December 4, 2018 at https://www.wheelessonline.com/ortho/radiographs_for_posterior_shoulder_dislocation.
3. Robinson CM, Aderinto J. Posterior shoulder dislocations and fracture-dislocations. J Bone Joint Surg Am 2005 Mar;87(3):639-650.

18. A 40-year-old, right-handed male presents with increasing right shoulder pain with overhead activities. He denies trauma but recently returned to playing softball. The pain is located over the lateral deltoid, is aching in nature, and disrupts sleeping on the right side. He presents with an MRI demonstrating supraspinatus tendinopathy. Which physical exam finding is most likely to be present in this patient?

    A. Pain with hornblower's test
    B. Pain with empty can test
    C. Pain with lift-off test
    D. Pain with resisted external rotation

Correct Answer: B. Pain with empty can test

The empty can test examines the supraspinatus muscle. This is the most commonly injured muscle of the rotator cuff. Hornblower's test examines the teres minor. This test is done with the arm abducted to 90 degrees in the scapular plane and the elbow flexed to 90 degrees. The patient attempts to externally rotate against resistance. The lift-off test is for the subscapularis. The patient places his hand in the small of the back and attempts to internally rotate, lifting his hand off of his back, against resistance. A positive test is weakness in comparison to the opposite side. Pain with resisted external rotation stresses the infraspinatus and teres minor. The arm is at the patient's side and the elbow is flexed to 90 degrees. The examiner attempts to internally rotate the arm.

1. Stovitz SD. Evaluation of the adult with shoulder complaints. UpToDate. Accessed December 4, 2018 at https://www.uptodate.com/contents/evaluation-of-the-adult-with-shoulder-complaints.
2. Malanga GA. Rotator cuff injury. Medscape. Accessed December 4, 2018 at https://emedicine.medscape.com/article/92814-overview.

19. A 40-year-old gentleman presents to his primary care physician for severe right shoulder pain. He awoke with pain three days ago, and has not improved with over-the-counter analgesics. Now, he is unable to reach overhead with his right arm. Which of the following advice is most appropriate for this patient?

   A. An electromyography should be performed immediately to evaluate his shoulder and neck
   B. Strenuous exercise and/or infections or immune triggers can predispose individuals to this condition
   C. Urgent orthopedic surgery referral is recommended, as surgery is usually necessary
   D. The loss of passive range of motion is usually the cause of the impaired shoulder function

Correct Answer: B. Strenuous exercise and/or infections or immune triggers can predispose individuals to this condition

Neurologic amyotrophy, or Parsonage-Turner Syndrome, classically presents with new onset of severe pain, often awakening a patient from sleep. Paresis in an irregular distribution develops hours to days after the onset of pain. The long thoracic nerve, suprascapular nerve, and anterior interosseous nerves are most commonly affected. The pain typically lasts two to three weeks. The exact pathophysiologic mechanism is thought to be due to a combination of environmental factors, such as infection or immune triggers; mechanical factors, such as repetitive or strenuous activity or exercise; and individual genetic susceptibility. An EMG is often used to evaluate for evidence of acute nerve injury. On the other hand, denervation is usually not present until three to four weeks after the onset of weakness, and would most likely be normal if performed immediately. Neurolysis and nerve transfers are performed for a subset of the more severe cases that do not recover strength. The differential diagnosis for shoulder pain and weakness would include a rotator cuff tear for which an orthopedic surgery referral is one of the treatment options. The loss of shoulder function results from pain and paresis in neurologic amyotrophy or Parsonage-Turner syndrome. The loss of passive range of motion is consistent with a diagnosis of adhesive capsulitis, which typically presents with a gradual onset of diffuse shoulder pain, followed by gradual progressive loss of passive range of motion.

   1. Van Eijk JJ, Groothuis JT, Van Alfen N. Neuralgic amyotrophy: an update on diagnosis, pathophysiology, and treatment. Muscle Nerve 2016 Mar;53(3):337-350. doi: 10.1002/mus.25008. Epub 2016 Jan 20.
   2. Roberts JR. Adhesive capsulitis. Medscape. Accessed December 4, 2018 at https://emedicine.medscape.com/article/1261598-overview.

20. Which of the following is required for a diagnosis of shoulder impingement?

    A. History and physical exam of the shoulder
    B. MRI of the shoulder with gadolinium contrast
    C. MRI of the shoulder without contrast
    D. X-rays of the shoulder

Correct Answer: A. History and physical exam of the shoulder

The general pathology of subacromial impingement relates to a chronic repetitive process in which the conjoint tendon of the rotator cuff undergoes repetitive compression and microtrauma as it passes under the coracoacromial arch. However, acute traumatic injuries may also lead to this condition. Diagnosis remains a clinical one. On the other hand, advances in imaging modalities have enabled clinicians to have an increased understanding of the pathological process. Ultrasound scanning appears to be a justifiable and cost-effective assessment tool following plain radiographs in the assessment of shoulder impingement, with MRI scans being reserved for more complex cases. The addition of intra-articular contrast to an MRI (MR arthrogram) is especially helpful to evaluate the labrum.

1. Holmes RE, Barfield WR, Woolf SK. Clinical evaluation of nonarthritic shoulder pain: diagnosis and treatment. Phys Sportsmed 2015 Jul;43(3):262-268. doi: 10.1080/00913847.2015.1005542. Epub 2015 Jan 26.
2. Diercks R, Bron C, Dorrestijn O, Meskers C, Naber R, de Ruiter T, et al. Guideline for diagnosis and treatment of subacromial pain syndrome: a multidisciplinary review by the Dutch Orthopaedic Association. Acta Orthop 2014 Jun;85(3):314-322. doi: 10.3109/17453674.2014.920991. Epub 2014 May 21.
3. Khan Y, Nagy MT, Malal J, Waseem M. The painful shoulder: shoulder impingement syndrome. Open Orthop J 2013 Sep 6;7:347-351. doi: 10.2174/1874325001307010347. eCollection 2013.

21. A seven-year-old male presents to your clinic after falling off the monkey bars at his school playground. He cannot remember how he landed on the ground, but is complaining of forearm pain. On clinical examination, you notice a bowed deformity to the forearm, but a normal elbow and wrist exam. You obtain a radiograph that reveals no obvious fracture, but you do see bowing of the radius that was apparent on exam. Using the Schemitsch and Richards method, you measure the bowing of the radius to be 25 degrees. What is your next step in treatment?

   A. This abnormality is called a plastic deformity and should be reduced to an acceptable angle of less than 20 degrees
   B. Since there is no fracture, you reassure the parents and do not provide any further treatment
   C. This abnormality is called a plastic deformity, but you do not need to reduce this injury, because the patient is less than 12 years old
   D. You send him to the radiology department for a stat CT scan, because that will assist you to create a treatment plan

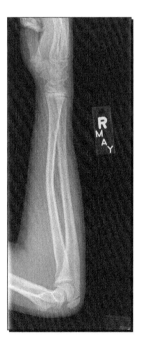
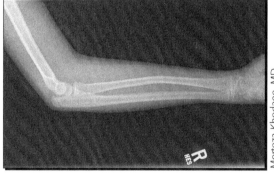

Correct Answer: A. This abnormality is called a plastic deformity and should be reduced to an acceptable angle of less than 20 degrees

Plastic deformities of the radius and ulna are common in pediatric forearm injuries. They need to be corrected if the patient is older than four years old and the bowing angle is greater than 20 degrees (using the Schemitsch and Richards method.) Answer B is incorrect, because a failure to recognize this injury will likely limit supination and pronation in this child. Accordingly, treatment is required. Answer C is incorrect, because proper remodeling will occur, without reduction, only if the patient is less than four years old. Answer D is incorrect, because a CT scan is not necessary to know how to proceed with the correct treatment option, and this will expose the child to unnecessary radiation exposure.

1. Firl M, Wunsch L. Measurement of bowing of the radius. J Bone Joint Surg Br 2004 Sep;86(7):1047-1049.
2. Sanders WE, Heckman JD. Traumatic plastic deformation of the radius and ulna. A closed method of correction of deformity. Clin Orthop Relat Res 1984 Sep;(188):58-67.
3. Murphy A, Jones J. Bowing fracture. Radiopaedia. Accessed December 4, 2018 at https://radiopaedia.org/articles/bowing-fracture.

22. You are finishing clinic for the day when a mom comes in with her two-year-old child. She relates that they were holding hands and about to cross the street when her son stepped forward toward traffic and she pulled him back by his right hand. Since then, he has refused to use his right arm and cries when his mother tries to move it. After an exam that confirms the most likely diagnosis, what is the most appropriate next step?

    A. X-ray of the elbow
    B. Surgical consult
    C. Long-arm cast
    D. Hyperpronation reduction

Correct Answer: D. Hyperpronation reduction

Nursemaid's elbow is one of the most common injuries in children under five years of age. It occurs when the child's hand is suddenly jerked up, forcing the elbow into extension and causing the radial head to slip out from the annular ligament. Diagnosis can be easily made with classic history, without the need for initial radiographs. Even in the absence of classic history, reduction can be attempted for a child with typical physical findings. Radiographs should be obtained if the history and exam does not clearly describe the nursemaid elbow. Reduction of radial head subluxation can be performed via either the supination/flexion or hyperpronation techniques. Meta analysis suggests that the hyperpronation technique is more successful and less painful.

1. Moore BR, Bothner J. Radial head subluxation (nursemaid's elbow). UpToDate. Accessed December 4, 2018 at https://www.uptodate.com/contents/radial-head-subluxation-nursemaids-elbow.
2. Krul M, van der Wouden JC, Kruithof EJ, van Suijlekom-Smit LW, Koes BW. Manipulative interventions for reducing pulled elbow in young children. Cochrane Database Syst Rev 2017 Jul 28;7:CD007759. doi: 10.1002/14651858.CD007759.pub4.

23. Which one of the following statements is correct regarding medial epicondylitis?

    A. The magnitude of grip strength impairment is greater than that seen in lateral epicondylitis
    B. Examination findings include pain with resisted wrist flexion, wrist pronation, and valgus stress testing
    C. Corticosteroid injections were shown to improve symptoms at six weeks, but showed no difference when compared with controls at three and 12 months
    D. Medial epicondylitis is more common than lateral epicondylitis in the general population

Correct Answer: C. Corticosteroid injections were shown to improve symptoms at six weeks, but showed no difference when compared with controls at three and 12 months

Grip strength impairment is greater in lateral epicondylitis than it is in medial epicondylitis. Valgus stress testing of the elbow would be more suggestive of ulnar collateral ligament insufficiency than medial epicondylitis. The prevalence of medial epicondylitis in the general population is less than 1%, compared to a prevalence of lateral epicondylitis of 1% to 2% annually in the general public.

1. Taylor SA, Hannafin JA. Evaluation and management of elbow tendinopathy. Sports Health 2012 Sep;4(5):384-393.
2. Jayanthi N. Epicondylitis (tennis and golf elbow). UpToDate. Accessed December 4, 2018 at https://www.uptodate.com/contents/epicondylitis-tennis-and-golf-elbow.
3. Sciascia A, Kibler B. The pediatric overhead athlete: what is the real problem? Clin J Sport Med 2006 Nov;16(6):471-477.

24. Which of the following statements is true regarding ulnar neuropathy in throwing athletes?

   A. Athletes with laxity of the ulnar collateral ligament are at increased risk for stretching the nerve
   B. The most common location of impingement is Guyon's canal
   C. These injuries may be treated by having the athlete wear braces that keep the elbow maximally flexed while sleeping
   D. Athletes often have a positive pronator compression test in which compression over the pronator teres reproduces symptoms

Correct Answer: A. Athletes with laxity of the ulnar collateral ligament are at increased risk for stretching the nerve

Athletes with laxity of the ulnar collateral ligament are at increased risk for stretching the ulnar nerve. Guyon's canal is a common location of ulnar nerve compression in bicyclists (handlebar palsy), but not in throwers. The fully flexed position tends to irritate ulnar cubital tunnel syndrome, and athletes are counseled to avoid this position as much as possible, particularly while sleeping. A positive pronator compression test is found in athletes with pronator syndrome, a condition that affects the median nerve.

1. Doherty TJ. Ulnar neuropathy at the elbow and wrist. UpToDate. Accessed December 4, 2018 at https://https://www.uptodate.com/contents/ulnar-neuropathy-at-the-elbow-and-wrist.
2. Young C. Throwing injuries of the upper extremity: clinical presentation and diagnostic approach. UpToDate. Accessed December 4, 2018 at https://www.uptodate.com/contents/throwing-injuries-of-the-upper-extremity-clinical-presentation-and-diagnostic-approach.
3. Petron DJ, Makovitch SA. Neurologic problems in the athlete. In: Madden CC, Putukian M, McCarty EC, Young CC (eds). Netter's Sports Medicine. 2nd ed. Philadelphia: Elsevier, 2018:265-279.

25. A 16-year-old high school football player impacts his right forearm against an opponent's helmet while tackling. He complains of pain over the point of impact at the dorsal lateral aspect of the proximal right forearm. He subsequently notes weakness with right wrist extension and finger extension, but no pain or tingling in his hand. His exam is remarkable for tenderness over the proximal edge of the supinator muscle, and diminished strength (4/5), with wrist extension and thumb and finger extension at metacarpal-phalangeal (MCP) joints. Diminished strength with forearm supination is also noted. Sensation is intact to light touch over radial and median distribution. X-ray of the right radius and ulna showed no fractures or dislocation. His most likely diagnosis is?

    A. Extensor tendon rupture
    B. Wartenberg syndrome
    C. Anterior interosseous nerve syndrome
    D. Posterior interosseous nerve syndrome

Correct Answer: D. Posterior interosseous nerve syndrome

The posterior interosseous nerve is a deep branch of the radial nerve, arising at the level of the lateral epicondyle of the humerus. It provides purely motor innervation to the extensor carpi radialis brevis (ECRB), extensor digitorum, extensor digiti minimi, extensor carpi ulnaris, supinator, abductor pollicis longus, extensor pollicis brevis, extensor pollicis longus, and extensor indicis. It does not innervate the triceps, anconeus, brachioradialis, or extensor carpi radialis longus (ECRL). Entrapment or injury to the nerve would result in weakness of wrist, thumb, and finger extension, as well as weakness in forearm supination. No sensory involvement is noted, however. Forearm extensor tendon rupture would result in loss of active extension of fingers. Wartenberg syndrome involves the superficial branch of radial nerve, which provides sensory innervation to the proximal dorsal three and one-half phalanges and dorsal hand. Patient presents with pain and decreased sensation over dorsoradial hand and dorsal thumb and index finger. No weakness of wrist or hand is noted. Etiology involves a tight band or clothing worn around the forearm. The anterior interosseous nerve is principally a motor nerve, arising from the median nerve, and traveling on the volar surface of the flexor digitorum profundus (FDP). It innervates the radial half of FDP, the flexor pollicis longus (FPL), and the pronator quadratus. Motor weakness is noted in radial half of FDP and FPL, with inability to make a circle with the index finger and thumb (OK sign).

1. Tennet TD, Woodgate A. Posterior interosseous nerve dysfunction in the radial tunnel. Current Orthopaedics 2008 Jun;22(3):226-232. doi.org/10.1016/j.cuor.2008.03.001.
2. Stanley J. Radial tunnel syndrome: a surgeon's perspective. J Hand Ther 2006 Apr-Jun;19(2):180-184.

26. During the preparticipation physical exam, an athlete has 20/20 vision in his left eye and 20/80 vision in his right eye. When is an athlete considered functionally monocular?

   A. When the best corrected vision in one eye is less than 20/40
   B. When the best uncorrected vision in one eye is less than 20/40
   C. When the best corrected vision in one eye is less than 20/80
   D. When the best uncorrected vision in one eye is less than 20/100

Correct Answer: A. When the best corrected vision in one eye is less than 20/40

Up to 90% of eye injuries in sports are preventable with proper protection. High-risk sports for eye injury include those with balls, pucks, and/or sticks. Many sports at highest risk for eye injury already mandate eye protection (hockey, lacrosse). All athletes should be made aware of the availability of eye protection in their respective sports. Certain athletes, however, are at higher risk for eye injury. Those at increased risk are athletes with high degrees of myopia and a history of retinal detachment, injury, infection, or eye surgery. Special care should be taken in athletes with significantly worse vision in one eye. These functionally monocular athletes would suffer significant disability with the loss of the better eye. Any athlete with the best corrected vision in one eye of less than 20/40 (with the other eye better than 20/40) should be considered functionally monocular. Mandatory eye protection is recommended for these athletes, and participation in sports in which eye protection cannot be used (e.g., boxing, full-contact martial arts) should be prohibited.

1. American Academy of Family Physicians, American Academy of Pediatrics, American College of Sports Medicine, American Medical Society for Sports Medicine, American Orthopaedic Society for Sports Medicine, American Osteopathic Academy of Sports Medicine. Bernhardt DT, Roberts WO (eds). Systems-based examination. Preparticipation Physical Evaluation. 4th ed. Elk Grove Village, IL: American Academy of Pediatrics, 2010:80-82.
2. Rodriguez JO, Lavina AM, Agarwal A. Prevention and treatment of common eye injuries in sports. Am Fam Physician 2003 Apr 1;67(7):1481-1488.

Test 2 Answers, Critiques, and References

27. A six-month-old child is brought to your office because he refuses to use his right hand. The child seems drowsy, but his mother states that she just gave him an OTC antihistamine/decongestant for an upper respiratory infection. The child weighs eight pounds, and his head circumference is 40 cm. He is sleepy, but awakens easily, and is non-toxic in appearance. His right wrist is swollen. You radiograph his right upper extremity and find a fracture, along with a partially calcified scaphoid bone. What is the most important next step?

   A. Reassure the child's mother that this type of fracture heals very well in a child of this age
   B. Immobilize the child's arm and wrist with a long-thumb spica cast
   C. Radiograph the opposite extremity and ask the child's mother some more questions about the mechanism of injury and any other injuries or illnesses that the child may have
   D. Consult an orthopedic surgeon comfortable treating patients in this age group

Correct Answer: C. Radiograph the opposite extremity and ask the child's mother some more questions about the mechanism of injury and any other injuries or illnesses that the child may have

This child's weight and head circumference are well under the fifth percentile for his age. This type of injury is almost unheard of in patients of this age. In addition, it is difficult to completely identify injuries of other carpal bones with plain radiographs, due to lack of calcification of the carpal bones in children of this age. These facts alone should alert you to dig deeper into the history for other disease processes. In your differential, you must entertain the possibility of child abuse or neglect. Even though this is the first time you examined the child, you have a duty to ask more questions and consider searching for other signs of neglect (recently there has been some controversy about repeating radiation to infants by the American Academy of Pediatrics). If there is no compelling explanation (e.g., chronic metabolic disease such as renal failure, osteopenia imperfecta) to explain this injury, child welfare officials should be notified.

   1. Prawer A. Radius and ulna fractures. In: Eiff MP, Hatch RL (eds). Fracture Management for Primary Care. 2nd ed. Philadelphia: Saunders, 2012:102-129.
   2. Toluwumi J. Forearm fractures in emergency medicine. Medscape. Accessed December 6, 2018 at https://emedicine.medscape.com/article/824949.

28. A 15-year-old female basketball player comes to the clinic after jamming her index finger trying to catch a basketball. On examination, she is tender at the DIP joint, and isolation of the DIP joint reveals an inability to actively extend the distal phalanx. Passive extension is intact. X-ray reveals a fracture of the proximal dorsal aspect of the distal phalanx. What is the proper treatment for this condition?

   A. Surgical referral within seven days
   B. Splinting the DIP joint in extension for eight weeks, followed by one month of night splinting
   C. Buddy taping the index finger to the middle finger
   D. Splinting the DIP joint with a clam-shell splint, with motion at DIP beginning after two to three weeks

Correct Answer: B. Splinting the DIP joint in extension for eight weeks, followed by one month of night splinting

This athlete has suffered a mallet finger, an injury occurring due to an axial load with a resultant disruption of the terminal extensor mechanism. It results in the patient being unable to actively extend at the DIP joint. Failure to treat properly could result in a permanent flexion deformity. The treatment for mallet finger involves splinting the DIP in extension for eight weeks, followed by one month of night splinting (Answer B). Jersey finger, an avulsion fracture involving the flexor digitorum profundus and its attachment to the palmar aspect of the distal phalanx, may result in tendon retraction and should be referred to a hand surgeon urgently (Answer A). Buddy taping is indicated for stable, non-displaced, extra-articular phalangeal fractures (Answer C). Clam-shell splints are indicated for phalangeal tuft fractures, in which the DIP is splinted only for a short time, and motion is allowed with protection after immobilization (Answer D).

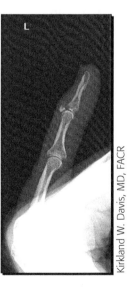

1. Borchers JR, Best TM. Common finger fractures and dislocations. Am Fam Physician 2012 Apr 15;85(8):805-810.
2. Oetgen ME, Dodds SD. Non-operative treatment of common finger injuries. Curr Rev Musculoskelet Med 2008 Jun;1(2):97-102. doi: 10.1007/s12178-007-9014-z.
3. Bowen JE. Phalangeal fractures treatment and management. Medscape. Accessed December 6, 2018 at https://emedicine.medscape.com/article/98322.

29. A 35-year-old, right-hand-dominant police officer presents to the emergency room after falling off his horse on an outstretched hand. He complains of severe pain in his wrist and numbness in his index finger and thumb. Radiographs reveal that he has a perilunate disassociation, Mayfield Classification Stage III. Which of the following is true?

   A. An emergent MRI arthrogram is required to confirm the diagnosis
   B. This patient requires immediate operative treatment of this condition
   C. The numbness in his hand is due to injury of the radial artery
   D. This condition is best treated by emergent closed reduction, followed by open reduction, ligament repair, fixation, and carpal tunnel release

Correct Answer: D. This condition is best treated by emergent closed reduction, followed by open reduction, ligament repair, fixation, and carpal tunnel release

A perilunate dislocation occurs with high energy injuries in which the wrist is extended and ulnarly deviated. In a perilunate dislocation, the lunate stays in position, and the carpus dislocates. This can cause an acute carpal tunnel syndrome. The treatment of choice for this injury is to emergently reduce the dislocation, and then, the patient should go to surgery for open reduction, ligament repair, fixation, and carpal tunnel release. The wrist should be reduced ASAP, and the treating practitioner should not wait until the patient is taken to the OR. Further imaging is not needed and leads to delay in treatment. The neurologic symptoms indicate median nerve entrapment in the carpal tunnel, not vascular compromise.

1. Melone CP Jr, Murphy MS, Raskin KB. Perilunate injuries repair by dual dorsal and volar approaches. Hand Clin 2000 Aug;16(3):439-448.
2. Kozin SH. Perilunate injuries diagnosis and treatment. JAAOS, 1998 Mar-Apr;6(2):114-120.

Test 2 Answers, Critiques, and References

30. A 20-year-old discus thrower presents to clinic after dropping the discus onto his left middle finger. On exam, he has diffuse swelling and pain of the distal aspect of his finger, with a large subungal hematoma involving the entire nail bed. The nail is still attached. He is neurovascularly intact, and the tendon function of his finger is intact. What is the most appropriate intervention at this time?

   A. Place him in an aluminum splint with a compression dressing and prescribe RICE therapy
   B. Trephinate the hematoma
   C. Obtain radiographs, and if no evidence of fracture, offer trephination
   D. Obtain radiographs, and if no evidence of fracture, removal of nail and drainage of hematoma

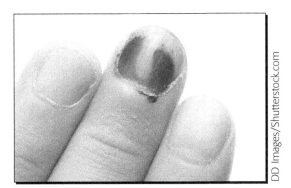

Correct Answer: C. Obtain radiographs, and if no evidence of fracture, offer trephination

Subungal hematomas that involve greater than 50% of the nail matrix are often associated with laceration of the nail bed. When there is a distal phalangeal fracture, the incidence of nail bed laceration is 94%. Historically, treatment of subungual hematoma of greater than 50% of the nail bed required removal of the nail to repair the nail bed. Outcomes have shown, however, that if the nail is still attached, even partially, or no displacement of the paronychia, no significant difference in outcomes with or without repair of nail bed were seen. Note, trephination is contraindicated when a fracture requires repair. Answers A and B are incorrect, because this injury should be radiographed to evaluate for fracture.

1. Sutijono D. Nailbed injuries. Medscape. Accessed December 6, 2018 at https://emedicine.medscape.com/article/827104.
2. Saladino RA, Antevy P. Management of fingertip injuries. UpToDate. Accessed December 6, 2018 at https://www.uptodate.com/contents/management-of-fingertip-injuries.

31. Which of the following is true regarding carpal tunnel syndrome?

   A. Patients have a positive Froment's sign
   B. Patients have numbness and tingling over the ulnar side of the ring finger and the fifth digit
   C. Nerve conduction studies are not helpful with diagnosis
   D. Patients typically complain of numbness and tingling affecting the first three digits and the radial side of the ring finger

Correct Answer: D. Patients typically complain of numbness and tingling affecting the first three digits and the radial side of the ring finger

The carpal bones and the transverse carpal ligament form the carpal tunnel. It contains the median nerve, as well as the finger flexor tendons (FDS and FDP) and flexor pollicis longus. Answer D is correct, because the medial nerve supplies sensation to the first three digits and the radial half of the fourth digit. Keep in mind that sometimes patients with pure carpal tunnel syndrome will still complain of symptoms in all the fingers, even though the ulnar nerve supplies the ulnar half of the ring finger and the fifth digit (small finger). Answer C is incorrect, because EMG studies usually show slowing of the nerve as it crosses the carpal tunnel. A positive Froment's sign is characteristic of ulnar neuropathy, specifically testing the adductor pollicis.

   1. LeBlanc KE, Cestia W. Carpal tunnel syndrome. Am Fam Physician 2011 Apr 15;83(8):952-958.
   2. Werner R. Electrodiagnostic evaluation of carpal tunnel syndrome and ulnar neuropathies. PM R 2013 May;5(5 Suppl):S14-S21. doi: 10.1016/j.pmrj.2013.03.027. Epub 2013 Mar 28.

32. A 33-year-old, right-hand-dominant male presents with complaint of right wrist pain. He is a competitive racquetball player and reports falling on his wrist during a match yesterday. He states the pain is worst over the ulnar side of the wrist, and he is especially concerned that he may have a fracture, because he has a "clicking" sensation when he moves his wrist. On physical exam, there is tenderness to palpation in the area between the ulnar styloid and pisiform. He has no tenderness with palpation of the hand or fingers. The pain is worsened with ulnar deviation of the wrist, as well as resisted pronation and supination. Patient is unable to lift the exam table with his wrist supinated, due to worsening pain. Given the physical exam findings, what is the most likely diagnosis?

   A. Ulnar styloid fracture
   B. Extensor carpi ulnaris tendinopathy
   C. Triangular fibrocartilage complex injury
   D. Scapholunate ligament disruption

Correct Answer: C. Triangular fibrocartilage complex injury

The triangular fibrocartilage complex (TFCC) is the major ligamentous structure of the distal radioulnar joint (DRUJ) and the ulnar carpus. Patients with TFCC injuries typically present with pain over the ulnar side of the wrist. Pain is often after a fall, but can be seen after repetitive use. Patients often complain of clicking or grinding sensation with range of motion. Examination often reveals tenderness between the ulnar styloid and pisiform ("fovea sign"). Ulnar deviation and resisted pronation/supination tend to reproduce the patient's symptoms. Answer A is incorrect, because while it may be possible for a fracture of the ulnar styloid to be present, the patient's presentation is more consistent with an injury to the TFCC. Answer B is incorrect, because the patient would likely have tenderness the entire length of the extensor carpi ulnaris tendon, including up to the insertion at the base of the fifth metacarpal. Answer D is incorrect, because the patient is tender on the ulnar side of the wrist and has pain with ulnar deviation as opposed to radial deviation, which would be more likely to be seen with disruption to the scapholunate ligament.

1. Verheyden JR. Triangular fibrocartilage complex injuries. Medscape. Accessed December 6, 2018 at https://emedicine.medscape.com/article/1240789.
2. Rettig AC. Athletic injuries of the wrist and hand part I: traumatic injuries of the wrist. Am J Sports Med 2003 Nov-Dec;31(6):1038-1048.

33. An 18-year-old male college freshman presents to your training room with right dorsal wrist pain. He denies any trauma or new activities. He is rowing in the freshman boat and is training for his spring racing season. The pain is located on the dorsal surface of his wrist, on the radial side, just proximal to the proximal carpal row. He states the pain is worse when he extends his wrist while he is feathering his oar. You diagnose him with intersection syndrome and place him in a thumb spica wrist splint. What does the second dorsal compartment of the wrist contain?

   A. Extensor pollicis longus and abductor pollicis longus
   B. Extensor pollicis brevis and abductor pollicis longus
   C. Extensor carpi radialis brevis and extensor carpi radialis longus
   D. Extensor carpi radialis brevis and extensor pollicis longus

Correct Answer: C. Extensor carpi radialis brevis and extensor carpi radialis longus

Intersection syndrome is a tenosynovitis, in which the first dorsal compartment crosses over the second dorsal compartment of the wrist. The first dorsal compartment contains the extensor pollicis brevis and abductor pollicis longus. The second dorsal compartment contains the extensor carpi radialis longus and extensor carpi radialis brevis. The third dorsal compartment contains the extensor pollicis longus. The fourth dorsal compartment contains the extensor digitorum and extensor indicis. The fifth dorsal compartment contains the extensor digiti minimi. The sixth dorsal compartment contains the extensor carpi ulnaris.

   1. Thompson JC. Hand. Netter's Concise Orthopaedic Anatomy. 2nd ed. Philadelphia: Saunders Elsevier, 2010:155.
   2. Steinberg DR. Intersection syndrome. Medscape. Accessed December 6, 2018 at https://emedicine.medscape.com/article/1242239.

34. Which of the following is true of De Quervain's tenosynovitis?

A. The two tendons involved are the abductor pollicis brevis and the extensor pollicis longus
B. The grind test is the most sensitive test for diagnosis
C. A corticosteroid injection into the tendon sheath of the second dorsal compartment has been shown to alleviate symptoms.
D. Splinting of the thumb and wrist can relieve symptoms

Correct Answer: D. Splinting of the thumb and wrist can relieve symptoms

While splinting of the thumb and wrist relieves symptoms, most patients find the loss of the thumb for functional activities too restrictive and do not consistently wear the splints. Answer A is incorrect, because the two tendons involved are the extensor pollicis brevis and the abductor pollicis longus. Answer B is incorrect, as the Finklestein's test is the most sensitive test for diagnosis. Answer C is incorrect, because a corticosteroid injection into the tendon sheath of the first (not second) dorsal compartment has been shown to alleviate symptoms.

1. Meals R. De Quervain tenosynovitis. Medscape. Accessed December 7, 2018 at https://emedicine.medscape.com/article/1243387.
2. Shehab R, Mirabelli M. Evaluation and diagnosis of wrist pain: a case-based approach. Am Fam Physician 2013 Apr 15;87(8):568-573.

35. You are working at a ski resort in Colorado when a skier comes in complaining of pain in his thumb after a fall. Following your examination, you suspect that he has suffered a gamekeeper's thumb or skier's thumb, without evidence of dislocation. What x-ray finding would prompt you to refer this patient to an orthopedic surgeon?

    A. Stener lesion
    B. Bankart lesion
    C. Segond fracture
    D. Bennett fracture

Correct Answer: A. Stener lesion

Stener lesions represent complete avulsion of the ulnar collateral ligament of the thumb and require surgical fixation. Not all bony avulsion fractures result in a Stener lesion. As a rule, only Stener lesions with attachments can be seen on an x-ray, and it may require ultrasound or MRI to be appreciated. A Bankart lesion is the detachment of the inferior glenohumeral ligament-labral complex from the anterior glenoid rim that can be seen with shoulder dislocation. A Segond fracture is an avulsion fracture of the lateral tibial condyle, and often a sign of ACL tear, though other ligament injuries can also be seen with it. A Bennett's fracture is a fracture of the base of the metacarpal extending into the CMC joint.

1. Bloom J. First (thumb) metacarpal fractures. UpToDate. Accessed December 7, 2018 at https://www.uptodate.com/contents/first-thumb-metacarpal-fractures.
2. Hannibal M. Gamekeeper's thumb. Medscape. Accessed December 7, 2018 at https://emedicine.medscape.com/article/97679.

Test 2 Answers, Critiques, and References

36. A 45-year-old man presents with sudden onset of severe right hip pain. His pain is mainly with weight-bearing. He denies any trauma or systemic symptoms. He had a similar episode of severe pain in his left hip three years ago, which resolved after several months. He did not have surgery. He has no risk factors for avascular necrosis. On examination, the patient is in distress and using crutches. He has preserved hip range of motion. His x-ray is below. What is his most likely diagnosis?

    A. Osteomyelitis
    B. Lumbar radiculopathy
    C. Avascular necrosis
    D. Transient osteoporosis of the hip
    E. Femoral neck fracture

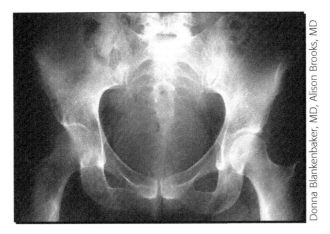

Correct Answer: D. Transient osteoporosis of the hip

The patient has transient osteoporosis of the hip (TOH). The patient has no systemic symptoms or risk factors (IV drug use, immunocompromised) to suggest osteomyelitis. Lumbar radiculopathy and avascular necrosis are possible sources of the patient's pain, but the osteoporosis in his right hip is evident on the x-ray. The right femoral head has lower bone density on plain film when compared to the left. X-ray findings of avascular necrosis (AVN) might include collapse of the cortex and local increases or decreases in bone density, but these typically affect only small areas of the cortex. MRI can differentiate between TOH and AVN. MRI shows edema in both problems, which tends to be more diffuse in TOH and more focal in the femoral head in AVN. AVN typically also shows subchondral changes. On physical exam, patients with AVN have limited hip rotation, whereas in TOH, ROM is typically preserved. TOH is treated with rest and non-weight-bearing. There is also some evidence that oral bisphosphonates may hasten recovery. It typically resolves within six months, but often recurs in either hip. TOH has been associated with low vitamin D, thyroid disease, and pregnancy, though is most commonly seen in middle-aged men.

1. Balakrishnan A, Schemitsch EH, Pearce D, McKee MD. Distinguishing transient osteoporosis of the hip from avascular necrosis. Can J Surg 2003;46(3):187-192.
2. Cahir JG, Toms AP. Regional migratory osteoporosis. Eur J Radiol 2008 Jul;67(1):2-10. doi: 10.1016/j.ejrad.2008.01.051. Epub 2008 Mar 20.
3. Kibbi L, Touma Z, Khoury N, Arayssi T. Oral bisphosphonates in treatment of transient osteoporosis. Clin Rheumatol 2008 Apr;27(4):529-532. Epub 2007 Oct 16.

37. Following hip replacement surgery, your patient was found to have an iatrogenic injury of the obturator nerve. Which of the following is true?

    A. Obturator nerve injury can be associated with quadriceps muscle weakness
    B. It innervates the adductor longus and brevis
    C. It originates from L5 and S1 nerve roots
    D. It innervates the vastus lateralis and the vastus intermedius

Correct Answer: B. It innervates the adductor longus and brevis

The obturator nerve originates from L2, L3, and L4, and can sustain an iatrogenic injury from traction of the hip during surgery. It innervates the adductor muscles of the leg, as well as provides sensation to the medial thigh. Recall that the adductor magnus also receives some innervation from the tibial nerve. All of the quadriceps muscles are innervated by the femoral nerve.

1. Stoller DW. Femoral nerve and obturator nerve. Stoller's Atlas of Orthopaedics and Sports Medicine. Philadelphia: Lippincott Williams & Wilkins, 2008:257.
2. Plowgian E, Pylwaka T. In: Daniels JM (ed). Common Musculoskeletal Problems: A Handbook. 2nd ed. New York: Springer, 2015:77-84.
3. Obturator nerve. Wheeless' Textbook of Orthopaedics. Accessed December 7, 2018 at http://www.wheelessonline.com/ortho/obturator_nerve.

38. An active 24-year-old female presents complaining of right hip pain associated with episodes of painful snapping. Which of the following is true about internal snapping hip?

   A. Physical therapy is not indicated
   B. Hip snapping is reproduced with extension of the hip from a flexed position
   C. A hip radiograph often confirms the diagnosis
   D. NSAIDs can be used for treatment, but corticosteroid injections are contraindicated

Correct Answer: B. Hip snapping is reproduced with extension of the hip from a flexed position

There are three types of snapping hip: external (iliotibial band over the greater trochanter), internal (iliopsoas over the femoral head or iliopectineal line), and intra-articular (often a labral tear). Internal hip snapping is often reproduced with extension of the hip from a flexed position, particularly if coming from an externally rotated and flexed position to an internally rotated and extended position. If painful, initial treatment options include physical therapy, NSAIDs, and corticosteroid injections. On the other hand, oftentimes, reassurance is all that is needed if it is non-painful. Surgical treatment should only be considered after failing non-operative treatments. Hip radiographs are often normal.

1. Ilizaliturri VM Jr, Camacho-Galindo J, Evia Ramirez AN, Gonzalez Ibarra YL, McMillan S, Busconi BD. Soft tissue pathology around the hip. Clin Sports Med 2011 Apr;30(2):391-415. doi: 10.1016/j.csm.2010.12.009.
2. Allen WC, Cope R. Coxa saltans: the snapping hip revisited. J Am Acad Orthop Surg 1995 Oct;3(5):303-308.

39. A 31-year-old man presents with a several month history of right knee pain and swelling. His pain has become severe with weight-bearing. There was no injury. He denies any other joint issues or any constitutional symptoms. On exam, his distal femur is tender and there is minimal soft tissue swelling. His x-ray reveals a cystic lesion in the distal femur, abutting the joint. His x-ray and MRI are below. What is the most likely diagnosis?

   A. Enchondroma
   B. Giant cell tumor of bone
   C. Nonossifying fibroma
   D. Intramedullary bone infarct

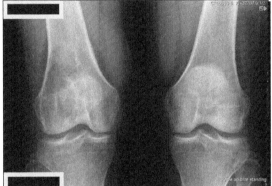

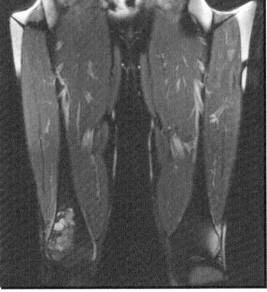

Correct Answer: B. Giant cell tumor of bone

Giant cell tumor of bone (GCT) is a cystic bone lesion that has the following features: narrow well-defined nonsclerotic transition zone, close epiphyses, eccentric lesion, and the lesion is epiphyseal and abuts the articular surface. GCT are benign but locally aggressive lesions with a 15% recurrence rate. They are treated by curettage and packing of the bone. Enchondroma (chondroid lesion) and intramedullary infarcts are sclerotic lesions. Nonossifying fibroma (fibroxanthoma, fibrous cortical defect) is a lytic lesion but does not cause pain.

1. Helms CA. Benign tumors. Fundamentals of Skeletal Radiology. 4th ed. Philadelphia: Elsevier, 2014:17-32.
2. Amanatullah DF, Clark TR, Lopez MJ, Borys D, Tamurian RM. Giant cell tumor of bone. Orthopedics 2014 Feb;37(2):112-120. doi: 10.3928/01477447-20140124-08.

40. A seven-year-old female soccer player presents to your office with pain in her left knee. The pain began during a soccer practice, and she was unable to walk after onset. On examination, she is acutely tender on the inferior aspect of her patella. She is unable to perform a straight-leg raise. What is the most likely diagnosis?

    A. Traction apophysitis of the tibial tubercle (Osgood-Schlatter's disease)
    B. Traction apophysitis of the distal patellar pole (Sindig-Larsen-Johansson disease)
    C. Patellofemoral dysfunction
    D. Patellar sleeve fracture

Correct Answer: D. Patellar sleeve fracture

A patellar sleeve fracture should be considered in children with open growth plates that present with acute onset of patellar pain during activity. The injury occurs due to excessive traction on the patellar apophysis and can be distinguished from Sindig-Larsen-Johansson disease by the inability of the patient to perform straight-leg raising (due to disruption of the knee-extensor mechanism). Because the process occurs mainly through cartilage, there may be little radiographic evidence of injury, so diagnosis is made on a clinical basis. Children with patellar sleeve fractures will require surgical repair by open reduction and internal fixation. In contrast, treatment of the more common traction apophysitis is conservative, with increased activity as tolerated. In addition, all of the other listed causes of knee pain in children tend to be more insidious in onset.

1. Chang D, Mandelbaum BR, Weiss JM. Special considerations in the pediatric and adolescent athlete. In: Frontera WR, Herring SA, Micheli LJ, Silver JK (eds). Clinical Sports Medicine, Medical Management and Rehabilitation. China: Elsevier, 2007:82-83.
2. Wright LB, Matchett WJ, Cruz CP, James CA, Culp WC, Eidt JF, et al. Popliteal artery disease: diagnosis & treatment. RadioGraphics 2004 Mar-Apr;24(2):467-479.

41. Which of the following is a dynamic stabilizer of the posterolateral corner of the knee?

    A. Fibular collateral ligament
    B. Popliteofibular ligament
    C. Popliteus tendon
    D. Arcuate ligament

Correct Answer: C. Popliteus tendon

The posterolateral corner of the knee is comprised of a complex group of tendons and ligaments which offer stability to this region. The arcuate ligament, fabellofibular ligament, fibular collateral ligament, popliteus tendon, and popliteofibular ligament make up the static stabilizers. Dynamic stabilizers consist of the popliteus muscle/tendon, biceps femoris, and lateral head of the gastrocnemius. The most important stabilizers among these are the fibular collateral ligament, popliteus tendon and muscle, and popliteofibular ligament.

1. Miller TT. Common tendon and muscle injuries: lower extremity. Ultrasound Clinics 2007:2(4);597-615. doi: 10.1016/j.cult.2007.11.005.
2. Stannard JP, Brown SL, Robinson JT, McGwin G Jr, Volgas DA. Reconstruction of the posterolateral corner of the knee. Arthroscopy 2005 Sep;21(9):1051-1059.

42. A 25-year-old male runner presents with bilateral lower extremity throbbing pain and numbness in the first web space of his feet that begins consistently after 10 minutes of intense exercise and is completely relieved with rest. He reports symptoms are brought on the following day in about half the time. What is the most likely explanation for this?

    A. His muscles are increasingly fatigued
    B. He has chronic exertional compartment syndrome and now has acute compartment syndrome
    C. He has increased muscle damage and necrosis, due to intense exercise
    D. He is experiencing the second-day phenomenon

Correct Answer: D. He is experiencing the second-day phenomenon

The patient is experiencing the second-day phenomenon, which occurs in patients with chronic exertional compartment syndrome (CECS). A patient will exercise intensely, and the following day has increased symptoms in a much shorter period of time. Muscle fatigue may occur, but is not the reason the symptoms are brought on sooner. Acute compartment syndrome occurs usually after trauma, and thus there is no reason why this patient should suddenly have acute compartment syndrome. There is no tissue necrosis, which occurs with CECS. Patients with CECS and second-day phenomenon usually have tissue ischemia, which causes the symptoms due to increased compartment pressures, but there is no tissue necrosis.

    1. Reid DC. Exercise-induced leg pain. Sports Injury Assessment and Rehabilitation. New York: Churchill Livingstone, 1992:269-300.
    2. Edmundsson D, Toolanen G, Sojka P. Chronic compartment syndrome also affects nonathletic subjects: a prospective study of 63 cases with exercise-induced lower leg pain. Acta Orthop 2007 Feb;78(1):136-142.
    3. Pedowitz RA, Hargens AR, Mubarak SJ, Gershuni DH. Modified criteria for the objective diagnosis of chronic compartment syndrome of the leg. Am J Sports Med 1990;18(1):35-40.

43. A 15-year-old tennis player presents to your office with an injury that has been present for two months. After examining him, you diagnose him with an overuse injury. He tells you that he has played tennis year-round for the last five years and trains at an elite tennis academy. He participates in weekly resistance training with a certified trainer while at the academy. You recall that you treated him successfully for a similar overuse injury one year ago. On chart review, you note that he has grown three inches in the last six months. Which of the following is true with regard to his risk factors for an overuse injury?

   A. Sport specialization at a young age has been shown to decrease injuries
   B. Resistance training leads to increased injuries in pediatric populations
   C. A history of a prior injury is an established risk factor for overuse injuries
   D. Injuries rarely occur during adolescent growth

Correct Answer: C. A history of a prior injury is an established risk factor for overuse injuries

Prior injury is a well-established risk factor for overuse injuries in this population. Early sports specialization is thought to be a risk for overuse injury and burnout. Early sports specialization is not recommended, with the exception of early entry sports, such as gymnastics or ice skating. Resistance training under proper supervision has been shown to be safe in pediatric populations. Injury risk appears to be increased during periods of rapid growth.

   1. DiFiori JP, Benjamin HJ, Brenner J, Gregory A, Jayanthi N, Landry GL, et al. Overuse injuries and burnout in youth sports: a position statement from the American Medical Society for Sports Medicine. Clin J Sport Med 2014 Jan;24(1):3-20. doi: 10.1097/JSM.0000000000000060.
   2. Roberts WO. Overuse injuries and burnout in youth sports. Clin J Sport Med 2014 Jan;24(1):1-2. doi: 10.1097/JSM.0000000000000061.

44. You are conducting preparticipation examinations for your local high school team. A 16-year-old female cross-country runner reports that her last menstrual period was approximately four months ago. Her menarche was at age 13, and her periods were regular until four months ago. She is not sexually active. She does not take any medications. There is no history of stress fractures, but she did see the athletic trainer for "shin splints" during both track and cross-country seasons last year. Body weight has been stable in the past year. Her BMI is 19. She follows a vegetarian diet but does not follow any other restrictions. The rest of her physical examination is normal. What is the next best step in management of this athlete?

   A. Refer for a DEXA
   B. Obtain more information regarding her diet history, exercise habits, and life stressors
   C. Initiate oral contraceptive pills to restore menses
   D. Order labs including beta HCG, complete blood count, basic chemistry, thyroid function tests, serum FSH, LH, and prolactin levels
   E. Instruct the athlete to add lean meats to her diet

Correct Answer: B. Obtain more information regarding her diet history, exercise habits, and life stressors

A more thorough dietary evaluation is indicated. This runner most likely has unintentionally low energy availability, but should also be screened for disordered eating. It would be inappropriate to advise adding meat to her diet, as she is a vegetarian. It is reasonable to rule out pregnancy in all cases of amenorrhea, but this patient is not sexually active. The other labs are indicated for secondary amenorrhea workup. In this case, however, more information is needed before pursuing further workup. The patient should not start oral contraceptives to stimulate menstruation without first having further workup. A DEXA scan is not indicated in this case, as the patient does not meet clinical criteria, which would include an abnormally low BMI, clinically significant fracture history, late menarche, diagnosed eating disorder, or less than six menstrual cycles over a 12-month period.

1. De Souza MJ, Nattiv A, Joy E, Misra M, Williams NI, Mallinson RJ, et al. Female athlete triad coalition consensus statement on treatment and return to play of the female athlete triad: 1st International Conference held in San Francisco, California, May 2012 and 2nd International Conference held in Indianapolis, Indiana, May 2013. Clin J Sport Med 2014 Mar;24(2):96-119. doi: 10.1097/JSM.0000000000000085.
2. Berz K, McCambridge T. Amenorrhea in the female athlete: what to do and when to worry. Pediatric Annals 2016 Mar;45(3):e97-e102. doi: 10.3928/00904481-20160210-03.

45. Which corticosteroid is most likely to cause hypopigmentation and subcutaneous fat atrophy when used for a soft-tissue injection?

   A. Betamethasone
   B. Triamcinolone
   C. Dexamethasone
   D. Hydrocortisone

Correct Answer: B. Triamcinolone

Corticosteroid injections have multiple potential complications, including infection, facial flushing, hypopigmentation, bleeding, tendon rupture, steroid flare, and soft-tissue atrophy. Hypopigmentation occurs in 1.3% to 4% of individuals undergoing steroid injections and often occurs within one to four months after the injection and resolves 6 to 30 months post-injection. Subcutaneous fat atrophy can resolve within 6 to 12 months after corticosteroid injection. More water-soluble steroid preparations, such as betamethasone, dexamethasone, and hydrocortisone, are associated with less hypopigmentation and subcutaneous fat atrophy. Of the corticosteroids listed, triamcinolone is the least water soluble and associated with the most hypopigmentation and subcutaneous fat atrophy.

1. MacMahon PJ, Eustace SJ, Kavanagh EC. Injectable corticosteroid and local anesthetic preparations: a review for radiologists. Radiology 2009;252(3):647-661. doi: 10.1148/radiol.2523081929.
2. Park S, Choi YS, Kim HJ. Hypopigmentation and subcutaneous fat, muscle atrophy after local corticosteroid injection. Korean J Anesthesiol 2013 Dec;65(6 Suppl):S59-S61. doi: 10.4097/kjae.2013.65.6S.S59.

46. While performing percutaneous needle aspiration of a knee effusion, which of the following best describes findings suggestive of an intra-articular fracture?

   A. Thin, turbid, serosanguinous fluid, with small white flecks of debris
   B. Thin, opaque, bloody fluid, with no discernible debris
   C. Thin, turbid, serosanguinous fluid, with white-cheesy clumps of debris
   D. Thin, opaque, bloody fluid, with greasy sheen or oil globules

Correct Answer: D. Thin, opaque, bloody fluid, with greasy sheen or oil globules

Synovial-lined joints feature secretory cells called synoviocytes, which produce matrix constituents, hyaluronic acid and salts, collagens, fibronectin, and synovial fluid. Synovial fluid reduces friction between bones during movement, and also provides the nutrients and lubrication for the joints. Biochemically, synovial fluid is an ultrafiltrate of plasma across the synovial membrane. In normal conditions, its biochemical composition is similar to that of plasma. While evaluating the injured and diseased joint, chemical analysis (glucose, total protein level, uric acid level) and microscopic evaluation (cell count and differential, crystal identification) can be very informative. Microbiologic, serologic, and cytologic laboratory evaluations may be indicated as well. However, physical examination of aspirated synovial fluid (appearance to include color, viscosity, other physical characteristics) can be performed at the point-of-care and provide quick and useful information. Viscosity can be empirically evaluated by forming a string of synovial fluid between the tips of the fingers. A string of 4-6 cm is considered normal. The mucin clot test can be used to evaluate viscosity, but it has little diagnostic information and is rarely used.

Normal synovial fluid is typically clear, highly viscous, colorless or faintly straw-colored, and of a small volume (a few milliliters). With articular cartilage loss, there may be small, soft, white flecks of debris. In inflammatory conditions, the synovial fluid obtained from an effused joint may appear cloudy or turbid, more densely yellow-colored, less viscous (thinner), and of a larger volume. If larger amounts of crystals are present, the fluid may appear milky or cloudy as well. In septic arthritis, the fluid may appear cloudy, yellow-green, more viscous, and occasionally with clumps of debris. In hemorrhagic conditions (hemarthrosis), the fluid may appear cloudy, reddish or brownish, and thin. Lipohemarthrosis occurs in approximately 40% of intra-articular knee fractures, and appears grossly as an oily or greasy sheen or globules floating on top of the aspirated bloody fluid. This results from leakage of marrow fat into the synovial fluid—and when tiny may take up to three hours to appear post-injury. Inspection for fat globules can be used to identify occult fractures not detected by plain radiography.

1. Dougados M. Synovial fluid cell analysis. Baillieres Clin Rheumatol 1996 Aug;10(3):519-534.
2. Johnson MW. Acute knee effusions: a systematic approach to diagnosis. Am Fam Physician 2000 Apr 15;61(8):2391-2400.
3. Aponte EM, Novik JI. Identification of lipohemarthrosis with point-of-care emergency ultrasonography: case report and brief literature review. J Emerg Med 2013 Feb;44(2):453-456. doi: 10.1016/j.jemermed.2012.07.062. Epub 2012 Sep 13.

47. Which of the following confirms the diagnosis of chronic exertional compartment syndrome (CECS)?

    A. One-minute post-exercise pressure of 28 mm Hg
    B. Pre-exercise pressure of 19 mm Hg
    C. Pre-exercise pressure of 14 mm Hg
    D. Five-minute post exercise pressure of 17 mm Hg

Correct Answer: B. Pre-exercise pressure of 19 mm Hg

The most widely used diagnostic criteria for CECS are the Pedowitz criteria, which states that CECS is present if one or more of the following intramuscular pressure criteria are met:
- Pre-exercise pressure ≥ 15 mm Hg
- One-minute post-exercise pressure ≥ 30 mm Hg
- ive-minute post-exercise pressure ≥ 20 mm Hg

1. Glorioso JE Jr, Wilckens JH. Compartment syndrome testing. In: Wilder RP, O'Connor FG, Magrum EM (eds). Running Medicine. 2nd ed. Monterey, CA: Healthy Learning, 2014:213-220.
2. Meehan WP, O'Brien MJ. Chronic exertional compartment syndrome. UpToDate. Accessed December 7, 2018 at https://www.uptodate.com/contents/chronic-exertional-compartment-syndrome.

48. You are the team physician for a youth club lacrosse team. One of the 15-year-old boys was struck in in the upper left abdominal area with an opponent's stick. Onfield evaluation demonstrates that he is hemodynamically stable, with point tenderness and early bruising to the left upper abdomen. He is also complaining of left shoulder pain. It is difficult to determine if he has true rebound tenderness on exam, although guarding is present. Given this scenario, if he remains hemodynamically stable, what is the next most important follow-up test/action?

   A. Laboratory tests: liver function and pancreatic enzymes
   B. Radiographs: plain upright films, KUB
   C. If he remains hemodynamically stable, no further study/exam is necessary other than serial observation and exams
   D. Ultrasound can reliably be used to determine free intraperitoneal blood

Correct Answer: D. Ultrasound can reliably be used to determine free intraperitoneal blood

This patient has worrisome mechanism and signs of blunt abdominal trauma (BAT). In particular, splenic injury is possible. In children, the solid organs (liver and spleen) are more exposed compared to adults. Furthermore, blunt trauma from a lacrosse stick to the upper left abdomen could cause this injury. Even though he is hemodynamically stable on the field, serial exams are needed to rule out delayed presentation of intraabdominal trauma and bleeding. In particular, splenic rupture needs to be ruled out and staged for optimal management. He has Kehr's sign (left shoulder pain with splenic injury), some guarding, and early ecchymosis on exam—which are signs of significant intraabdominal injury. In this scenario, at least a CT scan is needed before nonoperative management can successfully be utilized.

Laboratory exams have not been shown to significantly aid in algorithms for treating BAT. When positive, they are not diagnostic. Radiographs are usually not helpful in BAT. In the event of trauma to the torso or free air, they may be positive, but they are not often indicated in the early workup of BAT. CT, on the other hand, is indicated and useful for staging, especially if the patient is hemodynamically stable and nonoperative treatment is planned. Ultrasound has been shown to be very reliable for detecting free intraperitoneal blood. A FAST exam (focused assessment with sonography for trauma) has replaced the need for diagnostic peritoneal lavage and has been shown a specificity of 95%. FAST exam looks for free blood in Morison's pouch (perihepatic space/hepatorenal recess) and the space around the spleen, the pelvis, and the pericardium.

   1. Diercks DB, Clarke S. Initial evaluation and management of blunt abdominal trauma in adults. UpToDate. Accessed March 2, 2019 at https://www.uptodate.com/contents/initial-evaluation-and-management-of-blunt-abdominal-trauma-in-adults.
   2. Paul S, Bera S, Balcik B. Abdominal injuries. In: Miller M (ed). Orthopaedic Knowledge Update: Sports Medicine 5. Rosemont, IL: AAOS, 2016.

49. Which of the following is true regarding laryngotracheal (LT) injury?

    A. Stridor is the earliest symptom of LT injury
    B. MRI is the preferred diagnostic study for LT injury
    C. Flexible fiberoptic laryngoscopy should be performed immediately if the airway is unstable
    D. Intubation is essential to establish a secure airway in all suspected cases of LT injury
    E. The initial manifestations of LT injury may be subtle

Correct Answer: E. The initial manifestations of LT injury may be subtle

The most common and earliest symptoms of LT injury are variable but may include hoarseness and dyspnea. Stridor is a concerning, later finding that may be associated with progressive airway compromise (Answer A is incorrect). The foremost objective in managing a potential LT injury is to ensure a patent airway. The stable airway may be evaluated with flexible fiberoptic laryngoscopy and/or CT (Answers B and C are incorrect) and may be managed conservatively with close observation. Routine intubation can be hazardous and may further compromise or damage the airway, with underlying LT injury (Answer D is incorrect). The unstable airway should be managed with a tracheostomy, performed in a controlled setting by an experienced physician when possible.

1. Kim JD, Shuler FD, Mo B, Gibbs SR, Belmaggio T, Giangarra CE. Traumatic laryngeal fracture in a collegiate basketball player. Sports Health 2013 May;5(3):273-275. doi: 10.1177/1941738112473417.
2. Paluska SA, Lansford CD. Laryngeal trauma in sport. Curr Sports Med Rep 2008 Feb;7(1):16-21. doi: 10.1097/01.CSMR.0000308673.53182.72.

50. A 20-year-old female basketball player presents by EMS transport to the emergency department in respiratory distress that began acutely while scrimmaging at the end of basketball practice. She first started noticing intense urticaria of her upper torso and arms as the team started doing full-court drills. A few minutes later, one of her teammates noticed red raised wheals on both of her arms. She continued to play, and while they were scrimmaging, she started wheezing and had to stop due to severe difficulty breathing. EMS was then contacted, and she was taken to the nearest hospital. En route, she was placed into a partially reclined position, which was the position of comfort for her, and she was placed on oxygen. She was hypotensive with a blood pressure of 95/60, and therefore she was given a fluid bolus. She was also given a dose of epinephrine, which relieved her shortness of breath, and the wheals on her skin began clearing as well. Based on the most likely diagnosis for this athlete, what recommendations should be made for her long-term treatment?

A. Always exercise with a partner who is trained in administering epinephrine and basic life support, and carry an epinephrine auto-injector
B. Recommend athlete refrain from all exercise in the future to prevent another episode
C. Allergy testing should be performed; if athlete avoids any identified allergens, no further episodes should occur, and no other intervention is needed
D. Recommend taking a daily antihistamine to prevent future episodes

Correct Answer: A. Always exercise with a partner who is trained in administering epinephrine and basic life support, and carry an epinephrine auto-injector

This athlete had an episode of exercise-induced anaphylaxis. Athletes who have had an episode of exercise-induced anaphylaxis should undergo formal evaluation by an allergist for identification of specific food triggers (Answer C), but avoidance of that trigger has not been shown to be sufficient to prevent future episodes. It is recommended that specific triggers be avoided at least six hours prior to activity and that ingestion of any food be avoided at least two hours prior to activity. Current recommendations do not support the athlete refraining from all exercise in the future. Although administration of a daily antihistamine may reduce the number of episodes of exercise induced anaphylaxis, this intervention alone is not sufficient to prevent and treat further episodes. Answer A includes the current recommendations to allow an athlete to return to participation, while at the same time minimizing the risks of having a severe anaphylactic reaction. She should also avoid aspirin and NSAIDs before exercise, and should always carry an epinephrine auto-injector with her and use it if symptoms continue despite immediate cessation of physical exertion at the onset of symptoms. Most athletes recover fully within 30 minutes of cessation of exercise.

1. Hosey RG, Carek PJ, Goo A. Exercise-induced anaphylaxis and urticaria. Am Fam Physician 2001 Oct 15;64(8):1367-1372.
2. Schwartz LB, Delgado L, Craig T, Bonini S, Carlsen KH, Casale TB, et al. Exercise-induced hypersensitivity syndromes in recreational and competitive athletes: a PRACTALL consensus report (what the general practitioner should know about sports and allergy). Allergy 2008 Aug;63(8):953-961. doi: 10.1111/j.1398-9995.2008.01802.x.

51. A 17-year-old male comes to your office complaining of severe left lower quadrant pain that appeared six hours ago, which he believes is the result of strenuous physical activity before the symptoms started. Pain is described as achy and constant, with associated nausea and vomiting. He denies any other associated signs or symptoms or any positive medical, family, or surgical history. Vitals are within normal limits. On abdominal exam, you find that he has normal bowel sounds. The abdomen is soft, non-tender, and there is no rebound. All special tests for intraabdominal and abdominal wall conditions are negative too. What is your next step?

   A. Prescribe him a 10-day course of Ciprofloxacin and Metronidazole, with follow-up in one week
   B. Prescribe oral Tramadol prn pain and Promethazine prn nausea or vomiting, with follow-up in two days
   C. Order STAT complete blood count (CBC), comprehensive metabolic panel (CMP), Urinalysis UA), and a CT scan of the abdomen and pelvis
   D. Perform a testicular exam immediately

Correct Answer: D. Perform a testicular exam immediately

This athlete has testicular torsion. Patients classically present with an abrupt onset of severe testicular or scrotal pain, usually of less than 12 hours duration. However, inguinal or lower abdominal pain may be the presenting complaint. Nearly 90% of patients may have associated nausea and vomiting. The pain can be isolated to the scrotum or may radiate to the lower abdomen. The pain is constant unless the testicle is torsing and detorsing. On physical exam, the scrotum may be edematous, indurated, and erythematous, and the affected testis usually is tender, swollen, and slightly elevated because of shortening of the cord from twisting. The testis may be lying horizontally, displacing the epididymis from its normal posterolateral position. A reactive hydrocele may also be present. The cremasteric reflex (elevation of the testis in response to stroking of the upper inner thigh) is absent in nearly all cases of torsion, but it also may be absent in boys without torsion, particularly if they are younger than six months.

Prompt restoration of blood flow to the ischemic testicle is critical in cases of testicular torsion, and prompt referral to a urologist is recommended. There is typically a four- to eight-hour window before significant ischemic damage occurs, manifested by morphologic changes in testicular histopathology and deleterious effects on spermatogenesis. Altered semen parameters and potential decreased fertility secondary to increased permeability of the blood-testicle barrier may not normalize, even after blood flow has been successfully restored. In patients with a history and physical examination suggestive of torsion, imaging studies should not be performed; rather, these individuals should undergo immediate surgical exploration. The delay associated with performing imaging can extend the time of testicular ischemia, thereby decreasing testicular salvage rates. Negative surgical exploration is preferable to a missed diagnosis, because all imaging studies have a false-negative rate. Data provided by imaging studies are secondary to examination findings, and management should be based primarily on history and physical findings. Patients with physical findings strongly suggestive of testicular torsion should be referred for surgical exploration, regardless of ultrasound findings.

1. Sharp VJ, Kieran K, Arlen AM. Testicular torsion: diagnosis, evaluation, and management. Am Fam Physician 2013 Dec 15;88(12):835-840.
2. Van Heurn LW, Pakarinen MP, Wester T. Contemporary management of abdominal surgical emergencies in infants and children. Br J Surg 2014 Jan;101(1):e24-e33. doi: 10.1002/bjs.9335. Epub 2013 Nov 29.
3. Pogorelić Z, Mrklić I, Jurić I. Do not forget to include testicular torsion in differential diagnosis of lower acute abdominal pain in young males. J Pediatr Urol 2013 Dec;9(6 Pt B):1161-1165. doi: 10.1016/j.jpurol.2013.04.018. Epub 2013 Jun 3.

52. You are covering a high school track and field event. During one of the longer runs, you notice a thin young male who is suddenly slowing down, holding the right side of his chest. He keeps walking to finish the round, but when he arrives at the medical tent, he is pale and diaphoretic, complaining of right-sided chest pain and problems breathing. When you examine him, you notice a left deviation of his trachea, normal breath sounds over the left lung, and no breath sounds over the right lung. Hypertympany with percussion is noted over the right chest. You quickly make the diagnosis of spontaneous tension pneumothorax. Prior to the definite treatment of inserting a chest tube, which of the following would be the location of next best intervention?

   A. Fourth intercostal space, anterior axillary line
   B. Second intercostal space, midclavicular line
   C. Fifth intercostal space, anterior axillary line
   D. Fifth intercostal space, midaxillary line

Correct Answer: B. Second intercostal space, midclavicular line

This athlete has a spontaneous tension pneumothorax. While most cases of tension pneumothorax occur following trauma, they can also occur spontaneously. The fourth/fifth intercostal space at the anterior axillary line should be considered in trauma protocols as an alternative site for needle decompression, but it is not the first choice. The fifth intercostal space in the mid axillary line has shown to be highly efficient, with lower undesired effects, but this has not been studied on humans yet. The second intercostal space in midclavicular line is the only currently recommended location, as per current ATLS guidelines. As noted, definitive treatment is with a chest tube inserted at the fifth intercostal space (usually at the nipple level), just anterior to the midaxillary line, but needle decompression can be lifesaving when performed in the field.

1. Ben-Chetrit E, Merin O. Images in clinical medicine. Spontaneous tension pneumothorax. N Engl J Med 2010 Mar 25; 362(12):e43. doi: 10.1056/NEJMicm0901473.
2. Committee on Trauma, American College of Surgeons. Thoracic trauma. ATLS: Advanced Trauma Life Support—Student Course Manual. 9th ed. Chicago: American College of Surgeons, 2012:96-98.
3. Sanchez LD, Straszewski S, Saghir A, Khan A, Horn E, Fischer C, et al. Anterior versus lateral needle decompression of tension pneumothorax: comparison by computed tomography chest wall measurement. Acad Emerg Med 2011 Oct;18(10):1022-1026. doi: 10.1111/j.1553-2712.2011.01159.x. Epub 2011 Sep 26.

53. Which intravenous (IV) solution is usually preferred over other solutions for fluid resuscitation in anaphylaxis?

    A. Normal saline
    B. Lactated Ringer's
    C. Dextrose
    D. Colloid solutions

Correct Answer: A. Normal saline

Intravenous (IV) access should be obtained in all cases of anaphylaxis. Massive fluid shifts can occur rapidly, due to increased vascular permeability, with transfer of up to 35% of the intravascular volume into the extravascular space within minutes. Any patient whose hypotension does not respond promptly and completely to IM epinephrine should receive large volume fluid resuscitation. Normal saline is preferred over other solutions in most situations, because other solutions have potential disadvantages. For example, because Lactated Ringer's (LR) solution can potentially contribute to metabolic alkalosis, although large volumes of normal saline can cause hyperchloremic metabolic acidosis, some clinicians change from normal saline to LR if very large volumes are proving necessary. Dextrose is rapidly extravasated from the circulation into the interstitial tissues. Colloid solutions (e.g., albumin or hydroxyethyl starch) not only confer no survival advantage in patients with distributive shock, they are also costlier.

1. Lieberman P, Nicklas RA, Randolph C, Oppenheimer J, Bernstein D, Bernstein J, et al. Anaphylaxis—a practice parameter update 2015. Ann Allergy Asthma Immunol 2015 Nov;115(5):341-384. doi: 10.1016/j.anai.2015.07.019.
2. Simons FE, Ardusso LR, Bilò MB, El-Gamal YM, Ledford DK, Ring J, et al. World Allergy Organization anaphylaxis guidelines: summary. J Allergy Clin Immunol 2011 Mar;127(3):587-593.e1-22. doi: 10.1016/j.jaci.2011.01.038.
3. Perel P, Roberts I, Ker K. Colloids versus crystalloids for fluid resuscitation in critically ill patients. Cochrane Database Syst Rev 2013 Feb 28;(2):CD000567. doi: 10.1002/14651858.CD000567.pub6.

54. A 14-year-old male with Down syndrome presents with his parents, complaining of axial neck pain after falling one day prior on the tennis court. Pain is worsened with end ranges of flexion and extension. He denies any numbness, tingling, or weakness in his upper extremities. On exam, he has mild tenderness of his cervical paraspinal muscles. His range of motion is full in all directions, with pain at end ranges of flexion, extension, and bilateral rotation. His neurologic exam is intact. What condition must he be immediately evaluated for?

   A. Cervical stenosis
   B. Atlantoaxial (AA) instability
   C. Herniated disc
   D. Degenerative disc disease (DDD)

Correct Answer: B. Atlantoaxial (AA) instability

Patients with Down syndrome are at increased risk for AA instability. Therefore, appropriate cervical radiographs including AP, lateral and odontoid views should be obtained immediately. A separation of the odontoid and the atlas of greater than 4-5 mm is suggestive of atlantoaxial instability and requires immediate immobilization and referral to a spine specialist. If there is no abnormality on the aforementioned views, flexion/extension views can also be obtained. Cervical stenosis usually presents in older individuals, and symptoms may improve with flexion. He is at low risk for herniated disc, due to his age and lack of radicular symptoms. DDD usually presents in older individuals. AA instability is the only answer choice that requires immediate immobilization.

   1. Klenck C, Gebke K. Practical management: common medical problems in disabled athletes. CJSM 2007;17(1):55-60.
   2. Dedlow ER, Siddiqi S, Fillipps DJ, Kelly MN, Nackashi JA, Tuli SY. Symptomatic atlantoaxial instability in an adolescent with trisomy 21 (Down's syndrome). Clin Pediatr (Phila) 2013 Jul;52(7):633-638. doi: 10.1177/0009922813482178. Epub 2013 Apr 5.

55. Commotio cordis is the term used to describe ventricular fibrillation triggered by chest wall impact most commonly over what structure?

   A. Right atrium
   B. Right ventricle
   C. Left atrium
   D. Left ventricle

Correct Answer: D. Left ventricle

Ventricular fibrillation occurs following blunt trauma to the chest predominantly over the center of the left ventricle. Impact over precordial sites other than the left ventricle causes ventricular fibrillation less commonly. Ventricular fibrillation is most likely when the impact occurs 10 to 40 ms before the T wave peak.

1. Link MS. Commotio cordis: ventricular fibrillation triggered by chest impact-induced abnormalities in repolarization. Circ Arrhythm Electrophysiol 2012 Apr;5(2):425-432. doi: 10.1161/CIRCEP.111.962712.
2. Yabek SM. Commotio cordis. Medscape. Accessed December 7, 2018 at https://emedicine.medscape.com/article/902504-overview#a5.

Test 2 Answers, Critiques, and References

56. A professional basketball player comes off the court complaining of right-sided pleuritic chest pain and shortness of breath. He denies any injury. After a brief rest, his respiratory rate is 16 breaths per minute. He has slightly diminished breath sounds and absent tactile fremitus in his upper right lung field. A chest x-ray reveals a right-sided pneumothorax (PTX), with a 2 cm apex-cupola distance. What is the most appropriate action?

   A. Place a chest tube
   B. Send him home with his team, as long as he flies in a pressurized cabin
   C. Take him out of the game and repeat the x-ray in three hours
   D. Allow him back on the court, as long as his oxygenation is normal

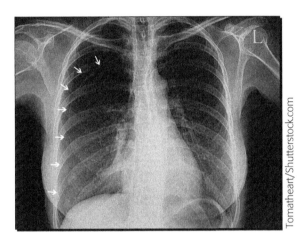

Correct Answer: C. Take him out of the game and repeat the x-ray in three hours

A chest tube is not necessary for a small PTX, defined as apex-cupola distance less than 3 cm. PTX is an absolute contraindication for flying. This restriction is typically observed for two weeks after radiographic resolution of the PTX. A patient with a small PTX should be observed for three to six hours, and chest x-ray repeated to insure stability. If stable at that point, a chest x-ray should be repeated in 24 to 48 hours. The player should not be allowed to play until there is radiographic resolution of the PTX. Beyond that, recommendations vary from 2 to 10 weeks, with most athletes returning after three to four weeks.

   1. Feden JP. Closed lung trauma. Clin Sports Med 2013 Apr;32(2):255-265. doi: 10.1016/j.csm.2012.12.003. Epub 2013 Jan 29.
   2. Hull JH, Ansley L, Robson-Ansley P, Parsons JP. Managing respiratory problems in athletes. Clin Med (Lond) 2012 Aug;12(4):351-356.

57. A 23-year-old college football player is taken off the field during practice on a hot and humid summer day after appearing to be confused and disoriented. He seems to be warm to the touch and is sweating profusely. You obtain a core rectal temperature that measures 105 degrees Fahrenheit (40.5 degrees Celsius). What is the most effective cooling method?

    A. Spray water over him while using a fan to cool him down
    B. Immediately give oral acetaminophen to bring his core temperature down below 102 degrees Fahrenheit (38.8 degrees Celsius)
    C. Place him in a bath of ice water
    D. Use cold packs at the neck, groin, and axillae

Correct Answer: C. Place him in a bath of ice water

Heat stroke is characterized by an elevated core body temperature that is > 104 degrees Fahrenheit (40 degrees Celsius). Heat stroke is also diagnosed in someone with altered mental status (AMS) and CNS abnormalities who is at risk for heat stroke but has not reached a core temperature of 104 degrees Fahrenheit (40 degrees Celsius) or greater. Often, the patient with heat stroke has both elevated core temperature (>104 degrees Fahrenheit [40 degrees Celsius]) and AMS and/or CNS deficits. Rapid cooling with fluid and electrolyte replacement with isotonic saline are essential in the management of heat stroke. Rapid cooling is the most important aspect in the management of heat stroke, as the longer the patient's temperature remains elevated, the greater the chance of permanent neurological damage or death. Placing cold packs at the neck, groin, and axillae or spraying water over patients while using a fan to cool him down are alternative methods of cooling, but not as efficient as cold-water immersion. Antipyretics, such as acetaminophen, have not been shown to be effective in the management of heat stroke.

1. Casa DJ, Armstrong LE, Kenny GP, O'Connor FG, Huggins RA. Exertional heat stroke: new concepts regarding cause and care. Curr Sports Med Rep 2012 May-Jun;11(3):115-123. doi: 10.1249/JSR.0b013e31825615cc.
2. Sloan BK, Kraft EM, Clark D, Schmeissing SW, Byrne BC, Rusyniak DE. On-site treatment of exertional heat stroke. Am J Sports Med 2015 Apr;43(4):823-829. doi: 10.1177/0363546514566194. Epub 2015 Jan 28.
3. Smith JE. Cooling methods used in the treatment of exertional heat illness. Br J Sports Med 2005 Aug;39(8):503-507; discussion 507.

58. While fielding a ground ball at second base, a 16-year-old African-American female softball player sustains a right eye injury when the ball bounces up and strikes her at the right orbital region. The patient complains of right periorbital pain, photophobia, and diminished visual acuity. Right eye exam reveals an intact globe, no enophthalmos or ptosis, and mild periorbital edema. Pen light exam shows blood at the inferior third of the anterior chamber. Initial medical treatment should include which of the following?

    A. Topical cycloplegic (atropine 1%), systemic and/or topical corticosteroid, rigid eye shield, reevaluate in three days
    B. Topical cycloplegic (atropine 1%), systemic and/or topical corticosteroid, rigid eye shield, restrict activities, and immediate referral to ophthalmology
    C. Topical cycloplegic (atropine 1%), systemic and/or topical corticosteroid, rigid eye shield, and return to play
    D. Topical cycloplegic (atropine 1%), systemic and/or topical corticosteroid, and may return to play if normal visual acuity

Correct Answer: B. Topical cycloplegic (atropine 1%), systemic and/or topical corticosteroid, rigid eye shield, restrict activities, and immediate referral to ophthalmology

The softball impact to the athlete's right eye caused a hyphema—blood in the anterior chamber from damage of peripheral blood vessels of the iris or ciliary body. Topical cycloplegics are muscarinic receptor blockers that help paralyze the ciliary muscle and reduce further injury. Systemic corticosteroids and topical corticosteroids may reduce risks of rebleeding through reduction of inflammation, stabilization of the blood-ocular barrier, and direct inhibition of fibrinolysis. Restriction of activities is recommended to reduce intra-ocular pressure. A rigid eye shield is used for protection of the injured eye. Immediate Ophthalmology referral is warranted to further evaluate for any concomitant injuries, measure and follow intraocular pressures, and monitor for recurrent hemorrhage. Patients should be followed up daily for three days in order to monitor intraocular pressures and check for rebleeding. Patient should not return to play the same day. Restriction of activities is recommended. African-American children tend to have increased risks for developing secondary bleeding. Sickle cell hemoglobinopathy was associated with increased intraocular pressure, but was not associated with increased risk of rebleeding.

1. Gharaibeh A, Savage HI, Scherer RW, Goldberg MF, Lindsley K. Medical interventions for traumatic hyphema. Cochrane Database Syst Rev 2013 Dec 3;(12):CD005431. doi: 10.1002/14651858.CD005431.pub3.
2. Lai JC, Fekrat S, Barrón Y, Goldberg MF. Traumatic hyphema in children: risk factors for complications. Arch Ophthalmol 2001 Jan;119(1):64-70.

59. You are evaluating a 20-year-old patient for a suspected concussion one hour ago during soccer practice. As part of your evaluation, you measure the near point convergence (NPC). What distance would be considered a normal NPC?

    A. 3 cm
    B. 6 cm
    C. 8 cm
    D. 10 cm

Correct Answer: A. 3 cm

Oculomotor problems are common after a sports-related concussion. One way of evaluating oculomotor problems is by evaluating for convergence insufficiency by measuring NPC. NPC is measured from the tip of the nose in cm. The patient holds a fixation stick with a letter in 12-point font at arm's length and slowly brings the stick towards the nose. The patient stops when they see two letters. The distance between the tip of the nose and the fixation stick is measured. A measurement of ≤ 5 cm is considered normal.

1. Pearce KL, Sufrinko A, Lau BC, Henry L, Collins MW, Kontos AP. Near point of convergence after a sport-related concussion: measurement reliability and relationship to neurocognitive impairment and symptoms. Am J Sports Med 2015 Dec;43(12):3055-3061. doi: 10.1177/0363546515606430. Epub 2015 Oct 9.
2. Kontos AP, Sufrinko A, Elbin RJ, Puskar A, Collins MW. Reliability and associated risk factors for performance on the Vestibular/Ocular Motor Screening (VOMS) tool in healthy collegiate athletes. Am J Sports Med 2016 Jun;44(6):1400-1406. doi: 10.1177/0363546516632754. Epub 2016 Mar 15.

60. A 37-year-old male is carried into the emergency department by his wife immediately after completing a marathon in Key West. He complains of severe muscle cramps in his legs. He reports that he drank fluids during the race, but probably not enough, and admits he hasn't urinated since before the race. His wife thinks he's running a temperature. On physical exam, his calves and thighs are in muscle spasms. Glascow Coma Scale score is 15, no loss of consciousness during or after race. Vitals normal, except temperature 100.1 degrees Fahrenheit (37.8 degrees Celsius). ECG shows peaked T waves. The blood work will likely show which of the following abnormalities?

   A. Increased serum creatinine kinase, increased serum potassium, increased serum lactate dehydrogenase, decreased serum calcium
   B. Increased serum creatinine kinase, increased serum potassium, decreased serum lactate dehydrogenase, increased serum calcium
   C. Increased serum creatinine kinase, decreased serum potassium, increased serum lactate dehydrogenase, increased serum calcium
   D. Decreased serum creatinine kinase, increased serum potassium, increased serum lactate dehydrogenase, increased serum calcium

Correct Answer: A. Increased serum creatinine kinase, increased serum potassium, increased serum lactate dehydrogenase, decreased serum calcium

From the clinical scenario, it can be determined the patient likely has rhabdomyolysis. The laboratory analysis in Answer A is to be expected with a patient presenting with acute rhabdomyolysis, and should be treated immediately with fluid hydration. Further laboratory analysis may include urine testing for presence of hemoglobin or myoglobin, and urine may characteristically appear brown or red.

1. Sauret JM, Marinides G, Wang GK. Rhabdomyolysis. Am Fam Physician 2002 Mar 1;65(5):907-912.
2. Bosch X, Poch E, Grau JM. Rhabdomyolysis and acute kidney injury. N Engl J Med 2009 Jul;361(1):62-72. doi: 10.1056/NEJMra0801327.

61. During a football game you are asked to evaluate a running back for a knee injury on the field. While running the ball, he states his foot was planted on the ground while a defender was holding his leg. As he tried to spin out of the tackle, a defensive lineman dove to tackle his legs, causing a heavy valgus load on the knee. He felt immediate pain and was unable to get up to walk off the field. On examination, you note normal alignment of the knee. However, he is unable to straighten it. There is a positive posterior sag sign. Both anterior and posterior drawer tests are grossly abnormal, and valgus stress reveals no endpoint. There appears to be an effusion forming, and all exam maneuvers are painful. Which of the following is true regarding the treatment of this patient?

A. The patient should be made non-weight-bearing to avoid completing an attached bucket handle tear of the medial meniscus
B. A majority of patellar dislocations are medial
C. Popliteal artery damage is the most serious complication of this injury
D. An intact knee extensor mechanism rules out an injury requiring emergent surgical repair
E. Peroneal nerve injury in this condition is rare, occurring in less than 5% of those affected

Correct Answer: C. Popliteal artery damage is the most serious complication of this injury

The most likely diagnosis in this case is a transient knee dislocation (tibio-femoral dislocation), as indicated by the exam demonstrating both cruciate ligaments and the MCL being disrupted. The mechanism of injury is consistent with this diagnosis as well, due to the twisting component. Knee dislocations involve injury to more than two of the four main stabilizing ligaments of the knee (ACL, PCL, MCL, LCL) and can be limb-threatening injuries, as the popliteal artery can be damaged. Thorough evaluation of the vascular status of the limb should be conducted in the hospital, and often involves angiography to evaluate for small tears or dissections. While it is recommended to make a patient with suspected bucket handle tears of the meniscus non-weight-bearing, that is not the most pressing concern in this patient. Most patellar dislocations are lateral, which is not the correct diagnosis in this case. In patellar fractures, an intact extensor mechanism is important, but again, that is not the diagnosis presented in this question. Peroneal nerve injuries with a knee dislocation are relatively common, occurring in up to 25% of patients.

1. Bedi A, Karunakar M. Patella fractures and extensor mechanism injuries. In: Bucholz R, Court-Brown CM, Heckman JD, Tornetta P III (eds). Rockwood and Green's Fractures in Adults. 7th ed. Philadelphia: Lippincott Williams & Wilkins, 2010:1752-1777.
2. Stannard JP, Schenck RC, Fanelli GC. Knee dislocations and fracture-dislocations. In: Bucholz R, Court-Brown CM, Heckman JD, Tornetta P III (eds). Rockwood and Green's Fractures in Adults. 7th ed. Philadelphia: Lippincott Williams & Wilkins, 2010:1832-1864.
3. Bachman MC. Knee (tibiofemoral) dislocation and reduction. UpToDate. Accessed December 8, 2018 at https://www.uptodate.com/contents/knee-tibiofemoral-dislocation-and-reduction.

62. A 25-year-old male presents to the emergency department with blunt ocular trauma after he was struck in the face with a baseball. Which of the following exam findings is associated with an ophthalmologic emergency requiring the most immediate attention?

   A. Restricted upgaze
   B. Proptosis
   C. Hyphema
   D. Constricted pupil

Correct Answer: B. Proptosis

Blunt ocular trauma is common in sports and encompasses a spectrum of injury severity. The most worrisome ocular injuries are those that can result in permanent loss of vision. Retrobulbar hemorrhage can produce a "compartment syndrome" of the orbit in which increasing intraocular pressures may rapidly compromise vision from injury to the optic nerve and central retinal artery. This condition may present with proptosis, limited extraocular movements, and a relative afferent pupillary defect. Emergent ophthalmology consultation and surgical decompression may be necessary to prevent loss of vision. Restricted upgaze is associated with inferior rectus entrapment and orbital floor fracture (orbital blowout fracture). In cases of entrapment, urgent ophthalmology consultation is indicated, but intervention is not as time-sensitive as retrobulbar hemorrhage. Blood in the anterior chamber from blunt trauma (hyphema) and pupillary constriction (traumatic iritis) also warrant prompt ophthalmology evaluation, but are not associated with rapidly progressive vision loss.

1. Aerni GA. Blunt visual trauma. Clin Sports Med 2013 Apr;32(2):289-301. doi: 10.1016/j.csm.2012.12.005.
2. Cass SP. Ocular injuries in sports. Curr Sports Med Rep 2012 Jan-Feb;11(1):11-15. doi: 10.1249/JSR.0b013e318240dc06.

63. You serve as a college team physician. While you do not receive any financial compensation for this position, you serve a formal role with regard to game coverage and return-to-play decisions. Which of the following statements best reflects how you manage this position?

   A. Due to competing pressures from other parties, this will alter how you counsel an athlete, since care is managed differently than the typical patient in the community
   B. Despite not receiving financial compensation from the team, Good Samaritan laws do not provide protection from malpractice litigation
   C. Since return-to-play decisions affect both the athlete and the team, the usual principles of informed consent and patient autonomy do not apply
   D. This position should be used as a significant part of marketing your practice

Correct Answer: B. Despite not receiving financial compensation from the team, Good Samaritan laws do not provide protection from malpractice litigation

Compensation can come in several ways (shirts, advertisements, etc.), and while serving in any formal position as a team physician, you are still held to the same standards as any other practicing physician, as outlined in the AMA Code for Medical Ethics. Answers A and C are incorrect, as "physicians should assist athletes to make informed decisions about their participation in amateur and professional contact sports which entail risks of bodily injury." Your decisions are held to the same standards as any other practicing physician. Answer D is incorrect, as the AAOS code of ethics state that physicians should not advertise based on "unmerited marks of quality," such as an appointment as a team physician.

1. Dunn WR, George MS, Churchill L, Spindler KP. Ethics in sports medicine. Am J Sports Med 2007 May;35(5):840-844. Epub 2007 Jan 11.
2. Holm S, McNamee MJ, Pigozzi F. Ethical practice and sports physician protection: a proposal. Br J Sports Med 2011 Dec;45(15):1170-1173. doi: 10.1136/bjsm.2011.086124. Epub 2011 Jun 3.

64. As part of your duties as team physician for a local NCAA Division II university, you perform a preparticipation examination on a 22-year-old defensive back, who is transferring to the university to play football. He informs you that 16 months ago, he had a surgical fusion of his fifth and sixth cervical vertebrae. He provides a letter, from a neurosurgeon at a prominent referral center, that states he can return to football without restrictions. You order a cervical MRI study and review the findings with the radiologist and the team neurosurgeon. The MRI findings demonstrate degenerative changes and disc space narrowing at the levels above and below his fusion. After extensive discussion with the athletic training staff, the team neurosurgeon, the athletic director, and the Vice President for Student Affairs, you decide not to clear this athlete to play football, because you and your team believe he is at high risk for another cervical spine injury. The athlete and his family are irate and threaten legal action against you and the university. Which of the following is the correct response to this situation?

A. The athlete should be allowed to play football, because he received clearance from a specialist at a highly regarded tertiary referral center
B. The university should have a standard waiver form for these situations that would allow athletes and parents to absolve the university of any responsibility for athletic participation
C. You and the university have the legal right to restrict this athlete from participation in football, as long as the decision is individualized and demonstrates sound medical judgment
D. The physician's risk is negligible is this situation, because Good Samaritan Laws protect physicians from liability in the performance of preparticipation physical examinations

Correct Answer: C. You and the university have the legal right to restrict this athlete from participation in football, as long as the decision is individualized and demonstrates sound medical judgment

There is legal precedent for restricting athletes from play, as long as the decision is individualized and represents sound medical judgment. The courts recognize that institutions may assess risk differently and have respected reasonable and ethical decisions. A standard waiver form is not as powerful as a written statement by the athlete and guardians of their understanding of the risks incurred by continuing to participate. Lastly, Good Samaritan Laws apply to volunteer work or emergency situations. The team physician has assumed a duty for comprehensive care of the university's athletes and would not be protected by these statutes.

1. American Academy of Family Physicians, American Academy of Pediatrics, American College of Sports Medicine, American Medical Society for Sports Medicine, American Orthopaedic Society for Sports Medicine, American Osteopathic Academy of Sports Medicine. Bernhardt DT, Roberts WO (eds). Administrative, ethical, and legal concerns. Preparticipation Physical Evaluation. 4th ed. Elk Grove, IL: American Academy of Pediatrics, 2010:23-25.
2. Rubin A. Legal issues in sports medicine. In: O'Connor FG, Casa DJ, Davis BA, St. Pierre P, Sallis RE, Wilder RP (eds). ACSM's Sports Medicine: A Comprehensive Review. Philadelphia: Lippincott Williams & Wilkins, 2013:9-13.

65. A 25-year-old female cyclist is training for her first century (100 miles) bicycle ride. She has been increasing her training mileage over the past two weeks. She complains of volar right ring finger and right little finger pain and tingling after her 20-mile bicycle ride. She also notes weakness with extension of her right ring finger. The examination of her right hand shows no atrophy. Mild weakness with extension of right ring finger and right little finger are noted. Decreased sensation to light touch is noted at the ulnar aspect of right ring finger and at right little finger compared to left side. Tinel's test over Guyon's canal is positive. Tinel's over flexor retinaculum at wrist and Phalen's test are negative. What is the most likely diagnosis?

   A. Wartenberg syndrome
   B. Carpal tunnel syndrome
   C. Radial tunnel syndrome
   D. Ulnar tunnel syndrome

Correct Answer: D. Ulnar tunnel syndrome

Ulnar tunnel syndrome (cyclist palsy) is secondary to compression of ulnar nerve at Guyon's canal from wrist pressure against the handle bar of the bicycle. The incidence between experienced and novice cyclists are similar, as well as between road and mountain cyclists. Some cyclists may experience carpal tunnel syndrome as well from compression of median nerve. If patient were to have tingling, pain, and weakness in the thumb, index finger, middle finger, and radial aspect of ring finger, carpal tunnel syndrome would be considered. Given a negative Tinel's test at wrist flexor retinaculum and a negative Phalen's test, carpal tunnel syndrome is unlikely. Radial tunnel syndrome and Wartenberg syndrome involve compression of the radial nerve at the level of the elbow and at the level of the superficial branch of the radial nerve in the forearm, respectively. The radial tunnel is the potential space between the lateral epicondyle and the supinator muscle. It may cause pain or aching distal to the lateral epicondyle that is worse after throwing or at night. Wartenberg syndrome may cause pain and decreased sensation over dorsal radial aspect of hand and dorsal aspect of thumb and index finger. It may be caused by tight clothing around forearm or by wearing a tight forearm band.

   1. Chen SH, Tsai TM. Ulnar tunnel syndrome. J Hand Surg Am 2014 Mar;39(3):571-579. doi: 10.1016/j.jhsa.2013.08.102.
   2. Akuthota V, Plastaras C, Lindberg K, Tobey J, Press J, Garvan C. The effect of long-distance bicycling on ulnar and median nerves: an electrophysiologic evaluation of cyclist palsy. Am J Sports Med 2005 Aug;33(8):1224-1230. Epub 2005 Jul 6.

66. Which injury can be associated with electrodiagnostic findings of denervation of the infraspinatus muscle?

    A. Quadrilateral space syndrome
    B. Posterior glenoid labral tear
    C. C7 radiculopathy
    D. Grade I AC joint separation

Correct Answer: B. Posterior glenoid labral tear

Patients with a posterior labral tear can develop a periarticular paralabral cyst that can cause a compression neuropathy of the suprascapular nerve as it travels through the spinoglenoid notch. This can cause denervation of the infraspinatus muscle. Quadrilateral space syndrome is associated compression of the neurovascular bundle within the quadrilateral space, which includes posterior humeral circumflex artery and/or the axillary nerve or one of its major branches. Compression neuropathy of the axillary nerve would result in denervation of the deltoid and teres minor muscles. The infraspinatus muscle is innervated by C5 and C6 primarily, with some contributions from C4. C7 does not have any contributions to the innervation of the infraspinatus muscle. An AC separation would not typically be associated with a nerve injury.

1. Trojian TH. Suprascapular neuropathy. Medscape. Accessed December 8, 2018 at https://emedicine.medscape.com/article/92672-overview.
2. Boykin RE, Friedman DJ, Higgins LD, Warner JJ. Suprascapular neuropathy. J Bone Joint Surg Am 2010 Oct 6;92(13):2348-2364. doi: 10.2106/JBJS.I.01743.

67. When evaluating the cardiovascular risks of a certain sport, the sports medicine physician must consider both the static and dynamic demands of the sport. What is an example of a sport with both high static and high dynamic demands?

   A. Rowing
   B. Long distance running
   C. Sprinting
   D. Baseball
   E. American football

Correct Answer: A. Rowing

Exercise or sport can be classified into two types: static (isometric) and dynamic (isotonic). Static exercise involves development of large intramuscular force, with little or no change in muscle length or joint movement. Dynamic exercise involves changes in muscle length and joint movement with relatively small intramuscular force. For example, a high-dynamic and low-static sport would be long distance running. Weightlifting would be an example of a low-dynamic, high-static sport. American football and sprinting would be a moderate-static and moderate-dynamic sport. Baseball would be a moderate-dynamic, low-static sport. Rowing is considered to be a high-dynamic, high-static sport.

   1. Mitchell JH, Haskell W, Snell P, Van Camp SP. Task Force 8: classification of sports. J Am Coll Cardiol 2005 Apr 19;45(8):1364-1367.

68. Which of the following is true regarding complex regional pain syndrome (CRPS)?

   A. MRI scans can demonstrate soft tissue changes in CRPS with high specificity but low sensitivity
   B. Three-phase bone scintigraphy can provide valuable information during the first year and is useful in differentiating CRPS from other pain syndromes
   C. Elevated ESR can confirm the diagnosis of CRPS
   D. A negative EMG can rule out the possible diagnosis of CRPS

Correct Answer: B. Three-phase bone scintigraphy can provide valuable information during the first year and is useful in differentiating CRPS from other pain syndromes

In CRPS, there is hypoperfusion in the first two phases and increased uptake in the third phase. MRI scans can demonstrate soft tissue changes in CRPS with low specificity and high sensitivity. An elevated ESR cannot confirm the diagnosis of CRPS, since, in general, this is a nonspecific finding. A negative EMG does not rule out the diagnosis of CRPS, and electrodiagnostics are generally used to rule in or out other competing diagnoses.

   1. Gupta G. Complex regional pain syndromes. Medscape. Accessed December 8, 2018 at https://emedicine.medscape.com/article/1145318-overview.

69. Which of the following is true with regard to strength training for pediatric athletes?

    A. Emerging evidence confirms that strength training in childhood is detrimental to bone health
    B. Although not contraindicated, pediatric athletes less than 10 years of age should be discouraged from strength training to minimize risk of injury
    C. To minimize the risk of growth or development disturbance, pediatric athletes should adhere to pediatric protocols based on one repetition maximum lifts
    D. There is no evidence-based minimum age for participation in a supervised strength training program

Correct Answer: D. There is no evidence based minimum age for participation in a supervised strength training program

Emerging evidence suggests childhood is an opportune time for the bone remodeling process to respond to tensile and compressive forces associated with resistance training. Motor performance skills are essential components of sport movements. Children have an opportunity to develop a base level of strength and power during this developmental period. There is not an agreed-upon minimum age for participation in a supervised strength training program. Furthermore, pediatric athletes of any age should not be discouraged from participating in a supervised strength training program. There is no evidence that strength training will cause growth or developmental disturbances. Pediatric one-rep protocols should be considered extreme, and there is evidence in adult weight lifters that extreme protocols increase risk of injury and maladaptive body mechanics.

    1. Faigenbaum AD, Lloyd RS, MacDonald J, Myer GD. Citius, Altius, Fortius: beneficial effects of resistance training for young athletes: narrative review. Br J Sports Med 2016 Jan;50(1):3-7. doi: 10.1136/bjsports-2015-094621. Epub 2015 Jun 18.
    2. Vehrs PR. Physical activity and strength training in children and adolescents: an overview. UpToDate. Accessed December 8, 2018 at https://www.uptodate.com/contents/physical-activity-and-strength-training-in-children-and-adolescents-an-overview.

70. According to the NCAA Drug Testing Program, every Division I athlete will be drug tested for performance-enhancing drugs at least once each academic year. If an athlete tests positive for a banned substance, without a previous offense, what is the penalty?

    A. Ineligibility for athletic competition for the remainder of the competition season, including the post-season
    B. Ineligibility for athletic competition for the remainder of the academic year
    C. Ineligibility for athletic competition for one calendar year from the date of notification
    D. Ineligibility for athletic competition for the remainder of their NCAA athletic career

Correct Answer: C. Ineligibility for athletic competition for one calendar year from the date of notification

According to the NCAA Drug Testing Program guidelines, if an athlete tests positive for a banned performance-enhancing substance, they are ineligible for athletic competition for one calendar year from the date of notification of the positive test. If an athlete tests positive on a second event for performance-enhancing drugs, they are ineligible for the remainder of their NCAA athletic career.

1. Frequently asked questions about drug testing. NCAA. Accessed December 14, 2018 at https://www.ncaa.org/health-and-safety/policy/frequently-asked-questions-about-drug-testing.
2. Drug testing program 2018-19. NCAA. Accessed December 14, 2018 at https://www.ncaa.org/sport-science-institute/ncaa-drug-testing-program.

71. An 18-year-old, right-hand-dominant offensive lineman complains of right wrist pain for several weeks. He denies any particular injury, just that it is getting worse. He denies numbness in the hand, but says when he tries to grab things, do pushups, or perform lineman drills, the pain gets worse. The pain is located in the middle of the wrist and does not radiate. An x-ray of the wrist, including clenched-fist views, is read as negative. An MRI of the wrist demonstrates a decrease in T1 weighted signal in the lunate. Which of the following is the most likely diagnosis?

    A. Scapholunate ligament disruption
    B. Lunate dislocation
    C. Disruption of the distal radial-ulnar joint
    D. Dietrich disease
    E. Kienbock's disease

Correct Answer: E. Kienbock's disease

Kienbock's disease is an osteonecrosis of the lunate bone. While the exact etiology is unclear, it is believed that it is caused by repetitive trauma to the lunate, resulting in sequential decrease in blood flow, leading to necrosis. It is more common in the dominant hand of those who repeatedly strike with the palm open (offensive linemen) or those with a negative ulnar variance of the wrist. There are four stages on x-ray for Kienbock's disease. Stage 1 is no change; stage 2 demonstrates density changes; stage 3 shows collapse of the lunate; and stage 4 shows collapse with associated carpal arthrosis. The following MRI images show decreased signal intensity of the lunate, which is in the early stages of Kienbock's disease. Scapholunate ligament disruption, lunate dislocation, and DRUJ disruption are more commonly seen as acute traumatic injuries, and you would expect findings on x-ray for each of these. Dietrich disease is osteonecrosis of the head of the metacarpals.

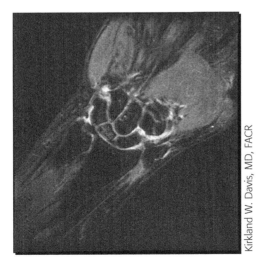

Kirkland W. Davis, MD, FACR

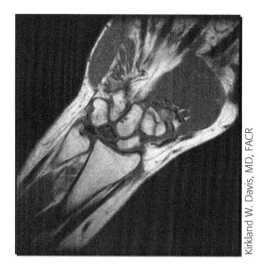

1. Turman KA, Hart JA, Miller MD. Cartilage problems in sports. In: Madden CC, Putukian M, Young CC, McCarty EC (eds). Netter's Sports Medicine. Philadelphia: Saunders Elsevier, 2010:438-444.
2. Boggess BR. Evaluation of the adult with subacute or chronic wrist pain. UpToDate. Accessed December 8, 2018 at https://www.uptodate.com/contents/evaluation-of-the-adult-with-subacute-or-chronic-wrist-pain.

72. Neuromuscular training that strengthens hip abductors and core strength, and that which improves knee control, has been an effective intervention in reducing anterior cruciate ligament injuries in female athletes. By increasing the frequency and duration of the neuromuscular training exercises, what has happened to the rate of anterior cruciate ligament injuries?

   A. Doubled
   B. Remained the same
   C. Increased
   D. Decreased

Correct Answer: D. Decreased

The increased frequency of neuromuscular training sessions and the increased duration of each session (greater than 20 minutes per session, at least two sessions per week) have been correlated with an inverse dose-response to anterior cruciate ligament injuries. Neuromuscular training exercises included single- and double-legged knee squats, lunges, jump landing, and pelvic tilt. The higher neuromuscular training volume resulted in a greater reduction in anterior cruciate ligament injuries than lower volume (less than 20 minutes per session, one session per week).

   1. Sugimoto D, Myer GD, Foss KD, Hewett TE. Dosage effects of neuromuscular training intervention to reduce anterior cruciate ligament injuries in female athletes: meta- and sub-group analyses. Sports Med 2014 Apr;44(4):551-562. doi: 10.1007/s40279-013-0135-9.
   2. Wingfield K. Neuromuscular training to prevent knee injuries in adolescent female soccer players. Clin J Sport Med 2013 Sep;23(5):407-408.

73. A nine-year-old pitcher comes to the office after pitching in a select tournament two weeks ago for one team, as well as pitching for his league team the next day. He complains of lateral elbow pain that did not occur on one pitch, but hurts only when he throws. He is having trouble completely extending the elbow. What is the most likely diagnosis?

   A. Osteochondritis dissecans of the capitellum
   B. Lateral epicondylitis
   C. Osteochondrosis of the capitellum (Panner's disease)
   D. Radial nerve entrapment at the arcade of Frohse
   E. Radial head fracture

Correct Answer: C. Osteochondrosis of the capitellum (Panner's disease)

Panner's disease is an osteochondrosis that usually occurs in young boys between the ages of five and 12 years of age in their dominant elbow. With the stress of throwing, the compressive force of the radial head into the capitellum can result in injury at this articulation. In a teenage patient, the diagnosis of osteochondritis dissecans is more likely. Lateral epicondylitis, with or without radial nerve entrapment, is not a common injury of throwers, especially ones in the pediatric population. Without specific trauma, radial head fracture is also less likely.

   1. Kobayashi K, Burton KJ, Rodner C, Smith B, Caputo AE. Lateral compression injuries in the pediatric elbow: Panner's disease and osteochondritis dissecans of the capitellum. J Am Acad Orthop Surg 2004 Jul-Aug;12(4):246-254.

74. Which of the following statements is true regarding the biomechanics of throwing?

    A. The primary generators of force in the throwing athlete are the shoulder girdle muscles
    B. Throwing athletes with open growth plates are at greater risk for ulnar collateral ligament tears, because with the smaller muscle mass, these athletes are unable to effectively dissipate the stress across the elbow
    C. In general, the biomechanics of youth pitchers are different from adult pitchers, due to the differences in lever arm length and muscle mass
    D. In theory, any pitch thrown at 80 miles/hour (130 km/hour) or faster has the potential to injure the ulnar collateral ligament

Correct Answer: D. In theory, any pitch thrown at 80 miles/hour (130 km/hour) or faster has the potential to injure the ulnar collateral ligament

Cadaveric studies suggest that the ulnar collateral ligament (UCL) is at risk for rupturing when subjected to torque greater than 32 Nm. A fastball thrown at 80 miles/hour (130 km/hour) generates approximately 64 Newton-meters (Nm) of torque, of which approximately half is transmitted to the UCL. Thus, in theory, any pitch thrown at 80 miles/hour (130 km/hour) or faster has the potential to injure the UCL. The primary generators of force for the throwing athlete are the large lower extremity and trunk muscles. Athletes with open growth plates actually have a lower incidence of UCL tears and a higher incidence of bony avulsions, since the ligament is usually stronger than the growth plate. In general, the biomechanics of youth pitchers are the same as for adults.

1. Fleisig GS, Andrews JR, Dillman CJ, Escamilla RF. Kinetics of baseball pitching with implications about injury mechanisms. Am J Sports Med 1995 Mar-Apr;23(2):233-239.
2. Fleisig GS, Barrentine SW, Zheng N, Escamilla RF, Andrews JR. Kinematic and kinetic comparison of baseball pitching among various levels of development. J Biomech 1999 Dec;32(12):1371-1375.
3. Young C. Throwing injuries: biomechanics and mechanism of injury. UpToDate. Accessed December 8, 2018 at https://www.uptodate.com/contents/throwing-injuries-biomechanics-and-mechanism-of-injury.

75. A patient presents with chronic forearm pain that she describes as a "deep ache" and associated with some weakness, but no loss of sensation. The pain is worse at night, and she points to an area distal to the lateral epicondyle. On physical exam, she has normal sensation, but the pain is reproduced with wrist extension and finger extension. You suspect a compression neuropathy, which of the following anatomical structures is the most likely source?

   A. Arcade of Frohse
   B. Arcade of Struthers
   C. Guyon's canal
   D. Two heads of pronator teres

Correct Answer: A. Arcade of Frohse

The scenario of forearm pain, especially at night, that is reproducible, with no sensory changes, describes radial tunnel syndrome. The most likely site of radial nerve compression in this syndrome is the Arcade of Frohse. The Arcade of Struthers is the site of ulnar nerve compression slightly above the elbow. Guyon's canal is the site of ulnar nerve compression in the ulnar tunnel at the wrist ("cyclist's palsy"). Median nerve compression may occur between the two heads of the pronator teres, and is associated with anterior interosseous nerve syndrome (AINS).

1. Keefe D, Lintner D. Nerve injuries in the throwing elbow. Clin Sports Med 2004 Oct;23(4):723-742, xi.
2. Neal S, Fields K. Peripheral nerve entrapment in the upper extremity. Am Fam Physician 2010 Jan 15;81(2):147-155.

76. A 13-year-old cross country runner complains of right anterior knee pain. He denies any trauma to the knee or specific injury. Pain worsens with running and prolonged walking, and improves with rest and ice. He denies locking or popping sensation. An x-ray of the right knee demonstrates a well-circumscribed, nondisplaced fragment of subchondral bone on the articular surface of the patella and no loose bodies. What is the next step in treatment of this condition?

   A. Obtain an MRI
   B. Stop running for six weeks and undergo rehab
   C. Stop running and undergo eccentric strengthening of the quadriceps
   D. Straight leg brace for two weeks

Correct Answer: A. Obtain an MRI

This lesion is characteristic of osteochondritis dissecans (OCD) in this adolescent. Cessation of aggravating activity and rehabilitation is appropriate for low-grade OCD lesions; however, they cannot be graded by plain radiographs. MRI is necessary to grade osteochondritis dissecans, and to determine if surgical treatment will be necessary. Eccentric strengthening of the quadriceps would be the treatment for patellar tendinopathy. Straight-leg bracing would be inappropriate in this situation.

1. Hixon A, Gibbs L. Osteochondritis dissecans: a diagnosis not to miss. Am Fam Physician 2000 Jan;61(1):151-156.
2. Jacobs BA. Knee osteochondritis dissecans. Medscape. Accessed December 8, 2018 at https://emedicine.medscape.com/article/89718.

77. What is the structure labeled on the sagittal and transverse imaging of the shoulder?

   A. Ulnar nerve
   B. Supraspinatus tendon
   C. Tendon of the long head of the biceps brachii
   D. Tendon of the short head of the biceps brachii
   E. Axillary nerve

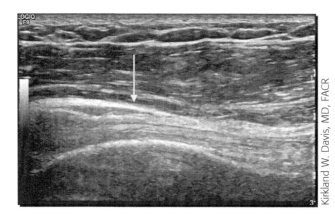

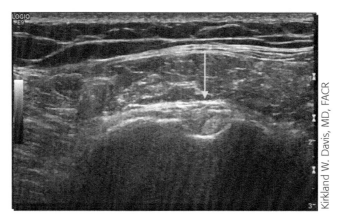

Correct Answer: C. Tendon of the long head of the biceps brachii

The first image is a sagittal image of the long head of the bicep brachii as it courses through the bicipital groove. The second image is transverse imaging over the bicipital groove with the transverse humeral ligament overlying the long head of the biceps brachii. The tendon should appear hyperechoic when the transducer is perpendicular to the course of the tendon. A well-defined humeral cortex in the floor of the bicipital groove indicates the sound beam is perpendicular to the overlying tendon.

1. Skendzel JG, Jacobson JA, Carpenter JE, Miller BS. Long head of biceps brachii tendon evaluation: accuracy of preoperative ultrasound. AJR Am J Roentgenol 2011 Oct;197(4):942-948. doi: 10.2214/AJR.10.5012.

78. A 12-year-old baseball player complains of worsening pain and swelling on the lateral aspect of his left foot for the past three to four weeks. He states that he notices it the most after he has played in a full baseball game or practice, or if he has just been very active that day. It generally has improved by the time he wakes up in the morning. He also states that his baseball cleats and other tight shoes cause pain. He has been wearing flip-flop-type shoes for relief. There is no known trauma to the area, and he has never had this before. Upon further questioning, his mother states that he has been growing quite a bit over the last few months. He has no other complaints of lower limb pain. Physical exam reveals tenderness to palpation directly over the base of the fifth metatarsal of the left foot and swelling at the same level on the lateral aspect of both feet. Below is a radiograph of the left foot. What is the diagnosis?

   A. Stress fracture
   B. Jones fracture
   C. Iselin's disease
   D. Kohler's disease

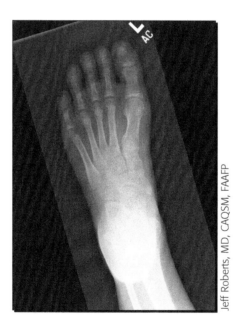

Correct Answer: C. Iselin's disease

The image of the left foot shows Iselin's disease, which is an apophysitis or traction-type injury to the growth plate of the base of the fifth metatarsal commonly seen in children. They complain of pain and swelling in the area, without a known trauma, which is aggravated by activity and tight-fitting shoes. Initial symptoms and recurrences are common in children during rapid periods of the growth. The peroneus brevis muscle attaches onto the base of the fifth metatarsal, causing the traction-type injury, and is generally classified as an overuse type injury. Treatment is relative rest; ice; padding the area, along with wearing looser fitting shoes; analgesic-type medicine, such as NSAIDS or Tylenol; and a short course of physical therapy, if severe. Kids can participate in sports as tolerated. Rarely, immobilization is needed for a short time. Iselin's is self-limited and will resolve once the physis is closed. A stress fracture is uncommon in this area in this age group. A Jones fracture will have a more horizontal appearance to the fracture line on radiographs. Kohler's disease is a self-limited osetochondrosis of the navicular bone in children ages six to nine.

1. Canale ST, Williams KD. Iselin's disease. J Pediatr Orthop 1992 Jan;12(1):90-93.
2. Gillespie H. Osteochondroses and apophyseal injuries of the foot in the young athlete. Curr Sports Med Rep 2010 Sep-Oct;9(5):265-268. doi: 10.1249/JSR.0b013e3181f19488.

79. During knee flexion, the primary restraints to medial and lateral translation of the patella change. When the knee is in 30 to 60 degrees of flexion, what is the primary restraint?

   A. Vastus medialis oblique (VMO)
   B. Medial patellofemoral ligament (MPFL)
   C. Femoral trochlear groove
   D. Lateral retinaculum

Correct Answer: C. Femoral trochlear groove

From 0 to 30 degrees of flexion, the primary restraint is the MPFL (Answer B). This ligament attaches from the medial patella to the medial femoral condyle. Secondary restraints are the VMO and lateral retinaculum. From 30 to 90 degrees of flexion, the patella has entered the trochlear groove, which is the primary restraint. Contact from the patella moves from inferior to superior poles of the patella. At 90 degrees, the patellar tendon contacts the trochlear groove and begins to absorb some of the compressive forces.

   1. Sherman SL, Plackis AC, Nuelle CW. Patellofemoral anatomy and biomechanics. Clin Sports Med 2014 Jul;33(3):389-401. doi: 10.1016/j.csm.2014.03.008. Epub 2014 May 17.
   2. Koh JL, Stewart C. Patellar instability. Clin Sports Med 2014 Jul;33(3):461-476. doi: 10.1016/j.csm.2014.03.011. Epub 2014 May 29.

80. Exercise has been found to be beneficial for those living with HIV. Which of the following measures is not a result of moderate exercise (aerobic and resistance training) in those infected with HIV?

    A. Increase in strength
    B. Decrease in resting heart rate
    C. Improved insulin sensitivity
    D. Decrease in lean tissue mass

Correct Answer: D. Decrease in lean tissue mass.

Several studies have demonstrated the beneficial effects of exercise in patients with HIV. This includes moderate aerobic and resistance training exercise routines. Some of the reported benefits include improvement in efficiency of oxygen consumption, insulin sensitivity, depression and other psychological symptoms, body composition, glucose levels, lipid levels, and CD4 counts. Studies have specifically demonstrated increase in strength, while showing a decrease in resting heart rate. Of interest, lean body mass has been shown to increase with exercise routine which is helpful, in particular, to the potential wasting effects of HIV infection.

1. Bessa A, Lopez JC, DiMasi F, Ferry F, Costa E, Silva G, et al. Lymphocyte CD4+ cell count, strength improvements, heart rate and body composition of HIV-positive patients during a 3-month strength training program. J Sports Med Phys Fitness 2017 Jul-Aug;57(7-8):1051-1056. doi: 10.23736/S0022-4707.16.06357-X. Epub 2016 Jul 19.
2. Dudgeon WD, Jaggers JR, Phillips KD, Durstine JL, Burgess SE, Lyerly GW, et al. Moderate-intensity exercise improves body composition and improves physiological markers of stress in HIV-infected men. ISRN AIDS 2012 Dec 11;2012:145127. doi: 10.5402/2012/145127. eCollection 2012.
3. Zanetti HR, da Cruz LG, Lourenço CL, Neves FF, Silva-Vergara ML, Mendes EL. Does nonlinear resistance training reduce metabolic syndrome in people living with HIV? A randomized clinical trial. J Sports Med Phys Fitness 2017 May;57(5):678-684. doi: 10.23736/S0022-4707.16.06294-0. Epub 2016 Apr 6.

81. A nine-year-old male fell on an outstretched left arm while skateboarding. He immediately had pain and a noticeable deformity of his left wrist. Radiographs show a displaced fracture of his distal radial metaphysis. He is in pain, but neurovascularly intact. Which of the following is true?

   A. He will need to be followed closely over the next few years for growth arrest of the radius
   B. He should be splinted and follow-up with orthopedic surgery in two weeks for further management
   C. He should undergo open reduction and immobilization
   D. Secondary to a significant degree of remodeling, incomplete reduction of distal radial metaphyseal fractures may yield successful outcomes in children

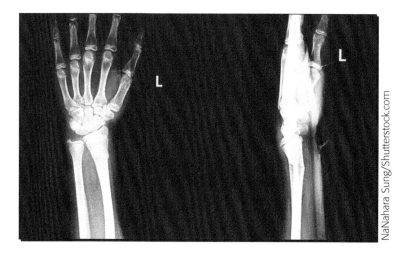

Correct Answer: D. Secondary to a significant degree of remodeling, incomplete reduction of distal radial metaphyseal fractures may yield successful outcomes in children

In children, high levels of remodeling can occur. He presents with a displaced metaphyseal fracture of the distal radius. He should be treated with closed reduction and immobilization. Though good reduction alignment is always desired, pediatric bone healing of metaphyseal/diaphyseal fractures allows for remodeling, a process which is much less robust or not even seen in skeletally mature adults. Another good example is mid-shaft clavicle fractures in children, and the degree of remodeling typically seen over the course of their healing. Because of the brisk healing response and rapid callous formation in children, any reduction should be completed as soon as possible to allow proper bone alignment and healing, which is why Answer B is incorrect. Closed reduction should be attempted first, unless there are other complicating factors, such as neurovascular compromise. Accordingly, Answer C is incorrect as an initial course of treatment for this fracture. This is not a physeal injury, and growth arrest is not a concern.

1. Crawford SN, Lee LS, Izuka BH. Closed treatment of overriding distal radial fractures without reduction in children. J Bone Joint Surg Am 2012 Feb 1;94(3):246-252. doi: 10.2106/JBJS.K.00163.
2. Pannu GS, Herman M. Distal radius-ulna fractures in children. Orthop Clin North Am 2015 Apr;46(2):235-248. doi: 10.1016/j.ocl.2014.11.003. Epub 2014 Dec 17.

82. You are working in a medical tent of a marathon in September. The wet bulb globe temperature on race day is 80 degrees Fahrenheit (26.7 degrees Celsius), and many runners are experiencing heat-related symptoms. A 42-year-old woman presents to your tent with vomiting, altered mental status, and cramping. On examination, her skin is hot and dry. Her rectal temperature is found to be 104 degrees Fahrenheit (40 degrees Celsius). You quickly treat her with cold water immersion in the medical tent. What concept of thermoregulation occurs during cold water immersion?

   A. Radiation
   B. Evaporation
   C. Convection
   D. Conduction

Correct Answer: D. Conduction

Conduction occurs when heat is transferred from a warmer surface to a cooler surface, such as when a patient is immersed in a cold bath of ice and water. The greater the surface area in contact with the cooler surface, the more effective the cooling. Radiation occurs when heat is absorbed or reflected without contact. This concept of cooling is demonstrated when wearing lighter-colored clothing to reflect heat. Evaporation is the process that cools the body during perspiration and becomes less effective during times of high humidity. When the body exchanges heat with the surrounding air, this is convection. This is how fans or the wind cool the body.

1. Armstrong LE, Casa DJ, Millard-Stafford M, Moran DS, Pyne SW, Roberts WO. American College of Sports Medicine position stand. Exertional heat illness during training and competition. Med Sci Sports Exerc 2007;39(3):556-572.
2. Becker JA, Stewart LK. Heat-related illness. Am Fam Physician 2011 Jun 1;83(11):1325-1330.

83. An 11-year-old male presents in clinic with his mother because he's complaining of pain in his right heel after basketball practice and games. At the end of games and practices, he appears to limp and continues to limp for the next hour or so afterwards. On inspection, he has no swelling about the foot or ankle, and normal appearance of both feet, with normal arches. He has tenderness to palpation at the posterior aspect of his calcaneus. Radiographs of both feet show no asymmetry, fracture, or bone cysts. What is the most likely diagnosis?

A. Calcaneal apophysitis
B. Os trigonum syndrome
C. Freiberg's disease
D. Köhler disease

Correct Answer: A. Calcaneal apophysitis

This patient presents with calcaneal apophysitis (Sever's disease). Pain develops and worsens with activity. This condition most commonly presents at the age of nine years in females and 11 years in males. Treatment consists of short-term modification or restriction of the precipitating activity. Shoe modifications, with heel-lift or Achilles tendon stretching, can also help. This is often self-limited. Os trigonum syndrome (posterior ankle impingement) causes posterolateral ankle pain, worsened with squatting, resisted plantarflexion, or dorsiflexion of the great toe, as these cause friction between the flexor hallucis longus as it passes over the talus. Freiberg's disease is avascular necrosis of the metatarsal head, most commonly the second metatarsal. A short period of immobilization is generally recommended. Kohler disease is an osteochondrosis of the navicular and generally requires a period of immobilization.

1. Chorley J. Heel pain in the active child or skeletally immature adolescent: overview of causes. UpToDate. Accessed December 8, 2018 at https://www.uptodate.com/contents/heel-pain-in-the-active-child-or-skeletally-immature-adolescent-overview-of-causes.

84. Normal growth and regeneration of muscle tissue in response to training or injury is controlled by satellite cells. Which of the following activates these satellite cells?

   A. Myosin
   B. Insulin-like growth factor-1 (IGF-1)
   C. Interleukin-7 (IL-7)
   D. Interleukin-3 (IL-3)

Correct Answer: B. Insulin-like growth factor-1 (IGF-1)

Insulin-like growth factor-1 (IGF-1) is a primary regulator of satellite cells. Myosin is a key muscle protein that helps constitute myofilaments and does not activate satellite cells. Interleukin-7 is involved in the differentiation and proliferation of lymphoid progenitor cells and increases pro inflammatory cytokines. Interleukin-3 activates hematopoietic stem cells and mast cells.

   1. Wilborn CD, Taylor LW, Greenwood M, Kreider RB, Willoughby DS. Effects of different intensities of resistance exercise on regulators of myogenesis. J Strength Cond Res 2009 Nov;23(8):2179-2187. doi: 10.1519/JSC.0b013e3181bab493.
   2. Zammit PS. All muscle satellite cells are equal, but are some more equal than others? J Cell Sci 2008 Sep 15;121(Pt 18):2975-2982. doi: 10.1242/jcs.019661.

85. A 16-year-old male football defensive end presents with left knee pain. He was rushing the quarterback at practice and felt a pop in his left knee. He has been unable to weight-bear. He reports no previous knee pain. Physical exam is notable for pain with knee flexion, and he cannot do a normal straight-leg raise against gravity. There is swelling over the tibial tubercle and across the proximal medial and lateral tibia. There does not appear to be a significant knee effusion. Ligament testing is deferred. X-rays are ordered. Based on this description, which of the following is the most likely injury?

   A. Osgood-Schlatter apophysitis
   B. Patellar tendon tear
   C. Patellar sleeve fracture
   D. Tibial tubercle avulsion fracture

Correct Answer: D. Tibial tubercle avulsion fracture

A tibial tubercle avulsion fracture is a fracture of the closing apophysis/physis. It occurs most often in adolescent males between 14 to 16 years old. There are several classifications, including the Ogden classification (see references for pictures). An important feature of the fracture, which starts at the tibial tubercle and extends superiorly, is whether the fracture extends into the joint line. This is best seen on a lateral x-ray. Fractures that extend into the joint line require surgical stabilization, while non-displaced fractures may be reduced and treated non-operatively. Advanced imaging with three-dimensional capacity, such as CT, may be necessary to determine if the fracture is adequately reduced. About 4% of these fractures develop compartment syndrome, so that must be clinically evaluated at the time of injury.

All of the choices listed involve an injury/disruption of the extensor mechanism. Osgood-Schlatter apophysitis is incorrect, because that usually presents in boys from 12 to 14 years old who have open physes, while a tibial tubercle avulsion fracture occurs in an older age group as the proximal tibial physis is closing. Osgood-Schlatter apophysitis is an injury but not a disruption of the extensor mechanism, although due to pain, some patients may not be able to demonstrate terminal extension on a straight-leg raise. It will also have a more insidious onset. A patellar sleeve fracture is an intra-articular fracture and, as such, would present with a joint effusion. Patellar tendon tear is possible, but most likely to occur with a completely closed physis seen in a fully grown individual, rather than a closing physis, making it less likely than a tibial tubercle avulsion fracture in this patient.

1. Pandya NK, Edmonds EW, Roocroft JH, Mubarak SJ. Tibial tubercle fractures: complications, classification, and the need for intra-articular assessment. J Pediatr Orthop 2012 Dec;32(8):749-759. doi: 10.1097/BPO.0b013e318271bb05.
2. Pretell-Mazzini J, Kelly DM, Sawyer JR, Esteban EM, Spence DD, Warner WC Jr, et al. Outcomes and complications of tibial tubercle fractures in pediatric patients: a systematic review of the literature. J Pediatr Orthop 2016 Jul-Aug;36(5):440-446. doi: 10.1097/BPO.0000000000000488.
3. Merrow AC, Reiter MP, Zbojniewicz AM, Laor T. Avulsion fractures of the pediatric knee. Pediatr Radiol 2014 Nov;44(11):1436-1445; quiz 1433-1436. doi: 10.1007/s00247-014-3126-6. Epub 2014 Oct 21.

86. What is the major contributor to the increased cardiac output in response to an acute bout of aerobic exercise in a well-trained athlete?

    A. Increase in heart rate
    B. Increase in stroke volume
    C. Increase in peripheral resistance
    D. Increase in the systolic blood pressure

Correct Answer: A. Increase in heart rate

Even in well-trained athletes, heart rate increases significantly in response to aerobic activity and is the major contributor to the increase in cardiac output. While other factors, like stroke volume and a-$\dot{V}O_2$ difference, contribute directly to cardiac output, the increase in these factors are modest. Aerobically trained athletes will increase stroke volume overall, which will blunt the heart rate response. Still this is modest. While systolic blood pressure increases with aerobic activity, this is modest and does not directly contribute to increased cardiac output. Peripheral resistance actually decreases in response to aerobic activity.

1. Kovacs R, Baggish AL. Cardiovascular adaptation in athletes. Trends Cardiovasc Med 2016 Jan;26(1):46-52. doi: 10.1016/j.tcm.2015.04.003. Epub 2015 Apr 10.
2. Asplund CA, Best T. Exercise physiology. In: Miller MD, Thompson SR (eds). DeLee & Drez's Orthopaedic Sports Medicine. 4th ed. Philadelphia: Saunders Elsevier, 2015:72-83.

87. A high school freshman baseball player presents to your office with the complaint of right elbow pain for two weeks. He describes sudden onset of pain on the medial aspect of the right elbow while throwing. Which of the following is the most likely injury in this patient?

    A. Golfer's elbow
    B. Ulnar collateral ligament (UCL) tear
    C. Medial epicondyle avulsion fracture
    D. Medial epicondyle apophysitis

Correct Answer: C. Medial epicondyle avulsion fracture

Medial elbow injuries in throwers follow predictable patterns, based on skeletal maturity. This patient is an adolescent, so the epiphysis is the weakest link in the kinetic chain. The sudden onset of pain indicates the possibility of an avulsion fracture. Golfer's elbow tends to occur in skeletally mature patients and is usually insidious in onset, associated with overuse. UCL tears also tend to occur in skeletally mature athletes. Medial epicondyle apophysitis is more common in younger children, while the ossification centers are still forming, and often presents with a more insidious onset of pain.

1. Jawetz ST, Shah PH, Potter HG. Imaging of physeal injury: overuse. Sports Health 2015 Mar;7(2):142-153. doi: 10.1177/1941738114559380.
2. Young C. Throwing injuries of the upper extremity: clinical presentation and diagnostic approach. UpToDate. Accessed December 1, 2018 at https://www.uptodate.com/contents/throwing-injuries-of-the-upper-extremity-clinical-presentation-and-diagnostic-approach.
3. Chorley J. Elbow injuries in active children or skeletally immature adolescents: approach. UpToDate. Accessed December 8, 2018 at https://www.uptodate.com/contents/elbow-injuries-in-active-children-or-skeletally-immature-adolescents-approach.

88. When using ultrasound to evaluate lateral hip pain, it is important to identify tendon insertions on bony landmarks. Which muscular groups have attachment sites on the greater trochanter of the femur?

   A. There are no muscles that attach to the greater trochanter of the femur
   B. The gluteus medius and gluteus maximus have attachment sites on the greater trochanter of the femur
   C. The gluteus medius and gluteus minimus have attachment sites on the greater trochanter of the femur
   D. The gluteus medius, gluteus minimus, and gluteus maxiumus have attachment sites on the greater trochanter of the femur

Correct Answer: C. The gluteus medius and gluteus minimus have attachment sites on the greater trochanter of the femur

The greater trochanter region is an important, easily found landmark with ultrasound. Both the gluteus medius and gluteus minimimus can be visualized. It is important to remember that the gluteus maxiumus crosses over this region, but has no attachment site there. In the following ultrasound image, the labeled structures are: (a) gluteus minimus, (b) gluteus medius, and (c) ITB.

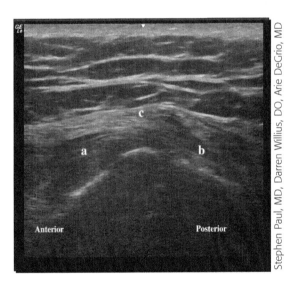

1. Thompson J. Pelvis. Netter's Concise Atlas of Orthopaedic Anatomy. Teterboro, NJ: Icon Learning Systems, 2002:182-190.
2. McEvoy JR, Lee KS, Blankenbaker DG, del Rio AM, Keene JS. Ultrasound-guided corticosteroid injections for treatment of greater trochanteric pain syndrome: greater trochanter bursa versus subgluteus medius bursa. AJR Am J Roentgenol 2013 Aug;201(2):W313-W317. doi: 10.2214/AJR.12.9443.

89. Which is true regarding vascular supply to the knee?

   A. With knee dislocations, the main concern is possible injury to the middle genicular artery
   B. The main blood supply to the ACL is from the superior medial genicular artery
   C. Regarding OCD in the knee, the medial femoral condyle is more often involved compared to the lateral femoral condyle, due to its relatively poor blood supply
   D. Regarding OCD in the knee, the lateral femoral condyle is more often involved compared to the medial femoral condyle, due to relatively poor blood supply

Correct Answer: C. Regarding OCD in the knee, the medial femoral condyle is more often involved compared to the lateral femoral condyle, due to its relatively poor blood supply

The blood supply to the medial femoral condyle (MFC) is primarily from branches of the superior medial genicular artery. Relative to the lateral femoral condyle (LFC), whose blood supply is primarily from the superior lateral genicular artery and an anastomotic branch from the inferior lateral genicular artery, the MFC has a relative watershed area, making it more vulnerable to vascular insults from trauma, surgery (AVN from incorrect ACL tunnel placement), and OCD. Answer A is incorrect, because injury to the popliteal artery should be considered in the setting of knee dislocation. Arteriography is the gold standard for evaluating suspected popliteal artery injury associated with knee dislocation. Answer B is incorrect, because the main blood supply to the ACL occurs via the middle genicular artery.

1. Natsuhara KM, Yeranosian MG, Cohen JR, Wang JC, McAllister DR, Petrigliano FA. What is the frequency of vascular injuries after knee dislocation? Clin Orthop Relat Res 2014 Sep;472(9):2615-2620.
2. Nicandri GT, Chamberlain AM, Wahl CJ. Practical management of knee dislocations: a selective angiography protocol to detect limb-threatening vascular injuries. Clin J Sport Med 2009 Mar;19(2):125-129. doi: 10.1097/JSM.0b013e31819cd37a.
3. Yamamoto H, Jones DB Jr, Moran SL, Bishop AT, Shin AY. The arterial anatomy of the medial femoral condyle and its clinical implications. J Hand Surg Eur Vol 2010 Sep;35(7):569-574. doi: 10.1177/1753193410364484. Epub 2010 Mar 17.

90. Which of the following muscles is correctly paired with the lower leg compartment in which it is found?

   A. Anterior compartment—extensor hallucis longus muscle
   B. Lateral compartment—flexor hallucis longus muscle
   C. Deep posterior compartment—soleus muscle
   D. Superficial posterior compartment—tibialis posterior muscle

Correct Answer: A. Anterior compartment—extensor hallucis longus muscle

The anterior compartment of the lower leg contains the extensor hallucis longus and extensor digitorum longus, along with the tibialis anterior muscle. The lateral compartment contains the peroneus (fibularis) longus and brevis muscles. The flexor hallucis longus is contained in the deep posterior compartment, along with the flexor digitorum longus and the tibialis posterior muscles. The soleus muscle and the gastrocnemius muscles are contained in the superficial posterior compartment of the lower leg.

   1. Netter FH. Atlas of Human Anatomy. 6th ed. Philadelphia: Saunders, 2014.

91. Your patient is a 32-year-old professional baseball player. He is African-American and had failed conservative management for uncomplicated hypertension. His BP is 145/98 mm Hg. What is the most appropriate first line drug choice?

    A. Amlodipine
    B. Valsartan
    C. Enalapril
    D. Hydrochlorothiazide

Correct Answer: A. Amlodipine

Amlodipine (a calcium channel blocker) and hydrochlorothiazide (a diuretic) would both be appropriate choices for an African-American patient. However, diuretics can cause salt and water losses that can be dangerous for athletes. Furthermore, diuretics are considered a masking agent by Major League Baseball. Because they can speed the excretion of banned substances, their presence constitutes a positive test. Valsartan (an ARB) and enalapril (an ACE inhibitor) would be reasonable choices for a white athlete in MLB.

1. Oliveira LP, Lawless CE. Hypertension update and cardiovascular risk reduction in physically active individuals and athletes. Phys Sports Med 2010 Apr;38(1):11-20. doi: 10.3810/psm.2010.04.1757.
2. Major League Baseball's Joint Drug Prevention and Treatment Program. Accessed December 8, 2018 at mlb.mlb.com/pa/pdf/jda.pdf.
3. James PA, Oparil S, Carter BL, Cushman WC, Dennison-Himmelfarb C, Handler J, et al. 2014 evidence-based guideline for the management of high blood pressure in adults: report from the panel members appointed to the Eighth Joint National Committee (JNC 8). JAMA 2014 Feb 5;311(5):507-520. doi: 10.1001/jama.2013.284427.

92. An aspiring bodybuilder inquires about anaerobic exercises in order to promote strength, speed, and power. Currently, he is more involved in doing aerobic exercises, and wishes to know more about what exercises lead to anaerobic energy expenditure, and what there is to expect once he starts doing more anaerobic exercises regularly. Which of the following is correct?

   A. Considerable anaerobic energy expenditure can be obtained with intense exercise, such as in a 10-mile race
   B. Greater performance in short-duration, high-intensity activities, lasting from seconds to about two minutes, has been observed in muscle energy systems trained using anaerobic exercise
   C. Recruitment of slow-twitch muscle fibers leads to increased anaerobic energy expenditure, as these operate using anaerobic metabolic systems
   D. The anaerobic system does not enable muscles to recover for the next burst in sports that require repeated short bursts of exercise
   E. The by-product of anaerobic glycolysis, lactate, may be detrimental to muscle function, and elevated muscle and blood lactate concentrations can be avoided by doing aerobic exercises in between, as these do not lead to lactate production

Correct Answer: B. Greater performance in short-duration, high-intensity activities, lasting from seconds to about two minutes, has been observed in muscle energy systems trained using anaerobic exercise

Muscle energy systems trained using anaerobic exercises perform better in short-duration, high-intensity activities. Answer A is incorrect, because intense exercise lasting upwards of about four minutes, such as in a one-mile race, leads to aerobic energy expenditure. Answer C is incorrect, because anaerobic energy expenditure is achieved through use of fast-twitch, not slow-twitch, fibers. Answer D is incorrect, because sports that require short bursts of exercise are, in fact, reliant on anaerobic systems. Answer E is incorrect, because elevated muscle and blood lactate concentrations can arise from both anaerobic and aerobic exercises.

1. Ciolac EG, Bocchi EA, Greve JM, Guimaraes GV. Heart rate response to exercise and cardiorespiratory fitness of young women at high familial risk for hypertension: effects of interval vs continuous training. Eur J Cardiovasc Prev Rehab 2011 Dec;18(6):824-830. doi: 10.1177/1741826711398426. Epub 2011 Feb 28.
2. Ellison GM, Waring CD, Vicinanza C, Torella D. Physiological cardiac remodeling in response to endurance exercise training: cellular and molecular mechanisms. Heart 2012 Jan;98(1):5-10. doi: 10.1136/heartjnl-2011-300639. Epub 2011 Aug 31.
3. Scott CB. Contribution of anaerobic energy expenditure to whole body thermogenesis. Nutr Metab 2005 Jun 15;2(1):14.

93. A 55-year-old male presents for evaluation of numbness and tingling in the thumb and radial aspect of the left hand. He is a mechanic and has known degenerative disc disease in his neck from previous radiographs. For further evaluation of his symptoms, an EMG/NCV test was performed that indicated the source of his symptoms was coming from his cervical spine. The nerve root likely being compressed exits between which two vertebrae?

   A. C4-5
   B. C5-6
   C. C6-7
   D. C7-T1

Correct Answer: B. C5-C6

There are eight cervical nerves and seven cervical vertebrae. The first seven cervical nerves exit the spine above the vertebra of the same number, whereas the eighth cervical nerve exits below C7 (between C7-T1). C6 nerve root is responsible for sensation to the thumb and radial aspect of the hand and forearm, and exits between C5-C6. Recall that in the lumbar spine, in contrast, the nerve exits below the vertebra of the same number (for example, the L5 nerve exits between L5-S1).

1. Childress MA, Becker BA. Nonoperative management of cervical radiculopathy. Am Fam Physician 2016;93(9):746-754.
2. Hansen JT. Netter's Clinical Anatomy. 3rd ed. Philadelphia: Saunders, 2014.

94. An 18-year-old male baseball pitcher presents to your office with a six-month history of medial-sided elbow pain aggravated by throwing. He has pain and some laxity when testing his ulnar collateral ligament. The transverse ligament (Cooper's ligament) contributes what percentage of ligamentous stability to valgus stress of the elbow?

   A. 0%
   B. 10%
   C. 25%
   D. 33%

Correct Answer: A. 0%

The transverse component of the ulnar collateral ligament (UCL) has no functional resistance to valgus load, as it originates and attaches to the same bone. The anterior bundle of the UCL is subdivided into anterior and posterior bands, which are reciprocally taut as the elbow moves through flexion and contribute most of the resistance to valgus load. The posterior bundle is only a restraint in flexion starting at > 55 degrees. In extension, the UCL provides 33% of stability, while bony restraint predominates. In contrast, while in flexion to 90 degrees, it provides 50% or more.

   1. Morrey BF, An KN. Articular and ligamentous contributions to the stability of the elbow joint. Am J Sports Med 1983;11(5):315-319.
   2. Alcid JG, Ahmad CS, Lee TQ. Elbow anatomy and structural biomechanics. Clin Sports Med 2004 Oct;23(4):503-517, vii.

95. A 10-year-old girl, level 8 gymnast, presents to your clinic with right greater than left wrist pain. She grew two inches in the past three months. Her 16-year-old sister, who is also a gymnast, presents with the same pain. Why might the younger gymnast's growth spurt put her at increased risk for physeal injury as compared to her older sister?

   A. Decreased physeal strength
   B. Increased bone mineralization
   C. Decreased muscle-tendon tightness
   D. Decreased strength of surrounding fibrous tissue

Correct Answer: A. Decreased physeal strength

Gymnasts are at risk for long-term wrist complications, given that these joints were not designed for extensive weight-bearing. As the physes are still open in a premenarchal young lady, the younger gymnast is at increased risk of growth plate injury, due to her decreased physeal strength. A younger gymnast, especially one going through a growth spurt, actually has decreased bone mineralization, increased muscle-tendon tightness, and increased strength of surrounding fibrous tissue.

1. Caine D, DiFiori J, Maffulli N. Physeal injuries in children's and youth sports: reasons for concern. Br J Sports Med 2006 Sep;40(9):749-760. Epub 2006 Jun 28.
2. Maffulli N, Longo UG, Gougoulias N, Loppini M, Denaro V. Long-term health outcomes of youth sports injuries. Br J Sports 2010 Jan;44(1):21-25. doi: 10.1136/bjsm.2009.069526. Epub 2009 Dec 1.

96. A 26-year-old male endurance athlete complains of weakness with pushing off with the toes of his left foot, as he tries to return to recreational running. Weakness is also noted with plantarflexion and inversion with running for the last few years, as well as slight numbness of the posterior calcaneus. In college, he recalls having lower leg pain with long runs that resulted in having a fasciotomy for chronic exertional compartment syndrome. What nerve may have been injured in the procedure?

   A. Deep peroneal nerve
   B. Superficial peroneal nerve
   C. Sural nerve
   D. Tibial nerve

Correct Answer: D. Tibial nerve

The deep peroneal nerve innervates the anterior compartment muscles, which dorsiflex the ankle and extend the toes, with sensation to the first dorsal web space. The superficial peroneal nerve innervates the lateral compartment muscles that aid in eversion of the foot, with some plantarflexion of the ankle and sensation to the dorsal lateral foot. The sural nerve provides sensory innervation to the posterolateral leg and lateral foot, without motor innervation. The tibial nerve was likely injured, given the sensory change to the calcaneus and the weakness with plantarflexion and inversion, as well as weakness with pushing off with toes. The tibial nerve innervates the muscles of the superficial and deep posterior compartments of the lower leg and travels in the deep posterior compartment.

   1. Rowdon GA. Chronic exertional compartment syndrome. Medscape. Accessed December 8, 2018 at https://emedicine.medscape.com/article/88014-overview.

97. Which of the following fractures involves only the physis and epiphysis, using the Salter-Harris fracture classification system?

   A. I
   B. II
   C. III
   D. IV
   E. V

Correct Answer: C. III

Salter-Harris type I fractures involve disruption of the physis only. Type II fractures involve the metaphysis and physis. Type III fractures involve the epiphysis and physis. Type IV fractures traverse the metaphysis, physis and epiphysis. Type V fractures involve crush injury to the physis only.

1. Eiff MP, Hatch RL, Calmbach WL (eds). Fracture Management for Primary Care. 2nd ed. Philadelphia: Saunders, 2002:28-35.
2. Young SJ, Barnett PL, Oakley EA. Fractures and minor head injuries: minor injuries in children II. Medl J Aust 2005;182(12):644-648.

98. A 33-year-old triathlete comes to your office to discuss his training for the upcoming triathlon season. He is trying to lose weight, but wants to ensure optimal performance as he continues to increase his aerobic endurance. He is interested in a ketogenic diet to help him meet his goals. How would you best describe a ketogenic diet?

- A. High in protein, low in carbohydrates
- B. Low in protein, high in carbohydrates
- C. High in fat, high in carbohydrates
- D. High in fat, low in carbohydrates

Correct Answer: D. High in fat, low in carbohydrates

A ketogenic diet is high in fat and low in carbohydrates, while keeping an adequate level of protein intake. These diets are gaining popularity with endurance athletes, especially cyclists and triathletes. Traditionally, these sports have utilized higher carbohydrate intake for energy availability. A ketogenic diet derives most of the energy from fat and protein intake. There are some encouraging data suggesting a role for a ketogenic diet in certain sports, especially those with weight categories and endurance sports. Sports physicians should be aware, however, of the strengths and limitations of this nutritional strategy. Strengths of the ketogenic diet are the potential to reduce body fat without causing excessive loss of lean body tissue, the potential to reduce body fat without reducing performance, and higher rates of whole body and muscle lipid utilization during submaximal aerobic exercise. The weaknesses are that this diet has not been shown to improve performance compared with a carbohydrate-rich diet, and there is a lot that is still now known about the effect of a ketogenic diet on strength performance.

1. Paoli A, Biano A, Grimaldi K. The ketogenic diet and sport: a possible marriage? Exerc Sport Sci Rev 2015 Jul;43(3):153-162. doi: 10.1249/JES.0000000000000050.
2. Zajac A, Poprzecki S, Maszczyk A, Czuba M, Michalczyk M, Zydek G. The effects of a ketogenic diet on exercise metabolism and physical performance in off-road cyclists. Nutrients 2014 Jun 27;6(7):2493-2508. doi: 10.3390/nu6072493.
3. Franchini E, Brito CJ, Artioli GG. Weight loss in combat sports: physiological, psychological, and performance effects. J Int Soc Sports Nutr 2012 Dec 13;9(1):52. doi: 10.1186/1550-2783-9-52.

99. A 24-year-old male is deep scuba diving with his friends. He starts swimming off course. His friends go after him, and he is not responding to them appropriately. They swim him to the surface. Within a few minutes, he is back to normal. Which gas is responsible for this reaction?

   A. Nitrogen
   B. Helium
   C. Oxygen
   D. Xenon

Correct Answer: A. Nitrogen

Nitrogen is the gas that is known for causing a narcotic effect and producing the aforementioned symptoms. It can cause confusion, disturbed coordination, lack of concentration, hallucinations, and/or unconsciousness, also known as rapture of the deep, while scuba diving at deeper depths. It is the gas in the highest concentration in the atmosphere. As the pressure increases at deeper depths, the solubility of gases in body tissues increases. The high level of nitrogen in the body causes the narcosis. Helium is the gas that is the least responsible for producing the aforementioned symptoms. Oxygen and ascent are used to treat the "nitrogen narcosis." Although Xenon has the highest narcotic strength, the levels in the atmosphere are not high enough to cause these symptoms.

1. Clark JE. Moving in extreme environments: inert gas narcosis and underwater activities. Extrem Physiol Med 2015 Feb 24;4:1. doi: 10.1186/s13728-014-0020-7. eCollection 2015.
2. Eichhorn L, Leyk D. Diving medicine in clinical practice. Dtsch Arztebl Int 2015 Feb 27;112(9):147-157; quiz 158. doi: 10.3238/arztebl.2015.0147.

100. Which of the following statements is true regarding exertional headache?

    A. Factors associated with increased risk of exertional headaches include hot weather and high altitude
    B. Exertional headaches are always benign
    C. Exertional headaches most commonly occur in young women
    D. The typical duration of exertional headaches is seconds to minutes

Correct Answer: A. Factors associated with increased risk of exertional headaches include hot weather and high altitude

Factors that increase the risk of exertional headache include hot weather, dehydration, and high altitude. Exertional headaches are not always benign, and can be related to intracranial bleeding, brain tumors, and myocardial infarction. Benign exertional headache occurs most frequently in men over 40 years old. Typically, exertional headaches last from five minutes to 24 hours. Headaches that are described as "the worst headache of my life" are suspicious for subarachnoid hemorrhage.

1. Putukian M. Headaches in the athlete. In: Mellion MB, Walsh WM, Madden C, Putukian M, Shelton GL (eds). Team Physician's Handbook. 3rd ed. Philadelphia: Hanley & Belfus, 2002:299-311.

101. A 31-year-old competitive triathlete training for the Ironman Triathlon presents with severe bilateral quadricep pain and swelling three days after completing an intense hill workout. Which of the following is the correct advice to give him regarding his training?

    A. Discontinue exercise and have lactic acid measurement performed
    B. Discontinue exercise until muscle soreness has been alleviated
    C. Continue exercise, with an intense warm-up
    D. Continue exercise, with pre- and post-exercise stretching

Correct Answer: C. Continue exercise, with an intense warm-up

This athlete is experiencing delayed-onset muscle soreness (DOMS). It is distinguished from immediate exercise-induced muscle soreness in that the symptoms, although similar, present 24 hours after exercise completion and peak within 72 hours. Answer A is incorrect, as lactic acid is not the only player in DOMS symptom production. In fact, six theories work in concert to explain the mechanism of DOMS: lactic acid accumulation, muscle spasm, microtrauma, connective tissue damage, inflammation, and electrolyte and enzyme efflux. The symptoms of DOMS slowly resolve over five to seven days, but waiting this long could hinder this athlete's training progress, making Answer B incorrect. It has been documented that further exercise before recovery from the original eccentric damage does not delay the rate of recovery, thus describing a "repeated bout" protective effect. In addition, there are reports that pain can be temporarily reduced by performing exercise. This exercise-induced analgesia (EIA) has been observed after prolonged aerobic exercise, as in cycling and running. The analgesic effect is greater for higher exercise intensities and occurs likely via increases in local blood flow and subsequent endorphin release. Answer C is therefore the correct choice. Evidence from randomized trials suggests that pre- and post-exercise stretching does not produce significant reductions in post-exercise soreness in healthy adults, thus Answer D is incorrect.

1. Lewis P, Ruby D, Bush-Joseph C. Muscle soreness and delayed onset muscle soreness. Clin Sports Med 2012 Apr;31(2):255-262. doi: 10.1016/j.csm.2011.09.009. Epub 2011 Nov 23.
2. Herbert RD, de Noronha M, Kamper SJ. Stretching to prevent or reduce muscle soreness after exercise. Cochrane Database Syst Rev 2011 Jul 6;(7):CD004577. doi: 10.1002/14651858.CD004577.pub3.
3. Sakamoto A, Maruyama T, Hisashi N, Sinclair P. Acute effects of high-intensity dumbbell exercise after isokinetic eccentric damage: interaction between altered pain perception and fatigue on static and dynamic muscle performance. J Strength Cond Res 2010 Aug;24(8):2042-2049. doi: 10.1519/JSC.0b013e3181d8e881.

102. In comparison to adult bone, how does pediatric bone differ?

    A. Pediatric bone is more dense
    B. Pediatric periosteum is thinner, and therefore more susceptible to fracture
    C. Pediatric bone is metabolically less active
    D. Pediatric bone is more cartilaginous

Correct Answer: D. Pediatric bone is more cartilaginous

Pediatric bone has distinct differences when compared to adult bone, allowing the bones in children to have unique fracture patterns such as buckle fractures and greenstick fractures. Pediatric bone is less dense than adult bone, having lower mineral content and being more porous (more flexible). The bone in children is more cartilaginous, therefore it is more pliable and has less tensile strength. The periosteum in pediatric bone is thicker, giving more strength to the bone and allowing for some bends and incomplete fracture patterns: bowing/plastic deformation, which is common to the ulna and associated with other fractures, and greenstick fractures, which are incomplete fractures due to a force perpendicular to shaft (side of incoming force has retained periosteum). Finally, pediatric bone is metabolically more active, which leads to more rapid callus formation, which allows rapid healing, rapid remodeling, and often shorter-term immobilization and quicker return to activities.

1. Carson S, Woolridge DP, Colletti J, Kilgore K. Pediatric upper extremity injuries. Pediatr Clin N Am 2006 Feb;53(1):41-67.
2. Arora R, Fichadia U, Hartwig E, Kannikeswaran N. Pediatric upper-extremity fractures. Pediatr Annals 2014;43(5):196-204.
3. Brooks A, Hammer E. Acute upper extremity injuries in young athletes. Clin Pediatr Emerg Med 2013;14(4):289-303.

103. A 12-year-old female presents to your clinic with a two-month history of generalized right foot pain and limping. The patient says her left foot hurts on occasion, as well. She cannot recall a specific injury, but this pain has started to make basketball practice somewhat difficult. On exam, you notice that she has rigid flat feet. You obtain bilateral, standing-foot radiographs and note an abnormality consistent with tarsal coalition. Which of the following is most true regarding the diagnosis and evaluation of tarsal coalition?

   A. On radiographs, beaking of the talar neck and widening of the talonavicular joint may be associated with tarsal coalition
   B. If a tarsal coalition is present, a radiograph should always be diagnostic, and a CT is rarely needed for diagnosis
   C. It would be unusual for this patient to have a tarsal coalition, as this condition typically presents around five years old
   D. Her right foot may have a tarsal coalition, but it is unlikely her left foot also has a tarsal coalition, because bilateral occurrence is extremely rare

Correct Answer: A. On radiographs, beaking of the talar neck and widening of the talonavicular joint may be associated with tarsal coalition

Radiographs can often be nondiagnostic, as the coalition can be fibrocartilaginous and not a true bony coalition. A noncontrast CT is considered the gold standard for diagnosis. This condition often presents in the second decade of life. 50% to 60% of coalitions are bilateral.

1. Benjamin HJ. The pediatric athlete. In: Madden CC, Putukian M, Young CC, McCarty EC (eds). Netter's Sports Medicine. Philadelphia: Saunders Elsevier, 2010:63-64.
2. Clark MC. Overview of the causes of limp in children. UpToDate. Accessed December 8, 2018 at https://www.uptodate.com/contents/overview-of-the-causes-of-limp-in-children.

104. A 45-year-old female presents to the office with chronic plantar heel pain. In considering a differential diagnosis, which of the following statements best describes tarsal tunnel syndrome?

   A. Tarsal tunnel syndrome does not co-exist with plantar fasciitis
   B. Tarsal tunnel syndrome causes "first-step" pain when rising from a resting position, and remits promptly with walking
   C. Tarsal tunnel syndrome causes pain with walking and gradually remits with rest
   D. Tarsal tunnel syndrome is associated with lateral ankle pain

Correct Answer: C. Tarsal tunnel syndrome causes pain with walking and gradually remits with rest

Tarsal tunnel syndrome describes an entrapment neuropathy affecting the posterior tibial nerve and its branches in the tarsal tunnel. The tarsal tunnel is bounded by medial malleolus, tibia, posterior process of the talus, calcaneus, abductor hallucis, and flexor retinaculum. The tunnel contains the tibial nerve, the flexor digitorum longus and flexor hallucis longus muscles, and the tibial artery and vein. Symptoms typically consist of pain in the medial aspect of the ankle and heel, which increases with activity. "First-step" pain is classically associated with plantar fasciitis. While tarsal tunnel syndrome is often misdiagnosed as plantar fasciitis, the two entities may co-exist.

1. Ferkel E, Davis WH, Ellington JK. Entrapment neuropathies of the foot and ankle. Clin Sports Med 2015 Oct;34(4):791-801. doi: 10.1016/j.csm.2015.06.002.
2. Gould JS. Tarsal tunnel syndrome. Foot Ankle Clin N Am 2011 Jun;16(2):275-286. doi: 10.1016/j.fcl.2011.01.008.

105. A 50-year-old female patient presents to your office with exertional pain in her right calf. She has noted the pain during exercise for the past several weeks. Which of the following historical and physical findings would you expect with a diagnosis of popliteal artery entrapment syndrome?

   A. Diminished foot pulses at rest
   B. Pain more closely associated with volume of exercise, rather than intensity of exercise
   C. Slow resolution of symptoms at conclusion of exercise
   D. Patients may have normal pulses that disappear or decrease with plantarflexion or dorsiflexion of the ankle
   E. Markedly elevated compartment pressure

Correct Answer: D. Patients may have normal pulses that disappear or decrease with plantarflexion or dorsiflexion of the ankle

Popliteal artery entrapment syndrome causes calf pain during exercise, due to compression of the popliteal artery by an abnormal relationship of the artery to the gastrocnemius and/or plantaris muscles. Unlike exertional compartment syndrome, symptoms are associated with intensity of exercise, rather than volume. In addition, symptoms tend to resolve quickly after the conclusion of exercise, until very late in the disease, when sclerosis of the artery creates a more chronic condition. Foot pulses tend to be normal at rest, but can be abnormal with dorsi- and plantarflexion of the ankle. For this reason, diagnostic workup for the disorder includes Doppler ultrasonography or angiography in neutral position, dorsiflexion, and plantarflexion. MRI and MR angiography can also be performed in provocative positions and can show the abnormal muscular or fibrous attachment. Compartment pressures are usually normal or slightly elevated. This disorder is usually treated by cessation of causative activities, followed by surgical release of the artery from the offending muscles. After surgical release, most patients can resume normal exercise.

1. Zetaruk M, Hyman J. Leg injuries. In: Frontera WR, Herring SA, Micheli LJ, Silver JK (eds). Clinical Sports Medicine, Medical Management and Rehabilitation. China: Elsevier, 2007:451.
2. Wright LB, Matchett WJ, Cruz CP, James CA, Culp WC, Eidt JF. Popliteal artery disease: diagnosis and treatment. Radiographics 2004 Mar-Apr;24(2):467-479.

Test 2 Answers, Critiques, and References

106. A 15-year-old gymnast presents to the office with back pain that has been present for several months, but she has not wanted to address the problem until the end of her competitive season. Her parents are very concerned that she has been complaining daily of back pain with all flipping skills, but became more concerned when she started having pain while lying supine. She has pain on extension of her back, but otherwise her exam is normal. You order x-rays, which are below. What would you tell her family?

  A. This is a normal back x-ray and she can take over-the-counter medications for pain. It will go away with time
  B. This is a vertebral crush injury and needs to be monitored very carefully, especially with the dynamics of gymnastics
  C. She needs an MRI, because this x-ray is non-diagnostic, and an MRI will give you the detail needed to appropriately address her findings
  D. She has a pars interarticularis fracture that has slipped forward (spondylolisthesis) and will need prolonged rest before a slow return to sport

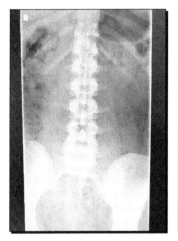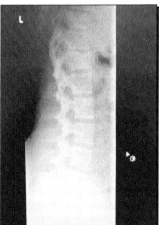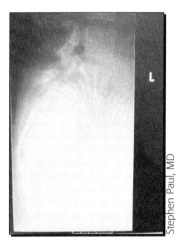

Correct Answer: D. She has a pars interarticularis fracture that has slipped forward (spondylolisthesis) and will need prolonged rest before a slow return to sport

This gymnast has a spondylolisthesis at L5-S1. The x-rays show AP, lateral, and spot views of L5-S1 of the lumbar spine, which demonstrates a bilateral break in the pars interarticularis or spondylolysis that allows the L5 vertebral body to slip forward on the S1 vertebral body: spondylolisthesis. This would be a grade I spondylolisthesis according to the Meyerding classification, which divides the superior endplate of the lower vertebrae into quarters. The grade is determined by percentage of overlap: grade I = 25% or less, grade II = 26% to 50%, grade III = 51% to 75%, grade IV = 76% to 100%, and grade 5 > 100%, which is defined as spondylolysis. Below are the oblique views which demonstrate bilateral "scottie dog," with a lucency in the neck at L5 demonstrating bilateral pars fracture.

A normal x-ray would not demonstrate slippage between L5 and S1. A vertebral crush injury is unlikely in a gymnast without a fall from substantial height, but it is more likely to be seen in an older patient. Vertebral crush injuries would also cause other symptoms of a fracture, rather than simply pain in gymnastics. In that event, most likely she would not have been able to continue with her season. MRIs are not always indicated in a spondylolisthesis injury. Oblique films and lateral films should demonstrate the injury, though oblique films are not generally ordered as often, since they are less reliable. Any athlete with a high suspicion for spondylolysis on history and exam, with negative x-rays, should undergo advanced imaging. There is current debate on ordering a bone scan, SPECT scan, or MRI, given radiation concerns, though bone scan with lumbar SPECT remains the most sensitive test.

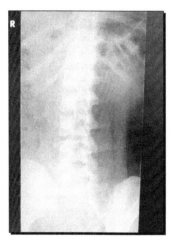
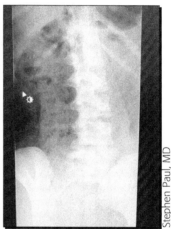

1. Cassas KJ, Cassettari-Wayhs A. Childhood and adolescent sports-related overuse injuries. Am Fam Physician 2006 Mar 15;73(6):1014-1022.
2. Standaert CJ, Herring SA. Expert opinion and controversies in sports and musculoskeletal medicine: the diagnosis and treatment of spondylolysis in adolescent athletes. Arch Phys Med Rehabil 2007 Apr;88(4):537-540.
3. Bernstein RM, Cozen H. Evaluation of back pain in children and adolescents. Am Fam Physician 2007 Dec 1;76(11):1669-1676.

107. A 35-year-old Paralympian with a T4 spinal cord injury is competing in wheelchair basketball at the national level when he is accused of "boosting." When evaluated just prior to the game, his heart rate is regular at 55 and his blood pressure is 195/100. By what mechanism is this patient able to achieve these parameters to improve his performance?

   A. Autonomic dysreflexia
   B. Amphetamine abuse
   C. Epogen injections
   D. Parasympathetic response

Correct Answer: A. Autonomic dysreflexia

Patients with spinal cord injuries (SCI) at or above the level of T6 have impaired control of their sympathetic nervous system below their injury level. They often develop a low resting blood pressure, orthostatic hypotension, and reflex bradycardia, due to the sympathetic nervous system (SNS) dysfunction. Autonomic dysreflexia occurs from a noxious stimulus present below the level of injury. This results in unopposed sympathetic outflow below the injury-producing hypertension, and a compensatory parasympathetic response produces bradycardia. These changes are relative to their baseline bradycardia and hypotension. "Boosting" involves intentional introduction of a noxious stimulus, such as a full bladder, for a performance advantage. While amphetamine abuse may cause hypertension, the patient would likely also have a higher heart rate, because illicit drug use causes systemic effects, while "boosting" specifically elicits an autonomic response in these individuals. Epogen will not impact HR and BP in these ways. Parasympathetic response is not a known entity in competitive cheating.

   1. Teasell RW, Arnold MO, Krassioukov A, Delaney GA. Cardiovascular consequences of loss of supraspinal control of the sympathetic nervous system after spinal cord injury. Arch Phys Med Rehabil 2000 Apr;81(4):506-516.
   2. Bhambhani Y, Mactavish J, Warren S, Thompson WR, Webborn A, Bressan E, et al. Boosting in athletes with high level spinal cord injury: knowledge, incidence, and attitudes of athletes in paralympic sport. Disabil Rehabil 2010;32(26):2172-2190. doi: 10.3109/09638288.2010.505678.

108. Which athlete with type 1 diabetes mellitus is at the most risk for developing hyperglycemia from a bout of exercise?

   A. 22-year-old cyclist racing in his first 150-mile event, with good glycemic control, who gave himself a pre-race bolus of regular insulin
   B. 18-year-old multi-event sprinter in the Texas state championship track meet, with elevated fasting blood sugars prior to the event, who pre-medicated with Lantus (insulin glargine)
   C. 19-year-old soccer player participating in early spring conditioning at 75% of her maximal heart rate, with hypoglycemia in the days leading up to her training
   D. 20-year-old rower performing drills in practice, who gave herself a pre-practice bolus of regular insulin, despite not eating that morning

Correct Answer: B. 18-year-old multi-event sprinter in the Texas state championship track meet, with elevated fasting blood sugars prior to the event, who pre-medicated with Lantus (insulin glargine)

Answer A is not the best choice, as the endurance activity is aerobic and generally leads to hypoglycemia. The absorption of subcutaneously injected insulin may be increased with exercise. The increase in subcutaneous and skeletal muscle blood flow resulting from exercise can be associated with a concurrent increase in insulin absorption and accelerated hypoglycemia. The athlete in Answer B participates in a highly anaerobic activity, which causes elevated blood sugar levels. His state track meet in Texas is likely to be held outdoors in the late spring. Individuals competing in warm and humid environments have higher blood glucose levels, due to exercise increases in plasma catecholamines, glucagon, cortisol, and growth hormone. In individuals with poor metabolic control, exercise can cause increases in blood glucose, due to exaggerated hepatic glucose production and impairment in exercise-induced glucose utilization. Finally, the psychological stress of competition is frequently associated with increases in blood glucose levels. Even though he gave himself insulin, exercise does not appear to alter insulin glargine absorption rate. Answer C is not correct, as her sport is soccer, which is an aerobic activity that generally leads to hypoglycemia. If the intensity increases to greater than 85% of maximal heart rate, the reverse may be true, due to elevations in catecholamines, free fatty acids, and ketone bodies. In addition, individuals who experience hypoglycemia on days preceding competition may have an elevated risk of hypoglycemia and autonomic counter-regulatory failure during exercise. Answer D is not correct, as her sport, rowing, is an aerobic activity that generally results in hypoglycemia. This will be increased by not eating, along with the increased absorption of insulin with exercise.

1. Riddell MC, Perkins BA. Type 1 diabetes and vigorous exercise: applications of exercise physiology to patient management. Can J Diabetes 2006;30(1):63-71.
2. Wilmore JH, Costill DL, Kenney WL. Obesity, diabetes, and physical activity. Physiology of Sport and Exercise. 4th ed. Champaign, IL: Human Kinetics, 2008:492-516.

109. An incoming freshman lacrosse player at an NCAA Division I university reports for his preparticipation evaluation. He is an asthmatic and uses an albuterol inhaler prior to exercise and as a rescue medication. He also uses an inhaled corticosteroid in the winter, as his symptoms tend to increase in cold weather. Which of the following statements is most accurate regarding his use of beta-2 agonists?

   A. He should switch to a long-acting beta agonist, given that short-acting beta agonists are banned by the NCAA
   B. He should switch to an inhaled corticosteroid year-round to avoid using a banned substance
   C. The NCAA should be notified of his use of a banned substance for therapeutic use
   D. Proper documentation of the verification of his diagnosis, treatment plan, and medication dose, as well as need for treatment, are sufficient for participation
   E. A request for exception to use a banned substance should be submitted to the NCAA

Correct Answer: D. Proper documentation of the verification of his diagnosis, treatment plan, and medication dose, as well as need for treatment, are sufficient for participation

The NCAA maintains a list of banned substances, which includes beta-2 agonists. However, there are exceptions for appropriate therapeutic use. For beta-2 agonists, the verification of diagnosis, medication, dose, and need for continued treatment should be documented in the patient's medical record, and is sufficient to allow for use of this medication. It is not necessary to apply for exception unless using an anabolic agent or peptide hormone. There is no difference in the status of long-acting versus short-acting beta-2 agonists, and appropriate treatment should take precedent. There is no need to notify the NCAA of the use of the beta-2 agonist. If requested, documentation may be sent to the NCAA regarding therapeutic use of a banned substance. Use of stimulant medication for ADHD requires the completion of a special form to be kept on file in the event of a positive drug screen, at which point the NCAA will request the documentation. Switching to an inhaled corticosteroid year-round to avoid use of a beta-2 agonist may help reduce the amount he uses the short-acting beta-2 agonist. It is, however, the gold standard for treatment of acute symptoms and should not be removed from his treatment plan. Also, use of a short-acting beta-2 agonist is the recommended treatment for symptoms that occur with exercise.

1. Medical exceptions procedures. NCAA Sports Science Institute. Accessed December 8, 2018 at http://www.ncaa.org/sport-science-institute/medical-exceptions-procedures.
2. Fanta CH. An overview of asthma management. UpToDate. Accessed December 8, 2018 at https://www.uptodate.com/contents/an-overview-of-asthma-management.

110. A 16-year-old female Junior Olympic javelin thrower presents with her father for her yearly sports physical. Her weight is 60 kg, she is feeling well, and her exam is normal. She has an international Junior Olympics competition coming up, and her father is concerned that she is drinking so much coffee that it would be considered illegal. The patient reports drinking an eight-ounce mug of regular coffee in the morning, and usually another in the mid-afternoon after school and before her workout. Regarding her caffeine intake, what is the most appropriate recommendations for this patient?

    A. She is consuming too much caffeine to legally compete in international competition, and should abstain from caffeine
    B. She should limit her coffee intake to eight ounces of regular coffee daily in order to avoid disqualification
    C. Inform them that caffeine is a legal performance enhancer, and intake is not enforced by the International Olympic Committee
    D. Inform them that her current intake is acceptable, but that caffeine is considered a performance-enhancing agent at high doses

Correct Answer: D. Inform them that her current intake is acceptable, but that caffeine is considered a performance-enhancing agent at high doses

Caffeine ingestion prior to performance is considered a performance enhancer for prolonged endurance events, as well as for certain short periods of intense exercise lasting approximately five minutes. The mechanism is not clearly understood. The NCAA and international Olympic committee have not banned use, but do specify allowable limits of 15 micrograms/mL and 12 micrograms/mL, respectively. This level can only be reached with excessive caffeine ingestion. For example, a 70 kg athlete could test positive if they rapidly consume five to six regular cups (three to four mugs) of regular coffee one hour before competition. Answer D is the most accurate advice given current recommendations. Answer A is incorrect, as the patient's caffeine ingestion is moderate and does not approach illegal levels. Answer B is incorrect, as it describes a quite low threshold for disqualification, which is not the case. Answer C is incorrect, as caffeine is monitored loosely by sports governing bodies, with established legal thresholds.

1. Spriett LL. Exercise and sport performance with low doses of caffeine. Sports Med 2014 Nov;44 Suppl 2:S175-S184. doi: 10.1007/s40279-014-0257-8.
2. Caffeine and Athletic Performance. Accessed December 8, 2018 at https://www.ncaa.org/.../Caffeine%20and%20Athletic%20Performance.pdf.

111. Which of the following is seen as an important aspect in the biomechanics of patellofemoral dysfunction that can respond to conservative treatments?

    A. Internal rotation of the femur at foot strike
    B. External rotation of the femur at foot strike
    C. Trochlear dysplasia
    D. Laterally displaced tibial tuberosity

Correct Answer: A. Internal rotation of the femur at foot strike

The functional significance of an internally rotated femur is that the trochlear groove can rotate beneath the patella, placing the patella in a relatively lateral position. If it is observed that the femur "collapses" into internal rotation during gait, and this motion appears to originate from the pelvis (as opposed to being influenced by tibial rotation), then strengthening of the external rotators, including gluteus maximus, gluteus medius, and the deep rotators, may be indicated. Trochlear dysplasia and a laterally displaced tibial tuberosity often require surgical interventions to correct, if needed for management.

1. Fredericson M, Powers C. Practical management of patellofemoral pain. Clin J Sport Med 2002 Jan;12(1):36-38.
2. Waryasz GR, McDermott AY. Patellofemoral pain syndrome (PFPS): a systematic review of anatomy and potential risk factors. Dyn Med 2008 Jun 26;7:9. doi: 10.1186/1476-5918-7-9.
3. Dutton RA, Khadavi MJ, Fredericson M. Update on rehabilitation of patellofemoral pain. Curr Sports Med Rep 2014 May-Jun;13(3):172-178. doi: 10.1249/JSR.0000000000000056.

112. The diagnosis of arrhythmogenic right ventricular cardiomyopathy (ARVC) can be challenging. Which of the following criteria suggest true ARVC, rather than changes that may occur within the normal athletic heart?

    A. Incomplete right bundle branch block
    B. Inverted T waves within the precordial leads
    C. Occasional premature ventricular complexes (two or less per 10 seconds)
    D. Bulging of the right ventricle or systolic dysfunction

Correct Answer: D. Bulging of the right ventricle or systolic dysfunction

Answers A-C are incorrect because they may also reflect the physiologic benign changes of the athletic heart. In the absence of obvious structural changes of the right ventricle, incomplete RBBB, frequent premature ventricular complexes, or inverted T waves in precordial leads can be benign. These changes are non-specific. On the other hand, caution is justified before considering these features as part of the athlete's heart syndrome. Further non-invasive investigations are advised to avoid the catastrophic consequences of a missed diagnosis. Physiological adaptations of the heart to training can obscure the diagnosis of ARVC. Right ventricular enlargement, ECG abnormalities, and arrhythmias are well documented in endurance athletes. Morphological criteria suggesting true ARVC, rather than physiological ventricular enlargement, include global right ventricular systolic dysfunction and regional wall motion abnormalities, such as bulging or aneurysm.

1. Basso C, Corrado D, Marcus FI, Nava A, Thiene G. Arrhythmogenic right ventricular cardiomyopathy. Lancet 2009 Apr 11;373(9671):1289-1300.
2. Myerburg RJ, Vetter VL. Electrocardiograms should be included in preparticipation screening of athletes. Circulation 2007 Nov 27;116(22):2616-2626; discussion 2626.
3. Drezner JA, Ackerman MJ, Anderson J, Ashley E, Asplund CA, Baggish AL, et al. Electrocardiographic interpretation in athletes: the 'Seattle criteria'. Br J Sports Med 2013 Feb;47(3):122-124. doi: 10.1136/bjsports-2012-092067.

113. A 40-year-old Caucasian male was admitted to the hospital after an episode of syncope that occurred while he was jogging. Witnesses reported that the patient began to swerve off of the jogging path into the adjacent bike lane, where he then passed out. In the emergency room, a 12-lead electrocardiogram was completely normal. A trans-thoracic echocardiogram was also completely normal. A two-hour postprandial glucose test was normal. An MRI of the brain was normal. Due to concerns about shortness of breath at the time of the incident, a ventilation-perfusion scan was performed, results: normal. A stress test (Bruce protocol) lasted 15 minutes, achieved 17 METs, a maximum blood pressure of 180/70 mm Hg, and a maximum heart rate of 184 beats per minute (100% of the maximal predicted value for age). A signal-averaged ECG revealed no abnormalities. After being released from the hospital, he had another pre-syncopal episode on a Holter monitor, which did not record any abnormalities. He said that his peripheral vision turned dark, and he became dizzy and experienced chest pressure. The patient reported that the Bruce protocol did not achieve the level of exertion necessary to produce his symptoms. Which of the following is your number one suspicion for his symptoms?

   A. Hypertrophic cardiomyopathy
   B. Acute myocarditis
   C. Cardiac aneurysm
   D. Coronary artery abnormality

Correct Answer: D. Coronary artery abnormality

In athletes > 35 years of age, coronary artery disease is the most common cause (85%) of sudden cardiac events. In younger athletes, hypertrophic cardiomyopathy is the leading cause of cardiac events (up to 30%), but even in this instance, a coronary artery anomaly is second as a cause for sudden cardiac events. Though not an uncommon cause for cardiac events in athletes, there are no signs or symptoms for acute myocarditis in this scenario. A cardiac aneurysm would have been seen on the echocardiogram.

   1. Rommel M, Griffin R, Harrison EE. Coronary anomalies: cardiac CT evaluation of the symptomatic adult athlete. Curr Sports Med Rep 2007 Apr;6(2):85-92.
   2. Wike J, Kernan M. Sudden cardiac death in the active adult: causes, screening, and preventive strategies. Curr Sports Med Rep 2005 Apr;4(2):76-82.

114. A 35-year-old Hispanic male cyclist presents to your clinic with continued concerns after being evaluated by cardiology. He was originally referred to cardiology after findings of sinus bradycardia of 45 bpm on ECG, as well as mild cardiomegaly on chest x-ray during a pre-operative evaluation prior to right knee arthroscopy. He has recovered from his knee surgery, but is now concerned that he is at risk for heart disease and asks your opinion on whether he should continue to cycle. You review his echocardiogram from three months ago. Which of the following is the most accurate recommendation?

   A. You recommend the patient should continue to cycle, because his findings of eccentric LV wall hypertrophy of 11 mm and left atrial enlargement are not uncommon findings with his sport and age
   B. You recommend the patient should continue to cycle, because isometric exercises can cause normal physiological changes to his heart, and he should not be concerned with a left ventricular hypertrophy of 16 mm, given the expected increase with exercise
   C. You recommend the patient should not continue to cycle, because the increase in his cardiac mass, along with the left ventricular end diastolic diameter of 55 mm, is consistent with cardiomyopathy
   D. You recommend the patient should not continue to cycle, because a second echo demonstrated decreasing cardiac mass, as well as decreasing left ventricular hypertrophy from 12 mm to 10 mm

Correct Answer: A. You recommend the patient should continue to cycle, because his findings of eccentric LV wall hypertrophy of 11 mm and left atrial enlargement are not uncommon findings with his sport and age

The patient has athletic heart syndrome, characterized by sinus bradycardia and mild cardiomegaly on ECG. Answer A is consistent with athletic heart with left ventricular hypertrophy < 13 mm, along with eccentric changes as expected with endurance sports, as compared to concentric with weight lifting sports. Given the patient's age of 35, it would not be uncommon to see left atrial enlargement, as compared to a younger athlete. Answer B is incorrect, because athletic heart should have left ventricular hypertrophy < 13 mm. With hypertrophy > 15 mm, you must be more worried about cardiomyopathies. Answer C is incorrect, because the patient should be allowed to continue to cycle, because there is no proven risk of athlete heart and sudden cardiac death or increased coronary artery disease. The diagnosis of athlete heart is supported with the left ventricular end diastolic diameter < 60 mm. Answer D is incorrect, because the echo finding of regression of the left ventricular hypertrophy supports athlete heart, and the athlete should not be restricted from exercise.

1. Baggish A, Wood M. Athlete's heart and cardiovascular care of the athlete: scientific and clinical update. Circulation 2011 Jun 14;123(23):2723-2735. doi: 10.1161/CIRCULATIONAHA.110.981571.
2. Marron B, Pelliccia A. The heart of trained athletes: cardiac remodeling and the risks of sports, including sudden death. Circulation 2006 Oct 10;114(15):1633-1644.

115. Which of the following findings on a preparticipation cardiovascular exam would be suspicious for a pathologic murmur and require further follow-up with a cardiologist prior to clearance?

    A. Crescendo-decrescendo murmur
    B. Murmur heard best over the pulmonic area
    C. Murmur that becomes louder with squatting
    D. Murmur that becomes louder with standing from a squatting position
    E. Murmur with musical or vibratory quality

Correct Answer: D. Murmur that becomes louder with standing from a squatting position

The murmur associated with hypertrophic cardiomyopathy becomes louder or longer with standing or during a Valsalva maneuver. In a normal heart, these actions cause decreased venous return, which also decreases left ventricular size and stroke volume. This decreased stroke volume should cause murmurs to become softer. However, if the opposite occurs, hypertrophic cardiomyopathy or possibly mitral valve prolapse should be suspected. Other concerning findings include: diastolic murmur, long duration or loud murmur (grade 3 or 4), and radiation to the axilla or carotids. Answers A, B, C, and E are all associated with benign murmurs. Other clues suggestive of a benign murmur include a soft murmur (grade 1 or 2) and normal splitting of S2, without extra heart sounds and best heard during early to mid-systolic phase.

1. Giese EA, O'Connor FG, Brennan FH, Depenbrock PJ, Oriscello RG. The athletic preparticipation evaluation: cardiovascular assessment. Am Fam Physician 2007 Apr 1;75(7):1008-1014.
2. Shah SN. Hypertrophic cardiomyopathy clinical presentation. Medscape. Accessed December 8, 2018 at https://emedicine.medscape.com/article/152913-clinical#a0256.

116. Which of the following findings on an ECG would NOT be considered a normal physiological adaptation to training in an athlete?

    A. Sinus bradycardia greater than or equal to 30 beats per minute
    B. QTc of 490 ms
    C. First degree AV block
    D. Incomplete right bundle branch block

Correct Answer: B. QTc of 490 ms

A QTc of greater than 470 ms in men and 480 ms in women is not considered a normal physiological adaptation to training in an athlete and needs further evaluation prior to sports clearance. A prolonged QTc, whether due to an inherited genetic mutation or drug-induced, can predispose athletes to tachyarrythmias, and, therefore, needs further evaluation. All of the other ECG findings are considered normal physiological adaptations to training in an athlete and are largely due to increased vagal tone and enlarged cardiac chamber size seen in response to regular exercise. They do not require further evaluation.

1. Uberoi A, Stein R, Perez MV, et al. Interpretation of the electrocardiogram of young athletes. Circulation 2011 Aug;124(6):746-757.
2. Drezner JA, Fischbach P, Froelicher V, Marek J, Pelliccia A, Prutkin JM, et al. Normal electrocardiographic findings: recognising physiological adaptations in athletes. Br J Sports Med 2013 Feb;47(3):125-136.

117. With regard to Brugada syndrome, which of the following statements is true?

   A. It is prompted by structural changes in the right ventricle, causing ventricular fibrillation and sudden death
   B. It is the same as early repolarization,.
   C. It is a channelopathy, characterized by a susceptibility to sudden death and associated with incomplete right bundle branch block and precordial ST elevations
   D. It is another name for short QT syndrome
   E. It cannot be identified on a preparticipation ECG

Correct Answer: C. It is a channelopathy, characterized by a susceptibility to sudden death and associated with incomplete right bundle branch block and precordial ST elevations

Brugada syndrome is a cause of sudden death in athletes. The ECG shows changes that can look like benign early repolarization, especially in African-American patients (elevated ST segment with an upward convexity ending in a negative T wave), but is clearly not just early repolarization. It is a channelopathy that involves early inactivation of the sodium channel. Brugada does cause susceptibility to ventricular fibrillation, but there is not a structural component by echocardiogram. It is not related to short QT. Fortunately, Brugada syndrome is rare, but is typically diagnosed by ECG, even in the absence of symptoms. The proponents of preparticipation ECG screening point to conditions like Brugada syndrome as reasons for using the ECG as a screening test.

1. Corrado D, Pelliccia A, Heidbuchel H, Sharma S, Link M, Basso C, et al. Recommendations for interpretation of 12-lead electrocardiogram in the athlete. Eur Heart J 2010 Jan;31(2):243-259. doi: 10.1093/eurheartj/ehp473. Epub 2009 Nov 20.
2. Uberoi A, Stein R, Perez MV, Freeman J, Wheeler M, Dewey F, et al. Interpretation of the electrocardiogram of young athletes. Circulation 2011 Aug 9;124(6):746-757. doi: 10.1161/CIRCULATIONAHA.110.013078.
3. Drezner J, Corrado D. Is there evidence for recommending electrocardiogram as part of the pre-participation examination? Clin J Sport Med 2011 Jan;21(1):18-24. doi: 10.1097/JSM.0b013e318205dfb2.

118. Which of the following is associated with the onset of shoulder adhesive capsulitis?

   A. Lumbar spondylolisthesis
   B. Aortic stenosis
   C. Renal disease
   D. Parkinson disease

Correct Answer: D. Parkinson disease

Hyperthyroidism, ischemic heart disease, diabetes mellitus, cervical spondylosis, Parkinson disease, stroke, hypertension, and malignancy have all been associated with the occurrence of adhesive capsulitis. Other conditions include trauma and surgery (especially those limiting mobility, e.g., neurosurgery, heart surgery). In the context of patients with these conditions and the development of a painful, stiff shoulder, adhesive capsulitis should be considered. On exam, loss of glenohumeral motion, especially passive external rotation and abduction, is noted. The prevalence of adhesive capsulitis has been estimated to be about 2% of the general population and 11% of those with diabetes mellitus. For those with type I diabetes mellitus, 40% will develop a frozen shoulder at some point in their lifetime. The etiology of adhesive capsulitis is unclear (and likely multifactorial), but has been associated with a number of chronic medical conditions, including diabetes mellitus, hyperlipidemia, hypertension, hypothyroidism, Parkinson's disease, and conditions involving a period of shoulder immobilization (e.g., post-surgical).

Adhesive capsulitis remains largely a clinical diagnosis, but there are a number of findings on imaging studies that have been proposed to aid in the diagnosis of a frozen shoulder. Typically, plain film radiographs have little to no degenerative arthritic changes to the glenohumeral joint—arthritic findings would suggest osteoarthrosis, rather than adhesive capsulitis. Because joint capsule thickening and contracture are thought to play a part in adhesive capsulitis, these may be evident on shoulder arthrography or MRI, particularly in the axillary recess. Kim et al. described a number of MRI findings commonly seen in patients with adhesive capsulitis, including thickening of the coracohumeral ligament greater than 2 mm, subcoracoid fatty infiltration, and thickening of the joint capsule in the axillary recess. Glenohumeral arthrography will show a joint volume around 13 to 15 mL in the normal adult shoulder, while in adhesive capsulitis, the joint volume can be reduced to as little as 5 to 8 mL. Binder et al. looked extensively at the clinical value of nuclear medicine bone scanning in adhesive capsulitis, and found that while very sensitive (up to 92%), there was very poor specificity in bone scanning. Ryu et al. evaluated the value of dynamic ultrasonography in the assessment of frozen shoulders and found continuous limitation of the sliding movement of the supraspinatus tendon against the acromion of the scapula to be a reliable test, with a sensitivity of 91% and a specificity of 100%.

1. Roberts JR. Adhesive capsulitis (frozen shoulder) treatment and management. Medscape. Accessed March 4, 2019 at http://emedicine.medscape.com/article/1261598-treatment#a28.
2. Tighe CB, Oakley WS Jr. The prevalence of a diabetic condition and adhesive capsulitis of the shoulder. South Med J 2008 Jun;101(6):591-595. doi: 10.1097/SMJ.0b013e3181705d39.
3. Kim YS, Kim JM, Lee YG, Hong OK, Kwon HS, Ji JH. Intercellular adhesion molecule-1 (ICAM-1, CD54) is increased in adhesive capsulitis. J Bone Joint Surg Am 2013 Feb 20;95(4):e181-e188.
4. Ryu KN, Lee SW, Rhee YG, Lim JH. Adhesive capsulitis of the shoulder joint: usefulness of dynamic sonography. J Ultrasound Med 1993;12:445-449.

119. A 15-year-old male athlete comes into your office for a sports physical. He appears to be in good shape. During the encounter, the patient's mother asks about a prior incident, in which the patient had passed out while playing basketball. The patient reports that during the incident he became very lightheaded and had tunnel vision just prior to syncope. Upon recovering, the patient experienced no confusion. Mom states the patient's older brother experienced this at a young age and was advised to stop intense physical activity. Upon examination, cardiac auscultation reveals a systolic ejection murmur at the left lower sternal border. The murmur associated with hypertrophic cardiomyopathy would be expected to increase with which of the following?

   A. Increased venous return
   B. Decreased venous return
   C. Increased systemic vascular resistance
   D. Increased afterload

Correct Answer: B. Decreased venous return

This patient may have hypertrophic cardiomyopathy. This is an autosomal dominant defect in sarcomere formation. It can be assumed that, due to the symptoms described by the patient (dizziness, tunnel vision, and no post confusion), this syncopal episode was not due to a seizure. Hypertrophic cardiomyopathy patients will likely have a systolic ejection murmur heard best at the left lower sternal border. This murmur will increase with standing and Valsalva, which cause decreased venous return. This murmur would decrease with squatting, which causes increased venous return. The murmur will also decrease with increased systemic vascular resistance and, thus, increased afterload.

1. Maron MS. Clinical manifestations, diagnosis, and evaluation of hypertrophic cardiomyopathy. UpToDate. Accessed December 9, 2018 at https://www.uptodate.com/contents/hypertrophic-cardiomyopathy-clinical-manifestations-diagnosis-and-evaluation.
2. Spirito P, Autore C, Rapezzi C, Bernabò P, Badagliacca R, Maron MS, et al. Syncope and risk of sudden death in hypertrophic cardiomyopathy. Circulation 2009 Apr 7;119(13):1703-1710. doi: 10.1161/CIRCULATIONAHA.108.798314. Epub 2009 Mar 23.

120. A 17-year-old female volleyball player presents for her first college preparticipation exam. You note that she is 6'4" with long thin limbs, arachnodactyly, scoliosis, and a pectus excavatum. Which of the following would be considered a major eye criteria in assisting in making the clinical diagnosis of Marfan syndrome?

    A. Ectopia lentis
    B. Flat cornea
    C. Myopia
    D. Retinal detachment

Correct Answer: A. Ectopia lentis

Marfan syndrome is currently diagnosed using criteria based on an evaluation of the family history, molecular data, and clinical evaluation. In 1995, a group of the world's leading clinicians and investigators in Marfan syndrome proposed revised diagnostic criteria. Known as the Ghent criteria, they identify major and minor diagnostic findings, which are largely based on clinical observation of various organ systems and on the family history. These criteria were revised in 2010. A major criterion is defined as one that carries high diagnostic precision because it is relatively infrequent in other conditions, as well as in the general population. The Ghent criteria were intended to serve as an international standard for clinical and molecular studies and for investigations of genetic heterogeneity and genotype-phenotype correlations. In the evaluation of the ocular system, the major criterion is ectopia lentis. About 50% of patients have lens dislocation. The dislocation is usually superior and temporal. This may present at birth or develop during childhood or adolescence. In the absence of family history, aortic root aneurysm and ectopia lentis are sufficient for a diagnosis. Flat cornea, myopia and retinal detachment are all minor criteria.

1. Defendi GL. Genetics of Marfan syndrome. Medscape. Accessed December 9, 2018 at https://emedicine.medscape.com/article/946315-overview.
2. Maron B, Ackerman M, Nishimura R, Pyeritz RE, Towbin JA, Udelson JE. Task Force 4: HCM and other cardiomyopathies, mitral valve prolapse, myocarditis, and Marfan syndrome. J Am Coll Cardiol 2005 Apr 19;45(8):1340-1345.

121. Morphologic adaptations of athlete's heart can closely resemble cardiovascular disease. Which of the following findings on ECG is abnormal and would be concerning in an athlete?

    A. First-degree AV block
    B. Early repolarization
    C. Incomplete RBBB
    D. Left-axis deviation

Correct Answer: D. Left-axis deviation

Left-axis deviation (-30 degrees to -90 degrees) is an abnormal finding on ECG. Answers A, B, and C are incorrect, as first-degree AV block, early repolarization, and incomplete RBBB are all common ECG findings in athletes.

1. Drezner JA. Standardised criteria for ECG interpretation in athletes: a practical tool. Br J Sports Med 2012 Nov;46 Suppl 1:i6-i8. doi: 10.1136/bjsports-2012-091703.
2. Pelliccia A, Zipes DP, Maron BJ. Bethesda Conference #36 and the European Society of Cardiology Consensus Recommendations revisited a comparison of U.S. and European criteria for eligibility and disqualification of competitive athletes with cardiovascular abnormalities. J Am Coll Cardiol 2008 Dec 9;52(24):1990-1996. doi: 10.1016/j.jacc.2008.08.055.
3. Drezner JA, Ackerman MJ, Anderson J, Ashley E, Asplund CA, Baggish AL, et al. Electrocardiographic interpretation in athletes: the 'Seattle criteria'. Br J Sports Med 2013 Feb;47(3):122-124. doi: 10.1136/bjsports-2012-092067.

122. An 18-year-old female lacrosse player presents for her annual preparticipation examination. In her history, she relates several episodes of "heart racing," accompanied by slight shortness of breath. Her physical examination, including vital signs, is normal. ECG testing was ordered and appears below. Which is true regarding her ECG?

   A. She has delta waves and a shortened PR interval, consistent with ventricular pre-excitation. She should be withheld from athletic participation and referred to a cardiologist for a diagnosis of Wolff-Parkinson-White syndrome
   B. She has atrial fibrillation and should be placed on anticoagulation after consultation with a cardiologist. She should be withheld from participation
   C. She has findings consistent with the athletic heart, and should be allowed full participation
   D. Normal ECG examination. Allow full participation

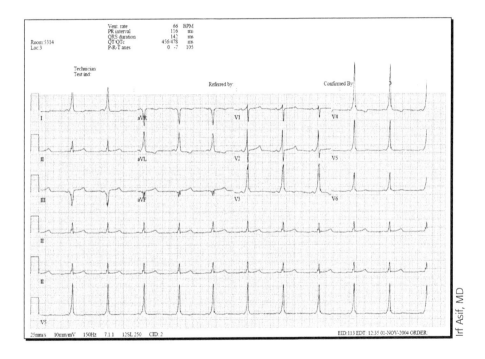

Correct Answer: A. She has delta waves and a shortened PR interval, consistent with ventricular pre-excitation. She should be withheld from athletic participation and referred to a cardiologist for a diagnosis of Wolff-Parkinson-White syndrome

A history of palpitations, chest pain, syncope, or unusual shortness of breath should prompt a cardiac evaluation, especially if these symptoms occur during exercise. Wolff-Parkinson-White (WPW) or pre-excitation syndromes involve an accessory pathway that can be induced with adrenaline states, such as exercise. This can produce a rapid heartbeat, and result in symptoms such as shortness of breath, dizziness, chest pain, or syncope. WPW occurs in 1.5 to 3/1000 persons, and is usually asymptomatic until adolescence or adulthood. When symptomatic, a referral to a cardiologist is appropriate to discuss treatment strategies. Atrial fibrillation will have an irregularly irregular heart rate, with absent P waves. The athletic heart ECG may have sinus bradycardia and even first-degree or type I second-degree heart block, but will not show a shortened PR interval or delta waves.

1. Saxena A, Chang CJ, Wang S. Wolff-Parkinson-White syndrome in athletes. Curr Sports Med Rep 2006 Sep;5(5):254-257.
2. West JJ, Mounsey JP. Wolff-Parkinson-White syndrome and asymptomatic ventricular pre-excitation: implications in sports cardiology. Curr Sports Med Rep 2008 Mar-Apr;7(2):93-99.

123. A 22-year-old female rower presents with the complaint of recurrent episodes of respiratory distress. These episodes are associated with inspiratory stridor, cough, choking sensations, and throat tightness. You suspect the diagnosis of vocal cord dysfunctions. Which of the following is a mainstay in the treatment of vocal cord dysfunction?

    A. Inhaled albuterol
    B. Speech therapy
    C. Inhaled corticosteroids
    D. Immediate administration of intramuscular epinephrine

Correct Answer: B. Speech therapy

Speech therapy is the mainstay of long-term management. Therapy that incorporates a variety of techniques, including relaxed-throat breathing, has been shown to improve symptoms of vocal cord dysfunction and reduce recurrences. Answers A and C are incorrect, as these are common treatments for asthma. Answer D is incorrect, as this is a treatment for anaphylaxis.

1. Deckert J, Deckert L. Vocal cord dysfunction. Am Fam Physician 2010 Jan 15;81(2):156-159.
2. Al-Alwan A, Kaminsky D. Vocal cord dysfunction in athletes: clinical presentation and review of the literature. Phys Sportsmed 2012 May;40(2):22-27. doi: 10.3810/psm.2012.05.1961.

124. A 15-year-old tennis player presents with wheezing and shortness of breath while playing. Criteria for moderate persistent asthma includes which of the following?

   A. Symptoms two to three times a week
   B. FEV1 of > 60% and < 80% of predicted
   C. Nighttime awakening three to four times per month
   D. Using short-acting beta agonist two to three times per day for symptoms control
   E. Minor limitation with normal activity

Correct Answer: B. FEV1 of > 60% and < 80% of predicted

According to NHLBI guidelines, moderate persistent asthma is characterized by daily symptoms; nighttime symptoms > once per week, but not nightly; FEV1 of > 60% and < 80% of predicted; some limitation with normal activity; and daily use of short-acting beta agonist for symptoms control.

1. National Heart, Lung, and Blood Institute, National Asthma Education and Prevention Program. Expert Panel Report 3: guidelines for the diagnosis and management of asthma. Summary report 2007. Accessed December 9, 2018 at https://www.nhlbi.nih.gov/guidelines/asthma/asthgdln.htm.
2. Pollart SM, Elward KS. Overview of changes to asthma guidelines: diagnosis and screening. Am Fam Physician 2009 May 1;79(9):761-767.

125. A female athlete comes to you for her NCAA preparticipation physical prior to her freshman year of college. She has had a successful career running cross country in high school, and was only held out for a period of weeks to allow for a tibial stress fracture to heal last year. She has since resumed running and is increasing her mileage in anticipation of the upcoming rigorous training schedule. She currently runs daily, approximately 55 miles weekly. Her only other notable finding on history is that she has missed her period for 16 months. When asked about this, she shrugs and states that she expected this due to her athletics. Menarche was at age 13. Vitals: BP: 110/62, pulse rate: 56, respirations: 11, BMI: 17.2 Kg/m2. You diagnose her with female athlete triad. What is the most successful intervention to reverse this condition?

   A. Prescribe oral contraceptives to regulate the menstrual cycle
   B. Prescribe 800 IU Vitamin D and 1200 mg Ca
   C. Refer her to sports psychology to manage the condition, as this is their specialty
   D. Referral to a nutritionist to develop a plan for a well-balanced diet ensuring sufficient caloric intake

Correct Answer: D. Referral to a nutritionist to develop a plan for a well-balanced diet ensuring sufficient caloric intake.

The female athlete triad is a syndrome that is comprised of three components: (1) low energy availability, (2) menstrual dysfunction, and (3) low bone mineral density. This athlete is demonstrating a concerning BMI, secondary amenorrhea, has suffered a stress fracture already, and will likely be increasing her training intensity even more at the collegiate level of training. The most important intervention is to increase her caloric intake, as this is the piece of the syndrome which drives the menstrual irregularities and an increased risk of bony injuries. A sport nutritionist is trained in understanding the complexities of calorie expenditure in athletes, and can help come up with a well-balanced dietary plan. Answer A is incorrect, as oral contraceptives do not reverse the condition. Although they may induce a withdrawal bleed, this is due to a false, exogenously-created condition from the medication, and does not indicate a correction of normal menstrual function. Answer B may be an important intervention later in the management of this condition, but will not reverse the syndrome. The root cause is an insufficient energy availability that needs to be addressed. Later, it may be indicated to further examine her bone health with labs and a DEXA scan, but not as an initial step. Answer C is incorrect, as this syndrome is a very difficult entity to tackle, and there is no one specialist that can manage all pieces. This condition requires a team approach, often involving medical doctors, psychologists, and nutritionists, as well as buy-in from family, friends, coaches, and teammates.

1. Joy E, De Souza MJ, Nattiv A, Misra M, Williams NI, Mallinson RJ, et al. 2014 female athlete triad coalition consensus statement on treatment and return to play of the female athlete triad. Curr Sports Med Rep 2014 Jul-Aug;13(4):219-232. doi: 10.1249/JSR.0000000000000077.

126. You have volunteered to help cover the local Paralympic training facility in town. You have heard that several players on the wheelchair basketball team have been clamping their urinary catheters (boosting) to gain a competitive advantage. What mechanism is giving them this advantage?

   A. Increased blood pressure from unopposed sympathetic discharge
   B. Decreased blood pressure from unopposed sympathetic discharge
   C. Increased blood pressure from unopposed parasympathetic discharge
   D. Decreased blood pressure from unopposed parasympathetic discharge

Correct Answer: A. Increased blood pressure from unopposed sympathetic discharge

Autonomic dysreflexia is a phenomenon that occurs in athletes who have sustained spinal cord injuries above the level of T6. It is the body's inability to control the sympathetic response to a stimulus. In order to increase the blood pressure, an athlete will inflict a noxious stimulus to themselves (e.g., bladder distention—clamping the catheter, using a tourniquet on the lower extremity, or breaking a toe). Autonomic dysreflexia can lead to seizure, stroke, or death. Symptoms include headache, flushing, emergent hypertension, and bradycardia.

1. Bhambhani Y, Mactavish J, Warren S, Thompson WR, Webborn A, Bressan E, et al. Boosting in athletes with high-level spinal cord injury: knowledge, incidence and attitudes of athletes in paralympic sport. Disabil Rehabil 2010;32(26):2172-2190. doi: 10.3109/09638288.2010.505678.
2. Blauwet CA, Benjamin-Laing H, Stomphorst J, Van de Vliet P, Pit-Grosheide P, Willick SE. Testing for boosting at the Paralympic games: policies, results and future directions. Br J Sports Med 2013 Sep;47(13):832-837. doi: 10.1136/bjsports-2012-092103. Epub 2013 May 16.

127. Which antidepressant is an activating agent and is on the World Anti-Doping Agency's (WADA) monitoring program list?

A. Nortriptyline
B. Venlafaxine
C. Paroxetine
D. Bupropion

Correct Answer: D. Bupropion

Prescribing physicians try to match side effect profiles of antidepressants to ameliorate bothersome symptoms of depression. Nortriptyline is a tricyclic antidepressant associated with anticholineric activity that can include drowsiness. Venlafaxine is a serotonin and norepiphrine reuptake inhibitor and is considered activating, but not as activating as bupropion. Paroxetine is a selective serotonin reuptake inhibitor and has some anticholineric activity, leading to potential drowsiness. Nortriptyline, venlafaxine, and paroxetine are not on the WADA drug-monitoring list. Bupropion is a norepinephrine and dopamine reuptake inhibitor and is one of the most activating antidepressants. It is listed by WADA as a stimulant, along with caffeine, nicotine, and phenylephrine, all of which are on the drug-monitoring list.

1. World Anti-Doping Agency. The World Anti-Doping Code International Standard Prohibited List January 2018. Accessed December 8, 2018 at https://www.wada-ama.org/sites/default/files/prohibited_list_2018_en.pdf.
2. Matching antidepressants to patients: selection dosing & cost. University of Michigan. Accessed December 9, 2018 at https://www.med.umich.edu/1info/FHP/practiceguides/depress/drugtable.pdf.

128. A 13-year-old male track and field athlete presents to clinic with a two-month history of decreased energy and anterior knee pain. His parents are concerned, because he seems depressed and tired all the time. He participates on his school's cross country and track team, and six months ago, he joined a community running team to help prepare for his first marathon. He used to be a member of the soccer and baseball teams but gave these up so that he could focus on becoming a better runner. Which statement is true regarding this athlete?

    A. He should not participate in endurance events like marathons because they may lead to overuse injuries
    B. He should avoid resistance training, as it may further increase his risk of injury
    C. He should avoid multi-sport participation, since he is already suffering from an overuse injury at the age of 13
    D. He is at risk of injury to his growth cartilage

Correct Answer: D. He is at risk of injury to his growth cartilage

The clinical scenario describes an example of overtraining syndrome, the opposite of a typical young, healthy athlete's profile. A "burnt-out" athlete can suffer from depression, but is also at significant risk of overuse injuries. While there is concern that participation in marathon running may be harmful to children and adolescents, there is no evidence to support this claim. It is generally accepted that a gradual increase in the amount and intensity of exercise is considered a safe practice. In the past, resistance training was discouraged in children and adolescents, because it was believed to be unsafe until the skeletal system matured. There is now sufficient evidence to show that resistance training is safe and may actually prevent injuries from occurring. Athletes who specialize in one sport are prone to overuse injuries and burnout. There is evidence that young athletes who participate in a variety of sports suffer from fewer injuries and stay active in sport longer. Athletes who participate in multiple sports all year long, without adequate rest between daily activities, are still at an increased risk of injury. Adequate periodization should be emphasized to encourage safe participation. Answer D is correct, as osteochondritis dissecans lesions commonly occur in the setting of overtraining. They affect the articular cartilage and subchondral bone and frequently occur at the knee, elbow, and ankle in active children and adolescents.

1. Carter CW, Micheli LJ. Training the child athlete for prevention, health promotion, and performance: how much is enough, how much is too much? Clin Sports Med 2011 Oct;30(4):679-690.
2. Brenner JS, Council on Sports Medicine and Fitness. Sports specialization and intensive training in young athletes. Pediatrics 2016 Sep;138(3). pii: e20162148. doi: 10.1542/peds.2016-2148.
3. Atanda A Jr, Shah SA, O'Brien K. Osteochondrosis: common causes of pain in growing bones. Am Fam Physician 2011 Feb 1;83(3):285-291.

129. A 45-year-old man from Colorado with no significant past medical history went with his friends to climb Pikes Peak (> 14,000 feet). He exercises regularly, without symptoms. He does not take any medications and is a non-smoker. After climbing to over 4000 m (13,000 feet) in one day, he developed headache, fatigue, nausea, and vomiting after setting up camp for the night. Upon closer examination, he appears slightly lethargic. His blood pressure is 138/72, pulse is 90/min, and respiratory rate is 20/min. The remainder of the general and neurological physical exam is unremarkable. The problem has slowly worsened overnight. What is the most appropriate next step?

   A. Ibuprofen and ondansetron
   B. Acetazolamide
   C. Dexamethasone
   D. Immediate descent

Correct Answer: D. Immediate descent

This patient has early signs of high altitude cerebral edema (HACE). The patient is already acclimatized to elevation, as he is a resident of Colorado. However, susceptibility to HACE can still occur. It is not necessarily related to physical condition. Although classically HACE presents with ataxia and/or altered mental status, he is in the early stages, with the development of mild lethargy. The other concern is that his condition seems to be deteriorating. Descent is the single best treatment for HACE, and would be the correct choice in this instance. Ibuprofen and ondansetron would only provide symptom management. Because HACE can be life-threatening, masking the symptoms would be deleterious. Acetazolamide is used in the prevention of acute mountain sickness (AMS) or HACE. It can also be used for the treatment of AMS. Dexamethasone can be used in the treatment of HACE and AMS. The most appropriate treatment for HACE, however, is immediate descent. Once descent has been made, it may be appropriate to give him dexamethasone. Dexamethasone can also be used for prophylaxis of AMS and HACE.

   1. Luks AM, McIntosh SE, Grissom CK, Auerbach PS, Rodway GW, Schoene RB, et al. Wilderness Medical Society practice guidelines for the prevention and treatment of acute altitude illness: 2014 update. Wilderness Environ Med 2014 Dec;25(4 Suppl):S4-S14. doi: 10.1016/j.wem.2014.06.017.
   2. Hackett PH, Roach RC. High altitude cerebral edema. High Alt Med Biol 2004 Summer;5(2):136-146.

130. A patient is brought into your clinic, accompanied by his friend, complaining of worsening generalized muscle and joint pains, shortness of breath, and dry cough upon return from a scuba diving excursion a few hours ago. The patient is a new diver, and his experienced friend is concerned he may have ascended too rapidly. You astutely diagnose the patient with decompression sickness (DCS) and begin treatment by giving 100% oxygen via NRB mask. Despite treatment, the patient shows no improvement, and you decide to treat with recompression therapy via a hyperbaric oxygen chamber. Which of the following accurately describes this mechanism of treatment?

   A. Compression of oxygen gas bubbles that caused the symptoms of DCS to diffuse into tissues and replacing them with oxygen
   B. Compression of nitrogen gas bubbles that caused the symptoms of DCS to diffuse into tissues and replacing them with oxygen
   C. Compression of nitrogen gas bubbles that caused the symptoms of DCS to diffuse into tissues and replacing them with nitrogen
   D. Compression of oxygen has bubbles that caused the symptoms of DCS to diffuse into tissues and replacing them with nitrogen

Correct Answer: B. Compression of nitrogen gas bubbles that caused the symptoms of DCS to diffuse into tissues and replacing them with oxygen

The compressive pressure of a hyperbaric oxygen chamber forces nitrogen gas bubbles (which cause symptoms of DCS) to dissipate into tissues to alleviate symptoms. Fresh oxygen is then used to replace the nitrogen. Treatment is administered based on established U.S. Navy treatment protocols.

1. St Leger Dowse M, Bryson P, Gunby A, Fife W. Comparative data from 2250 male and female sports divers: diving patterns and decompression sickness. Aviat Space Environ Med 2002 Aug;73(8):743-749.
2. Gill AL, Bell CN. Hyperbaric oxygen: its uses, mechanisms of action and outcomes. QJM 2004 Jul;97(7):385-395.

131. Exertional heat stroke (EHS) is the most severe form of heat illness. Which one of the following statements is true?

   A. Lowering the core body temperature to less than 104 degrees Fahrenheit (40 degrees Celsius) within 30 minutes should be the primary goal of EHS treatment
   B. Cool towels over the patient's head are sufficient to reduce the hyperthermia
   C. A body temperature of < 102.2 degrees Fahrenheit (39 degrees Celsius) by an oral thermometer can rule out EHS
   D. Altered mental status needs to be present to make the diagnosis of EHS

Correct Answer: A. Lowering the core body temperature to less than 104 degrees Fahrenheit (40 degrees Celsius) within 30 minutes should be the primary goal of EHS treatment

Any prolonged time remaining in an elevated temperature range could cause permanent end organ damage. Cool towels cannot cool down a patient in a sufficient time. A rectal thermometer is mandatory for accurate readings of the core temperature. Whole-body ice water immersion is the gold standard for rapid cooling, and lowering the core body temperature to less than 104 degrees Fahrenheit (40 degrees Celsius) within 30 minutes should be the primary goal of EHS treatment. Patients may simply complain of lethargy or dizziness, especially early in the course. In addition, consider IV fluids if the patient is dehydrated. The patient should be removed from the cold water immersion when core temperature reaches 102 degrees Fahrenheit (39 degrees Celsius).

   1. Armstrong LE, Casa DJ, Millard-Stafford M, Moran DS, Pyne SW, Roberts WO. American College of Sports Medicine position stand. Exertional heat illness during training and competition. Med Sci Sports Exerc 2007;39(3):556-572.
   2. Casa DJ, Anderson JM, Armstrong LE, Maresh CM. Survival strategy: acute treatment of exertional heat stroke. J Strength Cond Res 2006 Aug;20(3):462.
   3. Casa DJ, McDermott BP, Lee EC, Yeargin SW, Armstrong LE, Maresh CM. Cold water immersion: the gold standard for exertional heatstroke treatment. Exerc Sport Sci Rev 2007 Jul;35(3):141-149.

132. A 23-year-old cross country runner is complaining of a generalized papular itchy rash that occurs only during exercise. What would you recommend?

    A. Use sunscreen with PABA (para-aminobenzoic acid) at least 20 minutes prior to exercise
    B. Use topical steroids on the rash during exercise
    C. Take a hot shower the night before a long run or try an antihistamine tablet one hour prior to exercise.
    D. Desensitize with PUVA (Psoralen + UVA)

Correct Answer: C. Take a hot shower the night before a long run or try an antihistamine tablet one hour prior to exercise.

This athlete has cholinergic urticaria, which is characterized by papular wheals, with surrounding erythema, occurring during and after heat exposure or exercise. A hot shower prior to a long run may deplete histamine and provide a refractory period for the athlete. H1 antihistamines are effective when taken one hour prior to activity. Sunscreen with PABA or PUVA has no effect on cholinergic urticaria

1. O'Connor FG, Sallis RE, Wilder RP, St. Pierre P (eds). Sports Medicine: Just the Facts. New York: McGraw-Hill, 2005:152.
2. Montgomery SL. Cholinergic urticaria and exercise-induced anaphylaxis. Curr Sports Med Rep 2015 Jan;14(1):61-63. doi: 10.1249/JSR.0000000000000111.
3. Adams BB. Dermatologic disorders of the athlete. Sports Med 2002;32(5):309-321.

133. In 2008, the United States Department of Health and Human Services recommended comprehensive guidelines on physical activity for pregnant women. For healthy women (non-exercisers and moderate exercisers), what is the minimum recommended time per week of moderate-intensity aerobic activity during pregnancy?

   A. 90 minutes
   B. 150 minutes
   C. 300 minutes
   D. 225 minutes
   E. Only mild-intensity exercise is advised during pregnancy

Correct Answer: B. 150 minutes

It is recommended that pregnant women perform 150 minutes of moderate-intensity exercise per week. This number was arrived at by multiplying 30 minutes times five days per week, which equates to the definition of most days of the week. This is the same recommendation as for non-pregnant women.

1. Charlesworth S, Foulds HJ, Burr JF, Bredin SS. Evidence-based risk assessment and recommendations for physical activity clearance: pregnancy. Appl Physiol Nutr Metab 2011 Jul;36 Suppl 1:S33-S48. doi: 10.1139/h11-061.
2. Smith KM, Campbell CG. Physical activity during pregnancy: impact of applying different physical activity guidelines. J Pregnancy 2013;2013:165617. doi: 10.1155/2013/165617. Epub 2013 Feb 5.
3. Szymanski LM, Satin AJ. Exercise during pregnancy: fetal responses to current public health guidelines. Obstet Gynecol 2012 Mar;119(3):603-610. doi: 10.1097/AOG.0b013e31824760b5.

134. Which sport reports the highest incidence of urinary incontinence during participation among women?

   A. Softball
   B. Gymnastics
   C. Golf
   D. Swimming
   E. Cross country running

Correct Answer: B. Gymnastics

Prevalence of incontinence is the highest in high-impact sportswomen, such as trampolinists, gymnasts, hockey players, and ballet dancers. Gymnasts report more than 67% incidence of incontinence while participating in the sport. Other sports with high incidences of incontinence include basketball at 66%, tennis at 50%, field hockey at 42%, and track at 29%. Swimming reported 10% incidence, while volleyball and softball reported incidences of 9% and 6%, respectively. Golf had no reports of incontinence in the study.

1. Goldstick O, Constantini N. Urinary incontinence in physically active women and female athletes. Br J Sports Med 2014 Feb;48(4):296-298. doi: 10.1136/bjsports-2012-091880. Epub 2013 May 18.
2. Nygaard IE, Thompson FL, Svengalis SL, Albright JP. Urinary incontinence in elite nulliparous athletes. Obstet Gynecol 1994 Aug;84(2):183-187. Erratum in: Obstet Gynecol 1994 Sep;84(3):342.

135. A 17-year-old soccer player was diagnosed with infectious mononucleosis (IM) at an urgent care center 10 days ago. Her symptoms began approximately four days prior to diagnosis, so she is now two weeks from her onset of illness. She presents to you for follow-up regarding her return to play. She is no longer febrile, her pharyngitis has resolved, and she is well hydrated, but has continued complaints of fatigue. She is a starter for her high school team. Since they are in the middle of their competitive season, she is anxious to return to play. Which of the following is true regarding her return to contact sports?

   A. A short course of corticosteroids would be useful in helping her symptoms resolve and hastening her return to play
   B. Absence of splenomegaly on physical exam would allow for a safe return to contact sports
   C. In light of her persistent symptoms, she ought to be quarantined from her team to help prevent a spread to her teammates
   D. The athlete should to be afebrile, well hydrated, and asymptomatic before a return to play is considered

Correct Answer: D. The athlete should to be afebrile, well hydrated, and asymptomatic before a return to play is considered

The athlete must be afebrile, well hydrated, and asymptomatic before any return to play is considered. At that time, other factors, such as risk of splenic injury, may be considered in their return to play. Corticosteroids can be useful for acute symptoms, such as difficulty swallowing, but do not speed resolution of illness or return to sports. The presence or absence of splenomegaly would not be a determining factor in this athlete's return to play, as she remains symptomatic of IM. Furthermore, physical exam is inadequate to determine splenic enlargement. Epstein-Barr virus is the causative agent of IM and is transmitted through oral secretions. While she should be educated about not sharing things, like water bottles, there is no need to quarantine her from others.

1. Becker J, Smith J. Return to play after infectious mononucleosis. Sports Health 2014 May;6(3):232-238. doi: 10.1177/1941738114521984.
2. Putukian M, O'Connor FG, Stricker P, McGrew C, Hosey RG, Gordon SM, et al. Mononucleosis and athletic participation: an evidence-based subject review. Clin J Sport Med 2008 Jul;18(4):309-315. doi: 10.1097/JSM.0b013e31817e34f8.

136. A three-year-old male presents to your office with pain in his right hip and an inability to bear weight. His parents deny any acute injury or previous similar symptoms. Upon exam, he is febrile and appears acutely ill. He will not allow you to passively move his hip, which is held in flexion, abduction, and external rotation. Which of the following is the most likely diagnosis?

    A. Legg-Calve-Perthes Disease
    B. Juvenile rheumatoid arthritis
    C. Septic arthritis
    D. Leukemia

Correct Answer: C. Septic arthritis

Septic arthritis of the hip is a common musculoskeletal infection that is frequently missed initially, due to presentation with vague symptoms in young patients. Most patients with septic arthritis are infected via a hematogenous route, and causative organisms are usually Staphylococcus and Streptococcus species (H. influenza was a common causative organism prior to widespread immunization for that organism). Treatment involves incision and drainage of the affected synovial space, along with appropriate antibiotics. Legg-Calve-Perthes Disease is more common in older children, and fever should not present. Juvenile rheumatoid arthritis usually involves multiple joints, and fever is usually absent. Leukemia is in the differential diagnosis, but unlikely, due to monoarticular involvement and presence of a fever.

1. Shah SS. Abnormal gait in a child with fever: diagnosing septic arthritis of the hip. Pediatr Emerg Care 2005 May;21(5):336-341.
2. Leet AI, Skaggs DL. Evaluation of the acutely limping child. Am Fam Physician 2000 Feb 15;61(4):1011-1018.

137. Which of the following statements is true with respect to type 1 diabetic adults and exercise sessions of greater than one hour (endurance exercise)?

A. Insulin increases are recommended prior to initiation of exercise
B. Capillary glucose monitoring is only helpful in athletes who are using insulin pumps
C. Glucagon is the recommended choice to reverse exercise-induced mild hypoglycemia that may occur with exercise
D. Late-onset hypoglycemia related to prior exercise can be prevented by increasing carbohydrate intake and lowering longer-acting insulin dosages

Correct Answer: D. Late-onset hypoglycemia related to prior exercise can be prevented by increasing carbohydrate intake and lowering longer-acting insulin dosages

Generally speaking, insulin decreases (not increases) are recommended prior to endurance exercise. There are varying recommendations, depending on the exercise duration and intensity. Capillary glucose monitoring is useful in any diabetic athlete, regardless of their source of insulin. Checking glucose about every 30 minutes is recommended with endurance athletes during activity. There is no single recommended choice for reversing mild hypoglycemia, which is defined as 50 to 70 mg/dL. Sports drinks, which require approximately 250 mL to provide around 15 gm of carbohydrate, would work. Other sources of fluids, such as fruit juices or soda, contain higher concentrations of carbohydrate at lower volumes and would be just as efficacious. Hard candy and glucose tablets would also suffice. Glucagon, however, is reserved for severe hypoglycemia. Experience by the athlete is invaluable, and anticipation of the late-onset hypoglycemia during overnight sleeping is important to remember.

1. Lisle DK, Trojian TH. Managing the athlete with type 1 diabetes. Curr Sports Med Rep 2006 Apr;5(2):93-98.
2. Draznin MB. Managing the adolescent athlete with type 1 diabetes mellitus. Pediatr Clin N Am 2010 Jun;57(3):829-837. doi: 10.1016/j.pcl.2010.02.003.
3. Kirk SE. Hypoglycemia in athletes with diabetes. Clin Sports Med 2009;28(3):455-468.

138. A 12-year-old boy and his mother present to clinic for a preparticipation examination. The boy is healthy, but is known to have sickle cell trait. He has never played organized sports, but engages in active play on most days of the week. He is interested in trying out for various sports teams in his junior high school this year. His mother is concerned about any potential risks associated with his sickle cell trait. How do you counsel her?

   A. Her son should continue to be active and engage in moderate-intensity daily activity, but avoid competitive sports, where he may be subjected to high levels of physical exertion
   B. It is safe for her son to participate in sports characterized by intermittent bursts of intense exertion, but he should avoid sports that emphasize endurance or sustained activity
   C. It is safe for her son to participate in any sports of his choosing, as long as he follows universal precautions regarding hydration, acclimation to heat or altitude, and appropriate progression of exercise intensity
   D. Recommend hemoglobin electrophoresis testing for her son to determine the percentage of HbS, as this will determine if he can participate in sports

Correct Answer: C. It is safe for her son to participate in any sports of his choosing, as long as he follows universal precautions regarding hydration, acclimation to heat or altitude, and appropriate progression of exercise intensity

Current recommendations for athletes and military recruits with sickle cell trait (SCT) are based on the 2011 ACSM and CHAMP scientific summit meeting report. Guidelines are based on prior research and expert consensus, and recommend adherence to universal exercise precautions for participants with SCT. Attention to preparticipation conditioning, activity modification based on conditions, and maintaining adequate hydration have all been shown to significantly reduce the risk of exertional collapse and unexplained death in this population. There is no evidence to support avoidance of high-level activity or certain types of exercise in persons with SCT. Hemoglobin electrophoresis is sometimes required for specific military positions, but is not indicated for an asymptomatic athlete with SCT.

   1. Martin C, Pialoux V, Faes C, Charrin E, Skinner S, Connes P. Does physical activity increase or decrease the risk of sickle cell disease complications? Br J Sports Med 2018 Feb;52(4):214-218. doi: 10.1136/bjsports-2015-095317. Epub 2015 Dec 23.
   2. O'Connor FG, Bergeron MF, Cantrell J, Connes P, Harmon KG, Ivy E, et al. ACSM and CHAMP summit on sickle cell trait: mitigating risks for warfighters and athletes. Med Sci Sports Exerc 2012;44(11):2045-2056.

139. A 25-year-old female long distance runner presents to your office complaining of fatigue and poor performance. Her history and physical exam are consistent with anemia. Almost all lab work, including peripheral smear and serum iron and total iron binding capacity, are consistent with iron deficient anemia. The one exception is that the ferritin level is normal. What is the most likely explanation for a normal ferritin level in this athlete?

    A. Sickle cell trait
    B. Vitamin D malabsorption
    C. Hepatitis
    D. Volume depletion
    E. Malaria

Correct Answer: C. Hepatitis

A low serum iron and ferritin level, with an elevated TIBC, is typically diagnostic of iron deficiency. Because of its nature as an acute phase reactant, a normal or even elevated serum ferritin level can be seen in patients who are deficient in iron and have coexistent diseases, such as infection, chronic inflammation, malignancy, or conditions causing organ or tissue damage (e.g., arthritis, hepatitis). Sickle cell trait, vitamin D malabsorption, and volume depletion would not affect ferritin levels. Malaria should not cause her clinical picture, and peripheral smear was negative.

1. Harper JL. Iron deficiency anemia. Medscape. Accessed December 9, 2018 at https://emedicine.medscape.com/article/202333-overview.
2. Peng YY, Uprichard J. Ferritin and iron studies in anaemia and chronic disease. Ann Clin Biochem 2017 Jan;54(1):43-48. doi: 10.1177/0004563216675185. Epub 2016 Nov 7.
3. Clénin G, Cordes M, Huber A, Schumacher YO, Noack P, Scales J, et al. Iron deficiency in sports - definition, influence on performance and therapy. Swiss Med Wkly 2015 Oct 29;145:w14196. doi: 10.4414/smw.2015.14196.

140. You are starting a new position in the state of Colorado as a high school team physician. Towards the end of the first football practice of the year, during conditioning drills, an African-American football player collapses to the turf. He complains of severe pain in his bilateral quads and tells you that he is cramping. As the new team physician, you don't know the players yet. You ask the trainer about his medical history, and his response is that this athlete is a recent transfer student from Alabama, and he doesn't know him well. The athlete doesn't know any of his past medical history, other than to say that he's pretty healthy and doesn't know any of his family history. On exam, his muscles are soft, and there is no spasm. The cramps are spreading. He denies any new medications or drug use. He is lucid, alert, and oriented. What should your working diagnosis be, and what is your next step?

   A. Cramping from dehydration—start an IV or give him oral fluids
   B. Sickle cell trait—atart high flow oxygen and call 911
   C. Heat stroke—get him in a tub of cold water and call 911
   D. Not in shape—give him some water and let him sit on the sideline until he recovers, then let him go back to practice

Correct Answer: B. Sickle cell trait—start high flow oxygen and call 911

There are a few clues that would lead you to a diagnosis of sickle cell trait. First, the athlete has recently had a significant altitude change for training. Second, he collapsed to the turf, instead of pulled up limping. Most of the time with cramping from dehydration, the muscles spasm and "lock up." With sickle cell crisis, the muscles are soft, but severely painful from lack of oxygen. Third, there was no mention of it being a hot day, or the athlete being overheated, so even though heat stroke should be on your differential, it is not the most likely at this point.

1. Eichner ER. Sports medicine pearls and pitfalls—sickle cell trait and athletes: three clinical concerns. Curr Sports Med Rep 2007 Jun;6(3):134-135.
2. Schwellnus MP. Cause of exercise associated muscle cramps (EAMC)—altered neuromuscular control, dehydration or electrolyte depletion? Br J Sports Med 2009 Jun;43(6):401-408. doi: 10.1136/bjsm.2008.050401.

Test 2 Answers, Critiques, and References

141. A 19-year-old male Division I collegiate wrestler presented to you with a complaint of a painful rash on the right upper arm for the last day. Upon further inspection, it appears to look like a cluster of vesicles, with an erythematous base. You decide to withhold him from practice and treat the lesion. When can he resume participation in wrestling?

    A. He can return to play, as long as the lesion is covered with a non-permeable dressing and stretch tape
    B. After the lesion is treated with a topical steroid cream, and he has not developed any new lesions in the last 48 hours
    C. He has not developed any new lesions in the last 72 hours, all the lesions have a firm crust, and he has been on antiviral therapy for 120 hours
    D. He has no new lesions for 48 hours before a meet, has completed 72 hours of antibiotic therapy, and has no moist or draining lesions prior to competition
    E. The lesion has been treated with both topical therapy for 72 hours and a minimum of two weeks of oral therapy, and all lesions are adequately covered

Correct Answer: C. He has not developed any new lesions in the last 72 hours, all the lesions have a firm crust, and he has been on antiviral therapy for 120 hours

This is known as herpes gladiatorum, which is a herpes simplex virus infection of the skin of wrestlers. It is also called mat herpes. It is a skin eruption, identified as a cluster of vesicles on an erythematous base. This is common in wrestlers, due to skin-to-skin contact. Treatment is governed by an NCAA guideline. Active lesions are not permitted to be covered in order to allow participation. Antiviral therapy is required, not steroid cream or antibiotics.

1. Parsons JT. Skin infections. 2014-15 NCAA Sports Medicine Handbook. 25th ed. Indianapolis, IN: NCAA, 2014:65-71.
2. Mirfazaelian H, Daneshbod Y. Herpes gladiatorum. Emerg Med J 2013 Nov;30(11):892. doi: 10.1136/emermed-2013-202419. Epub 2013 Feb 14.

142. A 16-year-old high school football player comes to see you with a tender, red nodule on his leg. It is hot and swollen, and has been worsening for four days. There is some weeping of purulent fluid from the wound surface. Several members of his team have recently been diagnosed with methicillin-resistant staphylococcus aureus infections. Your exam shows a fluctuant area. See image below. What is the most appropriate treatment?

   A. Trimethoprim/sulfamethoxazole orally
   B. Amoxicillin orally
   C. Bactroban topically to the lesion
   D. Trimethoprim/sulfamethoxazole orally, with incision and drainage of the lesion
   E. Rifampin orally, with incision and drainage of the lesion

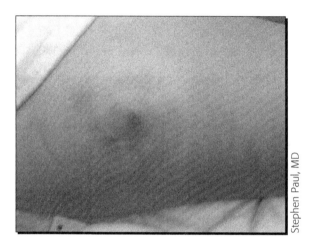

Correct Answer: D. Trimethoprim/sulfamethoxazole orally, with incision and drainage of the lesion

This patient has a classic skin abscess at high risk for community-acquired, methicillin-resistant staph aureus infection (MRSA). Recommended treatment includes proper antibiotic coverage, with prompt incision and drainage of all suspected abscesses. Neither topical medications nor rifampin alone are sufficient antibiotic coverage. Answer A is incorrect, because the antibiotic is proper, but does not include drainage of the abscess.

1. Liu C, Bayer A, Cosgrove SE, Daum RS, Fridkin SK, Gorwitz RJ, et al. Clinical practice guidelines by the Infectious Diseases Society of America for the treatment of methicillin-resistant Staphylococcus aureus infections in adults and children. Clin Infect Dis 2011 Feb 1;52(3):e18-e55. doi: 10.1093/cid/ciq146.
2. Lowy FD. Methicillin-resistant Staphylococcus aureus (MRSA) in adults: treatment of skin and soft tissue infections. UpToDate. Accessed December 15, 2018 at https://www.uptodate.com/contents/methicillin-resistant-staphylococcus-aureus-mrsa-in-adults-treatment-of-skin-and-soft-tissue-infections.

143. Which of the following is true regarding testicular torsion?

   A. Surgical detorsion and orchiopexy should be done within four to six hours of presentation
   B. Manual detorsion should be attempted, followed by observation if the color of the scrotum returns to normal
   C. Scrotal Doppler ultrasound is the test of choice and should be done before treatment is considered
   D. Testicular torsion is a problem seen only in adolescence

Correct Answer: A. Surgical detorsion and orchiopexy should be done within four to six hours of presentation

Testicular torsion is considered a surgical urgency. The longer the testicle is torsed, the greater the chance of losing viability. Most consider four to six, and at the outside eight, hours to save the viability of the testicle. Surgical detorsion, with orchiopexy, is considered the treatment of choice. Scrotal Doppler ultrasound is the method of choice to diagnose, but not if it will delay surgical release. If surgical release is not immediately available, manual detorsion may be tried. Testicular torsion is bimodal, with neonates having extravaginal torsion (the entire cord is twisted, including the processus vaginalis). Adolescents usually have intravaginal torsion, in which the testes twists within the tunica vaginalis.

1. Sharp VJ, Kieran K, Arlen AM. Testicular torsion: diagnosis, evaluation, and management. Am Fam Physician 2013 Dec 15;88(12):835-840.
2. Ogunyemi OI. Testicular torsion treatment and management. Medscape. Accessed June 29, 2018 at https://emedicine.medscape.com/article/2036003.

144. Gastroesophageal reflux disease (GERD) is a common diagnosis for runners who experience heartburn-type symptoms during activity. Which of the following is true?

    A. GERD symptoms occur because of the relaxation of the upper esophageal sphincter with activity
    B. Eating a large meal right before running will help relieve symptoms
    C. Certain foods, such as tomato sauce or orange juice, may exacerbate symptoms, while other foods, such as yogurt, may help decrease symptoms
    D. Over-the-counter and prescription treatments will provide no relief, and the only option is stopping all physical activity

Correct Answer: C. Certain foods, such as tomato sauce or orange juice, may exacerbate symptoms, while other foods, such as yogurt, may help decrease symptoms

Foods that are spicy or acidic often worsen symptoms, while soothing foods, such as yogurt, may help relieve symptoms. Symptoms occur because of relaxation of the lower esophageal sphincter. Eating a large meal is not recommended. Small meals 30 minutes to two hours before running are probably best. Often, over-the-counter medications, such as Tums, or even baking soda may help decrease stomach acid.

1. Herregods TV, van Hoeij FB, Oors JM, Bredenoord AJ, Smout AJ. Effect of running on gastroesophageal reflux and reflux mechanisms. Am J Gastroenterol 2016 Jul;111(7):940-946. doi: 10.1038/ajg.2016.122.
2. Leggit JC. Evaluation and treatment of GERD and upper GI complaints in athletes. Curr Sports Med Rep 2011 Mar-Apr;10(2):109-114. doi: 10.1249/JSR.0b013e31820f31ca.

145. Which of the following is not likely to be beneficial for osteoarthritis (OA) of the knee, based on available evidence-based literature?

   A. Physical therapy
   B. Taping of the knee
   C. Lateral wedge insoles for medial compartment OA
   D. Tai chi
   E. Exercise

Correct Answer: C. Lateral wedge insoles for medial compartment OA

The following have been shown to be effective treatments for OA of the knee: exercise, Tai chi, knee taping, and physical therapy. Effective medical management includes acetaminophen, although it is less effective than NSAIDs. Topical diclofenac and ketoprofen are moderately effective. The following have been shown to be ineffective for the treatment of OA of the knee: vitamin D and antioxidant supplements, shoes specifically designed for persons with OA, and lateral wedge insoles for medial knee OA, and arthroscopy. Corticosteroid intra-articular injections may be beneficial in the short term.

1. Ebell MH. Osteoarthritis: rapid evidence review. Am Fam Physician 2018 Apr 15;97(8):523-526.
2. Shaw KE, Charlton JM, Perry CKL, de Vries CM, Redekopp MJ, White JA, et al. The effects of shoe-worn insoles on gait biomechanics in people with knee osteoarthritis: a systematic review and meta-analysis. Br J Sports Med 2018 Feb;52(4):238-253. doi: 10.1136/bjsports-2016-097108. Epub 2017 Jul 6.
3. Rahlf AL, Braumann KM, Zech A. Kinesio taping improves perceptions of pain and function of patients with knee osteoarthritis. A randomized, controlled trial. J Sport Rehabil 2018 Feb 21:1-21. doi: 10.1123/jsr.2017-0306.

146. A healthy appearing 36-year-old white female runner presents to your office with a three-week history of left-sided sinus pain. She has been taking ibuprofen and pseudoephedrine for symptom relief. She continues with intermittent headache, despite the medications, which have given temporary relief of pain. Her pain is slightly increased with running and is mildly improved after running. Past medical history includes hospitalization for the birth of each of her three children. She has no other past medical problems. She takes estrogen/progesterone oral birth control pills, multivitamins, and fish oil. She has a family history of hypertension, CAD, and depression. On exam, her vital signs are as follows: height 5'4", weight 155 pounds, pulse 62, and blood pressure 170/100 mm Hg. She is awake and alert, with no significant distress. Heart and lung exam are within normal limits. What is the best initial choice for treating hypertension in this runner?

   A. Lisinopril
   B. Metoprolol
   C. Hydrochlorothiazide
   D. Lifestyle modification of weight loss, decreased alcohol intake, and decreased caffeine intake
   E. Discontinuation of birth control pills, ibuprofen, and pseudoephedrine

Correct Answer: E. Discontinuation of birth control pills, ibuprofen, and pseudoephedrine

Despite each answer being an appropriate choice for treatment of hypertension, the best answer is E. Identifying modifiable causes of hypertension should be the first goal of treatment. This patient is taking three medications, each of which can contribute to elevated blood pressure. The use of birth control in patients over the age of 35 years, especially if smokers, should be very closely monitored for elevation of blood pressure, as this can increase at any time while on the medication. Pseudoephedrine, which can raise blood pressure, should be used with caution in high-risk populations. Ibuprofen and other non-steroidal anti-inflammatory medication can cause elevated blood pressure in susceptible individuals. Lifestyle modifications should be used in patients with mild elevation of blood pressure. At 170/100 mm Hg, lifestyle modifications should be encouraged, but should not be the only treatment for this severe level of elevation. Hydrochlorothiazide is an excellent, affordable, effective treatment of blood pressure, but is a poor choice for athletes such as runners, as it can cause abnormalities in electrolytes and hypovolemia. Metoprolol is useful, especially when there is coexisting coronary artery disease. It is a poor choice in athletes, due to the control of heart rate and depressive effects. If needed, any beta blocker should be prescribed in conjunction with an alpha blocker to help manage the effects. Lisinopril is another good choice for blood pressure control, especially in athletes, and would be a good addition to this patient's treatment if blood pressure is not controlled by discontinuation of the likely aforementioned causes.

1. Niedfeldt M. Managing hypertension in athletes and physically active patients. Am Fam Physician 2002 Aug 1;66(3):445-453.
2. Onusko E. Diagnosing secondary hypertension. Am Fam Physician 2003 Jan 1;67(1):67-74.
3. James PA, Oparil S, Carter BL, Cushman WC, Dennison-Himmelfarb C, Handler J. 2014 evidence-based guideline for the management of high blood pressure in adults: report from the panel members appointed to the Eighth Joint National Committee (JNC 8). JAMA 2014 Feb 5;311(5):507-520. doi: 10.1001/jama.2013.284427.

147. The athletic heart syndrome includes which adaptive changes to exercise?

    A. Left ventricular wall thickness greater 15 mm
    B. Left ventricular cavity end diastolic diameter less than 45 mm
    C. Impaired left ventricular filling
    D. Interventricular septum to left ventricular posterior wall thickness ratio less than 1.3

Correct Answer: D. Interventricular septum to left ventricular posterior wall thickness ratio less than 1.3

Systematic training causes certain cardiac adaptations, including increasing left ventricular wall thickness and enlargement of the left ventricular cavity. Echocardiographic evidence suggestive of hypertrophic cardiomyopathy includes a left ventricular wall thickness greater than 15 mm, left ventricular cavity end-diastolic diameter less than 45 mm, and impaired left ventricular filling. Athletes often have interventricular septum to left ventricular posterior wall thickness ratio less than 1.3, because of eccentric hypertrophy related to dynamic exercise.

1. Maron BJ, Zipes DP. 36th Bethesda Conference: eligibility recommendations for competitive athletes with cardiovascular abnormalities. JACC 2005;45(8):1313-1375.
2. Rich BS, Havens SA. The athletic heart syndrome. Curr Sports Med Rep 2004 Apr;3(2):84-88.

148. A 26-year-old male marathon runner presents with a three-week history of progressive fatigue and exercise intolerance after a flu-like illness. His evaluation leads you to make the diagnosis of viral myocarditis. Per the 36th Bethesda guidelines, you recommend that he withdraw from competitive sports and undergo a prudent convalescent period of approximately?

   A. One month
   B. Three months
   C. Six months
   D. The athlete should never return to competitive sports

Correct Answer: C. Six months

There are currently no clinically accurate predictors of sudden death risk to guide return to play in athletes with myocarditis. The Bethesda guidelines are based on consensus/expert opinion. The Bethesda Guidelines further recommend athletes may return to training and competition after this six-month period of time if: a) LV function, wall motion, and cardiac dimensions return to normal (based on echocardiographic and/or radionuclide studies at rest and with exercise); b) clinically relevant arrhythmias, such as frequent and/or complex repetitive forms of ventricular or supraventricular ectopic activity, are absent on ambulatory Holter monitoring and graded exercise testing; c) serum markers of inflammation and heart failure have normalized; and d) the 12-lead ECG has normalized. Persistence of relatively minor ECG alterations, such as some ST-T changes, are not, per se, the basis for restriction from competition.

1. Maron B, Ackerman M, Nishimura R, Pyeritz RE, Towbin JA, Udelson JE. Task Force 4: HCM and other cardiomyopathies, mitral valve prolapse, myocarditis, and Marfan syndrome. J Am Coll Cardiol 2005 Apr 19;45(8):1340-1345.
2. McGrew C. What recommendations should be made concerning exercising with a fever and/or acute infection? In: MacAuley D, Best T (eds). Evidence-based Sports Medicine. 2nd ed. Malden, MA: Blackwell Publishing, 2007:107-119.
3. Anderson EL. Arrhythmogenic right ventricular dysplasia. Am Fam Physician 2006 Apr 15;73(8):1391-1398.

149. A 19-year-old female Division I collegiate cross-country athlete presents to the training room with complaints of fatigue and decreased performance. She is concerned she is anemic. Her BMI is 15 kg/m2. You ordered some labs, and her ferritin was 36 ng/ml with a hemoglobin of 12 g/dl. Upon further questioning, she reveals she hasn't had a menstrual period in four months, but she reports this is normal for her, since she rarely has one when she's in-season. Her first menstrual period was at 16 years of age. What is the recommended goal of treatment?

   A. Increase energy availability to 25 kcal/kg FFM
   B. Increase energy availability to 35 kcal/kg FFM
   C. Increase energy availability to 45 kcal/kg FFM
   D. Decrease energy availability, so that she can lose three to five pounds, which puts her at a better running weight

Correct Answer: C. Increase energy availability to 45 kcal/kg FFM

The underlying issue with relative energy deficiency in sport (RED-S) is an inadequacy of energy to support the range of body functions involved in optimal health and performance. Energy availability is calculated as energy intake minus the energy cost of exercise relative to fat-free mass (FFM). In healthy adults, a value of 45 kcal/kg FFM/day equates energy balance. Answers A and B are incorrect, as these energy availabilities are too low, and athletes with these numbers likely have amenorrhea or oligomenorrhea and RED-S. Answer D is incorrect, as this athlete already is not consuming enough energy to sustain her workload, and losing weight will further worsen the problem.

1. Mountjoy M, Sundgot-Borgen J, Burke L, Carter S, Constantini N, Lebrun C, et al. The IOC consensus statement: beyond the Female Athlete Triad—Relative Energy Deficiency in Sport (RED-S). Br J Sports Med 2014 Apr;48(7):491-497. doi: 10.1136/bjsports-2014-093502.
2. Loucks AB. Energy balance and body composition in sports and exercise. J Sports Sci 2004 Jan;22(1):1-14.
3. De Souza MJ, Nattiv A, Joy E, Misra M, Williams NI, Mallinson RJ, et al. Female athlete triad coalition consensus statement on treatment and return to play of the female athlete triad: 1st International Conference held in San Francisco, California, May 2012 and 2nd International Conference held in Indianapolis, Indiana, May 2013. Br J Sports Med 2014 Feb;48(4):289. doi: 10.1136/bjsports-2013-093218.

150. A 20-year-old college basketball player injures her knee while landing after pulling down a rebound. Her Lachman's test is positive, and there is concern that she tore her anterior cruciate ligament (ACL). Which of the following is thought to have made her more susceptible to this injury as compared to her male counterparts?

   A. Decreased femoral anteversion
   B. Smaller Q angle
   C. Greater amount of knee flexion while landing
   D. Greater quadriceps activation prior to landing

Correct Answer: D. Greater quadriceps activation prior to landing

Female athletes are at increased risk for noncontact ACL tears compared to male athletes—up to 3.5 times more likely in basketball and 2.67 times more likely in soccer. Gender-related biomechanical differences are thought to play a large role in this discrepancy. Females have a larger Q angle that may place more strain on the ACL. They also demonstrate greater femoral anteversion. Females tend to land in less knee flexion than their male counterparts. With landing, females tend to activate their quadriceps more in relation to the hamstrings, which may also place more strain on the ACL. There is thought that hormonal factors may play a role in this discrepancy, as the ACL contains estrogen and progesterone receptors, but the timing and role that these hormones play have not yet been established. Prevention strategies are aimed at improving neuromuscular control to decrease the strains placed on the ACL.

   1. Smith HC, Vacek P, Johnson RJ, Slauterbeck JR, Hashemi J, Shultz S, et al. Risk factors for anterior cruciate ligament injury: a review of the literature-part 2: hormonal, genetic, cognitive function, previous injury, and extrinsic risk factors. Sports Health 2012 Mar;4(2):155-161.
   2. Silvers HJ, Mandelbaum BR. Prevention of anterior cruciate ligament injury in the female athlete. Br J Sports Med 2007 Aug;41 Suppl 1:i52-i59. Epub 2007 Jul 3.

151. What is the most common cause of sudden death in older athletes (> 35 years old) while running the marathon?

    A. Exercise-associated hyponatremia
    B. Neurocardiogenic syncope
    C. Coronary artery disease
    D. Hypertrophic cardiomyopathy
    E. Cerebral vascular accident

Correct Answer: C. Coronary artery disease

Among older (>35 years old) athletes, available estimates suggest that the frequency of sudden cardiac death is in the range of one in 15,000 joggers per year or one in 50,000 participants in marathon per year, with a marked predominance of these deaths in men. Atherosclerotic coronary artery disease is the most common form of heart disease relevant to the older population as a cause of nonfatal or fatal cardiovascular events. Hypertrophic cardiomyopathy is the number one cause of sudden death in the younger athletic population, including marathons, for athletes under 35 years of age.

1. Franklin BA, Fern A, Voytas J. Training principles for elite senior athletes. Curr Sports Med Rep 2004 Jun;3(3):173-179.
2. Kim JH, Malhotra R, Chiampas G, d'Hemecourt P, Troyanos C, Cianca J, et al. Cardiac arrest during long-distance running races. N Engl J Med 2012 Jan 12;366(2):130-140. doi: 10.1056/NEJMoa1106468.

152. Which of the following is the most effective preventative measure for Lyme disease in athletes who spend a significant amount of time outdoors?

    A. Avoiding areas of high tick burdens
    B. Careful removal of ticks within 72 hours
    C. Immunization for those in high-risk or endemic areas
    D. Prophylaxis with amoxicillin for those who cannot take doxycycline

Correct Answer: A. Avoiding areas of high tick burdens

Avoiding areas with high tick burdens, such as grassy or wooded areas with a high deer population, is the best preventative measure that can be employed. For persons living in endemic areas, additional recommended measures include wearing light-colored protective clothing, using tick repellents, performing frequent body checks for ticks, bathing following outdoor activities, and instituting environmental landscape modifications to reduce the tick burden. Ticks must be removed within 24 hours to ensure prevention. The Lyme vaccine was taken off the market in 2002. Because amoxicillin has not shown the ability to reduce conversion to Lyme disease, prophylaxis is not recommended for those who cannot take doxycycline.

1. Clark RP, Hu LT. Prevention of Lyme disease and other tick-borne infections. Infect Dis Clin North Am 2008 Sep;22(3):381-396, vii. doi: 10.1016/j.idc.2008.03.007.
2. Wright WF, Riedel DJ, Talwani R, Gilliam B. Diagnosis and management of Lyme disease. Am Fam Physician 2012 Jun 1;85(11):1086-1093.

153. Which of the following is false regarding hepatitis B infection?

   A. Concurrent hepatitis D (delta) virus infection increases risk of fulminant infection
   B. Patients with positive HBsAb need immunization against hepatitis B virus
   C. Sexual contact increases the risk of transmission
   D. HBeAg positive status is of concern for possible transmission
   E. Symptoms begin two to four months post-exposure

Correct Answer: D. HBeAg positive status is of concern for possible transmission

Individuals with positive HBsAb are immune against hepatitis B virus, either by recovering from an infection or by immunization. While there is conflicting evidence regarding saliva as a mode of transmission, there is no question regarding blood, sharing needles, and sexual contact as known modes of transmission. Because hepatitis B has never been isolated from stool, enteric precautions are not necessary. Concurrent hepatitis D (delta) virus infection increases risk of fulminant infection. While the symptoms, including fever, malaise, jaundice, abdominal pain, nausea, vomiting, anorexia, and puritis, among others, may not start until two to four months, the chronic carrier who is HBeAg positive poses the greatest concern for transmission.

1. Kordi R, Wallace WA. Blood borne infections in sport: risks of transmission, methods of prevention, and recommendations for hepatitis B vaccination. Br J Sports Med 2004 Dec;38(6):678-684; discussion 678-684.
2. Wilkins T, Zimmerman D, Schade RR. Hepatitis B: diagnosis and treatment. Am Fam Physician 2010 Apr 15;81(8):965-972.

154. A 24-year-old professional soccer player came off the field during an exhibition match due to laceration to the scalp (see image below). There was head-to-head contact, and the opposing player left the field holding his mouth—no missing or loose teeth or blood noted. You bring the player with a scalp laceration to the training room. Which is the preferred treatment option?

    A. Irrigate with hydrogen peroxide, primary closure with hair apposition and adhesives (e.g., Dermabond)
    B. Irrigate with sterile saline, primary closure with tissue adhesives (e.g., Dermabond)
    C. Irrigate with sterile saline, primary closure with running suture
    D. Irrigate with tap water, allow secondary, delayed closure
    E. Irrigate with tap water, primary closure with staples

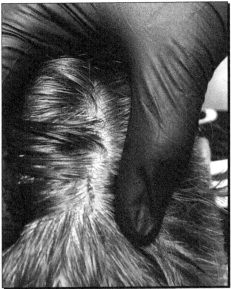

Correct Answer: E. Irrigate with tap water, primary closure with staples.

This case brings up several key points for proper wound closure for simple lacerations, as well as potential bite wounds. The evidence notes the following are effective for simple lacerations: irrigation with tap water and sterile saline are approved (in the absence of a potential bite wound or complicated laceration); and avoid hydrogen peroxide and betadine due to toxicity to fibroblasts and the increased potential for delayed healing. To close a simple laceration (no bite wound), all of the aforementioned choices are accepted for the scalp: staples and hair apposition with tissue adhesives (e.g., Dermabond). If there is no tissue tension on a simple laceration of the scalp, then the use of tissue adhesives (e.g., Dermabond) and sutures (absorbable or nonabsorbable) is appropriate.

With the potential for a wound caused by a human mouth (teeth) in this scenario, it changes the simple laceration to one that is more complicated and, hence, has complicated the closure methods. If the laceration is superficial and well irrigated, with good hemostasis, prophylactic antibiotics are not required, as long as the wound is not sealed (e.g., with tissue adhesives [e.g., Dermabond] or running suture). Therefore, answers A, B, and C are incorrect. These techniques will effectively seal the laceration and potentially harbor infection, even with the addition of oral antibiotics.

In general, with lacerations to the face and scalp, even if due to a bite, primary closure is preferred with the aforementioned techniques (caution to not seal the laceration with skin adhesive or running sutures if suspected bite wound) to achieve to better cosmetic results. If a laceration to the face or scalp is complicated by deep or large laceration, poor hemostasis, poor potential skin healing (delayed presentation, diabetes, drug or alcohol abuse, immunosuppressive use, or previous keloid formation), simple primary closure may not be ideal.

1. Hollander JE, Camacho M. Assessment and management of scalp lacerations. UpToDate. Accessed September 13, 2018 at https://www.uptodate.com/contents/assessment-and-management-of-scalp-lacerations.
2. Forsch RT. Essentials of skin laceration repair. Am Fam Physician 2008 Oct 15;78(8):945-951.
3. Harper M. Clinical manifestations and initial management of bite wounds. UpToDate. Accessed September 13, 2018 at https://www.uptodate.com/contents/clinical-manifestations-and-initial-management-of-bite-wounds.
4. Aukerman DF, Sebastianelli WJ, Nashelsky J. Clinical inquiries. How does tissue adhesive compare with suturing for superficial lacerations? J Fam Pract 2005 Apr;54(4):378.

155. A 67-year-old woman presents to your clinic with a persistent foot drop, after sustaining a fibular head fracture two years ago. What type of orthotic would you prescribe?

   A. Metatarsal bar
   B. Ankle foot orthosis (AFO)
   C. UCBL (University of CA Berkeley Lab) shoe insert
   D. Hinged knee brace
   E. Hip-knee-ankle-foot orthoses (HKAFO)

Correct Answer: B. Ankle foot orthosis (AFO).

This patient's foot drop is most likely due to a common peroneal (fibular) nerve injury, associated with her fibular head fracture. Due to loss of strength of ankle dorsiflexion strength and eversion, an ankle-foot orthosis (AFO) is the best option for her. A metatarsal bar will help relieve pressure off of the metatarsal heads of her foot, but will not address her foot drop. A University of California Berkeley Laboratory (UCBL) shoe insert can help with conditions such as pes planus, but not foot drop. Using a hinged knee brace does not address the patient's underlying ankle weakness. Hip-knee-ankle-foot orthoses (HKAFO) are used primarily with spinal cord injury in adults and children to stabilize the hip and pelvis, with assistive devices to aid in walking and standing.

1. Hennessey WJ, Johnson EW. Lower limb orthoses. In: Braddom RL (ed). Physical Medicine and Rehabilitation. Philadelphia: Saunders, 2000:326-352.
2. Gonzalez-Fernandez M, Taftian D, Hopkins M. Upper and lower limb orthoses and therapeutic footwear. PM&R Knowledge Now. Accessed December 21, 2018 at https://now.aapmr.org/upper-and-lower-limb-orthoses-and-therapeutic-footwear/.

156. In addition to descent, which of the following therapies is advised for the initial treatment of acute mountain sickness?

    A. Rest, ibuprofen, and magnesium sulfate
    B. Increased fluid intake and acetazolamide
    C. Alcohol in small amounts, hydrochlorothiazide, and propoxyphene
    D. Loop diuretics, beta-blockers, and calcium antagonists
    E. Oxygen, acetaminophen, and IV fluids

Correct Answer: B. Increased fluid intake and acetazolamide

Acute mountain sickness (AMS) is the mildest and the most common form of altitude sickness, and when severe symptoms occur, descent to a lower altitude is advised. Mild AMS can be managed by halting the ascent and waiting for acclimatization to improve. Fluids are necessary to replace fluids lost by hyperventilation of dry air. Acetazolamide is a carbonic anhydrase inhibitor that helps correct some of the respiratory alkalosis that occurs with rapid breathing, and can terminate AMS if given early. Diuretics, alcohol, and cathartics promote dehydration and are best avoided. Analgesics have little effect, and cardiac medications have no role in treatment of acute mountain sickness.

1. Fiore DC, Hall S, Shoja P. Altitude illness: risk factors, prevention, presentation, and treatment. Am Fam Physician 2010 Nov 1;82(9):1103-1110.
2. Eide RP, Asplund CA. Altitude illness: update on prevention and treatment. Curr Sports Med Rep 2012 May-Jun;11(3):124-130. doi: 10.1249/JSR.0b013e3182563e7a.

157. You are evaluating a 35-year-old soccer player with known HIV. His physical exam is normal. His HIV was discovered during an evaluation for penile discharge two years ago. Appropriate recommendations about clearance to play include which of the following?

    A. He may play without restriction as long as his CD4 count is > 200 cells/mm3
    B. He may play as long as his viral load is < 1000 IU/ml
    C. He may play without restriction for an abrasion as long as it can be covered
    D. He may not play unless he discloses his status to the team ATC

Correct Answer: C. He may play without restriction for an abrasion as long as it can be covered

Worldwide, there are an estimated 22 million persons infected with HIV. Nearly 25% are not aware of their infection, and one-third are in their twenties or younger. To date, there are not reported cases of HIV transmission in sports. Several studies have reviewed the influence of endurance and resistance exercise on immune function and activity of HIV and have failed to demonstrate any negative influence. Athletes are not required to disclose their personal HIV status. It is recommended that universal precautions always be practiced in an effort to reduce transmission. These precautions include: 1) existing wounds and skin rashes should be properly prepared; 2) equipment and supplies should be available for compliance with universal precautions; 3) those who have uncontrolled bleeding or an uncovered wound should be recognized and removed from competition, and blood-saturated clothing should be removed; 4) the athlete is responsible for wearing protective equipment; 5) minor cuts and abrasions should be cleaned and dressed; 6) care providers should follow universal precautions; 7) personal airway devices should be made available to care providers; 8) equipment contaminated with blood should be cleaned immediately with disinfecting solution; 9) wounds should be reevaluated post competition; and 10) HBV immunization should be considered for healthcare team members.

1. Clem KL, Borchers JR. HIV and the athlete. Clin Sports Med 2007 Jul;26(3):413-424.
2. McGrew C. Bloodborne pathogens and sports. UpToDate. Accessed December 15, 2018 at https://www.uptodate.com/contents/bloodborne-pathogens-and-sports.

158. A 25-year-old female presents to your office with the chief complaint of left thigh pain. She is not doing anything unusual, e.g.. training or workouts. She primarily does low-impact workouts, but did increase the frequency of them. She denies weight training. She denies any trauma. No pain at rest. Prior to her initial visit with you, she went to the ED and had negative radiographs. Your initial exam was unremarkable—no pain with IR, scour compression. A week later, she did a workout with weighted lunges and jump squats. On exam, she notes a bruise, as well as some pain to walk, causing a limp. She now has pain with figure 4, scour, IR, and compression, in addition to some pain with FADIR. She points to the lateral hip as the source of her pain. Palpation of the left thigh reveals a poorly localized area of pain in the midshaft of the femur. There is no difference in circumferential measurement of the right and left thighs. Strength testing of the right quadricep with resisted straight-leg raise does not exacerbate her pain. Radiographs performed in the office of the right hip and femur are negative (see below). What is the most likely diagnosis?

A. Quadriceps tear
B. Anterior superior iliac spine avulsion fracture
C. Femoral stress fracture
D. Myositis ossificans

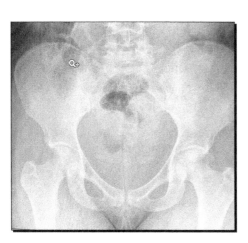
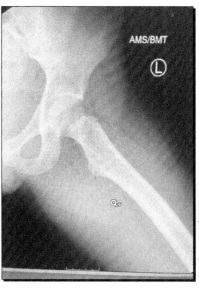

Correct Answer: C. Femoral stress fracture

This patient most likely has a femoral shaft stress fracture. She had an abrupt increase in her symptoms after adding jump squats, which resulted in a limp. Note, the initial radiographs were read and appear normal. The following radiographs after one week clearly show the femoral neck tension-side stress fracture. What is important is that the history is essential for diagnosing femoral neck fractures. Often, exam findings are not as reliable or predictable. What is interesting in this case is the progression of negative to positive findings on radiographs. The MRI clearly delineates the fracture site. She was sent for ORIF the same week.

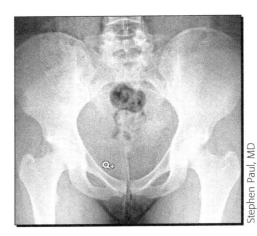

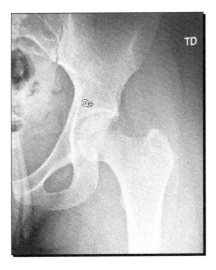

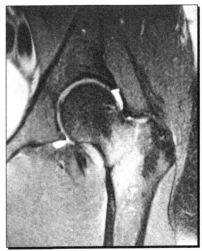

She reported no acute onset of pain during the race, which would have been more likely with an ASIS avulsion fracture. She would have tenderness to palpate at the ASIS, and hip flexion may provoke the sign. Furthermore, this patient at 25 years of age no longer has an open apophysis at the ASIS. A quadriceps tear would present with a discrete painful and swollen area in the thigh. Resisted strength testing would have revealed both pain and weakness. Range of motion would also have been limited with knee extension, and passive stretch would have reproduced pain. Likewise, myositis ossificans, representing heterotopic bone formation in muscle tissue, would have caused limited range of motion, especially with passive knee flexion with the patient in the prone position. A well-defined area of pain would have been palpated, and at three weeks, a firm mass in the area may have been felt as well.

1. DeFranco MJ, Recht M, Schils J, Parker RD. Stress fractures of the femur in athletes. Clin Sports Med 2006 Jan 31;25(1):89-103.
2. Walsh WM. Musculoskeletal injuries in sports. In: Mellion MB, Walsh WM, Madden C, Putukian M, Shelton GL (eds). Team Physician's Handbook. 3rd ed. Philadelphia: Hanley & Belfus, 2002.
3. Esposito PW. Pelvis, hip and thigh injuries. In: Mellion MB, Walsh WM, Madden C, Putukian M, Shelton GL (eds). Team Physician's Handbook. 3rd ed. Philadelphia: Hanley & Belfus, 2002.

159. A 15-year-old male football player presents to the sports medicine clinic complaining of left posterior thigh pain. Yesterday, he felt a pop at the posterior thigh while running, and this morning, he woke up with a stiff-legged gait and ecchymosis. What is the mechanism of action of this injury?

   A. Knee flexion and knee abduction/concentric contraction
   B. Hip flexion and knee extension/eccentric contraction
   C. Knee flexion and hip flexion/eccentric contraction
   D. Hip internal rotation and knee extension/pylometric contraction

Correct Answer: B. Hip flexion and knee extension/eccentric contraction

The diagnosis is a left hamstring injury. The hamstring muscle group spans both the hip and knee joints, producing potential for rapid and extreme muscle lengthening. Injury occurs most commonly during eccentric muscle contraction. During the last 25% of the swing phase, the hamstrings assist in proximal hip extension, while decelerating knee extension distally. The hamstrings remain active during the first half of the stance phase to produce hip extension and resist knee extension through a concentric contraction. Sprint mechanics research suggests that strain injury risk is greatest near the end of the swing phase, when the hamstrings reach maximal length and undergo eccentric contraction, just before heel strike. Most athletes experience acute, sharp pain in the posterior thigh, often with an audible or palpable pop, during an activity requiring a combination of sudden hip flexion and knee extension, as in running, jumping, and kicking sports. A smaller number note an insidious onset of progressive hamstring tightness, and some athletes may have an acute or chronic onset. A few athletes experience loss of hamstring flexibility, particularly with recurrent mild episodes of injury. Proximal avulsion injuries may cause discomfort with sitting. Athletes often describe difficulty in walking smoothly.

Inspection begins with an assessment of gait, with a "stiff-legged" gait pattern often noted, as the athlete attempts to avoid simultaneous hip flexion and knee extension. Most often, minimal ecchymosis is observed. However, broad ecchymosis along the posterior thigh may be encountered and may indicate a high-grade myotendinous injury or a proximal avulsion injury. In cases of a muscle belly rupture, a defect may be palpable. With either proximal or, more commonly, distal avulsion, a thickened area of subcutaneous tissue may be identified adjacent to the injury. Palpation of the injured posterior thigh from the ischial tuberosity to the posterior aspect of the knee localizes the injury by eliciting either tenderness or appreciating a defect.

1. Ahmad CS, Redler LH, Ciccotti MG, Maffulli N, Longo UG, Bradley J. Evaluation and management of hamstring injuries. Am J Sports Med 2013 Dec;41(12):2933-2947. doi: 10.1177/0363546513487063. Epub 2013 May 23.
2. Chan O, Del Buono A, Best TM, Maffulli N. Acute muscle strain injuries: a proposed new classification system. Knee Surg Sports Traumatol Arthrosc 2012 Nov;20(11):2356-2362. doi: 10.1007/s00167-012-2118-z. Epub 2012 Jul 7.
3. Clanton TO, Coupe KJ. Hamstring strains in athletes: diagnosis and treatment. J Am Acad Orthop Surg 1998 Jul-Aug;6(4):237-248.

160. Which of the following statements is true regarding hip flexor injury?

    A. In adolescents with the possible diagnosis of hip flexor pain and tenderness over the ischial tuberosity should have an x-ray to rule-out hip flexor origin avulsion
    B. A hop test with pain in the ipsilateral groin is indicative of a hip flexor strain
    C. Patients with large, palpable defects in the rectus femoris rarely need surgery
    D. Hip flexor strains are commonly accompanied by a tingling sensation in the anterior thigh because of irritation of the lateral femoral cutaneous nerve
    E. Significant weakness is usually seen on exam with hip flexor strains

Correct Answer: C. Patients with large, palpable defects in the rectus femoris rarely need surgery

Isolated deformities of the rectus femoris usually cause little to no functional disability and rarely need surgical intervention. The most common site of avulsion of hip flexors is the rectus femoris at the anterior inferior iliac spine (AIIS), not the ischial tuberosity, which is the origin of the hamstrings (a hip extensor). A positive hop test is suspicious for a femoral neck stress fracture. Meralgia paresthetica is a condition caused by irritation of the lateral femoral cutaneous nerve (often at the inguinal ligament), with symptoms over the lateral thigh. Meralgia paresthetica is not commonly associated with hip flexor strains. Because the hip flexors are very strong muscles, and there are a large number of hip flexors, most strains do not cause significant weakness, but instead have pain (and perhaps subtle weakness) with resistance testing.

1. Rosenberg J. Hip tendonitis and bursitis. Medscape. Accessed December 9, 2018 at https://emedicine.medscape.com/article/87169-overview.

161. A young female soccer player presents with hip pain and clicking. X-rays of the hip are negative, with no evidence of femoral acetabular impingement. What is the appropriate next step?

   A. Order a plain MRI of the hip
   B. Injection of the hip with corticosteroids
   C. Refer for arthroscopy
   D. Order an MR arthrogram of the hip

Correct Answer: D. Order an MR arthrogram of the hip

Likely this is consistent with a hip labral tear. X-ray of the hip can show FAI or osteoarthritis. The preferred method of evaluating the labrum is with MR arthrogram. Plain MRI has a much lower sensitivity and specificity compared to arthrogram. Arthroscopy is considered the gold standard for diagnosis of labral tear, but only after failed conservative management. Therapeutic injection of corticosteroid in the hip can be helpful if degenerative changes are present. However, in a young athlete, the risk of articular surface damage related to corticosteroid injection is a concern. Some individuals would advocate for a diagnostic injection with only anesthetic prior to MR arthrogram, to be sure that pain is truly intra-articular. On the other hand, the anesthetic must be chosen with care to prevent possible cartilage damage (typically ropivicaine is used).

   1. Hammoud S, Bedi A, Voos J, Mauro CS, Kelly BT. The recognition and evaluation of patterns of compensatory injury in patients with mechanical hip pain. Sports Health 2014 Mar;6(2):108-118. doi: 10.1177/1941738114522201.
   2. Tammareddi K, Morelli V, Reyes M. The athlete's hip and groin. Prim Care 2013 Jun;40(2):313-333. doi: 10.1016/j.pop.2013.02.005. Epub 2013 Mar 14.
   3. Prather H, Cheng A. Diagnosis and treatment of hip girdle pain in the athlete. PM R 2016 Mar;8(3 Suppl):S45-S60. doi: 10.1016/j.pmrj.2015.12.009.

162. An 18-year-old female freshman college soccer player presents to clinic with a two-month history of pubic and groin pain that began intermittently with activity and has progressively worsened. She originally noted some pubic and medial groin pain on her right side towards the end of practice. It gradually became more frequent, occurring when she kicked the ball or made a sudden twisting movement. Now, even jogging can trigger pain. Over the last six weeks, she has been treated by her trainer for a muscle strain with no benefit. On exam, her vitals are age-appropriate. She has pain with pelvic compression and tenderness to palpation of her pubic symphysis. There is no tenderness to palpation of the inguinal ligament or asymmetry in her musculature. Range of motion is slightly decreased on her right side, with pain noted on resisted hip flexion and adduction. No bulging is noted with Valsalva maneuvers. Thomas test is negative. She has difficulty standing on her right leg. Radiographs (see below) reveal widening of the pubic symphysis and some periarticular sclerosis. What is her most likely diagnosis?

A. Osteitis pubis
B. Adductor strain
C. Iliopsoas strain
D. Stress fracture of the pubic bone
E. Right indirect hernia

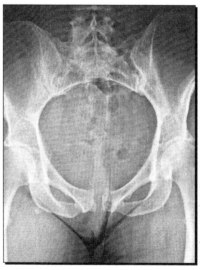

Correct Answer: A. Osteitis pubis

Groin pain is often difficult to diagnose. In this case, the most likely diagnosis, given her exam findings of tenderness of the pubic symphysis and pain with pelvic compression, as well as her radiograph with clear widening, is osteitis pubis. Adductor and iliopsoas strains are common and potential diagnoses, but the negative Thomas test and radiographic findings are more suggestive of osteitis pubis. A stress fracture is not seen on radiographic exam, and hernia is unlikely without bulging noted during Valsalva.

1. Holmich P. Long-standing groin pain in sports people falls into three primary patterns, a "clinical entity" approach: a prospective study of 207 patients. Br J Sports Med 2007 Apr;41(4):247-252; discussion 252. Epub 2007 Jan 29.
2. Mulhall KJ, McKenna J, Walsh A, McCormack D. Osteitis pubis in professional soccer players: a report of outcome with symphyseal curettage in cases refractory to conservative management. Clin J Sport Med 2002 May;12(3):179-181.
3. Rodriguez C, Miguel A, Lima H, Heinrichs K. Osteitis pubis syndrome in the professional soccer athlete: a case report. J Athl Train 2001 Dec;36(4):437-440.

163. A 17-year-old male high school football player injured his right knee after cutting while running. As he pivoted with the football, he stopped abruptly, hyperextended his right knee, and felt a "pop." He then felt excruciating pain in the anterior knee, as well as at the posterior lateral joint line. He rapidly developed an effusion and is now in your sports medicine clinic for rapid assessment of this injury. Examination of the patient is limited, secondary to pain and effusion. However, he does not appear to have an endpoint with anterior drawer. He does have a solid endpoint with posterior drawer, and a positive pivot shift test, and is stable to both valgus and varus stress. His dial test was negative. An x-ray taken in clinic of the right knee demonstrates a small avulsion fracture. Where is this fracture most likely located?

   A. The medial tibial plateau
   B. The medial aspect of the lateral femoral condyle
   C. The medial aspect of the medial femoral condyle
   D. The lateral tibial plateau

Correct Answer: D. The lateral tibial plateau

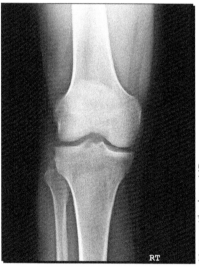

This vignette depicts the classic mechanism of an isolated anterior cruciate ligament (ACL) injury. The ACL is the predominant restraint to anterior tibial displacement. The mechanism of an isolated ACL injury usually entails cutting, deceleration, and hyperextension of the knee. Hyperextension typically develops much higher forces in the ACL, as opposed to the posterior cruciate ligament (PCL). Noncontact injury is the most common manner of ACL compromise. Contact injuries will often involve other structures as well (such as the terrible triad of ACL, MCL, and medial meniscus injuries, due to the attachment of the MCL to the medial meniscus). Were this injury a possible "terrible triad," the mechanism would have been by a valgus (contact) force as applied to a flexed and rotated knee, as opposed to one of hyperextension. A Segond fracture (small avulsion fracture at the lateral tibial condyle/plateau) is now known to be associated with ACL injuries, as demonstrated by the image above. A lateral tibial plateau avulsion will occur, due to excessive internal rotation and varus stress on the anterolateral ligament, after compromise of the ACL. More rarely, an avulsion fracture of the ACL insertion at the medial tibial eminence will be seen. The medial aspect of the lateral femoral condyle in the intercondylar notch is the anatomic origin of the ACL.

1. Claes S, Luyckx T, Vereecke E, Bellemans J. The Segond fracture: a bony injury of the anterolateral ligament of the knee. Arthroscopy 2014 Nov;30(11):1475-1482.
2. Evaluation of ACL tear. Wheeless' Textbook of Orthopaedics. Accessed December 9, 2018 at http://www.wheelessonline.com/ortho/evaluation_of_acl_tear.

164. A high school basketball athlete presents to the emergency department after sustaining a knee injury. He went up for a rebound and landed awkwardly on his right leg, while an opposing player fell into the lateral side of his knee, causing it to buckle. There was a gross deformity to the right knee. EMS states there was no dorsalis pedis pulse present initially at the scene, but after transferring the patient into the ambulance, the DP pulse returned, and the knee did not appear as deformed as before. The patient is complaining of severe pain. X-rays are taken and do not reveal any acute fracture. After adequate analgesia, you exam the knee and find significant laxity with Lachman test, posterior drawer test, and valgus stress test at 0 and 30 degrees of flexion. You are able to palpate a strong dorsalis pedis pulse and popliteal pulse on the right. The peroneal nerve appears intact. What is the next best step in the management of this injury?

A. Place the knee in a knee immobilizer and discharge
B. Place the knee in a hinged brace locked at 30 degrees, and discharge
C. Place the knee in a long-leg posterior splint and discharge with crutches
D. Measure compartment pressures in the lower leg
E. Perform ankle-brachial index

Correct Answer: E. Perform ankle-brachial index

This patient had a traumatic knee dislocation. Most knee dislocations spontaneously reduce prior to being evaluated by a physician. A popliteal artery injury occurs in 7% to 45% of all knee dislocations. All patients with knee dislocations should also be evaluated for vascular injury, even if strong pulses are palpated because of this risk. Failure to recognize a vascular injury can lead to limb ischemia and loss of limb. Workups for vascular injury include measuring the ankle-brachial index (ABI), performing Doppler studies, CT or MR angiography, or obtaining an arteriogram (the gold standard). Compartment syndrome can occur in the setting of a knee dislocation, but ABIs should be measured prior to compartment pressure testing.

1. Kelleher HB. Knee dislocation. Medscape. Accessed December 8, 2018 at https://emedicine.medscape.com/article/823589-overview.
2. Traumatic dislocations of the knee. Wheeless' Textbook of Orthopaedics. Accessed December 8, 2018 at https://www.wheelessonline.com/ortho/traumatic_dislocations_of_the_knee.

165. A 27-year-old female training for a 5K race presents with progressively worsening left lateral knee pain, ongoing for six weeks. She has steadily increased her mileage and has been running on the treadmill, as well as on pavement. Symptoms are exacerbated with running, climbing stairs, and squats. She denies any injury or prior knee problems. On exam, there is no joint effusion, normal and pain free range of motion, and no joint line tenderness or mechanical symptoms. Which of the following should be considered as initial treatment?

    A. Icing, stretching program, activity modification
    B. Referral to orthopaedic sports surgeon
    C. Corticosteroid injection
    D. Physical therapy

Correct Answer: A. Icing, stretching program, activity modification

Iliotibial band syndrome is a common cause of knee pain in runners. Excess friction from repetitive knee flexion and extension results in local inflammation of the distal iliotibial band as it slides over the lateral femoral condyle. The initial treatment goal is reduction of local inflammation (ice, NSAIDs, activity modification). The next step includes a targeted stretching program (iliotibial band, hip and plantar flexors) and strengthening program (gluteus medius and hip/pelvic stabilizers). Physical therapy can be beneficial. A local corticosteroid injection can be considered for persistent symptoms. For refractory cases, referral to an orthopaedic sports surgeon for surgical release of the iliotibial band may be indicated.

1. Calmbach WL, Hutchens M. Evaluation of patients presenting with knee pain: part II. Differential diagnosis. Am Fam Physician 2003 Sep 1;68(5):917-922.
2. Khaund R, Flynn SH. Iliotibial band syndrome: a common source of knee pain. Am Fam Physician 2005 Apr 15;71(8):1545-1550.

166. A 15-year-old female field hockey player cuts laterally to avoid an opponent and falls to the ground. She sits up, but cannot stand, and other players wave you onto the field. She has an obvious deformity to her anterior knee, and she states something "popped." Her knee is stable on testing, no effusion is present, and the neurovascular status of the leg is intact. Which of the following statements is correct regarding the athlete's injury?

   A. Reduce the injury, with the patient sitting, and send her to the hospital for angiography
   B. Reduction is best performed with the patient supine and hip extended
   C. Patients with genu valgum and increased Q angle are predisposed to this injury
   D. Sport specific activity should be continued in a couple of days to prevent deconditioning

Correct Answer: C. Patients with genu valgum and increased Q angle are predisposed to this injury

The athlete sustained a dislocated patella. This is more common in young females, and often is accompanied by a popping in the knee. Factors predisposing to dislocation of the patella include genu valgum, increased Q angle, shallow femoral groove, loose medial retinaculum, patella alta, and vastus medialis dysplasia. Patients do not require angiograpy, though evaluation of the vasculature is required with a knee (not patellar) dislocation. Reduction is best performed with the hip flexed and the knee in extension, with the patient seated. Rehabilitation starts with extension splinting of the knee and cryotherapy. Sport-specific activity is often delayed for six to eight weeks.

1. Cooper R, Morris H, Arendt L. Acute knee injuries. In: Brukner P, Khan K (eds). Clinical Sports Medicine. 3rd ed. Australia: McGraw-Hill, 2006:498-499.
2. Harner CD. Patellofemoral instability and malalignment. In: Griffin LY (ed). Essentials of Musculoskeletal Care. 3rd ed. Rosemont, IL: AAOS, 2005:541-545.

167. A 33-year-old male runner presents to your office with complaints of anterior right knee pain, worsening over the past month. He has just recently started training for a marathon that will take place in four months. On physical exam of the right knee, you find mild effusion, vague tenderness over the medial femoral condyle, and some swelling, just medial to the patellar border. With the patient in supine position, you apply pressure with the thumb over the inferior and medial aspect of the patellofemoral joint, and passively flex and extend the knee. The patient reports pain between 30 and 45 degrees, as well as a clicking sensation. Plain radiographs of both knees are unremarkable. What is the most likely cause of this patient's symptoms?

   A. Medial meniscal tear
   B. Osteoarthritis
   C. Patellofemoral pain syndrome
   D. Plica syndrome
   E. Pes anserinus pain syndrome

Correct Answer: D. Plica syndrome

Plica syndrome is the most likely cause of this patient's syndrome. The provocative maneuver described in this case is the medial patellar plica (MPP) test. The pain caused by this test supposedly is caused by the plica being pinched between the medial patellar facet and the medial condyle, and there may be a clicking or popping sensation. The diagnosis of plica syndrome is based on clinical features and is suggested by the history of anterior and medial knee pain after direct trauma, twisting injury, or repetitive injury. Other provocative maneuvers include the stutter test and the knee extension test (Hughston test). Arthroscopy provides a definitive diagnosis if a thickened, fibrotic plica is demonstrated. This patient did not report an acute inciting event to suspect meniscal tear. In addition, pain would be expected to be localized more to the joint line. Osteoarthritis is more common in the age group over 50, associated with morning stiffness, and would show a decrease in cartilage space on plain radiographs. Patellofemoral pain syndrome is not likely, due to a lack of effusion or synovitis and the fact that pain is not localized to the medial or lateral patellar facets. In pes anserinus sydrome, there is no clicking or popping, no catching or pseudo-locking, and on physical exam, the tenderness is over the insertion of the pes anserinus tendon at the medial proximal tibia.

1. Gregory AJM. Plica syndrome. UpToDate. Accessed December 9, 2018 at https://www.uptodate.com/contents/plica-syndrome.

168. A 62-year-old female presents to your office with increased right medial knee discomfort for one week, with no apparent injury. She has no swelling, and reports no locking or giving way episodes. She has had mild knee discomfort for 10 years. She has had no relief with anti-inflammatories. On exam, she has complete range of motion and no effusion, but does report medial joint line pain with palpation, and discomfort with McMurray's test. In-office x-rays performed show Kellgren-Lawrence grade III changes in the medial compartment. What is the next management step?

   A. MRI to confirm diagnosis
   B. Surgical referral for arthroscopy
   C. Surgical referral for total knee replacement
   D. Acetaminophen and physical therapy

Correct Answer: D. Acetaminophen and physical therapy

This patient likely has a degenerative meniscal tear. Conservative measures should always be attempted prior to other interventions. MRI is not necessary, only adds to expense, and does not change management in this situation. Surgical intervention for degenerative tears without mechanical symptoms has no benefit. Joint replacement is not needed with acute pain, and the patient has not failed conservative management for degenerative joint disease.

   1. Petron DJ, Greis PE, Aoki SK, Black S, Krete D, Sohagia KB, et al. Use of knee magnetic resonance imaging by primary care physicians in patients aged 40 years and older. Sports Health 2010 Sep;2(5):385-390.
   2. Moseley JB, O'Malley K, Petersen NJ, Menke TJ, Brody BA, Kuykendall DH, et al. A controlled trial of arthroscopic surgery for osteoarthritis of the knee. N Engl J Med 2002 Jul 11;347(2):81-88.

Test 2 Answers, Critiques, and References

169. A 21-year-old comes in for evaluation after an ankle injury. Using the Weber classification for lateral malleolus fractures, which of the following demonstrates a need for immediate evaluation?

    A. Weber A
    B. Weber B
    C. Weber C
    D. Both Weber A and B require consideration for surgical treatment

Correct Answer: C. Weber C

Weber classification refers to the level of fibular fracture relative to the syndesmosis. Weber A —generally no surgery. A CAM walker or splint may be used. The injury is below the syndesmosis. Weber B—if no medial swelling or tenderness to palpation, no surgery. The injury is at the level of the syndesmosis. Weber C with mortise disruption—unstable and almost always needs surgery, though depends on swelling. The patient should be sent for emergent evaluation. The injury is above the level of the syndesmosis.

1. Fractures. Wheeless' Textbook of Orthopaedics. Accessed December 10, 2018 at http://www.wheelessonline.com/ortho/weber_c_fractures.
2. Danis-Weber classification of ankle fractures. Orthopaedics One. Accessed December 10, 2018 at https://www.orthopaedicsone.com/x/iYUOBQ.

170. A 45-year-old overweight male presents with a complaint of pain in the left great toe. Recently, he started jogging two miles a day due to a desire to lose weight, but has not changed his diet. Patient reports drinking four cans of beer every night. The pain has developed over the last two weeks and is increased after running. Exam demonstrates a normal foot with tenderness and swelling of the medial plantar aspect of the left first metatarsophalangeal joint. Passive dorsiflexion of the toe causes pain in that area. Plantarflexion produces no discomfort, and no numbness can be appreciated. Which of the following is most likely his diagnosis?

    A. Cellulitis
    B. Gout
    C. Morton's neuroma
    D. Sesamoid fracture

Correct Answer: D. Sesamoid fracture

The first metatarsophalangeal (MTP) joint has two sesamoid bones, and injuries to these bones account for 12% of great-toe injuries. Overuse, a sharp blow, and sudden dorsiflexion are the most common mechanisms of injury. Sesamoiditis versus sesamoid fracture is difficult to diagnose. X-rays may not show a fracture. Treatment is similar, unless the fracture is open or widely displaced. Limit weight-bearing and flexion, but if pain persists at four to six weeks, reconsider the diagnosis. Cellulitis would present with erythema, rubor, and warmth. Gout may also present with those symptoms, in addition to joint swelling and exquisite tenderness over the joint. Morton's neuroma is felt in the plantar web space, most commonly between the third and fourth toes (third web space).

1. Sesamoid fractures. Wheeless' Textbook of Orthopaedics. Accessed December 10, 2018 at http://www.wheelessonline.com/ortho/sesamoid_fractures.
2. Wall J, Feller JF. Imaging of stress fractures in runners. Clin Sports Med 2006 Oct;25(4):781-802.

171. A 34-year-old male runner presents to your office with pain in the left Achilles region for the past six months. His pain has been worse over the past six weeks. He has had difficulty performing his six-mile runs, and yesterday, he could not run at all. Which of the following is true regarding Achilles tendinopathy?

    A. Achilles tendinopathy is a degenerative, as opposed to an inflammatory, condition
    B. Most patients fail non-operative measures, even if the condition is treated early
    C. Surgery is required in most cases involving decompression of the tendon by tenotomy and aggressive measures to improve the local circulation
    D. Surgery is recommended after non-operative methods of management have been tried for at least three months

Correct Answer: A. Achilles tendinopathy is a degenerative, as opposed to an inflammatory, condition

Most patients respond well with non-operative treatment if identified and treated early, but 24% to 45.5% of patients that do not respond to conservative care may go on to surgical treatment. Surgery may be recommended after exhausting non-operative methods of management, often tried for at least six months. Newer treatments, such as PRP and Tenex procedures, do not yet have strong literature supporting their use.

1. Kader D, Saxena A, Movin T, Maffulli N. Achilles tendinopathy: some aspects of basic science and clinical management. Br J Sports Med 2002;36(4):239-249.
2. Alfredson H, Pietilä T, Jonsson P, Lorentzon R. Heavy-load eccentric calf muscle training for the treatment of chronic Achilles tendinosis. Am J Sports Med 1998 May-Jun;26(3):360-366.

172. Which of the following statements is true regarding seizures and participation in water sports?

   A. Individuals with uncontrolled seizures should only be cleared for swimming activities when undertaken in the presence of a lifeguard
   B. Individuals with uncontrolled seizures may be cleared for non-swimming water sports with no restrictions
   C. Individuals who have been seizure-free for five years and are not taking anti-seizure medications may be allowed to participate in watersports
   D. Individuals with a history of epilepsy who are cleared for water sports should hyperventilate before entering the water, since this reduces the chance of seizures

Correct Answer: C. Individuals who have been seizure-free for five years and are not taking anti-seizure medications may be allowed to participate in watersports.

For individuals with seizure disorders, the risk of drowning is increased 15- to 19-fold compared to the general population. The general recommendations for individuals with uncontrolled seizures is no swimming and restrictions for non-swimming water sports (e.g., must wear life jacket). Hyperventilation may lower the seizure threshold and increase the risk of seizures.

1. Bell GS, Gaitatzis A, Bell CL, Johnson AL, Sander JW. Drowning in people with epilepsy. How great is the risk? Neurology 2008 Aug 19;71(8):578-582. doi: 10.1212/01.wnl.0000323813.36193.4d.
2. Greer HD. Neurologic consequences. In: Bove AA (ed). Bove and Davis' Diving Medicine. 3rd ed. Philadelphia: Saunders, 1997:258-269.
3. Nathanson AT, Young JM, Young CC. Preparticipation medical evaluation for adventure and wilderness watersports. Clin J Sport Med 2015 Sep;25(5):425-431. doi: 10.1097/JSM.0000000000000252.

173. What is the most common cause of weakness in entrapment syndromes?

    A. Neurapraxia
    B. Denervation
    C. Axonotmesis
    D. Neurotmesis
    E. Disuse atrophy

Correct Answer: A. Neurapraxia

Neurapraxia or conduction block is the most common pathology in entrapment or compression syndromes, followed by demyelination. Neurapraxia is the mildest type of focal nerve lesion that produces clinical deficits. Denervation is the complete loss of nerve supply. Axonotmesis is the interruption of the axons of a nerve, followed by complete degeneration of the peripheral segment, without severance of the supporting structure of the nerve. This can occur from pinching, crushing, or prolonged pressure on a nerve. Neurotmesis is a type of axon-loss lesion, resulting from focal peripheral nerve injury, in which the nerve stroma is damaged in addition to the axon and myelin, which degenerate from that point distally. Disuse atrophy is not a common cause of weakness with nerve entrapment syndrome.

1. Seddon HJ. A classification of nerve injuries. Br Med J 1942 Aug 29;2(4260):237-239.
2. O'Connor FG, Sallis RE, Wilder RP, St. Pierre P (eds). Sports Medicine: Just the Facts. New York: McGraw-Hill, 2005.
3. Nakano KK. Nerve entrapment syndromes. Curr Opin Rheumatol 1997 Mar;9(2):165-173.

174. You are consulted on a female track athlete with a known seizure disorder. Her favorite events are the middle distances, and she has never had a seizure training or in competition. She has not had a seizure in three years and has not changed medications. The school is concerned about whether she should be allowed to compete, due to her medical condition. Refraining from which of the following sports may be considered for this patient?

    A. Track
    B. Cycling
    C. Singles ice skating
    D. Football
    E. Swimming

Correct Answer: E. Swimming

There are no specific prohibitions regarding track. Aerobic activities, such as track, occasionally cause seizure exacerbations. However, on average, aerobic exercise decreases frequency. In the rare reports where seizures are triggered, patients readily identify the triggers. Medication can be adjusted for altered pharmacokinetics in aerobically conditioned athletes, if needed. Furthermore, a seizure occurring during the activity (running) does not pose life-threatening scenarios for other competitors, as in pistol shooting or automobile racing, and does not pose a life-threatening scenario for the athlete, as in sky diving or scuba diving. There are no restrictions for cycling, ice skating, or football. Swimming requires special consideration, and is most likely to be restricted, given that a seizure in the water could lead to drowning.

1. Fountain NB, May AC. Epilepsy and athletics. Clin Sports Med 2003 Jul;22(3):605-616, x-xi.
2. American Academy of Family Physicians, American Academy of Pediatrics, American College of Sports Medicine, American Medical Society for Sports Medicine, American Orthopaedic Society for Sports Medicine, American Osteopathic Academy of Sports Medicine. Bernhardt DT, Roberts WO (eds). Preparticipation Physical Evaluation. 4th ed. Elk Grove, IL: American Academy of Pediatrics, 2010.

175. Which of the following is an absolute contraindication to collision-sports participation?

  A. Torg-Pavlov Ratio < 0.8
  B. Recurrent cervical cord neuropraxia/transient quadriparesis
  C. Healed, non-displaced, stable fracture of C3-C4 at posterior ring
  D. Clay shoveler's fracture
  E. Healed cervical herniated disc

Correct Answer: B. Recurrent cervical cord neuropraxia/transient quadriparesis

Cervical cord neuropraxia/transient quadriparesis is defined as neurologic symptoms of at least two limbs that lasts less than 48 hours, which is typically caused by hyperflexion or hyperextension of the cervical spine. A Torg-Pavlov ratio is no longer used for clearance, as the preference is to look at functional reserve on an MRI when evaluating a patient for return to play. The listed fractures and disc herniation would not be severe enough for sport disqualification.

1. Cantu RC. Cervical spine injuries in the athlete. Semin Neurol 2000;20(2):173-178.
2. Torg JS, Guille JT, Jaffe S. Injuries to the cervical spine in American football players. J Bone Joint Surg Am 2002;84:112-122.
3. Concannon LG, Harrast MA, Herring SA. Radiating upper limb pain in the contact sport athlete: an update on transient quadriparesis and stingers. Curr Sports Med Rep 2012 Jan-Feb;11(1):28-34. doi: 10.1249/JSR.0b013e318240dc3f.

176. You are performing preparticipation physical exams at a local high school prior to the fall sports season. You examine a freshman male going out for football for the first time. His paperwork indicates that he is missing one of his testicles. After a little bit of questioning, he tells you his left testicle never came down and had to be surgically removed while he was a young child. You perform a physical exam and confirm the presence of only one testicle, which is on the right side. Which of the following is the best course of action for this young athlete?

A. Do not clear him for football, pending further evaluation by a urologist to determine if he can safely play
B. Restrict this athlete from playing football, but recommend trying out for golf or cross country as alternative sports for participation
C. Clear the athlete to play football without restriction, since studies have demonstrated there is a low risk of testicular injury in sports
D. Have a discussion with the athlete and his parents regarding the risk of injury to the lone testicle and review the use of protective equipment

Correct Answer: D. Have a discussion with the athlete and his parents regarding the risk of injury to the lone testicle and review the use of protective equipment

Since this athlete is a minor, including his parents in a discussion of the risks of participating in a contact sport with a solitary testicle is essential. Testicular injuries are uncommon in sports, but the risk must be carefully considered by athletes with one testicle. A serious injury to the remaining testicle could negatively impact fertility and endocrine function. Protective equipment can reduce, but not eliminate, that risk. Contact sports are not an absolute contraindication, however, if the athlete and their family have the opportunity to make a thoroughly informed decision. This is not a situation in which the expertise of a urologist is needed, unless specifically requested by the family.

1. American Academy of Family Physicians, American Academy of Pediatrics, American College of Sports Medicine, American Medical Society for Sports Medicine, American Orthopaedic Society for Sports Medicine, American Osteopathic Academy of Sports Medicine. Bernhardt DT, Roberts WO (eds). Systems-based examination—gastrointestinal/genitourinary. Preparticipation Physical Evaluation. 4th ed. Elk Grove Village, IL: American Academy of Pediatrics, 2010:97-100.
2. Hergenroeder AC. Sports participation in children and adolescents: the preparticipation physical evaluation. UpToDate. Accessed December 13, 2018 at https://www.uptodate.com/contents/sports-participation-in-children-and-adolescents-the-preparticipation-physical-evaluation.

177. Which of the following is correct regarding preparticipation decisions?

   A. An athlete with one congenitally missing kidney, who also has a polycystic remaining kidney, should be allowed to participate in football, as long as he has regular blood pressure monitoring and uses a kidney guard pad during practice and games
   B. An athlete with one testicle does not need to be counseled regarding the risk of losing his fertility during play if sport participants routinely use a protective cup (e.g., baseball and football)
   C. When an athlete has only one functional eye (with less than 20/40 corrected visual acuity), further evaluation by an ophthalmologist is recommended
   D. Athletes with only one functional eye can participate in boxing if the functional eye is ipsilateral to their dominant hand

Correct Answer: C. When an athlete has only one functional eye (with less than 20/40 corrected visual acuity), further evaluation by an ophthalmologist is recommended

Athletes with one single kidney that is polycystic or abnormally located are not allowed to participate in contact or collision sports. Athletes with one testicle need to use a protective cup during contact sports. The chance of injury and the subsequent possibility of loss of fertility should be discussed in counseling. Athletes with only one functional eye (with less than 20/40 corrected visual acuity) can participate only in sports (such as swimming, track and field, and gymnastics) that permit the use of protective eyewear and do not involve projected objects. Wrestling, boxing and martial arts are contraindicated sports in this scenario.

   1. Kurowski K, Chandran S. The preparticipation athletic evaluation. Am Fam Physician 2000 May 1;61(9):2683-2690, 2696-2698.
   2. Stock JG, Cornell FM. Prevention of sports-related eye injury. Am Fam Physician 1991 Aug;44(2):515-520.

178. A 14-year-old male with known solitary kidney, which is located in its normal anatomical location, presents to you for his preparticipation physical evaluation. He has played football for several years and wants to join his high school team this year. He and his parents report no known problems, hospitalizations, or concerns related to the kidney. His exam is normal. Which of the following recommendations best fits this athlete's clearance to play?

   A. This athlete should be cleared to play non-contact sports only
   B. This athlete may be cleared to play collision sports with a qualified yes, meaning that protective equipment must be worn
   C. This athlete may be cleared to play non-contact and limited contact sports only, but absolutely no collision sports
   D. This athlete should be cleared to play any sport without further recommendation

Correct Answer: B. This athlete may be cleared to play collision sports with a qualified yes, meaning that protective equipment must be worn

The absence of one kidney indicates that this athlete requires individual assessment at his preparticipation exam. Most athletes with single kidney can be cleared for contact, collision, and limited contact sports with a qualified yes, but discussion must be held regarding protective equipment to reduce risk of injury to the remaining kidney. Large trauma registries (two different registries of 15,000 and 50,000 patients each) show less than 5% of kidney injuries occur during contact sports, and no kidneys were lost in contact sports. It is important that the athlete and the guardians understand the potential risk and that the protective equipment must remain in place to be effective. The decision to participate in contact and collision sports with a single kidney is decided on an individual basis.

1. American Academy of Family Physicians, American Academy of Pediatrics, American College of Sports Medicine, American Medical Society for Sports Medicine, American Orthopaedic Society for Sports Medicine, American Osteopathic Academy of Sports Medicine. Bernhardt DT, Roberts WO (eds). Preparticipation Physical Evaluation. 4th ed. Elk Grove, IL: American Academy of Pediatrics, 2010:35.
2. Carter N. Renal trauma. In: Bracker MD (ed). The 5-Minute Sports Medicine Consult. 2nd ed. Philadelphia: Lippincott Williams & Wilkins, 2011:508-509.
3. Madden CC, Putukian M, Young CC, McCarty EC (eds). General medical problems in athletes: unilateral organ. Netter's Sports Medicine. Philadelphia: Saunders Elsevier, 2010:222.

179. A 30-year-old female computer worker presents with occupation-related forearm pain for several months. On physical exam, weakness is noted in the extensor carpi ulnaris and the distal extensors of the hand, but no sensory deficit is noted. You suspect which nerve syndrome?

   A. Posterior interosseus nerve syndrome
   B. Anterior interosseus nerve syndrome
   C. Carpal tunnel syndrome
   D. Tarsal tunnel syndrome
   E. Ulnar neuropathy

Correct Answer: A. Posterior interosseus nerve syndrome

The posterior interosseus nerve is a purely motor nerve branch of the radial nerve that innervates the extensor carpi ulnaris muscle. It is the deep branch of the radial nerve, coursing over the dorsum of the forearm lateral aspect of the radius.

   1. Sellards R, Kuebrich C. The elbow diagnosis and treatment of common injuries. Prim Care 2005 Mar;32(1):1-16.
   2. Lubahn JD, Cermak MB. Uncommon nerve compression syndromes of the upper extremity. J Am Acad Orthop Surg 1998 Nov-Dec;6(6):378-386.
   3. Stern M. Radial nerve entrapment. Medscape. Accessed December 4, 2018 at https://emedicine.medscape.com/article/1244110.

180. A 200-pound, first-string NCAA Division I quarterback reports to football camp after being diagnosed both clinically and by laboratory tests with mononucleosis three weeks ago. He is in excellent health, feels great, and brings with him a note from his internist that he is cleared for full contact. What facts can you count on when determining his return-safely-to-play status?

   A. There is no good evidence that return to play after clinical recovery from mononucleosis is particularly dangerous, but the risk is not zero
   B. His primary physician already signed off, and your exam is normal. This player is at no risk for splenic rupture now
   C. You have recently attended point-of-care ultrasound training. You ultrasound his abdomen. Because his spleen is not enlarged, you determine there is no risk for splenic rupture
   D. The patient and his family will sign a waiver exempting the medical staff and the university from any liability if he returns to play

Correct Answer: A. There is no good evidence that return to play after clinical recovery from mononucleosis is particularly dangerous, but the risk is not zero

Waivers signed by patients and family do not protect the medical staff and university from liability, even if the patient receives clearance from his personal physician. The team physician and staff must make the final decision about return to play based on the best evidence. What is known about mono and return to play is that if a patient is clinically improved, and three weeks have passed since the diagnosis was made, there is minimal risk for splenic rupture, but the risk is not at zero.

   1. Putukian M, O'Connor FG, Stricker PR, McGrew C, Hosey RG, Gordon SM, et al. Mononucleosis and athletic participation: an evidence-based subject review. Clin J Sport Med 2008 Jul;18(4):309-315. doi: 10.1097/JSM.0b013e31817e34f8.
   2. Herring SA, Kibler WB, Putukian M. Team physician consensus statement: 2013 update. Med Sci Sports Exerc 2013 Aug;45(8):1618-1622. doi: 10.1249/MSS.0b013e31829ba437.

181. In order to prevent exercise-induced bronchospasm (EIB) during competition, athletes with documented asthma would benefit from which of the following treatments?

    A. Pre-medicate with beta-adrenergic agonist
    B. Pre-medicate with corticosteroids
    C. Pre-medicate with inhaled corticosteroids
    D. Pre-medicate with anti-histamines
    E. Pre-medicate with nasal steroids

Correct Answer: A. Pre-medicate with beta-adrenergic agonist

The use of anti-asthma medications helps to control EIB in most asthmatics. For individuals with asthmatic symptoms associated only with exercise, the prophylactic use of a beta-2-agonist inhaler before exercise prevents EIB in most cases. Short-acting beta-2 agonists have the advantage of providing prevention and rescue therapy for EIB. Although long-acting beta-2 agonists provide a longer duration of EIB prophylaxis, they should not be used as a first-line treatment for EIB, because of their slow onset of action. Pre-treatment with corticosteroids is not indicated. Inhaled corticosteroids may be needed for moderate persistent asthmatics for control, but not an acute state as with exercise. Answers D and E both are control medications and may be part of the treatment for an asthmatic that also has allergic rhinitis. However, these are not the mainstay to prevent EIB.

1. Puffer JC. Twenty Common Problems in Sports Medicine. New York: McGraw-Hill, 2002:299-300.
2. Kynyk J, Parsons JP. Pulmonary medicine in the athlete: exercise-induced bronchospasm. In: Miller MD, Thompson SR (eds). DeLee & Drez's Orthopaedic Sports Medicine. 4th ed. Philadelphia: Saunders Elsevier, 2015:202-206.

182. A 17-year-old senior high school cross country runner with a history of two femoral neck stress fractures presents to your sports medicine clinic for persistent amenorrhea in the setting of decreased performance. She has not had her menstrual period for at least one year and also appears thin and frail. Her performance at recent track meets has suffered, as she was all-county last year, but has not even placed at her meets in quite some time. She says she feels a great deal of pressure as she applies for college, and badly wants an athletic scholarship. Which of the following is not a prudent next step in managing this patient?

    A. Educating the patient, her parents, and her coaches about the health risks of her diagnosis
    B. Supplementation with calcium/vitamin D and increasing caloric intake
    C. Limiting the time she spends running at her practice sessions
    D. Starting an oral contraceptive

Correct Answer: D. Starting an oral contraceptive

This is a case of female athlete triad syndrome, which is characterized by disordered eating (as evidenced by her frail appearance), menstrual disorders (amenorrhea), and osteoporosis/low bone mineral density (as evidenced by her history of multiple stress fractures). A prudent first step is to counsel the patient and those supporting her (parents, coaches, etc.) about the diagnosis. Simultaneously, it is reasonable to start nutritional supplements for her likely low bone mineral density in the setting of previous femoral neck stress fractures, as well as increasing her caloric intake in order to improve her energy level. It is likely that her baseline energy level is low, so it is also important to restrict energy expenditure on her part by limiting her practice sessions. An oral contraceptive may not be a wise next step, since by correcting her nutritional deficiencies and encouraging normal oral intake of food/nutrition, she stands a reasonable chance of improving. Simply returning menstruation by use of an oral contraceptive does nothing to treat the underlying problem.

1. De Souza MJ, Nattiv A, Joy E, Misra M, Williams NI, Mallinson RJ, et al. Female athlete triad coalition consensus statement on treatment and return to play of the female athlete triad: 1st International Conference held in San Francisco, California, May 2012 and 2nd International Conference held in Indianapolis, Indiana, May 2013. Clin J Sport Med 2014 Mar;24(2):96-119. doi: 10.1097/JSM.0000000000000085.

183. A 17-year-old female notes on her preparticipation physical that she has had regular menstrual periods over the past four years, until the last 10 months. During the last 10 months, she has had no menstrual periods. Her history reveals no obvious causes for this, other than her participation in cross-country and track. Her physical exam is unremarkable. Which of the following statements is the best statement that reflects her condition?

   A. She is suffering from exercise-related amenorrhea and should be counseled about starting on calcitonin to prevent osteoporosis
   B. She is suffering from oligomenorrhea and should be counseled to gain weight so that her menstrual cycles return to normal
   C. She is normal for her age and should wait one year to see if her menstrual cycle returns to normal
   D. She is suffering from an eating disorder and should be counseled to seek a mental health consultation
   E. She is suffering from amenorrhea and should be counseled to have laboratory testing to determine the cause

Correct Answer: E. She is suffering from amenorrhea and should be counseled to have laboratory testing to determine the cause

A history of amenorrhea is one of the easiest ways to detect the female athlete triad in its earliest stages. Evidence suggests that menstrual history may predict current bone density in female athletes. In a study of young female athletes, longer, more consistent patterns of amenorrhea were found to have a linear correlation with measures of bone density. Amenorrhea should not be discounted by the family physician as a benign consequence of athletic training. The vignette gives no indications of female athlete triad, other than amenorrhea. If after a thorough history and physical exam, including nutritional history, no obvious cause is found, further workup is indicated to evaluate for causes of secondary amenorrhea.

1. Ackerman KE, Misra M. Functional hypothalamic amenorrhea: evaluation and management. UpToDate. Accessed December 13, 2018 at https://www-uptodate-com.offcampus.lib.washington.edu/contents/functional-hypothalamic-amenorrhea-evaluation-and-management.
2. Hobart JA, Smucker DR. The female athlete triad. Am Fam Physician 2000 Jun 1;61(11):3357-3364, 3367.
3. Drinkwater BL, Bruemner B, Chesnut CH 3rd. Menstrual history as a determinant of current bone density in young athletes. JAMA 1990 Jan 26;263(4):545-548.

184. A defensive player on a collegiate football team has just come off the field after making a tackle. He tells the athletic trainer that the left side of his neck hurts, and he feels tingling and burning in his left shoulder. Sideline examination reveals decreased sensation over the lateral deltoid and weakness with abduction and elbow flexion. Spurling's maneuver is negative. After halftime, the symptoms abate. Of note, the player had one previous episode with similar symptoms two weeks prior. What is the next step in management of this player?

   A. Studies show that neck rolls and cowboy collars successfully prevent this type of injury
   B. He should not return to play and will need further imaging workup
   C. He should not return to play and requires an urgent nerve conduction study
   D. He should not return to play and should be withheld for the remainder of the season, since he has now had two injuries

Correct Answer: B. Should not return to play and will need further imaging workup

Stingers are a transient episode of unilateral pain and/or paresthesias in an upper extremity. There is a preponderance of C5 or C6 and upper trunk symptoms. Athletes must have resolution of all symptoms, with full, pain-free cervical ROM and full strength, along with an absence of any underlying risk factors for further injury, before they can return to play. An athlete who experiences a first stinger (or a second stinger in separate seasons), with rapid resolution and normal neurological examination, may return in the same game. All other scenarios will require further workup before the athlete may return to play. Any stinger with persisting neurological symptoms or signs requires evaluation before return to play. A history of three lifetime stingers, or two in the same season (even with rapid resolution) will require further evaluation. For a third stinger in the same season, with or without persisting symptoms or signs or a third stinger in separate seasons with persisting neurological symptoms or signs, recommendations include holding the athlete out for the season and considering restricting from contact sports. Nerve conduction studies will not be useful until at least three weeks after injury, since alteration in nerve conduction takes about three weeks for signs of denervation to be seen. There is no proven protective equipment to prevent stingers.

1. Concannon LG, Harrast MA, Herring SA. Radiating upper limb pain in the contact sport athlete: an update on transient quadriparesis and stingers. Curr Sports Med Rep 2012 Jan-Feb;11(1):28-34. doi: 10.1249/JSR.0b013e318240dc3f.
2. Standaert CJ, Herring SA. Expert opinion and controversies in musculoskeletal and sports medicine: stingers. Arch Phys Med Rehabil 2009 Mar;90(3):402-406. doi: 10.1016/j.apmr.2008.09.569.

185. You are working at a clinic in the Key West Florida and are asked to evaluate a group of scuba divers. They are planning to get certified for scuba diving and would like preparticipation clearance. Which one of the following patients has an absolute contraindication to scuba dive?

   A. 23-year-old female type 1 diabetic, who has been on an insulin pump for 12 years. She is a high-level triathlete. No recent episodes of ketoacidosis and no evidence of end organ damage. Her hemoglobin A1C is less than 7.5
   B. 28-year-old female with a recent past medical history of concussion while playing volleyball eight weeks ago. She completed her return-to-play protocol. She is thinking about getting pregnant
   C. 62-year-old male, former Navy diver, with a 12-year history of type 2 diabetes, who is on metformin. He was recently diagnosed with peripheral neuropathy and impaired low-glucose awareness. His last A1C was 9.1
   D. 22-year-old male with asthma. An albuterol inhaler is his only medication, and his last FEV1 was greater than 80% of predicted normal

Correct Answer: C. 62-year-old male, former Navy diver, with a 12-year history of type 2 diabetes, who is on metformin. He was recently diagnosed with peripheral neuropathy and impaired low-glucose awareness. His last A1C was 9.1

The long-standing diabetic who has lost the normal defense mechanism against hypoglycemia should not dive. The main risk to the diver is the occurrence of hypoglycemia that can manifest itself as confusion, sweating, rapid heartbeat, unconsciousness, and even death. DAN (Divers Alert Network) suggests that some diabetics may dive safely in controlled settings, when meeting certain criteria, for example, one year after initiation of insulin therapy, no episodes of hypoglycemia or hyperglycemia requiring intervention from a third party for at least one year, and age ≥ 18 years (16 years if in special training program). Recommendations for glucose management on the day of diving include blood glucose ≥ 150 mg/dL (8.3 mmol/L), which is stable or rising before entering the water. In addition, the individual should have completed a minimum of three pre-dive checks to evaluate blood glucose trends at 60 minutes, 30 minutes, and immediately prior to diving. Delay dive if glucose is 300 mg/dL (16.7 mmol/L). A history of concussion is not an absolute contraindication if an individual is neurologically normal and has completed a return-to-play protocol. There is no evidence of an increase in miscarriages or other problems in women who have been diving around the time of conception. Asthmatics may dive when the pulmonary function tests are normal at rest, though there may be minimal increased risk associated with diving for asthmatics.

   1. Frequently asked questions. Divers Alert Network. Accessed December 13, 2018 at https://www.diversalertnetwork.org/medical/faq/.
   2. Chandy D, Weinhouse GL. Complications of scuba diving. UpToDate. Accessed December 15, 2018 at https://www.uptodate.com/contents/complications-of-scuba-diving.

186. A mother brings her 13-year-old boy with Down syndrome to your office for medical clearance to participate in Special Olympics. Which of the following statements is true regarding sports participation in this athlete?

    A. Athletes with Down syndrome should never participate in sports such as equestrian, diving, high jump, or alpine skiing
    B. There is a congenital absence or laxity of the transverse atlas ligament in 10% to 30 % of patients with Down syndrome
    C. Cervical spine manipulation is frequently recommended for patients with Down syndrome
    D. Routine yearly x-rays are recommended to evaluate for atlantoaxial instability

Correct Answer: B. There is a congenital absence or laxity of the transverse atlas ligament in 10% to 30 % of patients with Down syndrome

The use of screening cervical spine x-rays, with flexion and extension, is controversial, but is often recommended around age eight, as well as in adolescents, to screen for atlantoaxial instability. Yearly x-rays are not recommended. Serial neurologic examinations is also recommend, particularly in athletes. The Special Olympics requires that athletes with Down syndrome either 1) are cleared by a physician with normal cervical spine x-rays with flexion and extension, or 2) if atlantoaxial instability is present, they submit written certifications from two physicians, with an acknowledgment of risks signed by the adult athlete or their parent or guardian to participate in sports at higher risk (e.g., butterfly stroke and diving starts in swimming, diving, pentathlon, high jump, equestrian sports, artistic gymnastics, soccer, alpine skiing). Cervical spine manipulation should be avoided in all patients who have a risk of atlantoaxial instability.

1. Alvarez N. Atlantoaxial instability in Down syndrome. Medscape. Accessed December 13, 2018 at https://emedicine.medscape.com/article/1180354-overview#a9.
2. Tassone JC, Duey-Holtz A. Spine concerns in the Special Olympian with Down syndrome. Sports Med Arthrosc Rev 2008 Mar;16(1):55-60. doi: 10.1097/JSA.0b013e3181629ac4.
3. El-Khouri M, Mourão MA, Tobo A, Battistella LR, Herrero CF, Riberto M. Prevalence of atlanto-occipital and atlantoaxial instability in adults with Down syndrome. World Neurosurg 2014 Jul-Aug;82(1-2):215-218. doi: 10.1016/j.wneu.2014.02.006. Epub 2014 Feb 14.

187. A 15-year-old male with Down syndrome presents to your clinic for his preparticipation examination. He will be participating in judo. Per Special Olympics guidelines, the patient will require a lateral cervical spine x-ray, with flexion and extension views, to rule out atlantoaxial instability (AAI). These x-rays will be used to assess the atlanto-dens interval (ADI), which is the space between the posterior aspect of the anterior arch of the atlas and the odontoid. Which measurement of the atlanto-dens interval (ADI) would disqualify the athlete from competing in a high-risk sport such as judo?

    A. Greater than 1.5 mm
    B. Greater than 2.5 mm
    C. Greater than 3.5 mm
    D. Greater than 4.5 mm

Correct Answer: D. Greater than 4.5 mm

Despite the lack of evidence confirming the value of these radiographs in asymptomatic athletes with Down syndrome, the Special Olympics requires this study before competing in certain sports. The Special Olympics has chosen an atlanto-dens interval (ADI) greater than 4.5 mm for the diagnosis of atlantoaxial instability in children. The events for which a radiologic evaluation is required include judo, equestrian sports, gymnastics, diving, pentathlon, butterfly stroke, swimming that involves a diving start, high jump, alpine skiing, snowboarding, squat lift, and soccer. The AAP Committee on Genetics recommends obtaining lateral plain cervical spine radiographs in the neutral position, with odontoid and anterior-posterior (A-P) views, to examine for evidence of AAI or subluxation in patients with myelopathic signs or symptoms. Nearly all people with AAI who have suffered a catastrophic injury to the spinal cord have had preceding neurologic symptoms. Despite this, the Special Olympics requires screening neck radiographs in all children with Down syndrome before participation.

1. American Academy of Family Physicians, American Academy of Pediatrics, American College of Sports Medicine, American Medical Society for Sports Medicine, American Orthopaedic Society for Sports Medicine, American Osteopathic Academy of Sports Medicine. Bernhardt DT, Roberts WO (eds). The athlete with special needs. Preparticipation Physical Evaluation. 4th ed. Elk Grove, IL: American Academy of Pediatrics, 2010:131-139.
2. Ostermaier KK. Down syndrome: management. UpToDate. Accessed December 13, 2018 at https://www.uptodate.com/contents/down-syndrome-management.

188. A 26-year-old male soccer player consults with you about groin injuries. He has had a number of groin injuries in the course of sports participation, usually diagnosed as "groin strains" by his team's athletic trainers. His last injury was about eight months ago, and while he is currently asymptomatic, he asks you if there was any way to potentially prevent recurrence of this injury, while still allowing him to participate in soccer. His physical examination shows no areas of tenderness to palpation, full normal range-of-motion, and roughly equal adductor and abductor muscle strength bilaterally. What do you recommend as part of a training strategy to prevent athletic groin strains?

    A. Strengthen the hip adductors to increase the adductor: abductor strength ratio
    B. Strengthen the hip abductors to increase the abductor: adductor strength ratio
    C. Strengthen the hip flexors to increase the flexor: extensor strength ratio
    D. Strengthen the hip extensors to increase the extensor: flexor strength ratio

Correct Answer: A. Strengthen the hip adductors to increase the adductor: abductor strength ratio

Athletic-related groin injuries are a significant cause of missed practice and playing time for many athletes, as well as, unfortunately, premature termination of athletic careers. An estimated 13% of soccer injuries are groin-related, which tend to recur. In 2007, Holmich and colleagues reported that 58% of athletes with long-standing groin pain had adductor-related pathology, while 35% had iliopsoas-related pathology. Reported modifiable risk factors include reduced adduction strength, reduced hip internal rotation and bent knee fallout, heavier athletes, and overload or overuse. Tyler et al. reported a significantly higher risk of adductor injuries in a cohort of professional ice hockey players with a hip adductor muscle strength less than 80% of the hip abductors. Off-season training of abdominal and adductor muscles saw a two-thirds reduction of this risk. Based on available evidence, Holmich et al. provided the following prevention measures for groin-injury prevention in turf athletes in 2007: gradual introduction of cutting and pubic shearing movements, especially in heavy athletes; avoid adductor and lower abdominal overstraining; early emphasis on pelvic core stability strengthening; dynamic cross-motion training; agility drills as routine part of warm-up; and adductor strengthening, with a goal of an adductor:abductor strength ratio of 1.3 (4:3).

1. Emery CA, Meeuwisse WH. Risk factors for groin injuries in hockey. Med Sci Sports Exerc 2001 Sep;33(9):1423-1433.
2. Tyler T, Nicholas SJ, Campbell RJ, Donellan S, McHugh MP. The effectiveness of a preseason exercise program to prevent adductor muscle strains in professional ice hockey players. Am J Sports Med 2002 Sep-Oct;30(5):680-683.
3. Holmich P. Long-standing groin pain in sportspeople falls into three primary patterns, a "clinical entity" approach: a prospective study of 207 patients. Br J Sports Med 2007 Apr;41(4):247-252; discussion 252. Epub 2007 Jan 29.

189. Overtraining syndrome (OTS) is a poorly understood condition characterized by the following symptoms: mood changes, fatigue, and decreased performance, accompanied by increased achiness and more frequent injuries. What is the best explanation of the pathophysiology?

    A. Branched-chain amino acid (BCAA) deficiency
    B. Glycogen depletion
    C. Cytokine overload
    D. Hypothalamic dysregulation
    E. Overtraining syndrome involves a complex, poorly understood pathophysiology, likely involving multiple pathways

Correct Answer: E. Overtraining syndrome involves a complex, poorly understood pathophysiology, likely involving multiple pathways

While all other answers have theoretical capabilities to explain overtraining, none has sufficient evidence as the unifying cause. The pathophysiology is thought to involve these pathways and likely others, which are poorly understood. Tryptophan, the serotonin (5-HT) precursor, competes with BCAA for the same carrier in the blood-brain barrier. This hypothesis proposes that decreased BCAA levels ultimately allow more tryptophan into the brain, which drastically elevates central 5-HT concentration. This requires the amount of 5-HT to rise so high as to induce a state of fatigue in the individual, as well as other OTS symptoms, like mood and sleep disturbances. Low muscle glycogen can have a negative effect on training and performance by not providing enough energy for the high workload. However, studies have shown that athletes who consume inadequate carbohydrates may fatigue more quickly, but do not meet the requirements to diagnose OTS. In addition, athletes who maintain normal glycogen levels through increased carbohydrate consumption during heavy training may still develop OTS.

The cytokine hypothesis is the most inclusive explanation for OTS. It explains why OTS occurs by presenting a primary cause with effects all over the body that correlate with the symptoms of over trained athletes. Training induces trauma and stimulates an acute local inflammatory response and cytokine recruitment. Prolonged activation of muscles and joints, without adequate rest, can shift local acute inflammation to chronic inflammation, thus stimulating an amplified inflammatory response with correlated pathology. Despite this hypothesis explaining the etiology of OTS, limitations still remain, given that little evidence exists that shows elevated cytokines in overtrained athletes.

Another mechanism that may potentially cause OTS is dysregulation of the hypothalamus and its axes. Specifically, the hypothalamic-pituitary-adrenal (HPA) and hypothalamic-pituitary-gonadal axes would account for many of the symptoms seen in over trained athletes. These athletes can have drastic changes primarily in cortisol, adrenocorticotropic hormone (ACTH), testosterone, and subsequently estrogen levels. Unfortunately, studies that quantify these hormone levels in athletes have varied widely.

1. Carfagno DF, Hendrix JC 3rd. Overtraining syndrome in the athlete: current clinical practice. Curr Sports Med Rep 2014 Jan-Feb;13(1):45-51. doi: 10.1249/JSR.0000000000000027.
2. Meeusen R, Duclos M, Foster C, Fry A, Gleeson M, Nieman D, et al. Prevention, diagnosis, and treatment of the overtraining syndrome: joint consensus statement of the European College of Sport Science and the American College of Sports Medicine. Med Sci Sports Exerc 2013 Jan;45(1):186-205. doi: 10.1249/MSS.0b013e318279a10a.

190. A 28-year-old male endurance runner complains of symptoms of fatigue as he increases his training runs in preparation for an upcoming marathon. He also mentions that his mile split times have worsened, which is causing him a lot of anxiety. His wife is concerned that he has grown more irritable and has not been eating well lately. What do you recommend?

   A. Start a selective serotonin reuptake inhibitor (SSRI)
   B. Try drinking a caffeinated beverage 30 minutes to an hour prior to his training runs
   C. Take a break from running until his symptoms resolve
   D. Start iron and vitamin C supplementation
   E. Be sure to plan for carbohydrate ingestion (either a carbohydrate-electrolyte solution or sports gel containing glucose and fructose) during his longer training runs

Correct Answer: C. Take a break from running until his symptoms resolve

This athlete's symptoms are most consistent with overtraining as he prepares for his upcoming endurance event. The best treatment for overtraining is rest from sport, along with an emphasis on good dietary habits and perhaps even psychological support. While symptoms of overtraining can be difficult to distinguish from those of clinical depression, use of SSRIs has not yet been proven effective in overtraining syndrome. Caffeine and proper carbohydrate replacement can improve exercise performance, but would not help with this athlete's more serious condition. Finally, anemia can cause symptoms of fatigue and decreased exercise tolerance, but usually is not associated with psychological changes. Thus, empiric treatment with iron supplementation for supposed iron-deficiency anemia would not be the best option.

   1. Armstrong LE, VanHeest JL. The unknown mechanism of the overtraining syndrome: clues from depression and psychoneuroimmunology. Sports Med 2002;32(3):185-209.
   2. Mackinnon LT, Hooper SL. Overtraining and overreaching: causes, effects, and prevention. In: Garrett WE, Kirkendall DT (eds). Exercise and Sports Science. Philadelphia: Lippincott Williams & Wilkins, 2000:487-498.
   3. Meeusen R, Duclos M, Foster C, Fry A, Gleeson M, Nieman D, et al. Prevention, diagnosis, and treatment of the overtraining syndrome: joint consensus statement of the European College of Sport Science and the American College of Sports Medicine. Med Sci Sports Exerc 2013 Jan;45(1):186-205. doi: 10.1249/MSS.0b013e318279a10a.

191. A 15-year-old female elite figure skater presents to your clinic with her sixth injury in six months. Review of history reveals fatigue, loss of appetite, decrease in athletic performance, sleep disturbance, and worsening school grades. In addition to treating her current injury, you diagnose her with overtraining and burnout. One strategy for preventing overtraining/burnout is periodization. What is periodization?

    A. A process of slowly progressing workout intensity and workload
    B. A process of periodically evaluating an athlete for symptoms and signs of overtraining
    C. A process of emphasizing proper technique and mechanics to prevent chronic or acute injuries
    D. A process of cyclically varying the training stimulus in phases throughout the calendar year

Correct Answer: D. A process of cyclically varying the training stimulus in phases throughout the calendar year

Periodization is a process of varying the training stimulus in cycles to promote long-term fitness gains and avoid overtraining. The year as a whole is taken into consideration and divided up into phases. In each phase, the workout emphasizes a specific type of training. Periodization can also be undertaken in the span of a single week. Answers A, B, and C are all appropriate techniques to prevent overtraining and burnout, but are not periodization by definition.

   1. Brenner JS, American Academy of Pediatrics Council on Sports Medicine and Fitness. Overuse injuries, overtraining, and burnout in child and adolescent athletes. Pediatrics 2007 Jun;119(6):1242-1245.

192. A running group that is currently developing their training regimen for an upcoming marathon in six months has asked you to speak to them about the effects of altitude training on running performance. Which of the following is the most appropriate general recommendation?

    A. Training at altitude does not seem to improve performance in endurance events and is generally not thought to be effective
    B. Best available evidence suggests that living at moderate altitude then training and competing at low altitude does improve performance in endurance events
    C. Current recommendation is to live and train at high altitude as often as possible, regardless of the altitude of the competition site
    D. Encourage the participants to live at low altitude and train at high altitude to maximize performance

Correct Answer: B. Best available evidence suggests that living at moderate altitude then training and competing at low altitude does improve performance in endurance events

Despite a large amount of theoretical evidence, there are a paucity of studies on the appropriate utilization of altitude training to maximize athletic performance. The few studies and multiple case reports that are available suggest that living and sleeping at moderate altitude (~2500 meters), while training at low altitude, affords for maximal performance in endurance events. Interestingly, training at high altitude can have adverse effects on training, due to lack of exercise tolerance. Answer A is incorrect, since there seems to be clear consensus that altitude training has positive effects on sports performance. Answer C is incorrect, as training at high altitude is not currently recommended, due to possible adverse effects on performance. Answer D is incorrect for the same reasons as Answer C, and is the opposite of current recommendations.

1. Girard O, Amann M, Aughey R, Billaut F, Bishop DJ, Bourdon P, et al. Position statement—altitude training for improving team-sport players' performance: current knowledge and unresolved issues. Br J Sports Med 2013 Dec;47 Suppl 1:i8-i16. doi: 10.1136/bjsports-2013-093109.
2. Lundby C, Millet GP, Calbet JA, Bärtsch P, Subudhi AW. Does 'altitude training' increase exercise performance in elite athletes? Br J Sports Med 2012 Sep;46(11):792-795. doi: 10.1136/bjsports-2012-091231. Epub 2012 Jul 14.
3. Levine BD, Stray-Gundersen J. "Living high-training low": effect of moderate-altitude acclimatization with low-altitude training on performance. J Appl Physiol (1985) 1997 Jul;83(1):102-112.

193. You are the medical director for a large youth soccer tournament that will be played in hot weather. Which of the following is correct about pediatric patients exercising in hot weather?

   A. Pediatric patients who are well hydrated and acclimated to heat are able to exercise in the heat at no greater risk than adult patients
   B. Pediatric patients have similar sweat volumes compared to adults
   C. Pediatric patients have the same number of sweat glands compared to adults
   D. Pediatric patients have a similar body surface area-to-mass ratio and a similar heat gain from the environment compared to adults

Correct Answer: A. Pediatric patients who are well hydrated and acclimated to heat are able to exercise in the heat at no greater risk then adult patients

Children are able to compensate for their lower number of sweat glands and lower sweat rates by increasing cutaneous blood flow to increase convective heat loss during exercise. Pediatric patients have increased body surface area-to-mass ratio compared to adults. Theoretically, they could have increased heat gain from the environment, but clinically, this has not been a problem. Previous reports of having lower cardiac outputs during exercise has been demonstrated not to be accurate when adjusted for body size and relative cardiac intensity. However, if they are not well hydrated, their adaptive mechanics may not be adequate for heat dispersion. Accordingly, adequate hydration is critical for pediatric athletes. This is especially problematic at weekend tournaments with multiple games played throughout the day. Clinicians involved in planning events should ensure that pediatric athletes have adequate time between events to rehydrate.

1. Council on Sports Medicine and Fitness and Council on School Health, Bergeron MF, Devore C, Rice SG, American Academy of Pediatrics. Policy statement—climatic heat stress and exercising children and adolescents. Pediatrics 2011 Sep;128(3):e741-e747. doi: 10.1542/peds.2011-1664. Epub 2011 Aug 8.
2. Rowland T. Thermoregulation during exercise in the heat in children: old concepts revisited. J Appl Physiol (1985) 2008 Aug;105(2):718-724. Epub 2007 Dec 13.
3. Bergeron MF. Training and competing in the heat in youth sports: no sweat? Br J Sports Med 2015 Jul;49(13):837-839. doi: 10.1136/bjsports-2015-094662.

194. Which of the following is true of resistance training in the pediatric population?

   A. Resistance training can result in increased strength without muscle hypertrophy or changes in body composition
   B. Strength gains are not lost during detraining
   C. Resistance training is generally discouraged in children and adolescents, due to safety concerns
   D. Growth in height and weight of preadolescents can be influenced by resistance training

Correct Answer: A. Resistance training can result in increased strength without muscle hypertrophy or changes in body composition

Resistance training in children and adolescents has been shown to increase muscular strength significantly, independent of body composition changes or muscle hypertrophy. Strength gains are lost in the detraining period. Growth in height or weight are not influenced by resistance training. Resistance training is generally thought to be safe when properly supervised.

   1. Malina RM. Weight training in youth-growth, maturation, and safety: an evidence-based review. Clin J Sport Med 2006 Nov;16(6):478-487.

195. You are one of several first responders on the scene of an unresponsive 17-year-old female with witnessed collapsed during basketball practice. CPR is begun, EMS activated, and the AED placed. Shock is advised. What is the next step?

    A. Give three consecutive shocks, followed by resumption of CPR
    B. Give one shock, and then check pulse/rhythm and immediately reshock if advised
    C. Give one shock, and then resume CPR for five cycles before rechecking rhythm
    D. Give two rescue breaths and five cycles of CPR before proceeding with shock

Correct Answer: C. Give one shock, and then resume CPR for five cycles before rechecking rhythm

The 2005 AHA adult CPR guidelines for CPR and Emergency Cardiac Care in the case of a witnessed collapse recommend immediate CPR, EMS activation, and AED placement as soon as possible. If the AED advises to shock, shock once and resume CPR immediately, without checking the pulse or rhythm until five cycles of CPR have been completed. Previous protocols have involved a sequence of three shocks. Because this has been found to cause a delay of up to 37 seconds between delivery of shock and chest compressions, it is therefore no longer recommended. If the collapse is unwitnessed, providers should consider giving two rescue breaths and five cycles of CPR before defibrillation. If the collapse is witnessed, however, the AED should be placed as quickly as possible, with CPR interrupted if shock advised.

1. Drezner JA, Courson RW, Roberts WO, Mosesso VN, Link MS, Maron BJ. Inter-association task force recommendations on emergency preparedness and management of sudden cardiac arrest in high school and college athletic programs: a consensus statement. J Athl Train 2007;42(1):143-158.
2. ECC Committee, Subcommittees and Task Forces of the American Heart Association. 2005 American Heart Association Guidelines for Cardiopulmonary Resuscitation and Emergency Cardiovascular Care. Circulation 2005 Dec 13;112(24 Suppl):IV1-IV203. Epub 2005 Nov 28.

196. Which of the following is a correct statement about burnout and overtraining in youth sports?

    A. Most young athletes who drop out of sports are burned out
    B. Most youth who discontinue a sport do so as a result of poor coaching
    C. To reduce the likelihood of burnout, an emphasis should be placed on competition more than skill development
    D. Symptoms may include fatigue, lack of enthusiasm about practice or competition, or difficulty with successfully completing usual routines

Correct Answer: D. Symptoms may include fatigue, lack of enthusiasm about practice or competition, or difficulty with successfully completing usual routines

Burnout, especially in youth sports, is considered part of a spectrum that includes overtraining and overreaching in sport. Often, it is a result of too early sport specialization. As noted, some of the symptoms can be somatic, such as fatigue, or difficulty with successfully completing usual routines. The chronic stress of the sport participation can lead to lack of enthusiasm about practice or competition, boredom, and eventually dropping the sport. Poor coaching has not been cited as a major contributor to sport dropout, although there is a greater psychological component to burnout in youth sports with adult supervision. Most youth who drop out of a sport often do so due to other interests, time conflicts, or trying out a new or different sport. To reduce the likelihood of burnout, an emphasis should be placed on skill development, rather than competition or winning. Data suggests that by making the practice and sport fun, reducing the required time and days (depending on age and maturation), and reducing sport specialization, burnout and overtraining, as well as overuse injuries, may be reduced.

1. DiFiori JP, Benjamin HJ, Brenner J, Gregory A, Jayanthi N, Landry GL, et al. Overuse injuries and burnout in youth sports: a position statement from the American Medical Society for Sports Medicine. Clin J Sport Med 2014 Jan;24(1):3-20. doi: 10.1097/JSM.0000000000000060.
2. Brenner JS. Sports specialization and intensive training in young athletes. Pediatrics 2016 Sep;138(3). pii: e20162148. doi: 10.1542/peds.2016-2148.
3. Brenner JS, The Council on Sports Medicine and Fitness. Overuse injuries, overtraining, and burnout in adolescent athletes. Pediatrics 2007 Jun;119(6):1242-1245.

197. A 14-year-old male patient presents to your office for a preparticipation physical exam. The patient's mother and brother have Marfan syndrome. The family has been tested for the genetic mutation for Marfan syndrome. This patient was found to be negative and cleared for all sports in the past. What is the mutation that is tested for?

   A. Prothrombin gene mutation
   B. Trisomy 21
   C. Sarcomeric mutation
   D. BRCA1 gene
   E. Fibrillin 1 mutation

Correct Answer: E. Fibrillin 1 mutation

Answer A is a mutation leading to a hypercoaguable state. Answer B is a genetic mutation leading to Down syndrome. Answer C is a mutation that leads to hypertrophic cardiomyopathies. Answer D is a gene that is a risk for breast cancer.

1. Pelliccia A, Zipes DP, Maron BJ. Bethesda Conference #36 and the European Society of Cardiology Consensus Recommendations revisited a comparison of U.S. and European criteria for eligibility and disqualification of competitive athletes with cardiovascular abnormalities. J Am Coll Cardiol 2008 Dec 9;52(24):1990-1996.
2. Halabchi F, Seif-Barghi T, Mazaheri R. Sudden cardiac death in young athletes; a literature review and special considerations in Asia. Asian J Sports Med 2011 Mar;2(1):1-15.
3. Türk UO, Alioğlu E, Nalbantgil S, Nart D. Catastrophic cardiovascular consequences of weight lifting in a family with Marfan syndrome. Turk Kardiyol Dern Ars 2008 Jan;36(1):32-34.

198. A 14-year-old football player at the 25th percentile for height and 100th percentile for weight has a persistent blood pressure of 145/80 mm Hg during his preparticipation physical, with an otherwise normal cardiovascular exam. Which of the following is true regarding sports clearance for this athlete?

    A. Clearance for sports with no further evaluation required
    B. Clearance for sports with recommendation of repeat blood pressure measurement in six months
    C. Clearance for sports after the athlete has lost 10% of his extra weight
    D. Clearance for sports after blood pressure is controlled

Correct Answer: D. Clearance for sports after blood pressure is controlled

Blood pressure in children is categorized by severity, using sex and percentage of height. Using The Fourth Report on the Diagnosis, Evaluation, and Treatment of High Blood Pressure in Children and Adolescents, this athlete's blood pressure is stage 2 (higher than 5 mm Hg above the 99th percentile). If the athlete's blood pressure was in the prehypertension range, it is recommended for the blood pressure to be checked in six months, without sporting restrictions. Using the Bethesda guidelines, an athlete with sustained blood pressure elevation should have an evaluation for etiology and end organ damage, and should undergo at least an electrocardiogram and echocardiogram to rule out left ventricular hypertrophy. If the athlete is found to have stage 2 hypertension, even without end organ damage, per the Bethesda guidelines, it is recommended to control the blood pressure with lifestyle modifications, with or without medications, prior to participation in competitive sports. As this athlete's percentage of weight is dramatically much higher than his percentage of height, he likely has obesity-associated hypertension and would benefit from weight loss. His sporting clearance is dependent on his blood pressure control and not on achieving a particular percentage of weight loss.

1. Riley M, Bluhm B. High blood pressure in children and adolescents. Am Fam Physician 2012 Apr 1;85(7):693-700.
2. American Academy of Family Physicians, American Academy of Pediatrics, American College of Sports Medicine, American Medical Society for Sports Medicine, American Orthopaedic Society for Sports Medicine, American Osteopathic Academy of Sports Medicine. Bernhardt DT, Roberts WO (eds). Preparticipation Physical Evaluation. 4th ed. Elk Grove, IL: American Academy of Pediatrics, 2010.
3. Maron BJ, Zipes DP. 36th Bethesda Conference: eligibility recommendations for competitive athletes with cardiovascular abnormalities. JACC 2005;45(8):1313-1375.
4. National High Blood Pressure Education Program Working Group on High Blood Pressure in Children and Adolescents. The fourth report on the diagnosis, evaluation, and treatment of high blood pressure in children and adolescents. Pediatrics 2004 Aug;114(2 Suppl 4th Report):555-576.

199. Which of the following is a current American Heart Association (AHA) recommendation regarding cardiac evaluation during the preparticipation exam?

A. Auscultate for heart murmur during provocative maneuvers
B. Palpate bilateral brachial pulses
C. Obtain bilateral brachial blood pressure with the athlete standing
D. Perform electrocardiogram on all athletes

Correct Answer: A. Auscultate for heart murmur during provocative maneuvers

In addition to the preparticipation medical and family history screening, the current AHA recommendations for the cardiovascular screening physical exam include recognition of physical stigmata related to Marfan syndrome, seated brachial blood pressure, palpation of radial and femoral pulses, and auscultatory cardiac exam, including provocative maneuvers for murmurs. ECG remains optional and is usually reserved for those found to have abnormal findings on screening history or exam.

1. Maron B, Thompson PD, Ackerman MJ, Balady G, Berger S, Cohen D, et al. Recommendations and considerations related to preparticipation screening for cardiovascular abnormalities in competitive athletes: 2007 update: a scientific statement from the American Heart Association Council on Nutrition, Physical Activity, and Metabolism: endorsed by the American College of Cardiology Foundation. Circulation 2007 Mar 27;115(12):1643-1655. Epub 2007 Mar 12.

200. A 16-year-old male presents for his preparticipation physical evaluation. On exam, he is found to have corrected right eye visual acuity of 20/20, but corrected left eye visual acuity of only 20/200. Mom explains that the left eye vision loss was due to a childhood injury at age two. He has just recently been seen for his yearly eye exam with an eyecare professional, who did not suggest any change in his correction or any eye protection for this athlete's sports of choice, which are football, wrestling, sprinting events, and full-contact martial arts. Which of the following is the correct protective eyewear recommendation for the associated activity for this athlete?

   A. Track: normal street-wear frames with 2 mm polycarbonate lenses
   B. Football: helmet with wire face mask
   C. Baseball: normal street-wear frames with 2 mm polycarbonate lenses
   D. Full-contact martial arts: custom made sport goggles

Correct Answer: A. Track: normal street-wear frames with 2 mm polycarbonate lenses

The athlete is deemed functionally one-eyed if the loss of the better eye would result in a significant change in lifestyle. Consequently, those with best corrected vision in one eye less than 20/40 should be considered functionally one-eyed. The evidence for eye protection is all consensus and expert opinion. The American Society for Testing and Materials requires all safety sports eyewear to conform to ASTM standard F803 for most high- and moderate-risk sports, with a few exceptions, such as youth baseball batter/runner, paintball, skiing, and ice hockey, which have higher standard specifications. Street-wear frames meeting the American National Standards Institute (ANSI) standard or safety eyewear meeting ANSI standards and mandated by Occupational Safety and Health Administration (OSHA) are not satisfactory for sports. Polycarbonate is the recommended material because it is the most shatter resistant clear lens material. A functionally one-eyed person should wear protective lenses, such as street-wear frames with 2 mm polycarbonate lenses, at all times to protect from non-sports related trauma.

Sports are categorized based on risk of eye injury to the unprotected player in the following categories: high risk (sub-classified by "small, fast projectiles" or "hard projectiles, sticks, close contact" or "intentional injury"), moderate risk, low risk, and eye-safe. This athlete's choice of sports includes football (moderate risk), baseball (moderate risk), sprints in track (eye-safe), and full-contact martial arts (high risk, intentional injury). These sports have the following recommendations for eye protection: football—polycarbonate eye shield attached to helmet-mounted wire face mask (in addition sports goggles are also strongly recommended); baseball—polycarbonate face guard attached to the helmet for batting and baserunning, with sports goggles with polycarbonate frames for fielding; sprints in track—considered eye-safe and only daily wear is suggested, which for this functionally one-eyed athlete should be a street-wear frame with a 2 mm polycarbonate lens; full-contact martial arts—given that no protective eyewear is permitted in this sport, participation by a functionally one-eyed athlete is contraindicated.

1. American Academy of Family Physicians, American Academy of Pediatrics, American College of Sports Medicine, American Medical Society for Sports Medicine, American Orthopaedic Society for Sports Medicine, American Osteopathic Academy of Sports Medicine. Wappes JR (ed). Preparticipation Physical Evaluation. 3rd ed. Minneapolis, MN: McGraw Hill, 2005:32-33, 46-47, 70-72.
2. American Academy of Pediatrics Committee on Sports Medicine and Fitness. Protective eyewear for young athletes. Pediatrics 2004 Mar;113(3 Pt 1):619-622.
3. Rodriguez JO, Lavina AM, Agarwal A. Prevention and treatment of common eye injuries in sports. Am Fam Physician 2003 Apr 1:67(7):1481-1488.

Appendix

Case Studies

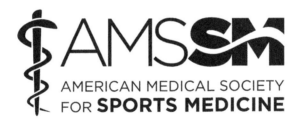

CASE STUDY #1: CERVICAL NEUROPRAXIA

Patient Presentation

A 23-year-old male special teams football player with no history of prior neck injuries complaining of bilateral "stingers"

History

While attempting to make a tackle in a game, he hit his head, causing hyperextension of his neck. After coming off of the field, he complained of bilateral numbness and tingling throughout his arms that he described as "stingers." Physical examination on the sideline revealed full strength and range of motion bilaterally. No Nexus* criteria were met. He was removed from the game due to his discomfort. He was seen for follow-up two days later, at which time he reported continued dysesthesias in his bilateral shoulders, described as "burning" elicited by light touch, such as contact between his shirt and skin or water from the shower. He denied any radiation, numbness, or tingling. He also complained of neck stiffness, but denied any neck pain.

Physical Examination

- ❑ Neurological: Alert and oriented to person, place, and time
- ❑ Neck: Full range of motion of the cervical spine, no midline tenderness. Spurling's test was negative.
- ❑ Extremities: Tenderness to light touch along the clavicles and trapezius bilaterally. Otherwise, full range of motion, 5/5 strength and 2+ DTRs in the bilateral upper extremities.

Differential Diagnosis

- Brachial plexopathy
- Cervical fracture/dislocation
- Cervical disc herniation
- Cervical strain/sprain

---

* NEXUS criteria: Cervical spine imaging is indicated if any of the following are present:
- Focal neurologic deficit
- Midline spinal tenderness
- Altered level of consciousness
- Intoxication
- A distracting injury is present

Other Studies

❑ MRI of the cervical spine was significant for mild circumferential disc bulge, resulting in moderate central canal stenosis, with suspected central and right-sided cord edema at C3-C4.

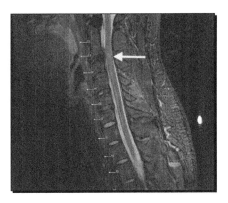

Working Diagnosis: Spinal cord contusion, central canal stenosis, secondary to disc bulge.

Treatment

The athlete was given a short course of oral steroids. His pain was controlled with acetaminophen. Tramadol was given for breakthrough pain and pregabalin for neurogenic pain. He was referred for physical therapy and worked on gentle range of motion of his cervical spine, as well as strengthening.

Outcome

Over the next month, his shoulder dysesthesias decreased to "minimal." He eventually required no further medications for pain. However, he decided to medically retire from football.

Author's Comments

Spinal cord contusion injuries can be mistaken for the more common and transient peripheral nerve stingers. Proper evaluation of patient history and physical examination may help to prevent potentially catastrophic spinal cord re-injury due to premature re-entry into athletic competition.

Editor's Comments

Transient neurapraxia or cervical cord neurapraxia is known to occur in collision sports, including football. It is thought to be due to reversible deformation of the spinal cord due to trauma. Spinal stenosis has been implicated as a risk factor, but is not considered an absolute contraindication to participation in collision sports. In general, the injury is thought to occur from a pincer-like mechanism between two adjacent vertebrae when the spine is in either a flexed or extended position. Symptoms can include motor symptoms ranging from mild weakness to frank paralysis (transient paraplegia or quadriplegia). However, it more commonly manifests as a disruption in sensation, such as burning, numbness, or tingling. In contrast to a stinger or burner, symptoms are bilateral. Symptoms most commonly last less than 15 minutes, but have been described as lasting as long as 36 to 48 hours. In this case, the patient's symptoms were more protracted than is typical for cervical cord neurapraxia. This was most likely due to the fact that he also had a bulging disc in the cervical spine. It is difficult to determine whether this disc pathology was an acute injury occurring at the time he tackled his opponent or was more chronic in nature and created a predisposition to cervical cord neurapraxia.

References

1. Dailey A, Harrop JS, France JC. High-energy contact sports and cervical spine neurapraxia injuries: what are the criteria for return to participation? Spine Oct 1;35(21 Suppl):S193-S201.
2. Torg JS, Corcoran TA, Thibault LE, Pavlov H, Sennett BJ, Naranja RJ Jr, et al. Cervical cord neurapraxia: classification, pathomechanics, morbidity, and management guidelines. J Neurosurg 1997 Dec;87(6):843-850.

AMSSM Case Title: Bilateral Stingers

- ❏ AMSSM Case Category: Cervical neurapraxia
- ❏ Author: Trent Tamate, BA
- ❏ Editor: Christian Fulmer, DO
- ❏ Board Review Book Reference Question: 1-10, Cervical neurapraxia

CASE STUDY #2: EXERTIONAL COMPARTMENT SYNDROME

Patient Presentation

Chronic bilateral exertional lower leg pain

History

A 16-year-old elite soccer player was referred by her pediatrician to the orthopedic office for consultation of chronic bilateral exertional lower leg pain. The pain was non-bony and diffuse, described as tightness around the calves. Her pain was worse with exertion and completely resolved with rest. Her review of systems was positive for excessive fatigue with exercise and feeling abnormally cold.

Physical Examination

- Inspection: No obvious deformity, atrophy, swelling, or fascial herniation noted in bilateral legs
- Palpation: No bony or muscle tenderness to palpation in the bilateral legs
- Range of motion: Full range of motion of her knees and ankles bilaterally
- Neurological: Motor—5/5 strength in all motions, no foot drop bilaterally, normal reflexes bilaterally

Differential Diagnosis

- Stress fracture/periostitis
- Popliteal artery claudication
- Chronic exertional compartment syndrome
- Neurogenic claudication
- Exertional myopathy

Lab Studies

- CBC, CMP, UA, lyme, vitamin D, and ESR normal/negative
- C-reactive protein 6.2 mg/L (0.0-4.9)
- TSH 131.100 uIU/mL (0.450-4.500), free T4 0.19 mg/dL (0.93-1.60), thyroid peroxidase (TPO) antibody 329 IU/mL (0-26)

Other Studies

- ❏ MRI calves: No stress fracture
- ❏ Compartment pressures:

	Compartment							
	Anterior		Lateral		Superficial Posterior		Deep Posterior	
	Pre-Exercise Pressure (mm Hg)	Post-Exercise Pressure (mm Hg)	Pre-Exercise Pressure (mm Hg)	Post-Exercise Pressure (mm Hg)	Pre-Exercise Pressure (mm Hg)	Post-Exercise Pressure (mm Hg)	Pre-Exercise Pressure (mm Hg)	Post-Exercise Pressure (mm Hg)
Left Leg	16	50	22	25	17	37	25	61
Right Leg	21	48	17	26	13	25	24	30

Consultation

She was seen by the clinical director of the division of endocrinology and started on synthroid. Based on the duration of her fatigue and laboratory findings, she was thought to have had severe, undiagnosed hypothyroidism for approximately a year.

Working Diagnosis: Chronic exertional compartment syndrome secondary to chronic hypothyroidism

Treatment

She underwent bilateral tri-compartmental decompressive fasciotomies and subsequent physical therapy for rehabilitation.

Outcome

She progressed well, and six weeks after surgery, she was cleared to return to sport without limitations. This is consistent with prior studies showing a majority of athletes status post-decompressive fasciotomy were able to return to their elite level of sport at a mean of 10.6 weeks post-operatively. After a couple of months of treatment, her TSH normalized, and she no longer felt fatigued.

Author's Comments

This patient's presentation of bilateral exertional lower extremity pain that resolved with rest is classic for chronic exertional compartment syndrome (CECS). Her lab findings of an elevated TSH, suppressed free T4, and an elevated thyroid peroxidase antibody level are consistent with a diagnosis of Hashimoto's thyroiditis. In a review of literature, the first case report linking hypothyroidism to compartment syndrome was published in 1993. Since then, there have only been a handful of publications linking the two conditions, all involving adults with acute compartment syndrome (ACS) presenting with foot drop or severe, crippling pain. To our knowledge, this is the first case linking hypothyroidism to chronic exertional compartment syndrome. Of note, she was only discovered to be hypothyroid after she had received the fasciotomy. Had it been determined earlier, we would have treated the hypothyroidism first, and would have only done surgery had her symptoms not resolved.

Editor's Comments

The incidence of CECS has been estimated to be between 14% and 27% in athletes with leg pain. It has an equal distribution in males and females. It more commonly affects the young, endurance athlete, typically runners. Of the four compartments in the leg, the anterior compartment is the most commonly affected, with the deep posterior being a close second. The lateral and superficial compartments are rarely affected. The condition is characterized by reversible ischemia that occurs during exercise and is relieved by rest. Several mechanisms have been proposed as the pathophysiologic mechanism of this condition including: inherent noncompliance of the fascial tissue, exaggerated increase in volume of muscle due blood flow or edema, and aberrant muscle hypertrophy. When conservative treatment methods fail, fasciotomy or fasciectomy of the involved compartment(s) is considered to be the choice for definitive treatment.

References

1. Barnes M. Diagnosis and management of chronic compartment syndromes: a review of the literature. Br J Sports Med 1997 Mar;31(1):21-27.
2. Rajasekaran S, Finnoff JT. Exertional leg pain. Phys Med Rehabil Clin N Am 2016 Feb;27(1):91-119. doi: 10.1016/j.pmr.2015.08.012.

AMSSM Case Title: Chronic Bilateral Exertional Lower Leg Pain and Fatigue in a 16-Year-Old Soccer Player

- ❏ AMSSM Case Category: Metabolic disorders
- ❏ Author: Adam Lyons, MD
- ❏ Editor: Christian Fulmer, DO
- ❏ Board Review Book Reference Question: 1-108, Exertional compartment syndrome

CASE STUDY #3: FRACTURE, ISCHIAL TUBEROSITY

Patient Presentation

A 19-year-old male football player presented to the orthopedic office for chronic left hip pain.

History

A 19-year-old male complaining of left hip pain for over two years, after he hurt it while playing football. The patient also recalled having a left hip injury while playing football in the eighth grade. He could not remember the exact mechanism of injury, but his pain was located in the left proximal hamstring and gluteus region. He was diagnosed with a hamstring injury at that time, which was treated non-operatively. At time of presentation, he was able to walk and jog, however, any explosive activities, such as sprinting, made the pain worse. He also had pain with prolonged sitting.

Physical Examination

- ❑ General: Alert and oriented; in no acute distress. He had an antalgic gait.
- ❑ Musculoskeletal: Tenderness over the left ischial tuberosity. Hip exam revealed normal range of motion, although with prolonged extension of the hip, he had some pain at the ischial tuberosity. There was no bruising and no other skin changes noted.

Differential Diagnosis

- Hamstring strain or avulsion
- Ischial apophysis avulsion
- Gluteal muscle strain or avulsion
- Piriformis syndrome
- Sacroiliac joint dysfunction

Other Studies

- ❑ X-rays of the pelvis, including inlet and outlet views, demonstrated a nonunion of the ischial tuberosity.

Case Studies

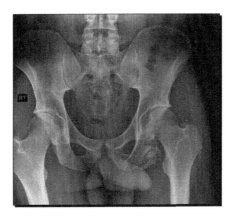

- ❏ CT scan of the hips/pelvis revealed heterotopic ossification on the left compared to the right.

Consultation

- Orthopedic surgery

Working Diagnosis: Nonunion of the left ischial tuberosity

Treatment

The patient underwent reconstruction of his left proximal hamstring and open reduction and internal fixation of the chronic left ischial tuberosity nonunion.

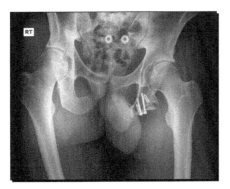

Outcome

The patient followed up after his left proximal hamstring reconstruction and open reduction and internal fixation of the chronic left ischial tuberosity nonunion. He was doing well after surgery and was non-weight-bearing for six weeks post-op.

Author's Comments

This case was particularly interesting because of the rarity of ischial tuberosity avulsion fractures compared to mid-hamstring strains. In this case, the patient had the original injury over two years prior to presentation and was treated non-operatively. However, he continued to have persistent pain, which was affecting his daily activities. Avulsion fractures of the ischial tuberosity can be missed in young athletes because the secondary ossification center fuses in late adolescence. During this time, the apophysis is at its weakest and ischial tuberosity avulsions occur instead of mid-hamstring ruptures.

Editor's Comments

The ischial tuberosity serves as the origin of the hamstring muscles, including the semitendinosus, semimembranosus, and the long head of the biceps femoris. The injuries to the ischial tuberosity are the result of a "sudden forceful flexion of the hip joint with an extended knee joint and contracted hamstring muscles."[1] Workup typically starts with pelvis radiographs. Conservative management consists of six weeks of partial weight-bearing and physical therapy. Patients with less than 15 mm of displacement are best treated non-operatively, and those with greater displacement benefit from surgical intervention.[1] When treating hamstring strains, It is essential to keep a broad differential diagnosis and consider imaging to look for bone pathology, especially when symptoms are not improving despite appropriate treatment.

References

1. Ferlic P, Sadoghi P, Singer G, Kraus T, Eberl R. Treatment for ischial tuberosity avulsion fractures in adolescent athletes. Knee Surg Sports Traumatol Arthrosc 2014 Apr;22(4):893-897.

AMSSM Case Title: Chronic Hip Pain in a 19-Year-Old Football Player

- ❏ AMSSM Case Category: Ischeal tuberosity apophyseal injury
- ❏ Author: Yaqoob Sayed, DO
- ❏ Editor: Namita Bhardwaj, MD
- ❏ Senior Editor: Mandeep Ghuman, MD
- ❏ Board Review Book Reference Question: 1-144, Fracture, ischial tuberosity

CASE STUDY #4: FRACTURE, TARSO-NAVICULAR

Patient Presentation

An 18-year-old male baseball player presented with left mid-foot pain.

History

The patient reported that while running the magnetic bases, he suffered a mid-foot dorsiflexion injury after stepping on a base. Despite the injury, he continued playing for six weeks. He self-treated the injury with ice, and wore an ankle brace. The patient reported minimal temporary relief of pain, but overall the pain worsened.

Physical Examination

- ❑ Right foot: Full active range of motion; mid-arch height
- ❑ Left foot: Full active range of motion. Pes planus with loss of arch height present prior to injury. Tender to palpation over the navicular body and tuberosity. Pain with resisted plantarflexion, dorsiflexion, and adduction; no pain with resisted abduction.

Differential Diagnosis

- Subacute navicular fracture
- Midfoot contusion
- Tarsal coalition
- Lisfranc dislocation or sprain
- Posterior tibial tendon injury or tear

Other Studies

- ❑ Radiographs of the left foot
  - Medial oblique: Wedge-shaped navicular with medial protuberance, narrow lateral border, and subtle lucency between the medial and lateral portions

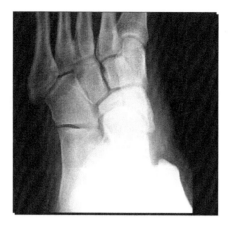

- Lateral: Irregular navicular with an oblique cleft and dorsal prominence

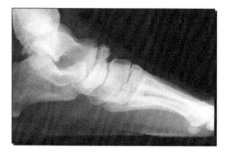

- MRI of the left foot showed the navicular to be comprised of three parts, each well corticated and demonstrating marrow edema.

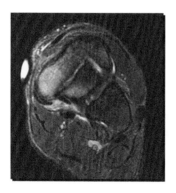
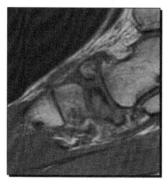
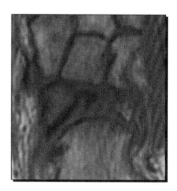

- CT of the left foot again showed the navicular comprised of three parts, each well corticated. Superior and inferior portions well-approximated and joined by a thin, osseous bridge at the medial aspect. The lateral portion is irregularly shaped, more displaced, and containing areas of lucency within the marrow.

Case Studies

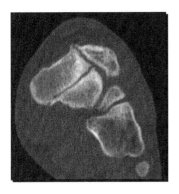 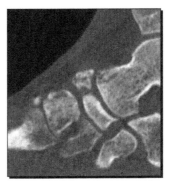 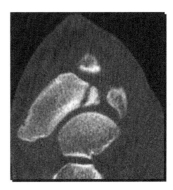

Consultation

A podiatrist was consulted after imaging demonstrated displacement and developing osteonecrosis.

Working Diagnosis: Bipartite navicular with subacute fracture concerning for developing osteonecrosis

Treatment

Initially, the athlete was managed non-operatively with non-weight-bearing status and immobilized in a walking boot. Surgical management included debridement of the sclerotic regions along the fracture site, placement of a bone auto-graft, and fixation. No arthrodesis was performed.

Outcome

At 12 weeks post-op, the athlete progressed to running, limited jumping/foot contacts, and baseball activities. Post-op radiograph of the left foot showed navicular fixation with screws and fracture plate. The athlete was expected to return to baseball at his previous level of functioning.

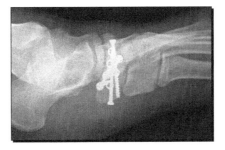

Author's Comments

A bipartite navicular can cause pes planus and promote osteoarthritic change of the talo-navicular joint. If non-operative management fails to treat arthritis, arthrodesis can be considered, with potential for restricted mid-tarsal motion. Navicular fractures commonly result from trauma or chronic overload, and are susceptible to osteonecrosis and arthrosis of surrounding joints.

Editor's Comments

The navicular bone is the keystone of the medial column of the foot, and it bears the majority of the load when weight-bearing. Weight-bearing radiographs can help to rule out unstable injuries of the mid-tarsal joint complex. Advanced imaging can also help rule out soft-tissue injuries that can present with fractures.

Accessory navicular bones are the most common accessory ossification center in the foot. They appear during adolescence and most are found incidentally and are asymptomatic. Most common issues with accessory naviculars include traumatic pain, chronic irritation/overuse, and as the posterior tibialis tendon inserts on the navicular athletes may present with posterior tibialis pain and dysfunction. Stress fractures of the navicular are often not visible on plain films and are under diagnosed. Delay to diagnosis is common. Navicular stress fractures are at risk for avascular necrosis and thus considered a high-risk stress fracture. Complications to be aware of including non-union and delay of union.

References

1. Ramadorai MU, Beuchel MW, Sangeorzan BJ. Fractures and dislocations of the tarsal navicular. J Am Acad Orthop Surg 2016 Jun;24(6):379-389. doi: 10.5435/JAAOS-D-14-00442.
2. Coulibaly MO, Jones CB, Sietsema DL, Schildhauer TA. Results and complications of operative and non-operative navicular fracture treatment. Injury 2015 Aug:46(8):1669-1677. doi: 10.1016/j.injury.2015.04.033.
3. Tanaka Y, Takakura Y, Omokawa S, Kumai T, Sugimoto K. Crank-shaped arthrodesis for a flatfoot with a bipartite navicular: a case report. Foot Ankle Int 2006 Sep;27(9):734-737.
4. Brukner P, Bradshaw C, Khan KM, White S, Crossley K. Stress fractures: a review of 180 cases. Clin J Sport Med 1996 Apr;6(2):85-89.

AMSSM Case Title: 18-Year-Old Male Athlete With Foot Pain

- ❏ AMSSM Case Category: Foot and ankle
- ❏ Author: Rathna Nuti, MD
- ❏ Editor: Caitlyn Mooney, MD
- ❏ Senior Editor: Margaret E Gibson, MD
- ❏ Board Review Book Reference Question: 1-157, Fracture, tarso-navicular

CASE STUDY #5: FRACTURE, TIBIAL STRESS

Patient Presentation

The patient reported left anterior mid-tibia pain for one month.

History

A 17-year-old healthy male presented with a one-month history of left anterior mid-tibia, dull, achy pain that was aggravated with running. He reported an increase in his training volume, with most of his runs occurring on concrete, when his leg pain began. His pain rapidly increased after he was "cleated" during a track practice, and his pain began to radiate to his knee as well. He denied any prior treatment for his pain.

Physical Examination

- ❏ General: No acute distress
- ❏ HEENT: Atraumatic
- ❏ Musculoskeletal: Left knee with full range of motion. No swelling was noted, but he had point tenderness along the left anterior mid tibia. He had a negative anterior draw test and McMurray's test.
- ❏ Neurological: Sensation was intact, with no gross focal deficits

Differential Diagnosis

- Tibial stress syndrome
- Stress injury
- Bone contusion
- Stress fracture
- Knee sprain

Other Studies

- ❏ Radiographs were obtained, indicating an anterior tibial stress fracture.

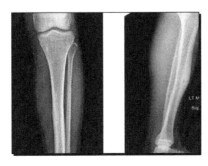

Working Diagnosis: Tibial stress fracture

Treatment

He was placed in a long leg cast and asked to use axillary crutches to maintain a non-weight-bearing status for four weeks. He was then transitioned to a short-leg cast with progressive weight-bearing for an additional four weeks. After eight total weeks of casting, he was transitioned to a walking boot for an additional four weeks.

Outcome

Four months after his original injury, he continued to have pain during ambulation and a fracture line on his radiographs. Therefore, his vitamin D level was checked and found to be 9. After aggressive replacement of vitamin D, he began to show signs of healing on his radiographs (b) at six months since his original presentation.

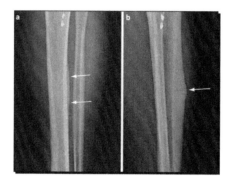

Author's Comments

Vitamin D is involved in calcium and bone metabolism, with vitamin D deficiency associated with increased bone loss and fractures. Sunlight exposure is the greatest source of vitamin D. However, as there is an increased awareness of the risk of skin cancer with sunlight exposure, more people are avoiding sunlight exposure, which has increased the incidence of vitamin D deficiency in the Sun Belt states. If there is delayed bone healing, it is worth checking the vitamin D level, even in the Sun Belt states.

Editor's Comments

Stress reactions and stress fractures are common injuries in athletes, with treatment dictated based on the fracture site's biomechanical environment. Stress injuries found to have high amount of load bearing and a poor natural healing history are considered high-risk injuries. Tibial stress fractures are among the most common stress injuries in the body and can be divided into either the two low-risk stress fractures, posteromedial (compression) side stress fracture and longitudinal stress fracture, or the high-risk anterior tibial stress fracture. As seen in this case, the anterior tibial stress fracture (dreaded black line) is considered high risk, as the fracture is along the tension side of the tibia, predisposing the fracture to delayed or nonunion. High-risk stress fractures should be made non-weight-bearing, or even placed in a cast, to allow bony healing to exceed the rate of continued damage at the fracture site. Return to play may dictate early surgical consideration for high-risk fractures, but optimization of bone health must be considered if delayed healing is noted.

References

1. Kaeding CC, Yu JR, Wright R, Amendola A, Spindler KP. Management and return to play of stress fractures. Clin J Sport Med 2005 Nov;15(6):442-447.
2. Liem BC, Truswell HJ, Harrast MA. Rehabilitation and return to running after lower limb stress fractures. Curr Sports Med Rep 2013 May-Jun;12(3):200-207. doi: 10.1249/JSR.0b013e3182913cbe.

AMSSM Case Title: Is Increased Training and Running on Concrete Causing Tibial Pain?

- ❏ AMSSM Case Category: Fractures and dislocations
- ❏ Author: Annie Casta, MD
- ❏ Editor: Adam Lewno, DO
- ❏ Senior Editor: Margaret E Gibson, MD
- ❏ Board Review Book Reference Question: 1-102, Tibial stress fracture

CASE STUDY #6: HEAD INJURY, INTRACRANIAL PATHOLOGY

Patient Presentation

A 17-year-old male high school football player presented with repetitive head injuries.

History

A 17-year-old male high school football player made hard helmet-to-helmet contact with another player and immediately experienced headache, photophobia, and dizziness. He did not report the symptoms and continued to play. Shortly thereafter, he suffered a second blow to the head in a collision with another player and experienced increased symptom severity. He reported his symptoms to his coach and was removed from competition. He returned home under the supervision of his parents, where his symptoms continued to worsen. He subsequently developed nausea, vomiting, and pressure behind his right eye. He was brought to the emergency department by the parents for further evaluation.

Physical Examination

- ❏ General: Somnolent but arousable and cooperative
- ❏ Neurological: Alert and oriented x 3. Cranial nerves II-XII intact. 5/5 strength in bilateral upper and lower extremities. Normal cerebellar function. Normal sensation throughout. No spinal tenderness and had full range of motion of his spine.

Differential Diagnosis

- Concussion
- Epidural hematoma
- Subdural hematoma
- Subarachnoid hemorrhage
- Skull fracture

Other Studies

- ❏ CT brain without contrast: 3 mm right subdural hematoma and an adjacent subarachnoid hemorrhage, with associated 3 mm of right-to-left midline shift. No underlying skull fractures identified.

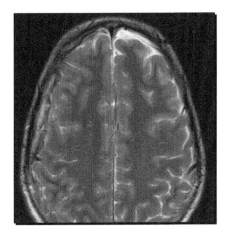

- MRI brain without contrast: 5 mm right subdural hematoma with adjacent subarachnoid hemorrhage better appreciated on CT associated with 3 mm of right-to-left midline shift.

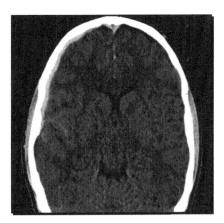

Consultation

- Neurosurgery

Working Diagnosis: Subdural hematoma, subarachnoid hemorrhage

Treatment

The patient received 1 g bolus of levetiracetam for seizure prophylaxis, and continued on 500 mg BID.

Outcome

The patient was admitted to the pediatric intensive care unit (PICU) for neurologic monitoring and supportive care. On hospital day two, he developed two generalized tonic-clonic seizures, each lasting approximately 60 seconds. The seizures were self-limiting, and he did not require any abortive medications. One seizure did result in cyanosis, with an SpO_2 in the 60s, requiring bag-valve-mask ventilation. The Levetiracetam dose was increased, and he was started on phenytoin. Repeat brain imaging showed stable intracranial pathology. He remained seizure-free and was discharged home on hospital day eight with a seizure prophylaxis regimen consisting of levetiracetam and phenytoin, as well as a pain control regimen of oxycodone and gabapentin.

Three weeks post-injury, he had not yet returned to school, due to persistent headaches and concentration difficulties. At that time, he was taking daily narcotics and gabapentin for headache pain control. Concern at that time was that his headaches were due to analgesic overuse. Therefore, he was instructed to wean off the narcotic pain medication and gabapentin, as tolerated, until seen in concussion clinic the following week. At four weeks post-injury, the patient had successfully weaned off pain medication within forty-eight hours of his previous visit and was able to return to school. At that time, he had returned to his neurological baseline. He also began implementing physical activity back into his routine, under the guidance of a physical therapist. Repeat CT at this time showed improvement of his subdural hematoma and resolution of his subarachnoid hemorrhage.

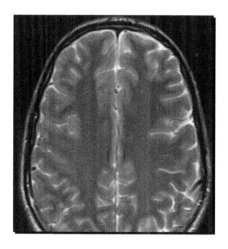

He was held out of contact and collision sports (i.e., basketball) until four months post-injury, at which time the MRI was repeated to evaluate for gliosis. There was no evidence of gliosis, however there was dural enhancement consistent with a resolving subdural hematoma. At that time, we advised to avoid collision sports until the end of the school year. We advised that he could return to full basketball participation during the summer months. He has remained seizure-free during this time period and has been able to wean off of his antiepileptic medications, under the guidance of a pediatric neurologist.

Author's Comments

This case highlights the importance of identifying on-the-field head injuries of athletes. This case is also a reminder that overuse of analgesic medications in post-concussive headaches can prolong symptoms. Proper management of athletes with concussions post-injury is essential in return to daily activities, as well as return to play.

Editor's Comments

Although this is not a classic case of second-impact syndrome, the repeat head trauma certainly aggravated the athlete's symptoms and highlights the importance of removing the athlete from play after a concerning head injury. This case also illustrates the value of serial examinations and close observation, since symptoms can be progressive. Narcotics are not generally used in concussion management, and may have contributed to prolonged school absence. Weaning off clearly helped the patient.

References

1. Baandrup L, Jensen R. Chronic post-traumatic headache—a clinical analysis in relation to the International Headache Classification 2nd Edition. Cephalalgia 2005 Feb 1;25(2):132-138.
2. Lane JC, Arciniegas DB. Post-traumatic headache. Curr Treat Options Neurol 2002 Feb;4(1):89-104.
3. Kinnaman KA, Mannix RC, Comstock RD, Meehan WP. Management strategies and medication use for treating paediatric patients with concussions. Acta Paediatr 2013 Sep;102(9):e424-e428.

AMSSM Case Title: A Feared, but Uncommon Injury in a High School Football Player

- ❏ AMSSM Case Category: Neurology
- ❏ Author: Mathew Negaard, MD
- ❏ Editor: Rebecca Martinie, MD
- ❏ Senior Editor: Margaret E Gibson, MD
- ❏ Board Review Book Reference Question: 1-9, Head injury, intracranial pathology

CASE STUDY #7: HEAT STROKE

Patient Presentation

A 17-year-old male had increased work of breathing and a syncopal episode after football practice in September.

History

A 17-year-old offensive lineman began breathing heavily and then collapsed, becoming unresponsive, after a September football practice when the temperature was 85 degrees Fahrenheit (29.4 degrees Celsius). EMS was called and arrived on the scene, where the patient appeared to be in a tonic-clonic state. Seizures, lasting 8 to 10 minutes, were unbroken until the patient was brought to ED and given an IV dose of Valium (5 mg). The patient was noted to be cool, pale, and diaphoretic, with a core temperature of 104.9 degrees Fahrenheit (40.5 degrees Celsius). He subsequently had an episode of vomiting and then began more tonic-clonic movements. He was then given a 1 mg dose of Ativan and intubated. He was transferred to a cooling bed and received 1 l of IV fluids rapidly. Labs were then drawn, head CT was obtained, and the patient was admitted to pediatric ICU. Additional tonic-clonic activity was noted in route to PICU.

Physical Examination

- Vitals: Temp 100.9 degrees Fahrenheit (38.3 degrees Celsius), pulse 117, respirations 22, blood pressure 104/49, and O_2 99% on ventilator
- General: Sedated and unresponsive to verbal stimuli, withdraws to painful stimuli
- HEENT: Pupils were reactive to light and had a positive corneal reflex.
- Cardiovascular: Hyperdynamic precordium, with strong pulses and tachycardia, capillary refill less than two seconds, no murmurs
- Pulmonary: Lungs were clear to auscultation bilaterally, with no wheezes, rhonchi, or rales.
- Abdomen: Soft with no hepatosplenomegaly, positive bowel sounds, with multiple foul-smelling liquid bowel movements during the exam, bright red blood per rectum
- GU: Foley in place, no scrotal edema
- Extremities: No edema, no clubbing, no cyanosis
- Neurological: Deep tendon reflexes 1+
- Skin: Rash under bilateral pectoralis muscles from shoulder pads

Differential Diagnosis

- Exercise-induced hyponatremia
- Diabetic ketoacidosis
- Status epilepticus
- Cardiac arrhythmia
- Heat stroke

Lab Studies

- Admission lab studies: BUN/Cr: 20/2.18; potassium: 5.1; LFTs: within normal limits; CBC: within normal limits; lactate: 8.1; urine: negative for ketones; thyroid panel: negative; UDS: negative; ABG pH 7.32, pCO_2 33, pO_2 269, $HCO3$ 17.0; C diff: negative; occult blood: negative.
- Follow-up lab studies: First 18 hours: Platelets dropped to 61. BUN increased to 22. ALT/AST/CK elevated to 10x upper limit of normal. D-Dimer 763. Fibrinogen 315. Uric acid 9.8. 18-42 hours: Platelets 38. 42-66 hours: Platelets 30. LFTS improved to 2x normal. Creatinine 1.4.

Other Studies

- CT head without contrast: No acute process
- EEG: Within normal limits
- EKG: Within normal limits
- Echocardiogram: Within normal limits

Consultation

- Pediatric hematology and oncology
- Pediatric neurology

Working Diagnosis: Exertional heat stroke, with disseminated intravascular coagulation

Treatment

The patient remained intubated in the PICU to protect his airway for 48 hours and was started on Keppra for seizure prophylaxis. Patient labs were monitored closely until improvement was noticed while he was on maintenance IVF.

Outcome

The patient returned to school the following week. Anti-epileptic medication was continued for six weeks. He was not able to participate in exercise until completion of anti-epileptic course. He was followed by hematology until his platelets returned to baseline.

Author's Comments

Heat stroke is the leading cause of death in young athletes each year, with the incidence increasing annually. The highest incidence of heat stroke occurs in American football players, with 4.5 cases per 100,000. Morbidity and mortality of a heat stroke are directly related to duration of the athlete's temperature elevation; therefore, it is imperative to cool the patient down as fast as possible. Early recognition and immediate treatment are critical. The best way to cool an athlete is with rapid cooling within the first 30 minutes via cold water immersion until the core temperature reaches 101 degrees Fahrenheit (38.3 degrees Celsius). This should be done before transportation, unless onsite cooling is not available or the patient is having seizures. The main complications to be concerned about with patients are electrolyte abnormalities, seizures, delirium, acute respiratory distress syndrome, rhabdomyolysis, acute kidney injury, hepatic injury, disseminated intravascular coagulation (our patient), ischemic bowel, and myocardial injury. The treatment of heat stroke, besides rapid cooling, is mostly supportive and correction of aforementioned abnormalities. Prevention strategies include: allowing the athletes time for acclimatization to the heat (which should take between 7 to 14 days), allow frequent breaks for cooling and hydration (6 mL per kg every two to three hours), avoid vigorous exercise in severe heat or humidity, pay close attention to obese athletes, and minimize equipment and clothing that hinders heat loss. Educating coaches and staff on the prevention, recognition, and treatment of heat illness is essential.

Editor's Comments

The author identifies the key points in treatment of exertional heat stroke (EHS), which are early recognition and immediate cooling on-site prior to transport. More importantly, heat stroke is a preventable disease. The following conditions increase the risk of EHS or exertional heat exhaustion: obesity, low physical fitness level, lack of heat acclimatization, dehydration, history of EHS, sleep deprivation, sweat gland dysfunction, sunburn, viral illness, diarrhea, and certain medications. Proper education of athletes and coaches, as well as awareness of these conditions by the medical staff, is extremely important. In addition, monitoring the environmental conditions using a wet bulb globe temperature (WBGT) is useful, as a WBGT over 82 degrees Fahrenheit (27.8 degrees Celsius) places athletes at risk of developing such an event. When returning athletes with significant heat illness to sports, it is important to make sure that heat tolerance has returned. Gradual return to activity and possibly additional testing and management at a center specializing in heat illness should be considered.

References

1. Bouchama A, Knochel JP. Heat stroke. N Engl J Med 2002 Jun 20;346(25):1978-1988.
2. Heled Y, Rav-Acha M, Shani Y, Epstein Y, Moran DS. The "golden hour" for heatstroke treatment. Mil Med 2004 Mar;169(3):184-186.

3. Centers for Disease Control and Prevention (CDC). Heat-related deaths—United States, 1999-2003. MMWR Morb Mortal Wkly Rep 2006 Jul 28;55(29):796-798.
4. Khosla R, Guntupalli KK. Heat-related illnesses. Crit Care Clin 1999 Apr; 15(2):251-263.
5. Bouchama A, Bridey F, Hammami MM, Lacombe C, al-Shail E, al-Ohali Y, et al. Activation of coagulation and fibrinolysis in heatstroke. Thromb Haemost 1996 Dec;76(6):909-915.
6. Smith JE, Wallis L. Cooling methods used in the treatment of exertional heat illness. Br J Sports Med 2005 Aug;39(8):503-507.
7. Krohn AR, Sikka R, Olson DE. Heat illness in football: current concepts. Curr Sports Med Rep 2015 Nov-Dec;14(6):463-471. doi: 10.1249/JSR.0000000000000212.

AMSSM Case Title: 17-Year-Old Athlete Drops to the Ground, Not for Pushups

- AMSSM Case Category: Metabolic disorders
- Author: Jeffrey Ham, DO
- Editor: Charlie Michaudet, MD
- Senior Editor: Margaret E Gibson, MD
- Board Review Book Reference Question: 1-189, Heat stroke

CASE STUDY #8: HYPERTROPHIC CARDIOMYOPATHY (HOCM)

Patient Presentation

An asymptomatic 13-year-old African-American male was evaluated during a large, station-based pre-participation physical evaluation (PPE).

History

He is a talented, high-intensity athlete, and otherwise healthy. He was asymptomatic and specifically denied chest pain (CP), shortness of breath (SOB), palpitations, lightheadedness, or syncope. The patient reported a family history of cardiovascular disease (grandparents) and hypertension (both parents), but denied a family history of structural cardiac abnormalities or premature sudden cardiac death. He also mentioned a personal history of occasional high blood pressure readings. During a later chart review, BPs ranging from 146-166/62-76 were noted over the preceding two years. Despite this, he denied all other medical conditions, medicine use aside from an occasional over-the-counter medication (NSAID/Tylenol), the use of alcohol, illicit drugs, steroids, or tobacco. He also denied prior restrictions on sports participation.

Physical Examination

The patient was afebrile (T 98). Although he was large for his age, with both height (6'0") and weight (172 pounds) being greater than the 99th percentiles for age, he was a healthy weight per BMI (22). Pulse (60) and RR (14) were WNL, but blood pressure (140/76) was noticeably elevated, especially when compared to age-related normative values.

In general, the patient was well-appearing and devoid of any obvious dysmorphic features. His cardiac exam did reveal a grade 3/6 crescendo-decrescendo systolic murmur heard best at the left upper sternal border. Murmur increased with Valsalva maneuver. Lungs, abdomen, genitourinary, and extremity exams were unremarkable.

Blood Pressure Levels for Boys by Age and Height Percentile														
		Systolic BP (mm Hg) Percentile of Height						Diastolic BP (mm Hg) Percentile of Height						
Age (Year)	BP Percentile	5th	10th	25th	50th	75th	90th	95th	5th	10th	25th	50th	75th	90th	95th
13	50th	104	105	106	108	110	111	112	60	60	61	62	63	64	64
	90th	117	118	120	122	124	125	126	75	75	76	77	78	79	(79)
	95th	121	122	124	126	128	129	130	79	79	80	81	82	83	83
	99th	128	130	131	133	135	136	(137)	87	87	88	89	90	91	91

Differential Diagnosis

- Pediatric hypertrophic cardiomyopathy (HCM) due to a sarcomeric defect
- Athlete's heart (physiologic adaptation to exercise)
- Primary hypertensive, with left ventricular hypertrophy (LVH)
- Secondary hypertension (e.g., renal disease, anabolic steroid use, coarctation of the aorta)
- Aortic stenosis

Lab Studies

- ❏ CBC, CMP, thyroid function panel, and urinalysis were WNL.
- ❏ GeneDx hypertrophic cardiomyopathy (HCM) panel: No disease-causing gene mutation was detected.

Other Studies

- ❏ EKG: Sinus rhythm, prominent precordial voltage, "dome-shaped" convex ST segment elevations in the anterior precordial leads (V1-V2), and diffuse T wave inversions (most notably in the inferolateral leads).

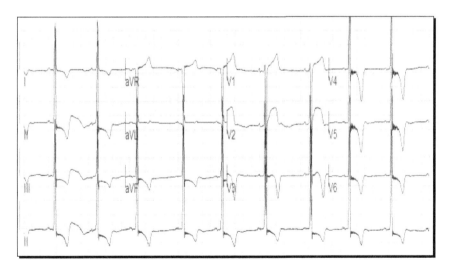

- 2D Echo: Concentric LVH (maximal wall thickness of 1.6 cm), with speckled appearance of myocardium. Hyperdynamic global systolic function (EF > 75%). No LV outflow obstruction or systolic anterior motion of the mitral valve.

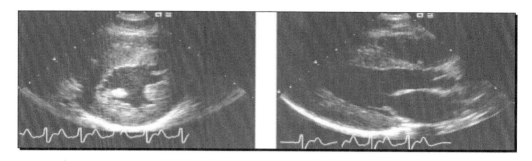

- Cardiac MRI: Abnormal LV myocardial mass at 125 g/m² (47-87 g/m²). Concentric LV thickening, with slightly more prominent apical involvement (1.6 cm in anterior basilar septum and basilar inferolateral wall). No abnormal uptake of gadolinium was noted.

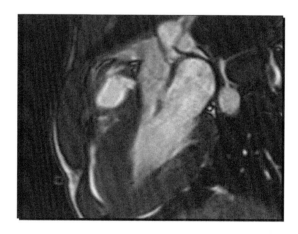

- Stress ECHO: Standard Bruce protocol: Achieved predicted maximal HR without CP or SOB. Hypertensive response to exercise (baseline BP 152/73, HR 71; peak BP 220/60, HR 84), widespread repolarization abnormalities, and dynamic LV outflow tract obstruction

Case Studies

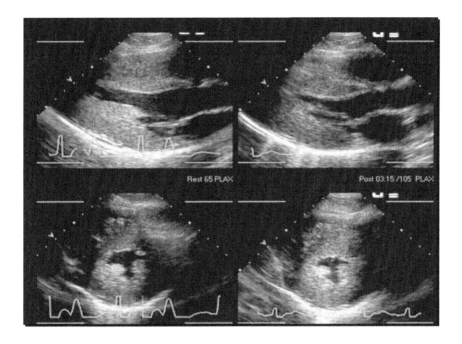

Working Diagnosis: Hypertrophic cardiomyopathy

Treatment

Internal cardiac defibrillator (ICD) placement was not deemed necessary, but the patient was given a home automatic external defibrillator (AED) and instructed to avoid competitive sports. He was also offered counseling to help cope with the suspected diagnosis of HCM and exclusion from competitive sports. After three months of rest, the repeat EKG and ECHO were unchanged, and resting blood pressures remained markedly elevated (146-168/62-74). After this observation, he was started on Atenolol 25 mg twice a day for improved blood pressure control and to see if cardiac mass resolution would be achieved once his target BP (<125/75) was maintained. At a subsequent visit, BP remained markedly elevated, and the Atenolol dosage was increased to 50 mg twice a day. A daily dose of Hydrochlorothiazide 12.5 mg was also added.

Outcome

The cardiac murmur, screening EKG, ECHO, and cardiac MRI were suggestive of hypertrophic cardiomyopathy; however, genetic testing was negative. Disqualification was made from participation in competitive sports due to suspicion of HCM. Deconditioning for three months did not result in resolution of his cardiac mass. Patient was diagnosed with stage 1/2 hypertension and started on two antihypertensive agents. He has remained asymptomatic since his initial evaluation and disqualification.

Author's Comments

HCM is the most common cause of sudden cardiac death (SCD) in sports[1], largely affects males (9:1, M:F), and results in a disproportionately higher rate of death among African-Americans.[2] While the prevalence of HCM is > 1:500 in adults,[3] it is much less common in children (0.3 to 0.5 per 100,000).[4] Athlete's Heart results in increased LV wall thickness due to systematic training, but usually resolves with a period of deconditioning.[5] Systemic hypertension-induced LVH can also present similarly to HCM, but regression of LV wall thickening often occurs with adequate blood pressure control.[6] Genetic testing of sarcomere protein genes identifies a disease-causing mutation in up to 60% of HCM cases[4]; therefore, a negative test does not exclude diagnosis. HCM patients with sarcomere mutations usually present earlier and have a higher prevalence of SCD.[7] To reduce risk of SCD in HCM: (1) Exercise restriction and (2) ICD placement if patient experiences life-threatening ventricular arrhythmias or ≥2 major risk factors (severe LVH, syncope, NSVT, or family history of SCD).[4]

Editor's Comments

This case underscores the importance of cardiac auscultation in a quiet environment during the pre-participation physical examination, and the need for appropriate workup when a possibly pathologic murmur is noted.

References

1. Harmon KG, Asif IM, Klossner D, Drezner JA. Incidence of sudden cardiac death in National Collegiate Athletic Association athletes. Circulation 2011 Apr 19;123(15):1594-1600. doi: 10.1161/CIRCULATIONAHA.110.004622.
2. Maron BJ, Pelliccia A. The heart of trained athletes: cardiac remodeling and the risks of sports, including sudden death. Circulation 2006 Oct 10;114(15):1633-1644.
3. Semsarian C, Ingles J, Maron MS, Maron BJ. New perspectives on the prevalence of hypertrophic cardiomyopathy. J Am Coll Cardiol 2015 Mar 31;65(12):1249-1254. doi: 10.1016/j.jacc.2015.01.019.
4. Elliott PM, Anastasakis A, Borger MA, Borggrefe M, Cecchi F, Charron P, et al. 2014 ESC Guidelines on diagnosis and management of hypertrophic cardiomyopathy: the Task Force for the Diagnosis and Management of Hypertrophic Cardiomyopathy of the European Society of Cardiology (ESC). Eur Heart J 2014 Oct 14;35(39):2733-2779. doi: 10.1093/eurheartj/ehu284.

5. Maron BJ, Pelliccia A, Spataro A, Granata M. Reduction in left ventricular wall thickness after deconditioning in highly trained Olympic athletes. Br Heart J 1993 Feb;69(2):125-128.
6. Fagard RH, Celis H, Thijs L, Wouters S. Regression of left ventricular mass by antihypertensive treatment: a meta-analysis of randomized comparative studies. Hypertension 2009 Nov;54(5):1084-1091. doi: 10.1161/HYPERTENSIONAHA.109.136655.
7. Olivotto I, Girolami F, Ackerman MJ, Nistri S, Bos JM, Zachara E, et al. Myofilament protein gene mutation screening and outcome of patients with hypertrophic cardiomyopathy. Mayo Clin Proc 2008 Jun;83(6):630-638. doi: 10.4065/83.6.630.

AMSSM Case Title: Pre-Participation Screening Detects Cardiac Disease in an Asymptomatic Preadolescent Athlete

- ❏ AMSSM Case Category: Cardiac
- ❏ Author: Jeremy Coleman, MD
- ❏ Editor: Rebecca Carl, MD
- ❏ Board Review Book Reference Questions: 1-71, 1-78, 2-119, Hypertrophic cardiomyopathy (HOCM)

CASE STUDY #9: KNEE DISLOCATION

Patient Presentation

A 33-year-old African-American female with a medical history of severe obesity presented to the ED with right knee pain status post a hyperextension injury.

History

While at work, the patient had bent forward to pick up a 15-pound box from the floor, when she felt her right knee lock up. Immediately afterward, the patient was unable to bear weight on the affected leg. She denied numbness, tingling, weakness, or a prior injury to that lower leg.

Physical Examination

BMI 61, patient in mild distress. Deformity of the proximal tibia was present, with pronounced swelling of the right knee. The patient was unable to flex or extend the right knee. Full range of motion and 5/5 strength of the ankle and hip joints. Special tests were unable to be performed. Neurovascularly, she was intact with +2 pulses and normal sensation of the lower extremities bilaterally. The remainder of the physical exam was within normal limits.

Differential Diagnosis

- Tibial plateau fracture
- Tibial dislocation
- Patellar dislocation
- Ligament tear
- Meniscal injury

Other Studies

- ❏ X-ray right knee: Anterior tibial dislocation
- ❏ X-ray right knee: Post-reduction film with improved alignment

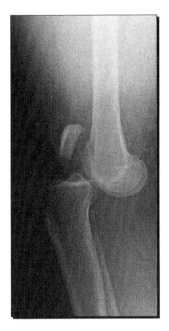 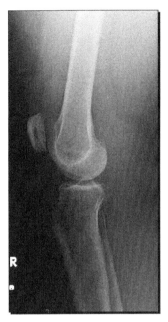

- MRI right knee: Lateral displacement of patella with surrounding effusion, grade 3 ACL and LCL tear, extensive grade 2 PCL sprain, grade 1 MCL sprain, posterolateral corner injury

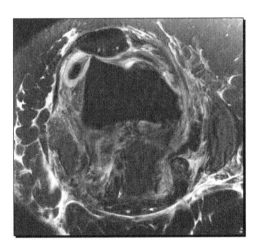 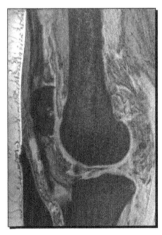

- ABI: Before and after manual reduction 0.94
- Arterial doppler study of lower extremity showed patent femoral and popliteal arteries

Consultation

- Orthopedic surgery

Working Diagnosis: Anterior tibial dislocation, grade 3 ACL and LCL tears, extensive grade 2 PCL sprain, grade 1 MCL sprain, posterolateral corner injuries

Treatment

Manual reduction in the emergency room, followed by staged surgical repair of the ACL, PCL, MCL, LCL.

Outcome

Patient underwent manual reduction on presentation to the emergency room. Orthopedic surgeon subsequently performed a right-knee posterolateral corner reconstruction. Post-operatively, the patient worked with physical therapy and was cleared for discharge home, with 24- hour assist and a bariatric rolling walker. She was instructed to follow up with orthopedic surgery as an outpatient for planning of staged ACL and PCL reconstruction.

Author's Comments

Knee injury is common, but knee dislocation is rare, and accounts for less than 0.2% of orthopedic injuries. Dislocation requires multi-ligament injury and a force typically associated with high-velocity trauma. However, damaging forces may also be achieved with smaller accelerations if the patient has a large body mass. This is concerning, because it requires clinicians to approach their obese patients cautiously when evaluating knee pain after seemingly minor injuries.

Editor's Comments

True knee dislocation (not to be confused with patellar dislocation) can only result from multi-ligamentous injury and typically requires high force, but unusually can happen with large body mass, as illustrated in this case. Knee dislocation is considered a musculoskeletal emergency, and vascular status must be carefully evaluated to rule out popliteal artery injury. The patient in this case was fortunate in that she did not have a vascular injury. If she had a vascular injury, she would have required emergency vascular surgery, which would have taken priority over orthopedic knee reconstruction.

References

1. Robertson A, Nutton RW, Keating JF. Dislocation of the knee. J Bone Joint Surg Br 2006;88(6):706-711.
2. Nickless J, Chandran S, Mohan V. Recognition to rehabilitation: treating traumatic knee injuries. Consultant 2015;55(8):601-613.
3. Georgiadis AG, Mohammad F, Mizerik KT, Nypaver TJ, Shepard AD. Changing presentation of knee dislocation and vascular injury from high-energy trauma to low-energy falls in the morbidly obese. J Vasc Surg 2013;57(5):1196-1203.

AMSSM Case Title: Surprisingly Severe Knee Injury in an Obese Female

- ❏ AMSSM Case Category: Fractures and dislocations, knee
- ❏ Author: Valerie Rygiel, DO
- ❏ Editor: Kelly Wilkinson, MD
- ❏ Senior Editor: Kristine Karlson, MD
- ❏ Board Review Book Reference Question: 1-196, Knee dislocation

CASE STUDY #10: KNEE, POSTEROLATERAL COMPLEX

Patient Presentation

A 16-year-old male football player presented due to right knee pain.

History

A 16-year-old male high school football fullback with no previous knee injury was struck in the anterior right knee by a helmet during the first two minutes of the game. He had immediate onset of knee pain and needed assistance to ambulate off the field. Within a couple of minutes on the sideline, he was ambulating without assistance, and he was quickly able to sprint, backpedal, and perform lateral cutting maneuvers without pain or instability. He was allowed to return to play, and during the remainder of the game, his only complaint was right hamstring tightness, late in the fourth quarter. Later that evening, he noticed knee swelling. He began noticing popping, stiffness, and tightness, which developed over the next several days. On reexamination by his athletic trainer, there was concern about possible varus laxity, with persistent effusion, and he was referred for further evaluation.

Physical Examination

- ❑ Musculoskeletal: There was a mild effusion in the right knee, with tenderness over the lateral joint line and lateral patellar facet. Active range of motion was 0 to 130 degrees. 2+ laxity with varus stressing at 30 degrees of flexion was noted. Negative dial, Lachman, anterior drawer and posterior drawer. Negative sag sign. Positive McMurray's, Apley Grind, and Thessaly's testing. There was mild pain on patellar apprehension testing.

Differential Diagnosis

- Lateral meniscal tear
- Lateral collateral ligament (LCL) sprain
- Patellar subluxation
- Osteochondral lesion
- Other posterolateral corner (PLC) injury

Case Studies

Other Studies

❏ X-rays of the right knee revealed a mild effusion without acute bony abnormality.

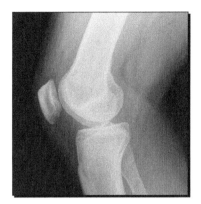
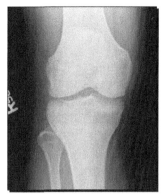

❏ MRI of the right knee revealed a full-thickness tear of the LCL, a contusion or impaction fracture of the medial femoral condyle, a minor contusion of the lateral femoral condyle, and a mild joint effusion.

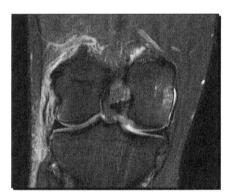
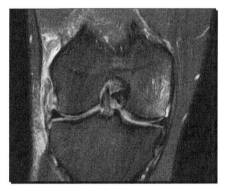

Consultation

- Orthopedic surgery

Working Diagnosis: Third-degree LCL sprain

Treatment

The athlete was prescribed a stabilizing knee brace and permitted to weight-bear, as tolerated, for the first two weeks. Over the next four weeks, he was progressed to activity, as tolerated, with the exclusion of cutting, twisting, pivoting, and impact movements.

Outcome

By seven weeks after diagnosis, he was able to fully participate in athletics without pain or limitation.

Author's Comments

LCL injuries only account for 1% to 8% of all acute ligamentous injuries of the knee.[2,3] The large majority of these are associated with other ligamentous or meniscal injuries. This case is an exception, as it involves an isolated complete LCL tear. The limited recent studies available exploring treatment options for this injury pattern seem to support non-operative management, with a quicker return to play and similar functional outcomes when compared to operative management.[1] What makes this case unusual is the minimal degree of symptoms in the athlete, allowing him to participate in nearly a full game of football after the initial injury. With this degree of functional stability and lack of associated injury, he was a great candidate for conservative treatment.

Editor's Comments

The LCL originates on the lateral femoral condyle and inserts along with the biceps femoris on the fibular head as part of the conjoined tendon. Clinically, it is best palpated with the patient supine with 90 degrees of knee flexion. LCL stability is tested with the application of varus stress with the knee at full extension, along with 30 degrees of flexion. Injury in isolation is very rare.[4] Hence, it is crucial, when evaluating a potential LCL sprain, to perform a complete examination of the structures of the posterior lateral corner, along with the posterior cruciate ligament and anterior cruciate ligament. Treatment is guided by injury severity and knee stability. Grade 1 or 2 sprains are treated conservatively, with a period of non-weight-bearing, then progressing to weight-bearing, with bracing for support.[2] Typical recovery time is six to eight weeks. Traditionally, grade 3 sprains have required surgical intervention, since the vast majority involve associated ligamentous or soft tissue injuries and instability. However, when the injury is in isolation and the knee is functionally stable, it is appropriate to treat non-operatively, which more recent evidence has suggested can lead to a quicker recovery time.[1]

References

1. Bushnell BD, Bitting SS, Crain JM, Boublik M, Schlegel TF. Treatment of magnetic resonance imaging-documented isolated grade III lateral collateral ligament injuries in National Football League athletes. Am J Sports Med 2010;38(1):86-91.
2. Majewski M, Susanne H, Klaus S. Epidemiology of athletic knee injuries: a 10-year study. Knee 2006;13(3):184-188.
3. Swenson DM, Collins CL, Best TM, Flanigan DC, Fields SK, Comstock RD. Epidemiology of knee injuries among U.S. high school athletes, 2005/2006-2010/2011. Med Sci Sports Exerc 2013;45(3):462-469.

4. Levy BA, Stuart MJ, Whelan DB. Posterolateral instability of the knee: evaluation, treatment, results. Sports Med Arthrosc 2010;18(4):254-262.
5. LaPrade RF, Wentorf F. Diagnosis and treatment of posterolateral knee injuries. Clin Orthop Relat Res 2002 Sep;(402):110-121.

AMSSM Case Title: Unusual Injury Pattern Causing Lateral Knee Pain: A Case Report

- ❏ AMSSM Case Category: Knee, posterior lateral complex
- ❏ Author: Richard Pearson, MD
- ❏ Editor: Eric Schub, DO
- ❏ Senior Editor: Mandeep Ghuman, MD
- ❏ Board Review Book Reference Question: 1-98, Knee, posterolateral complex

CASE STUDY #11: OSTEOID OSTEOMA

Patient Presentation

A 20-year-old male NCAA Division II collegiate basketball player presented to clinic with atraumatic right knee pain for six months.

History

A 20-year-old male NCAA Division II collegiate basketball player presented with chronic right knee pain for six months. The pain was described as "deep to the bone," located over the anterior proximal tibia and radiating down his lateral calf. It was noted both at rest and with activity. The athlete denied swelling or mechanical symptoms, trauma, fevers, chills, or weight loss. Four months prior to presentation, he was diagnosed with a right proximal tibial stress fracture by MRI. There was also a lesion noted at medial aspect of proximal tibia, benign in appearance. After three months of rest, the pain returned with the initiation of exercise.

Physical Examination

The athlete's vital signs were normal. Right knee exam: no effusion noted, mild vague tenderness over the lateral proximal tibia, but otherwise no other bony tenderness; full flexion and extension; normal strength; neurologic and vascular exams were normal. Provocative maneuvers including: varus/valgus stress, Lachman's, anterior/posterior drawer, McMurray's, bounce home, patellar grind, Ober's, and Noble's were all negative.

Differential Diagnosis

- Patellofemoral syndrome
- Patellar tendonitis
- Iliotibial band syndrome
- Stress fracture of proximal tibia
- Meniscal tear
- Osteomyelitis
- Bone tumor
    - ✓ Benign: Osteoid osteoma, non-ossifying fibroma
    - ✓ Malignant: Osteosarcoma, Ewing sarcoma

Lab Studies

A complete blood count showed mild anemia (Hgb 11.7); comprehensive metabolic panel and coagulation panel were within normal limits; LDH (186) and uric acid (7.2) were moderately elevated.

Other Studies

❑ The initial x-rays (June 2015) were reported as negative. MRI right knee without contrast (June 30, 2015) showed a proximal tibial stress reaction, benign-appearing lesion in proximal medial tibia.

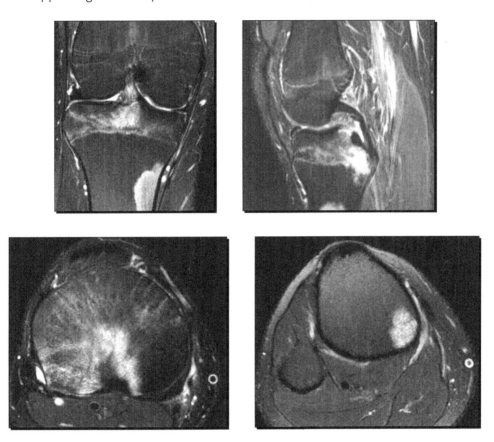

❑ CT right lower extremity without contrast (Jan. 15, 2016): Lateral proximal tibial lesion consistent with an osteoid osteoma.

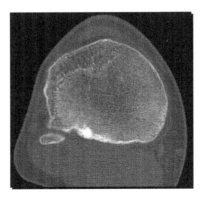

- Bone scan (Jan. 22, 2016): Radiotracer uptake throughout right tibial plateau

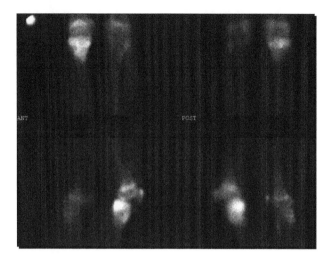

- Bone biopsy (Feb. 9, 2016):
  - Lateral lesion: Osteoid osteoma
  - Medial lesion: Primary bone large B cell lymphoma

Consultation

- Orthopedics
- Orthopedic oncology
- Hematology/oncology

Working Diagnosis: Osteoid osteoma in lateral lesion, diffuse large B cell lymphoma in medial lesion

Treatment

- Osteoid osteoma (lateral lesion): Radiofrequency ablation treatment
- Diffuse large B cell lymphoma (medial lesion): Chemotherapy (Rituximab, Cyclophosphamide, Doxorubicin, Vincristine, and Prednisolone 9R-CHOP), six cycles; after chemotherapy, 17 rounds of radiation treatment

Outcome

- Post-treatment MRI right knee without contrast (Sep. 25, 2016): Post-treatment changes; new marrow signal alteration and enhancement, concerning for recurrent disease

Case Studies

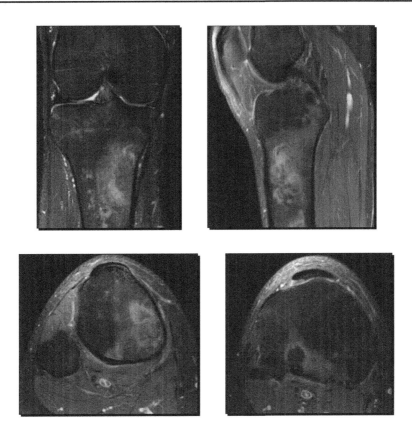

- Bone biopsy (Oct. 11, 2016): Negative for malignancy
- Return to basketball protocol: After chemotherapy and radiation treatment was completed, he progressed through closed-chain lower body strength exercises, functional strengthening, plyometrics, stationary bike, and alter-G running. Fourteen months after diagnosis and six months after remission, he returned to unrestricted basketball.

Author's Comments

Advanced imaging should be considered in patients with persistent or undifferentiated symptoms, despite negative initial imaging. Both benign and malignant bone tumors can cause pain. A multidisciplinary approach, involving physicians and athletic training staff, is crucial for expedited diagnostic, therapeutic interventions, and return to play when evaluating and treating athletes with cancer.

Editor's Comments

Osteoid osteoma is most common in the lower extremity of males in their second decade. The proximal femur is the most common location, with the tibia being second. Patients most often present with chronic, nighttime pain unrelated to activity.

References

1. Tis JE. Nonmalignant bone lesions in children and adolescents. UpToDate. Accessed March 22, 2019 at https://www.uptodate.com/contents/nonmalignant-bone-lesions-in-children-and-adolescents.

AMSSM Case Title: Second Shot at Life

- ❑ AMSSM Case Category: Oncology, osteoid osteoma
- ❑ Author: Marcia Faustin, MD
- ❑ Editor: Marc Hilgers, MD, PhD
- ❑ Board Review Book Reference Question: 1-112, Osteoid osteoma

CASE STUDY #12: OVERUSE INJURY, PEDIATRICS

Patient Presentation

A 15-year-old male presented with right elbow pain and weakness.

History

A 15-year-old male, right-hand-dominant catcher presented with insidious onset of right elbow pain. There was no trauma or specific injury he could recall. Nine months prior to presentation, he was diagnosed with a non-displaced medial epicondyle avulsion fracture by an outside provider. At that time, he stopped all throwing activities, but did not complete a throwing program before returning to his high school baseball team after six months of rest. Upon his return, he experienced intermittent pain throughout the throwing cycle, diffusely about his elbow. He also began to experience numbness and tingling in his right forearm. Symptoms improved with rest and worsened with throwing. He had tried ice, acetaminophen, and non-steroidal anti-inflammatory medications, without improvement.

Physical Examination

- ❑ Musculoskeletal: Normal active range of motion of his shoulder and elbow. Tenderness to palpation over the ante-cubital fossa, as well as just medial and lateral to this region. Slight weakness with wrist flexion and radial deviation. Finger flexion, pronation, and supination strength was normal, though there was mild pain with resisted pronation. Sensory examination was normal throughout the right upper extremity and symmetric to the left arm.

Differential Diagnosis

- Flexor mass strain
- Medial epicondylitis
- Medial epicondyle fracture
- Pronator syndrome
- Radial tunnel syndrome
- Traction apophysitis
- Ulnar collateral ligament injury

Other Studies

- ❏ Initial anterior-posterior and lateral elbow radiographs were normal, with the medial epicondyle physis still open. A stress radiograph was normal. MRI revealed marrow edema concerning for a non-displaced fracture of the distal metaphysis from lateral to medial in the supracondylar region.

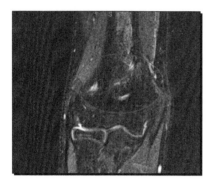 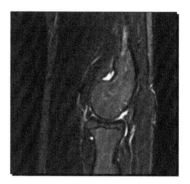

- ❏ An electromyography (EMG) and nerve conduction study (NCS) was performed, which revealed decreased conduction velocity in the median motor nerve at the elbow and wrist, with decreased conduction amplitudes and mild acute-on-chronic neurogenic changes in the pronator teres, as well as chronic neurogenic changes in the abductor pollicis brevis and flexor pollicis longus muscles.

Consultation

- Orthopedic surgery

Working Diagnosis: Distal humeral stress fracture with concomitant pronator syndrome

Treatment

The patient was made non-throwing for four weeks. On follow-up, he endorsed continued pain and occasional tingling in his forearm, but he had not adhered to medical recommendations for rest. Thus, he was put into a long-arm cast with elbow at 90 degrees in neutral position for a period of three weeks. After casting, the patient had complete resolution of his pain and neurological symptoms. A repeat MRI to assess for healing, however, revealed increased marrow edema along the capitellum and extending into the trochlea, without a discrete fracture line.

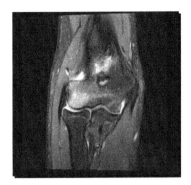 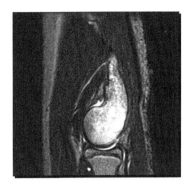

Based on this, the patient was referred to an orthopedic surgeon for a second opinion. On the surgeon's examination, the patient was asymptomatic, with full active and passive range of motion without pain. A complete motor and sensory examination was normal and symmetric to the contralateral side. Given these findings, the patient was instructed to begin physical therapy and to progress to a light throwing program.

Outcome

The patient returned to full unrestricted activity prior to the start of his high school baseball season after completing a progressive throwing program without difficulty.

Author's Comments

Overuse throwing injuries can manifest in a variety of pathology. What is consistent is that repeated microtrauma to the throwing arm may result in a significant injury, regardless of competition level. In order to prevent significant injuries, providers must continue to emphasize to throwing athletes that they should not throw in pain. Furthermore, if an athlete has recovered from a throwing injury, it is imperative for them to participate in a throwing program prior to full competition to prevent a recurrence of injuries.

In this case, in order to develop a successful treatment plan, it was necessary to repeat advanced imaging (MRI) to aid in treatment by assessing bony healing. Visualizing resolution of stress reactions and fractures in athletes' throwing arms can help prevent additional development of injury or delayed recovery due to early return. As the bony edema resolved, the patient's neurological symptoms improved. Thus, once the patient was asymptomatic at rest, he then began an appropriate rehabilitative program and progressed to a throwing program without difficulty.

Editor's Comments

Humeral stress fractures occur when excessive torque while throwing or lifting is placed on immature or unconditioned bone.[6,7] It is during the late cocking and early acceleration phases of throwing that the trauma due to repetitive use occurs. Axial loads produced by the biceps and triceps during pitching are protective to the arm, but fatigue diminishes the benefit. Initial imaging should consist of radiographs. If initial imaging is negative, but clinical suspicion remains high, MRI is the imaging modality of choice.[8] Uncomplicated stress fractures can be managed conservatively with rest, acetaminophen, and sling for at least three weeks before attempting graduated return to play involving a throwing program. The presence of neurovascular symptoms should raise the suspicion of a more complicated injury, with a low threshold for orthopedic referral. In this instance, symptoms were likely from compression of the median nerve between the humeral head and pronator teres.[9] Typically, when this form of median nerve impingement occurs, numbness and pain involving the thenar eminence, lateral palm, and forearm are the predominate symptoms. In prolonged or severe cases, however, weakness can also be present. Treatment involves avoiding provocative maneuvers, use of anti-inflammatory medication, and a progressive return to throwing.

References

1. Gonzalez-Zapata A, Familiari F, McFarland EG. Stress reaction of the humerus in a high school baseball player. J Orthop Sports Phys Ther 2014 Dec;44(12):998. doi: 10.2519/jospt.2014.0414.
2. Fleisig GS, Andrews JR, Dillman CJ, Escamilla RF. Kinetics of baseball pitching with implications about injury mechanisms. Am J Sports Med 1995 Mar-Apr;23(2):233-239.
3. Mautner BK, Blazuk J. Overuse throwing injuries in skeletally immature athletes—diagnosis, treatment, and prevention. Curr Sports Med Rep 2015 May-Jun;14(3):209-214.
4. McFarland EG, Wasik M. Epidemiology of collegiate baseball injuries. Clin J Sport Med 1998 Jan;8(1):10-13.
5. McFarland EG, Ireland ML. Rehabilitation programs and prevention strategies in adolescent throwing athletes. Instr Course Lect 2003;52:37-42.
6. Linn RM, Kriegshauser LA. Ball thrower's fracture of the humerus. A case report. Am J Sports Med 1991 Mar-Apr;19(2):194-197.
7. Pehlivan O, Kiral A, Akmaz I, Solakoglu C, Arpacioglu O, Kaplan H. Humeral shaft fractures secondary to throwing. Orthopedics 2003 Nov;26(11):1139-1141.
8. Jones GL. Upper extremity stress fractures. Clin Sports Med 2006 Jan;25(1):159-174.
9. Lee MJ, LaStayo PC. Pronator syndrome and other nerve compressions that mimic carpal tunnel syndrome. J Orthop Sports Phys Ther 2004 Oct;34(10):601-609.

AMSSM Case Title: 15-Year-Old With Elbow Pain and Weakness

- ❏ AMSSM Case Category: Overuse injuries
- ❏ Author: Jason Zaremesky, MD
- ❏ Editor: Eric Schub, DO
- ❏ Senior Editor: Mandeep Ghuman, MD
- ❏ Board Review Book Reference Question: 1-36, Overuse injury, pediatrics

CASE STUDY #13: PATELLOFEMORAL PAIN DYSFUNCTION

Patient Presentation

A 23-year-old female recreational runner came into sports medicine clinic with a chief complaint of recurring and ongoing right knee pain for eight months.

History

The pain started eight months ago after a hyperextension of her right knee while catching herself from tripping. She used to run one to two miles every other day, but has stopped due to pain. The pain is dull, localized to her right knee, with a severity of 8/10, and progressing. It is most painful when she transitions from a long period of sitting to standing. She has noted worsening swelling around her patella, as well. The patient has tried home exercises, as well as ice, bracing, and ibuprofen, with no improvement. Her past medical history is negative for any previous knee injuries or surgeries.

Physical Examination

- Vitals: Height 5'3", weight 100 pounds, body mass index 17.7
- General: Alert, no acute distress
- Psychiatric: Bright affect
- Cardiovascular: Capillary refill less than two seconds
- Respiratory: Non-labored breathing, no dyspnea
- Skin: No rash, no edema
- Right knee exam: 1+ effusion
- Medial joint line tenderness
- No patellar tenderness on palpation
- Full active flexion and extension (0 to 135 degrees)
- Pain on end range of motion
- No patellar instability
- Lachman's test: Negative
- McMurray's test: Negative
- Varus/valgus testing: Negative
- Clarke's inhibition test: Positive
- J sign: Positive
- Patellar compression test: Negative

Differential Diagnosis

- Patellofemoral pain syndrome
- Quadriceps tendinopathy
- Hemangioma
- Patella fracture
- Anterior cruciate ligament tear
- Posterior cruciate ligament tear
- Meniscus tear
- Osteochondritis dissecans

Other Studies

- ❑ Right knee x-rays: Negative
- ❑ MRI of the right knee: There is a lobulated region of fluid signal, with thin septations, a fluid-fluid level, and multiple filling defects at the superomedial aspect of the patella, which appears to be above the suprapatellar plica in the suprapatellar recess. There are no filling defects which show significant hyperintense or fatty marrow signal. The patella is in a normal position, and the patellofemoral cartilage is intact. Menisci and cruciate ligaments are intact. No fracture or bone marrow edema are noted.

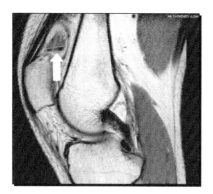
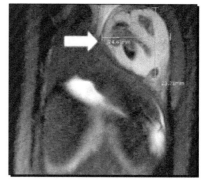

Consultation

The patient was referred for orthopedic consultation. Excision versus needle biopsy were discussed. Patient opted for excision. Resultant pathology showed a soft tissue mass, with numerous small and large vascular structures, lined by bland endothelial cells, consistent with synovial hemangioma. No was no evidence of malignancy.

Working Diagnosis: Synovial hemangioma of the knee

Treatment

Excisional biopsy of the mass

Outcome

The patient recovered fully and returned to unrestricted activity.

Author's Comments

This case initially appears like a seemingly clear-cut example of patellofemoral pain syndrome. This case, however, was just a bit different, as the patient's knee pain progressively worsened, despite discontinuing running. Synovial hemangiomas are often difficult to diagnose, resulting in delayed treatment.[1] They are rare and benign tumors that are often found in the knee[1,2] and represent less than 1% of all hemangiomas.[2] Normally a diagnosis in the young adult population, synovial hemangiomas may cause unexplained pain and joint effusions, as demonstrated in this case. This mass was unilateral, as most synovial hemangiomas are. Most synovial hemangiomas arise in the knee, but other joints may include the elbow, wrist, or ankle.[3] A palpable mass may be found, along with a limitation of motion. Current treatment is surgical excision.[4] Failure to treat may lead to loss of range of motion and early joint degeneration.[1]

Editor's Comments

This case is a good example of the importance of looking further into a patient's symptoms when they fail to respond to therapy or the symptoms don't fit the initial working diagnosis. Not every patient with knee pain needs an MRI, but in this case, the persistence of symptoms, failure to respond to treatment, and recurrent effusions warranted further imaging, even though the initial x-ray was negative. The hemangioma would likely be visualized on diagnostic ultrasound, but MRI would still be needed to adequately visual the meniscal and articular cartilage.

References

1. Tahmasbi MN, Sobhan MR, Bashti K, Ariamanesh AS. Synovial hemangioma of the knee with recurrent effusion and pain: a case report. Acta Med Iran 2014;52(8):644-646.
2. Arslan H, İslamoğlu N, Akdemir Z, Adanas C. Synovial hemangioma in the knee: MRI findings. J Clin Imaging Sci 2015 Apr 30;5:23. doi: 10.4103/2156-7514.156129.
3. Llauger J, Monill JM, Palmer J, Clotet M. Synovial hemangioma of the knee: MRI findings in two cases. Skeletal Radiol 1995 Nov;24(8):579-581.
4. Price NJ, Cundy PJ. Synovial hemangioma of the knee. J Pediatr Orthop 1997 Jan-Feb;17(1):74-77.

AMSSM Case Title: Not the Average Runner's Knee

- AMSSM Case Category: Patellofemoral pain
- Author: Eri Yamaguchi, BA
- Editor: Michael Henehan, DO
- Board Review Book Reference Questions: 1-4, 1-7, 1-94, 2-7, Patellofemoral pain dysfunction

CASE STUDY #14: PERONEAL NEUROPATHY

Patient Presentation

Acute right foot drop

History

An 11-year-old girl was referred to the sports medicine clinic for evaluation of a right foot drop for six weeks. She denied any preceding injury. She complained of right foot weakness and numbness on the dorsum of the foot, extending up the lateral leg to the knee. She reported difficulty going up stairs and had a fall in the past week, due to weakness. She reported achy right thigh pain. She was a dancer and a cross-country athlete. She denied any fever/chills or myalgias. She denied significant past medical history, and there is no family history of cancer or autoimmune disease.

Physical Examination

- General: Thin-appearing, weight 88 pounds (BMI 16 kg/m2)
- Musculoskeletal: No atrophy or fasciculation
- Strength exam:
    - RLE—5/5 knee flexion, 5/5 knee extension, 1/5 ankle dorsiflexion, 1/5 extensor hallucis longus, 5/5 ankle plantarflexion, 3/5 peroneals
    - LLE—5/5 knee flexion, 5/5 knee extension, 5/5 ankle dorsiflexion, 5/5 extensor hallucis longus, 5/5 ankle plantarflexion, 5/5 peroneals
- Neurological: Sensation to light touch decreased at the right distal lateral leg, dorsum of the foot, and the webspace between the great and second toe.
- Gait: Significant increase in right hip flexion, with hip circumduction to clear her foot.

Differential Diagnosis

- Peroneal neuropathy
- Lumbosacral plexopathy
- Lumbar radiculopathy, L5
- Tibialis anterior tendinopathy
- Mass lesion/cancer

Other Studies

- Right knee x-ray: AP and lateral views demonstrated no abnormalities.

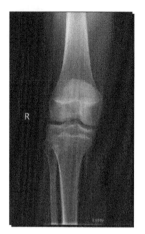
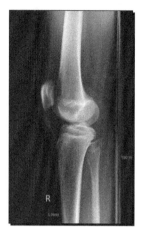

- Right knee MRI: Coronal T2 image showed a cystic lesion within the proximal tibiofibular joint, measuring 1.3 cm. Axial T2 image showed edema-like signal within the anterior compartment musculature of the leg consistent with denervation injury.

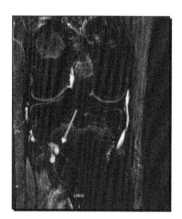
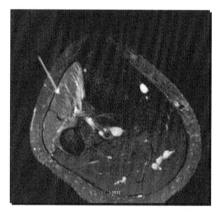

- EMG: Revealed electrodiagnostic evidence of a moderate to severe right peroneal neuropathy at the knee; incomplete injury with motor units recruited in tibialis anterior and peroneus longus.

Motor NCS						
Nerve/Sites	Rec. Site	Lat ms	Amp mV	Rel Amp %	Dist. cm	Vel m/s
R COMM PERONEAL-EDB						
Ankle	EDB	3.95	0.2	100	8	
Fib Head	EDB	10.5	0.8	435	31	47.3
Knee	EDB	12.7	4.3	2244	8	36.4

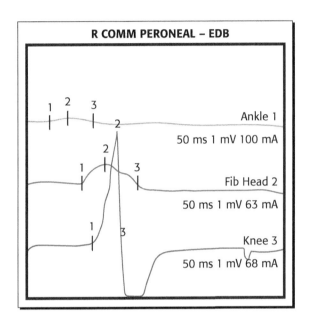

Consultation

- Orthopedic surgery

Working Diagnosis: Right peroneal neuropathy

Treatment

The patient was prescribed an ankle-foot orthosis. She was advised to avoid sitting cross-legged and recommended to refrain from gym class, dance, and running. At four weeks follow-up, the patient reported a recent diagnosis of anorexia nervosa. On chart review, her initial weight was 103 pounds (BMI 19.5 kg/m2), and over the course of several months, she had dropped to 88 pounds (BMI 16 kg/m2). The onset of the acute foot drop coincided with this significant weight loss. She was enrolled in a comprehensive pediatric eating disorder clinic for further treatment. She had an orthopaedic surgical consult at six weeks from her initial sports medicine consultation. Her weight had increased, and her symptoms were improving. Conservative management was recommended, as it was unlikely that the cystic lesion visualized on MRI was contributing to her symptoms.

Outcome

At four weeks follow-up, the patient reported improvement in her gait with use of the ankle-foot orthosis, and the thigh pain had resolved. However, she still had significant weakness with ankle dorsiflexion and persistent numbness. At three months follow-up, she reported significant return of strength and only required the ankle-foot orthosis during gym class. She continued treatment in the comprehensive pediatric eating disorder clinic with continued weight gain, although she was not yet weighing herself. She was not yet allowed to return to running or dance. At four months follow-up, she only had mild weakness of ankle dorsiflexion and a small area of numbness on the distal lateral leg. At six months follow-up, she had only subtle weakness, and had returned to her prior weight of 103 pounds (BMI 18.4 kg/m2). She was cleared from wearing the ankle-foot orthosis. She continued active treatment of her anorexia. With the okay from her psychologist, she was progressed back to running and dance.

Author's Comments

This case illustrates an acute peroneal neuropathy as a rare manifestation of anorexia nervosa.[1,2] Not only is this atypical, but it also highlights the importance of treating the patient as a whole, including diet and lifestyle factors.

Editor's Comments

While this case highlighted anorexia nervosa as a contributing cause, issues with less severe disordered eating leading to poor energy availability should always be considered in both female and male athletes. Oftentimes, training levels are so high that even the best-intentioned athlete may have difficulty maintaining appropriate caloric intake to meet their energy needs. RED-S (relative energy deficiency in sport) describes this issue in male and female athletes.[3]

References

1. Lutte I, Rhys C, Hubert C, Brion F, Boland B, Peeters A, et al. Peroneal neuropathy palsy in anorexia nervosa. Acta Neurol Belg 1997 Dec;97(4):251-254.
2. MacKenzie JR, LaBan MM, Sackeyfio AH. The prevalence of peripheral neuropathy in patients with anorexia nervosa. Arch Phys Med Rehabil 1989 Nov;70(12):827-830.
3. Mountjoy M, Sundgot-Borgen JK, Burke LM, Ackerman KE, Blauwet C, Constantini N, et al. IOC consensus statement on relative energy deficiency in sport (RED-S): 2018 update. Br J Sports Med 2018 Jun;52(11):687-697. doi: 10.1136/bjsports-2018-099193.

AMSSM Case Title: Foot Drop in a Young Female Athlete

- ❏ AMSSM Case Category: Nerve, peroneal
- ❏ Author: Carrie Miller, MD
- ❏ Editor: Tracy Zaslow, MD
- ❏ Senior Editor: Kristine Karlson, MD
- ❏ Board Review Book Reference Question: 1-134, Peroneal neuropathy

CASE STUDY #15: PNEUMOTHORAX

Patient Presentation

A 50-year-old male presented with shortness of breath and chest pain after being hit in the left upper chest by another player's shoulder while trying to head the ball during a soccer game.

History

He stated that symptoms began immediately after he was hit. He had sharp, stabbing left upper chest pain rated at 6 out of 10 that increased with inspiration and coughing. He also complained of shortness of breath, abdominal cramping, nausea, and palpitations. He had a pertinent medical history of asthma, though he denied that his symptoms were similar to an asthma exacerbation. He denied any loss of consciousness or head injury.

Physical Examination

On inspection, there was localized swelling and blanchable erythema in the left upper chest, just inferior to the clavicle, two to three inches lateral of the sternum. There was no subcutaneous emphysema or palpable deformity. The patient was tender over the third and fourth ribs, near the left sternal border and mid-axillary line. He was tachypneic with a respiratory rate of 30 without obvious distress. There were clear and equal breath sounds in all lung fields, and normal heart rate and rhythm without murmurs, rubs, or gallops.

Differential Diagnosis

- Chest wall contusion
- Rib fracture
- Asthma exacerbation
- Myocardial infarction
- Traumatic pneumothorax

Lab Studies

Lab results, including complete blood count, basic metabolic panel, troponin, d-dimer, and CK, were normal.

Other Studies

- Initial chest x-ray showed no fractures or pneumothorax.

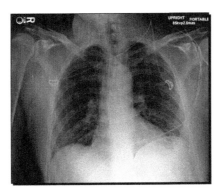

- A chest CT scan with IV contrast showed a small left apical pneumothorax (CT images of a similar case). An abdominal CT scan with IV contrast was unremarkable.

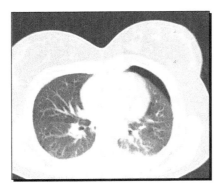

Working Diagnosis: Left apical traumatic pneumothorax

Treatment

After initial evaluation, the patient was admitted to the hospital for observation overnight. There was a stable appearance of his pneumothorax on x-ray, and his vital signs were stable overnight. His pain was improved, and he was breathing comfortably by the morning. He was discharged home from the hospital, with instructions to avoid flying, contact activity, or any moderate physical activity until seen in follow-up. He was also advised to use the incentive spirometer for three to four days, and then as needed.

Outcome

The patient was seen for follow-up 10 days after discharge from the hospital and had resolution of his shortness of breath, with pain improved to 2 out of 10 with deep breathing and twisting. He also had migrating chest pain that gradually improved. He was instructed to continue to avoid physical activity and air travel for the next two to four weeks. At three weeks, he was symptom-free, with a normal chest x-ray. He was provided with a plan for a gradual return to physical activity over a week as long as he remained symptom-free. There were no further complications, and he was able to resume full physical activity.

Author's Comments

Traumatic pneumothorax is an uncommon injury during athletic events, although it could lead to significant morbidity if overlooked. While most athletes with acute chest trauma typically have contusions or rib fractures, it is important to consider a traumatic pneumothorax within the differential, along with other serious diagnoses, such as cardiac arrest or arrhythmias. If unnoticed, patients could deteriorate quickly. Thankfully, this patient did not need significant interventions after his injury.

Editor's Comments

Rib fractures, pneumothorax, tension pneumothorax, hemothorax, flail chest, steronoclavicular joint dislocation, pulmonary contusions, and cardiac contusions can occur during sporting activities. In order to make the correct diagnosis, one must consider all of these diagnoses. More common in higher energy traumatic injuries involving motor vehicle accidents, these can occur in sports as well. A missed pneumothorax can lead to cardiorespiratory arrest and death.

References

1. Curtin SM, Tucker AM, Gens DR. Pneumothorax in sports: issues in recognition and follow-up care. Phys Sportsmed 2000 Aug:28(8):23-32.

AMSSM Case Title: A Rare Presentation of Chest Pain in an Athlete

- ❏ AMSSM Case Category: Chest trauma, pneumothorax
- ❏ Author: Mark DeFord, MD
- ❏ Editor: Benjamin Hasan, MD
- ❏ Senior Editor: Kristine Karlson, MD
- ❏ Board Review Book Reference Question: 1-195, Pneumothorax

CASE STUDY #16: RHABDOMYOLYSIS

Patient Presentation

Dark urine and intense leg pain

History

The patient is a 26-year-old incarcerated African-American male with no significant past medical or surgical history who presented to the emergency department with a one-day history of intense bilateral leg pain and dark urine. The patient states that the previous day he completed an air squat pyramid workout (started at one and progressed to 50, increasing his squat total by one each time) that totaled about 1225 air squats over a two-hour period. He drank only a little water during the workout and felt fine afterwards, with only some mild soreness in his quadriceps. He states that he woke up the next morning with extreme pain in both of his thighs. He also had dark, ginger-ale-colored urine, without seeing any blood. He went to the jail infirmary, where he was given Naproxen and Prednisolone. His urine showed excessive blood fragments. He was immediately sent to the emergency room for further workup. He smokes marijuana socially and takes Alprazolam for sleep at night. In the emergency room, the patient was afebrile, normotensive, and had a normal heart rate and normal respiratory rate on room air. His creatine phosphokinase level was greater than 40,000 and was given 1 l bolus of normal saline. The patient was admitted to the hospital for further management and care.

Physical Examination

- ❏ Constitutional: Oriented to person, place, and time, and well-developed, well-nourished, and in no distress
- ❏ Head: Normocephalic and atraumatic
- ❏ Eyes: Conjunctivae, EOM are normal; pupils are equal, round, and reactive to light.
- ❏ Neck: Normal range of motion; neck supple
- ❏ Cardiovascular: Normal rate, regular rhythm, and normal heart sounds
- ❏ Pulmonary/chest: Effort normal and breath sounds normal.
- ❏ Abdominal: Soft; bowel sounds are normal.
- ❏ Musculoskeletal: Examination of the thighs showed tenderness bilaterally. Range of motion was normal. No edema or sensory abnormalities were noted. Pulses in the lower extremities were 2+. Deep tendon reflexes were normal.

Differential Diagnosis

- Exercise-induced rhabdomyolysis
- Myositis
- Drug-induced myositis

Lab Studies

- ❑ Creatine phosphokinase trended over his stay in the hospital, from 40,000 to 19,857 to 7,997.
- ❑ Chest x-ray showed no acute cardiopulmonary abnormality. Urine myoglobin 21,508, Serum Myoglobin 6340, AST 1037, ALT 174, normal creatinine. Urine dip was positive for blood.

Other Studies

- ❑ Urine drug screen was negative.

Working Diagnosis: Exercise-induced rhabdomyolysis

Treatment

The patient remained in the hospital for three days. Over his hospital course, the patient was started on a bicarbonate drip at 150cc/hour, as well as normal saline for 100cc/hour. The patient was allowed a regular diet during his stay, and physical therapy and occupational therapy were ordered for evaluation before he was discharged.

Outcome

The patient was able to return to normal activity and was given education on rhabdomyolysis and signs to look out for. Advised to continue increased daily oral fluids and to limit intense workouts.

Editor's Comments

Classical presentation in an uncommon setting. Emphasis is on rehydration measures and kidney protection.

References

1. Grau JM, Poch E. Pathophysiology and management of rhabdomyolysis. In: Webb A, Angus D, Finfer S, Gattinoni L, Singer M (eds). Oxford Textbook of Critical Care. 2nd ed. Oxford Medicine Online: Oxford University Press, 2016. doi: 10.1093/med/9780199600830.003.0355.
2. Lin AC, Lin CM, Wang TL, Leu JG. Rhabdomyolysis in 119 students after repetitive exercise. Br J Sports Med 2005 Jan;39(1):e3. doi: 10.1136/bjsm.2004.013235.

AMSSM Case Title: Dark Urine and Intense Leg Pain After an Air Squat Workout

- ❏ AMSSM Case Category: Exertional rhabdomyolysis
- ❏ Author: Aaron Tracy, MD
- ❏ Editor: Marc Hilgers, MD, PhD
- ❏ Board Review Book Reference Question: 1-101, Rhabdomyolysis

About the Editors

Stephen Paul, MD, CAQSM, is an associate professor at the University of Arizona, where he is a staff physician and coordinator for sports medicine at Campus Health Service, head team physician for club sports, and assistant team physician for intercollegiate sports medicine. He started and was program director for the University of Arizona Sports Medicine Fellowship for 10 years until he took a year-long sabbatical to live in Chile with his family in 2015. Dr. Paul graduated from the University of Texas Health Science Centers at Houston in 1987. He completed his fellowship in sports medicine at the Center for Sports Medicine and Orthopedics in Phoenix in 1996. He is board-certified in family medicine and holds a Certificate of Added Qualifications in Sports Medicine. He has worked with professional, intercollegiate, club sports, and recreational athletes. He has published in *Athletic Training & Sports Health Care, Sports Health, The 5-Minute Sports Medicine Consult, Clinical Journal of Sport Medicine, Saunders Manual of Medical Practice,* and *Orthopedic Knowledge Update: Sports Medicine.* He worked with the AMSSM to develop the first sports medicine In-Training Exam and is past chair of the AMSSM In-Training Exam subcommittee. He is past programming chair for the AMSSM Annual Meeting 2014 in New Orleans. He served as the chair of the AMSSM 25th Anniversary/Founders/History Video ad hoc committee and helped prepare the video which was presented at the 2016 annual meeting. Dr. Paul has been a member of the AMSSM board of directors, chairing the Publications Committee since 2015, and has recently been elected an AMSSM officer (secretary/treasurer). He has also been selected to co-guest-author the AMSSM-BJSM joint issue for 2020. He lives in Tucson, Arizona, with his wife Janice and children Nika and Stryder.

Leah G. Concannon, MD is a clinical associate professor in the Department of Rehabilitation Medicine, Sports and Spine Division, at the University of Washington. She has worked with intercollegiate, high school, club sports, and recreational athletes, including event coverage for international elite-level gymnasts. Dr. Concannon earned her medical degree at the University of Illinois-Chicago, and completed residency and fellowship training at the University of Washington. She is board-certified in physical medicine and rehabilitation, with subspecialty certification in sports medicine. She has a clinical focus on sports concussion and has written several articles and book chapters on the subject. She is actively involved in the Physical Medicine and Rehabilitation residency and fellowship training programs at the University of Washington. She currently serves as co-chair of the AMSSM In-Training Exam subcommittee. She lives in Seattle, Washington with her family.

Morteza Khodaee, MD, MPH, FACSM, FAAFP, is an associate professor at the University of Colorado School of Medicine. He is the head primary care team physician for the Denver Nuggets and the team physician for the University of Denver Pioneers. He is also a volunteer physician for USA Swimming. Dr. Khodaee earned his medical degree from Islamic Azad University in Tehran, Iran. He completed his family medicine residency and sports medicine fellowship at the University of Michigan. He is board-certified in family medicine and has earned a CAQ in sports medicine. Dr. Khodaee is passionate about teaching and promoting scholarly activities among young learners. He is the co-chair of the AMSSM In-Training Exam subcommittee. He lives in Denver, Colorado, with his wife Atousa and children Arshia and Kimia.

Michael Henehan, DO, CAQSM, FAOASM, is an adjunct clinical professor at Stanford University. He is program director of the Stanford Health Care Primary Care Sports Medicine Fellowship program at O'Connor Hospital in San Jose, California and is a faculty member in the affiliated family medicine residency program. Dr. Henehan graduated from the Chicago College of Osteopathic Medicine and completed his residency in family medicine at the Stanford-affiliated San Jose Medical Center program. He is currently a team physician at San Jose State University and has been the team physician for the San Jose Earthquakes professional soccer team, USA Water Polo team, and SaberCats arena football team. Dr. Henehan is past president of the American Osteopathic Academy of Sports Medicine (AOASM) and a former AMSSM board member and chairman of the Fellowship Committee. He has also been an active member of the AMSSM Education Committee and is developing the AMSSM Case Studies Library. He has published in the *Clinical Journal of Sport Medicine, Journal of Emergency Medicine,* and *Physician and Sportsmedicine* and has written multiple book chapters. He lives in Palo Alto, California, with his wife Barbara and has two children.

About the Contributors

IMAGE CONTRIBUTORS

Irfan M. Asif, MD
Professor and Chair, Department of Family and Community Medicine, University of Alabama Birmingham (UAB) School of Medicine
Birmingham, AL

Donna G. Blankenbaker, MD
Medical Director, Outpatient Radiology
Co-Director, Medical Student Radiology Education
Professor, Department of Radiology
University of Wisconsin-Madison School of Medicine & Public Health
Madison, WI

Susannah M. Briskin, MD
Director, University Hospitals Sports Medicine Institute Primary Care Sports Medicine Fellowship
Co-Director, University Hospitals Cleveland Medical Center Concussion Program
Associate Professor of Pediatrics, Division of Pediatric Sports Medicine
Rainbow Babies and Children's Hospital/University Hospitals Cleveland Medical Center
Cleveland, OH

Alison Brooks, MD, MPH
Associate Professor
Team Physician, Sports Medicine
Department of Orthopedics, University of Wisconsin-Madison
Madison, WI

Kirkland W. Davis, MD, FACR
Professor, Department of Radiology, University of Wisconsin School of Medicine and Public Health
Madison, WI

Arie DeGrio, MD
Family Medicine Resident, HonorHealth
Phoenix, AZ

Jonathan Drezner, MD
Professor, Department of Family Medicine
Director, Center for Sports Cardiology
University of Washington
Seattle, WA

Matthew Grady, MD
Director, Sports Medicine Fellowship
Member, Department of Pediatrics and Orthopedics
Children's Hospital of Philadelphia
Associate Professor of Clinical Pediatrics, University of Pennsylvania Perelman School of Medicine
Philadelphia, PA

Barry E. Kenneally, MD
Sports Medicine and Orthopedic Oncology, Rothman Institute
Sidney Kimmel Medical College, Thomas Jefferson University
Team Physician, Philadelphia 76ers
Philadelphia, PA

Stephen R. Paul, MD, CAQSM, MA
Associate Professor, Department of Family and Community Medicine
Assistant Professor, Department of Orthopedics
Assistant Team Physician, Intercollegiate Athletics
Coordinator for Sports Medicine, Campus Health Service
The University of Arizona
Tucson, AZ

Jeff Roberts, MD, CAQSM, FAAFP
Program Director, VCU-St. Francis Primary Care Sports Medicine Fellowship Program
Associate Clinical Professor, VCU Department of Family Medicine and Population Health
St. Francis Family Medicine Center and Residency Program
Bon Secours Sports Medicine
Midlothian, VA

Darren Willius, DO
Fellow, University of Arizona Sports Medicine Fellowship 2018-2019
Tucson, AZ

Eliot J. Young, MD, FAAFP, CAQSM
Director, Primary Care Sports Medicine Fellowship
Sports Medicine Associates of San Antonio
Team Physician, San Antonio Spurs/San Antonio Rampage/San Antonio FC
San Antonio, TX

TEXT CONTRIBUTORS

Andrea Aagesen, DO, MS
Clinical Assistant Professor, Department of Physical Medicine and Rehabilitation
Team Physician
Michigan Medicine
University of Michigan
Ann Arbor, MI
Team Physician, Eastern Michigan University
Ypsilanti, MI

Irfan M. Asif, MD
Professor and Chair, Department of Family and Community Medicine, University of Alabama Birmingham (UAB) School of Medicine
Birmingham, AL

Matthew B. Baird, MD, CAQSM
Associate Program Director, Primary Care Sports Medicine Fellowship Program
Assistant Professor of Emergency and Sports Medicine
Greenville Health Systems, University of South Carolina School of Medicine – Greenville
Steadman Hawkins Clinic of the Carolinas
Greenville, SC

Robert J. Baker, MD, PhD
Director, Primary Care Sports Medicine Fellowship
Professor, Department of Family & Community Medicine
Professor, Department of Orthopedic Surgery
Western Michigan University Homer Stryker MD School of Medicine
Team Physician, Western Michigan University
Kalamazoo, MI

Jonathan Becker, MD
Chair, Department of Family and Geriatric Medicine
Professor, School of Medicine
Team Physician
University of Louisville
Louisville, KY

Barbara Brandon, DO, CAQSM
Associate Program Director, Sports Medicine Fellowship Spokane
Clinical Assistant Professor, University of Washington Department of Family Medicine
Team Physician, Spokane Indians Baseball
Team Physician, Whitworth University
Spokane, WA

Susannah M. Briskin, MD
Director, University Hospitals Sports Medicine Institute Primary Care Sports Medicine Fellowship
Co-Director, University Hospitals Cleveland Medical Center Concussion Program
Associate Professor of Pediatrics, Division of Pediatric Sports Medicine
Rainbow Babies and Children's Hospital/University Hospitals Cleveland Medical Center
Cleveland, OH

Joseph Chorley, MD
Associate Professor of Pediatrics, Section of Adolescent Medicine and Sports Medicine
Fellowship Director, Primary Care Sports Medicine
Baylor College of Medicine
Associate Medical Director, Chevron Houston Marathon
Texas Children's Hospital Sports Medicine Group
Houston, TX

Rachel Coel

Nailah Coleman, MD, FAAP, FACSM
Associate Professor of Pediatrics, The George Washington University
Pediatrician and Sports Medicine Physician, Children's National Health System
Washington, DC

Gerardo Miranda Comos

Leah G. Concannon, MD
Clinical Associate Professor, Department of Rehabilitation Medicine, University of Washington
Seattle, WA

Jennifer Daily, MD
Assistant Professor, Department of Family and Geriatric Medicine
Associate Program Director, Sports Medicine Fellowship
Team Physician
University of Louisville
Louisville, KY

James M. Daniels, MD, MPH
Vice Chair, Department of Family and Community Medicine
Director, Sports Medicine Fellowship
Professor of Family and Community Medicine and Orthopedic Surgery
Southern Illinois University School of Medicine
Quincy, IL

Brian Donohue, DO
Associate Director, Sports Medicine Fellowship
Associate Director, Family Medicine Residency
Presence Resurrection Medical Center
Chicago, IL

Ted A. Farrar, MD, FAAFP
Director, Primary Care Sports Medicine Fellowship
Assistant Director, Family Medicine Residency
USF/Morton Plant Mease Healthcare
Affiliate Assistant Professor, Department of Family Medicine, USF Morsani College of Medicine
Tampa, FL

Jeffrey Feden, MD
Associate Professor (Clinical), Department of Emergency Medicine, Alpert Medical School of Brown University
Providence, RI

Robert Flannery, MD
Assistant Professor, Division of Sports Medicine, Department of Orthopedic Surgery, Case Western Reserve University School of Medicine
Assistant Medical Physician, Cleveland Browns
Lead Medical Physician, Oberlin College
University Hospitals Cleveland
Cleveland, OH

Michael K. Fong, MD
Associate Director, Sports Medicine Fellowship
Assistant Physician in Charge, Division of Sports Medicine
Kaiser Los Angeles Medical Center
Team Physician, California State University Los Angeles
Los Angeles, CA

Margaret E. Gibson, MD
Director, Sports Medicine Fellowship
Associate Professor
University of Missouri Kansas City
Kansas City, MO

Andrew H. Gordon, MD, PhD
Faculty, Department of Physical Medicine and Rehabilitation, MedStar Georgetown University Hospital
MedStar National Rehabilitation Network
Washington, DC

Matthew Grady, MD
Director, Sports Medicine Fellowship
Member, Department of Pediatrics and Orthopedics
Children's Hospital of Philadelphia
Associate Professor of Clinical Pediatrics, University of Pennsylvania Perelman School of Medicine
Philadelphia, PA

Sunny Gupta, DO
Clinical Assistant Professor, Department of Family and Community Medicine, Sidney Kimmel Medical College at Thomas Jefferson University
Sports Medicine, Rothman Orthopaedic Institute
Philadelphia, PA

Benjamin A. Hasan, MD
Team Physician, USA Triathlon
Family Medicine and Sports Medicine Practice
Director, NCH Back and Spine Clinic
NCH Medical Group, Northwest Community Hospital
Arlington Heights, IL
Instructor, Department of Family and Community Medicine, Feinberg School of Medicine, Northwestern University
Assistant Professor of Clinical Family Medicine, University of Illinois College of Medicine
Chicago, IL

Daniel Herman, MD, PhD, FACSM, FAAPMR, CAQSM
Assistant Professor, Department of Orthopedics and Rehabilitation, University of Florida
Gainesville, FL

Marc P. Hilgers, MD, PhD, FAAFP
Medical Director – Sports Medicine, Advocate Aurora Health
Aurora, IL

Crystal L. Hnatko, DO, CAQSM
Director, Napa-Solano Pediatric Sports Concussion Clinic
Vacaville, CA
Clinical Professor, Napa-Solano Kaiser Permanente Family Medicine Residency
Vallejo, CA
Clinical Professor, David Grant Medical Center Family Medicine Residency
Travis Air Force Base, CA

Garry W. K. Ho, MD, FACSM, FAAFP, RMSK, CIC
Program Director, VCU/Fairfax Family Practice Sports Medicine Fellowship Program
Associate Professor, Department of Family Medicine, VCU School of Medicine
Richmond, VA
Associate Professor, Department of Family Medicine, Georgetown University School of Medicine
Washington, DC
Assistant Professor, Department of Family Medicine, Uniformed Services University of the Health Sciences
Bethesda, MD
Team Physician, George Mason University
Fairfax, VA
Team Physician, DC Divas Football
Landover, MD
Team Physician, Potomac Nationals Baseball
Woodbridge, VA

Eugene Hong, MD
Professor and Chief Physician Executive, MUSC Health and MUSC Physicians
Charleston, SC

Thomas Howard

Yao-Wen Eliot Hu, MD, MBA, FAAFP
Faculty, Sports Medicine Fellowship
Civilian Sports Medicine Physician
Naval Hospital Camp Pendleton
Oceanside, CA

Dominic A. Jacobelli, MD
Mercy Health Sports Medicine Northwest Arkansas
Rogers, AR

Rajat Jain, MD
Team Physician, Northwestern University
Clinical Instructor of Pediatrics and Internal Medicine, Northwestern Feinberg School of Medicine
Evanston, IL

Kimberly Kaiser, MD
Assistant Professor, Department of Orthopaedic Surgery and Sports Medicine
Assistant Professor, Department of Family and Community Medicine
Team Physician
University of Kentucky
Lexington, KY
Head Team Physician, Eastern Kentucky University
Richmond, KY

Rahul Kapur, MD, CAQSM
Assistant Professor, Department of Family Medicine and Community Health
St. John's Family Medicine Residency Program
University of Minnesota Sports Medicine
St. Paul, MN
Team Physician, US Lacrosse

Barry E. Kenneally, MD
Sports Medicine and Orthopedic Oncology, Rothman Institute
Sidney Kimmel Medical College, Thomas Jefferson University
Team Physician, Philadelphia 76ers
Philadelphia, PA

Jeremy Kent

Julie Kerr

Morteza Khodaee, MD, MPH, FACSM, FAAFP
Associate Professor, Department of Family Medicine & Orthopedics, Division of Sports Medicine, University of Colorado School of Medicine
Head Primary Care Team Physician, Denver Nuggets
Team Physician, University of Denver Pioneers Men Soccer
Denver, CO

Charles A. Lascano, MD, CAQSM
Sports Medicine, Sanitas Medical Centers
Clinical Assistant Professor, Florida International University, Herbert Wertheim College of Medicine (FIU-HWCOM)
Miami, FL

Justin Lee

Matthew S. Leiszler, MD
Football Team Physician, University of Notre Dame
Notre Dame, IN

Amy Leu, DO, FAAFP
Associate Clinical Professor, Department of Family Medicine and Public Health
Assistant Director, Primary Care Sports Medicine Fellowship
Team Physician, Intercollegiate Athletics and Sports Clubs
University of California, San Diego
Team Physician, US Figure Skating
Team Physician, San Diego Padres
San Diego, CA

Jeff Manning

Scott Marberry

Bobby Masocol, MD, FAAFP
Clinical Assistant Professor, Department of Family Medicine, Greenville Health System, University of South Carolina School of Medicine Greenville
Greenville, SC

Todd May

Christopher McGrew, MD
Director, Primary Care Sports Medicine Fellowship
Professor, Department of Family and Community Medicine
Professor, Department of Orthopedics and Rehabilitation
University of New Mexico Health Sciences Center
Assistant Team Physician, University of New Mexico
Albuquerque, NM

Jonathan D. McKrell, MD
Associate Director, Heritage Valley Family Medicine Residency Program
Beaver Falls, PA

Christopher M. Miles, MD
Associate Program Director, Sports Medicine Fellowship
Assistant Professor, Department of Family and Community Medicine
Wake Forest University School of Medicine
Winston-Salem, NC

David Millward, MD, MSc
Assistant Head Team Physician
Clinical Assistant Professor, Family and Community Medicine
The University of Arizona
Tucson, AZ

Jason A. Mogonye, MD
Assistant Program Director, JPS Sports Medicine Fellowship
Arlington, TX
Team Physician, TCU
Fort Worth, TX

Guy W. Nicolette, MD, CAQSM
Director, Sports Medicine Fellowship
Director, Student Health Services
University of Florida
Gainesville, FL

Richard A. Okragly, MD
Director, TriHealth Primary Care Sports Medicine Fellowship
Team Physician, Xavier University and Mount St. Joseph University
Cincinnati, OH

Luis Palacio

Stacey Pappas, MD, CAQSM
Staff Physician, University of Rhode Island Health Services
Team Physician, University of Rhode Island
Kingston, RI
Ringside Physician, USA Boxing
Colorado Springs, CO
Assistant Clinical Professor, Department of Family Medicine, Brown University
Providence, RI

Stephen R. Paul, MD, CAQSM, MA
Associate Professor, Department of Family and Community Medicine
Assistant Professor, Department of Orthopedics
Assistant Team Physician, Intercollegiate Athletics
Coordinator for Sports Medicine, Campus Health Service
The University of Arizona
Tucson, AZ

Jennifer Payne

Bernadette Pendergraph, MD
Sports Medicine Fellowship Director, Harbor-UCLA/Team to Win Sports Medicine Fellowship
Torrance, CA
Associate Professor, Department of Family Medicine, David Geffen School of Medicine
Los Angeles, CA

Ryan Petering

Ziva Petrin, MD
Salt Lake City, UT

Thomas L. Pommering, DO, FAAFP
Team Physician, Ohio Dominican University
Division Chief for Sports Medicine, Nationwide Children's Hospital
Associate Professor, Departments of Pediatrics and Family Medicine, The Ohio State University College of Medicine
Columbus, OH

Jason Pothast

George G.A. Pujalte, MD, FACSM
Vice Chair for Academics, Department of Family Medicine
Associate Program Director, Mayo Clinic Florida Sports Medicine Fellowship Program
Assistant Professor
Mayo Clinic College of Medicine and Science
Consultant, Family Medicine and Sports Medicine, Mayo Clinic
Jacksonville, FL
Team Physician, USA Taekwondo

Scott E. Rand, MD, FAAFP, CAQSM
Director, Primary Care Sports Medicine Fellowship, Houston Methodist Orthopedics and Sports Medicine
Houston, TX

Edward Reisman, MD, CAQSM
Program Director, Sports Medicine Fellowship Spokane
Activity Sports and Exercise Medicine, Kaiser Permanente Spokane
Clinical Assistant Professor, University of Washington Department of Family Medicine
Team Physician, Whitworth University
Spokane, WA

Mark F. Riederer, MD
Clinical Assistant Professor of Pediatrics and Orthopaedic Surgery, University of Michigan, Michigan Medicine
Ann Arbor, MI

Jeff Roberts, MD, CAQSM, FAAFP
Program Director, VCU-St. Francis Primary Care Sports Medicine Fellowship Program
Associate Clinical Professor, VCU Department of Family Medicine and Population Health
St. Francis Family Medicine Center and Residency Program
Bon Secours Sports Medicine
Midlothian, VA

Richard E. Rodenberg, MD
Program Director, Sports Medicine Fellowship, Nationwide Children's Hospital
Associate Professor of Pediatrics, The Ohio State University College of Medicine
Columbus, OH

David S. Ross, MD
Director, Geisinger Northeast Primary Care Sports Medicine Fellowship
Clinical Professor, Geisinger Commonwealth School of Medicine
Wilkes-Barre, PA

Jack Spittler, MD, MS
Associate Director, Sports Medicine Fellowship
Assistant Professor, Family Medicine and Orthopedics
University of Colorado
Denver, CO

Siobhan M. Statuta, MD
Team Physician, UVA Sports Medicine
Director, Primary Care Sports Medicine Fellowship
Associate Professor, Departments of Family Medicine and Physical Medicine & Rehabilitation
University of Virginia Health System
Charlottesville, VA

Mark Stovak, MD
Professor, University of Nevada, Reno School of Medicine, Department of Family & Community Medicine
Team Physician, University of Nevada, Reno Athletics
Reno, NV

Irvin Sulapas, MD, FAAFP
Assistant Professor, Department of Family & Community Medicine, Baylor College of Medicine
Houston, TX

Poonam P. Thaker, MD, FACSM
Program Director, Sports Medicine Fellowship
Associate Program Director, Family Medicine Residency
AMITA Health Resurrection Medical Center
Chicago, IL

Saif Usman, MD, FAAFP
Sports Medicine, Facey Medical Group
Valencia, CA

Marissa S. Vasquez, MD, MBA, CAQSM, FAAFP
Program Director, Sports Medicine Fellowship
Division of Sports Medicine Physician in Charge
Kaiser Permanente Los Angeles Medical Center
Clinical Instructor, UCLA-Family Medicine
Team Physician, Occidental College
Los Angeles, CA

Gerardo Vazquez, MD
Assistant Professor, CAQ Sports Medicine
Assistant Program Director, Family Medicine Residency
TTUHSC-El Paso
El Paso, TX

Anna L. Waterbrook, MD, FACEP, CAQSM
Associate Professor, Department of Emergency Medicine
Associate Program Director, South Campus Residency Program
Associate Program Director, Sports Medicine Fellowship
Assistant Team Physician, Intercollegiate Athletics
The University of Arizona
Tucson, AZ

David Webner, MD
Director, Sports Medicine Fellowship, Crozer-Keystone Health System
Adjunct Associate Professor, Drexel University College of Medicine
Team Physician, Widener University
Philadelphia, PA

David N. Westerdahl, MD, FAAFP, RMSK
PMG Bridgeport Sports Medicine
Tigard, OR

Jason P. Womack, MD
Assistant Professor, Department of Family Medicine & Community Health
Director, Sports Medicine Fellowship
Rutgers University – Robert Wood Johnson Medical School
Rutgers Athletics Assistant Team Physician
New Brunswick, NJ

Justin M. Wright, MD
Associate Professor, Department of Family and Community Medicine
Program Director, Sports Medicine Fellowship Program
Program Director, Family Medicine Residency Program
Texas Tech University Health Sciences Center – El Paso
El Paso, TX

Velyn Wu, MD, FAAFP
Assistant Director, Sports Medicine
Lynchburg Family Medicine Residency Program
Centra Medical Group
Team Physician, Sweet Briar College
Team Physician, Lynchburg Hillcats – Cleveland Indians High A
Lynchburg, VA

Craig C. Young, MD
Professor of Orthopaedic Surgery & Community and Family Medicine, Medical College of Wisconsin
Milwaukee, WI
Team Physician, Milwaukee Brewers, Milwaukee Bucks, Milwaukee Ballet, US Ski & Snowboard

Jason L. Zaremski, MD, CAQSM, FACSM, FAAPMR
Associate Professor, Divisions of PM&R, Sports Medicine, and Research
Co-Medical Director, Adolescent and High School Sports Medicine Outreach Program
Department of Orthopaedics and Rehabilitation, UF Health, University of Florida College of Medicine
Gainesville, FL

About the Case Study Contributors

CASE STUDY AUTHORS

Annie Casta, MD, FAAFP
Nonoperative Orthopedic Specialist, Nicklaus Children's Hospital
Miami, FL

Jeremy L. Coleman, MD, CAQSM
Assistant Professor, Primary Care Sports Medicine, University of Florida College of Medicine – Jacksonville
Jacksonville, FL

Mark DeFord, MD
Sports Medicine Fellow, Kettering Medical Center
Kettering, OH

Marcia Faustin, MD, CAQSM
Associate Physician Primary Care Network and Department of Sports Medicine, University of California
Davis, CA

Jeffrey Ham, DO
Fellow, Sports Medicine, Atrium Health
Belmont, NC

Adam Lyons, MD
Department of Family Medicine and Community Health, Hospital of the University of Pennsylvania
Philadelphia, PA

Carrie Miller, MD
Resident, Physical Medicine and Rehabilitation, Medical College of Wisconsin
Milwaukee, WI

Matthew Negaard, MD
Resident, Department of Emergency Medicine, University of Iowa Hospitals and Clinics
Iowa City, IA

Rathna Nuti, MD
Texas Metroplex Institute for Sports Medicine and Orthopedic Surgery
Arlington, TX

Richard Pearson, MD
Metro Health – University of Michigan Health
Wyoming, MI

Valerie Rygiel, DO
Fellow, Sports Medicine, University of Chicago
Chicago, IL

Yaqoob Syed, DO
Primary Care Sports Medicine, Northwest Community Healthcare
Arlington Heights, IL

Trent Tamate, MD
Orthopedic Surgery Resident, University of Hawai'i
Honolulu, HI

Aaron Tracy, MD, MHMS
Resident Physician, Department of Family and Community Medicine, The University of Texas Health Science Center at Houston
Houston, TX

Eri Yamaguchi, BA
John A. Burns School of Medicine, University of Hawai'i
Honolulu, HI

Jason L. Zaremski, MD, CAQSM, FACSM, FAAPMR
Associate Professor, Divisions of PM&R, Sports Medicine, and Research
Co-Medical Director, Adolescent and High School Sports Medicine Outreach Program
Department of Orthopaedics and Rehabilitation, UF Health, University of Florida College of Medicine
Gainesville, FL

CASE STUDY EDITORS

Namita Bhardway, MD
Assistant Professor and Director of Sports Medicine, Department of Family Medicine
Clinical Assistant Professor, Department of Orthopaedics and Rehabilitation
The University of Texas Medical Branch
Galveston, TX

Rebecca L Carl, MD, MSCI
Assistant Professor of Pediatrics, Northwestern Feinberg School of Medicine
Ann & Robert H. Lurie Children's Hospital of Chicago

Christian Fulmer, DO
Clinical Assistant Professor, Division of Primary Care and Population Health, Department of Medicine, Stanford University School of Medicine
Palo Alto, CA

Mandeep Ghuman, MD
Director, Dignity Health Primary Care Sports Medicine Fellowship Program
Northridge, CA

Margaret E. Gibson, MD, CAQSM
Associate Professor, Department of Community and Family Medicine, TMC Lakewood
UMKC Sports Medicine Fellowship Program Director
University of Missouri
Department of Orthopedics, Children's Mercy Hospital and Clinics
Kansas City, MO

Benjamin Hasan, MD
Family and Sports Medicine, NCH Medical Group
Rolling Hills, IL

Michael Henehan, DO
Adjunct Clinical Professor, Division of Primary Care and Population Health, Department of Medicine, Stanford University School of Medicine
Palo Alto, CA

Marc P. Hilgers, MD, PhD, FAAFP
Medical Director, Sports Medicine, Advocate Aurora Health
Aurora, IL

Kristine Karlson, MD, FACSM
Associate Professor, Community and Family Medicine and Orthopaedics, Geisel School of Medicine at Dartmouth
Lebanon, NH

Adam Lewno, DO
Assistant Professor, University of Michigan
Ann Arbor, MI

Rebecca Martinie, MD
Assistant Professor, Baylor College of Medicine
Attending Physician, Texas Children's Urgent Care
Houston, TX

Charlie Michaudet, MD, CAQSM
Clinical Assistant Professor, Department of Community Health and Family Medicine, University of Florida
Gainesville, FL

Caitlyn Mooney, MD
Adjunct Professor, University of Texas at San Antonio, Pediatrics
San Antonio, TX

Eric Schub, DO
Fellow, Sports Medicine, Dignity Health Primary Care Sports Medicine Fellowship
Northridge, CA

Kelly Wilkinson, MD
Sports Medicine, Primary Health Medical Group
Boise, ID

Tracy Zaslow, MD
Director, Children's Orthopaedic Center (COC) Sports Concussion Program
Medical Director, COC Sports Medicine Program
Children's Hospital Los Angeles
Los Angeles, CA

Index

Note: Question numbers are denoted using the test number (1 or 2) and sequence number (1 through 200), as follows: 1-1, 1-2, 2-1, 2-2, etc. Each question number is followed in parentheses by the two page numbers that the question appears on (i.e., the page number of the question, and the page number of the answer, critique, and references).

Abdominal trauma, liver, 1-17 (18, 189)
Abdominal trauma, spleen, 1-18 (19, 191)
Abdominal wall muscle strain, 1-16 (18, 188)
Abnormal ECG, 2-121 (138, 532)
Achilles tendinopathy, 2-171 (160, 589)
Achilles tendinopathy, rehabilitation, 1-5 (14, 177), 2-5 (93, 402)
ACL, rehabilitation, neuromuscular training, 2-72 (118, 477)
ACL tear, risk factors, 2-150 (150, 563)
ACL tear, Segond fracture, 2-163 (157, 580)
Acute compartment syndrome, 1-193 (87, 387)
Acute mountain sickness, 1-152 (73, 342), 1-194 (88, 389), 2-156 (153, 570)
Adductor strain, treatment, 2-188 (166, 606)
Adhesive capsulitis, 2-118 (137, 528)
Altitude, 1-49 (30, 225), 1-171 (79, 361), 2-192 (168, 611)
Altitude, conditioning and training, 1-50 (30, 226)
Amenorrhea, 2-183 (164, 601)
Anaerobic exercise, 2-92 (127, 501)
Anaphylaxis, 1-191 (86, 385), 2-53 (111, 456)
Anatomy, blood supply, knee, 2-89 (126, 498)
Anatomy, cervical spine, 1-179 (82, 370)
Anatomy, forearm, intersection syndrome, 1-178 (81, 369)
Anatomy, hamstring, 1-154 (74, 344)
Anatomy, hip-pelvis, 1-177 (81, 368)
Anatomy, lower leg, 1-159 (75, 349), 2-90 (126, 499)
Anatomy, muscle fiber type, 1-143 (70, 333)
Anatomy, nerve, C6, 1-148 (72, 338)
Anatomy, nerve, lumbar radiculopathy, 1-151 (73, 341)
Anatomy, nerve, suprascapular, 1-174 (80, 365)
Anatomy, patella, 2-79 (122, 486)
Anatomy, pectoralis muscle, 1-149 (72, 339)

Anatomy, posterior-lateral corner, 2-41 (107, 442)
Anatomy, quadrilateral space, 1-140 (70, 330)
Anatomy, ulnar collateral ligament, elbow, 2-94 (127, 503)
Anatomy, ultrasound, biceps tendon, 2-77 (120, 482)
Anatomy, ultrasound, hip, 2-88 (126, 497)
Anemia, hepatitis, 2-139 (146, 551)
Anemia, iron deficiency, 1-122 (60, 308)
Anemia, physiologic, 1-123 (61, 309)
Ankle, rehabilitation, 2-3 (92, 400), 2-4 (92, 401)
Ankle sprain, syndesmotic sprain, 1-121 (60, 307)
Aortic stenosis, 1-68 (36, 244)
Apophysitis, AIIS, 1-76 (40, 254)
Apophysitis, calcaneal (Sever's disease), 2-83 (124, 491)
Apophysitis, Iselin's disease, 2-78 (121, 484)
Apophysitis, medial elbow, 1-147 (72, 337)
Arrhythmogenic right ventricular dysplasia, 1-69 (37, 245), 2-112 (135, 522)
Asthma, 2-124 (140, 536)
Asthma, exercise-induced, 1-82 (43, 262), 1-89 (46, 271), 2-181 (164, 599)
Athletic heart syndrome, 2-114 (136, 524), 2-147 (149, 560)
Atlantoaxial instability, Down syndrome, 2-54 (111, 457)
Atrial septal defect, 1-73 (39, 251)
Autonomic dysreflexia, 1-55 (32, 231), 2-107 (133, 517), 2-126 (141, 538)
Back, scoliosis, 1-119 (59, 305), 2-14 (96, 411)
Battle's sign, 1-187 (85, 381)
Biomechanics, barefoot running, 1-175 (80, 366)
Biomechanics, patella function, 2-111 (134, 521)
Biomechanics, posterior corner, knee, 1-176 (81, 367)
Biomechanics, throwing motion, 1-162 (76, 352), 2-74 (119, 479)
Blunt abdominal trauma, liver, 1-17 (18, 189)
Blunt abdominal trauma, splenic rupture, 1-18 (19, 191), 2-48 (109, 449)
Blunt ocular trauma, 2-62 (115, 465)
Brugada syndrome, 2-117 (137, 527)
Cardiac contusion, 1-12 (16, 184)
Cardiac output, 2-86 (125, 495)
Carpal tunnel syndrome, 2-31 (102, 430)
Casting, distal radius fracture, 1-185 (84, 378)
Cervical neuropraxia, 1-10 (16, 182), 1-11 (16, 183), 2-175 (161, 593), 2-184 (165, 602)
Cervical spine, anatomy, 1-179 (82, 370)
Cervical spine injury, sideline management, 1-199 (90, 394)
Child abuse, 2-27 (100, 425)

Chronic exertional compartment syndrome, 1-108 (54, 291), 1-138 (69, 326), 2-42 (107, 443), 2-47 (109, 448)
Commotio cordis, 1-197 (89, 392), 2-55 (112, 458)
Complex regional pain syndrome, 2-68 (117, 472)
Concussion, 1-195 (88, 390)
Concussion, oculomotor, 2-59 (113, 462)
Concussion, risk factor, 2-10 (94, 407)
Conditioning and training, cardiorespiratory, 1-50 (30, 226)
Conditioning and training, intensity, 1-46 (29, 222)
Conditioning and training, periodization, 2-191 (167, 610)
Conditioning and training, stretching, 1-47 (29, 223)
Conditioning and training, weight training, 1-48 (30, 224)
Congenital coronary artery anomalies, 1-77 (40, 255)
Corticosteroids, 2-45 (108, 446)
Creatine, pharmacology, 1-166 (78, 356)
Cystic fibrosis, 1-67 (35, 243)
De Quervain's tenosynovitis, 2-34 (103, 433)
Decompression sickness, 2-130 (142, 542)
Delayed onset muscle soreness, 2-101 (129, 510)
Dental trauma, 2-11 (95, 408)
Depression, 1-129 (64, 317)
Depression, medication drug testing, 2-127 (141, 539)
Depression, reactive, 1-43 (28, 219)
Dermatologic, bacterial infection, 1-118 (59, 304)
Dermatologic, exercise-induced urticaria, 2-132 (143, 544)
Dermatologic, herpes gladiatorum, 2-141 (147, 553)
Dermatologic, lacerations, 1-105 (52, 28), 1-106 (53, 289)
Dermatologic, molluscum contagiousum, 1-116 (58, 301)
Dermatologic, MRSA (methicillin-resistant staph aureus), 2-142 (147, 554)
Dermatologic, nail, 1-104 (52, 287)
Dermatologic, tinea capitis, 1-110 (54, 294)
Dermatologic, tinea corporis, 1-111 (55, 295)
Diabetes, exercise, 1-57 (32, 233), 1-200 (90, 395), 2-108 (133, 518), 2-137 (145, 549), 2-155 (152, 569)
Diabetes, medication side effect, 1-133 (66, 321)
Down syndrome, atlantoaxial instability, 2-54 (111, 457)
Down syndrome, preparticipation exam, 1-45 (29, 221), 2-186 (166, 604), 2-187 (166, 605)
Drug testing, 2-70 (118, 474), 2-109 (133, 519)
Drug testing, depression medication, 2-127 (141, 539)
Ehlers-Danlos, clearance, 1-40 (27, 216)
Elbow, ulnar collateral ligament, 1-31 (23, 205)

Elbow, valgus extension overload, 1-30 (23, 204)
Electrocardiogram, prolonged QT, 2-116 (136, 526)
Emergency assessment and care, witnessed collapse, 2-195 (169, 614)
Environmental, thermoregulation, 2-82 (124, 490)
Epicondylitis, medial, 2-23 (99, 421)
Epidemiology, marathon mortality, 1-61 (33, 237)
Epidemiology, pediatric injuries, 1-64 (34, 240)
Event administration, inclement weather, 1-62 (34, 238)
Event administration, mass casualties, 1-63 (34, 239)
Exercise, diabetes, 1-57 (32, 233), 1-200 (90, 395), 2-108 (133, 518), 2-137 (145, 549)
Exercise, osteoporosis, 1-59 (33, 235)
Exercise, pediatric strength training, 1-92 (47, 274)
Exercise, pregnancy, 1-58 (33, 234), 2-133 (143, 545)
Exercise, training response, 1-107 (53, 290)
Exercise-induced anaphylaxis, 2-50 (110, 451)
Exercise-induced asthma, 1-82 (43, 262), 1-89 (46, 271), 2-181 (164, 599)
Exercise-induced bronchospasm, 1-82 (43, 262), 1-89 (46, 271)
Exercise-induced urticaria, 2-132 (143, 544)
Exercise physiology, muscle regeneration, 2-84 (124, 492)
Exercise physiology, muscle, 1-172 (79, 362)
Exercise physiology, respiratory system, 1-173 (80, 364)
Exercise prescription, 1-54 (31, 230)
Exercise prescription, obesity, 1-56 (32, 232)
Exercise response, HIV, 2-80 (122, 487)
Exertional headache, 2-100 (129, 509)
Exertional heat stroke, 1-189 (86, 383), 2-57 (113, 460), 2-131 (143, 543)
Exertional rhabdomyolysis, 1-96 (49, 279), 1-101 (51, 284)
Eye, blunt ocular trauma, 2-62 (115, 465)
Female athlete triad, 2-44 (108, 445), 2-125 (140, 537), 2-182 (164, 600)
Femoral acetabular impingement, 1-84 (44, 264)
Femoral stress fracture, 2-158 (154, 572)
Fracture, ankle, Weber classification, 2-169 (159, 587)
Fracture, avulsion ASIS, 1-132 (66, 320)
Fracture, avulsion ischial tuberosity, 1-144 (71, 334)
Fracture, avulsion medial epicondyle, 2-87 (125, 496)
Fracture, avulsion rectus femoris, 1-124 (61, 310)
Fracture, avulsion tibial tubercle, 2-85 (125, 493)
Fracture, calcaneal apophysitis, 1-139 (69, 328)
Fracture, distal radius, 1-33 (24, 208), 2-81 (123, 488)
Fracture, distal radius, casting, 1-185 (84, 378)
Fracture, femoral neck, 1-1 (12, 172)

Fracture, femoral stress, 2-158 (154, 572)
Fracture, femur, giant cell tumor, 2-39 (106, 439)
Fracture, humeral neck, 2-16 (96, 413)
Fracture, mallet finger, 1-34 (25, 209), 2-28 (101, 426)
Fracture, metacarpal, 1-32 (24, 206)
Fracture, patellar sleeve, 2-40 (107, 441)
Fracture, pubic rami stress, 1-86 (45, 267)
Fracture, radius, bowed, 2-21 (98, 418)
Fracture, Salter-Harris classification, 1-156 (74, 346), 2-97 (128, 506)
Fracture, Segond, ACL tear, 2-163 (157, 580)
Fracture, sesamoid, 2-170 (160, 588)
Fracture, skull, 2-9 (94, 406)
Fracture, stress, rib, 2-12 (95, 409)
Fracture, stress, tibia, 1-102 (51, 285)
Fracture, supracondylar (median nerve injury), 1-28 (22, 201)
Fracture, tarsal navicular, 1-157 (75, 347)
Fracture, tibial plateau, 1-163 (77, 353)
Fracture, tibial stress, 2-13 (95, 410)
Gastrointestinal, GERD (gastroesophageal reflux disease), 2-144 (148, 556)
Hamstring, rehabilitation, 1-6 (14, 178)
Hamstring strain, 1-87 (45, 269), 2-159 (155, 575)
Head injury, 1-9 (15, 181)
Head trauma, Battle's sign, 1-187 (85, 381)
Headache, exertional, 2-100 (129, 509)
Heat acclimation, pediatric, 2-194 (168, 613)
Herpes gladiatorum, 2-141 (147, 553)
High altitude cerebral edema, 2-129 (142, 541)
High ankle sprain, syndesmotic sprain, 1-121 (60, 307)
Hip, labral tear, 2-161 (155, 577)
Hip, septic arthritis, 2-136 (144, 548)
Hip, transient osteoporosis, 2-36 (104, 435)
Hip flexors, 2-160 (155, 576)
HIV (human immunodeficiency virus), 1-135 (67, 323), 2-152 (151, 565), 2-157 (153, 571)
HSV (herpes simplex virus), 1-115 (57, 300), 1-145 (71, 335)
Human growth hormone (hGH), 1-168 (78, 358)
Hydration, 1-75 (39, 253)
Hypertension, 1-38 (26, 214), 1-180 (82, 371), 2-91 (126, 500), 2-146 (149, 558), 2-198 (170, 617)
Hypertension, pharmacology, 2-91 (126, 500)
Hypertension, preparticipation exam, 2-198 (170, 617)
Hypertension, youth, 1-38 (26, 214)

Hypertrophic cardiomyopathy (HOCM), 1-71 (38, 249), 1-78 (40, 256), 2-119 (137, 530)
Hyphema, 1-186 (85, 379), 2-8 (94, 405), 2-58 (113, 461)
Iliotibial band syndrome, 1-90 (46, 272), 2-165 (158, 583)
Infectious mononucleosis, 1-141 (70, 331), 2-135 (144, 547), 2-180 (163, 598)
Injection technique, 1-181 (82, 373), 1-182 (83, 374)
Injury prevention, 1-60 (33, 236), 1-65 (35, 241)
Intersection syndrome, 1-35 (25, 210), 1-178 (81, 369), 2-33 (103, 432)
Iselin's disease, 2-78 (121, 484)
Juvenile idiopathic arthritis, 1-125 (61, 311)
Ketogenic diet, 2-98 (129, 507)
Kienbock's disease, 2-71 (118, 475)
Knee, biomechanics, 1-113 (56, 298)
Knee, dislocated patella, 2-166 (158, 584)
Knee, meniscus, 1-155 (74, 345), 2-168 (159, 586)
Knee, patellofemoral pain syndrome, 1-4 (13, 176), 1-7 (15, 179), 1-94 (49, 277), 2-7 (93, 404)
Knee, popliteus tendinopathy, 1-161 (76, 351)
Knee, posterior lateral complex, 1-98 (50, 281)
Knee aspiration, intraarticular fracture, 2-46 (109, 447)
Knee dislocation, 1-196 (88, 391), 2-61 (114, 464), 2-164 (157, 582)
Laceration repair, 2-154 (152, 567)
Laryngotracheal injury, 2-49 (109, 450)
Legg-Calve-Perthes disease, 1-136 (68, 324)
Little League shoulder, 1-130 (64, 318), 2-15 (96, 412)
Liver, abdominal trauma, 1-17 (18, 189)
Long QT syndrome, 1-81 (43, 261)
Low back pain, 1-19 (19, 192), 1-22 (20, 195)
Lyme disease, 1-137 (68, 325), 2-153 (151, 566)
Marfan syndrome, 1-79 (41, 257)
Marfan syndrome, preparticipation exam, 1-72 (38, 250), 2-120 (138, 531), 2-197 (169, 616)
Mobitz type II block, 1-70 (38, 247)
Molluscum contagiousum, 1-116 (58, 301)
Morton's neuroma, 1-117 (58, 303)
MRSA (methicillin-resistant staph aureus), 2-142 (147, 554)
Murmurs, 2-199 (170, 618)
Myocarditis, viral, 2-148 (149, 561)
Nerve, C6 anatomy, 1-148 (72, 338)
Nerve, entrapment syndromes, 2-173 (161, 591)
Nerve, median, 1-28 (22, 201), 1-103 (52, 286)
Nerve, obturator, 2-37 (105, 437)
Nerve, peroneal, 1-134 (67, 322), 2-155 (152, 569)
Nerve, posterior interosseous, 1-29 (23, 203), 2-25 (100, 423), 2-179 (163, 597)

Nerve, pudendal neuropathy, 1-100 (51, 283)
Nerve, quadrilateral space syndrome (axillary nerve), 1-24 (21, 197)
Nerve, radial tunnel, 1-184 (84, 377)
Nerve, roots, cervical spine, 2-93 (127, 502)
Nerve, saphenous, 1-114 (57, 299)
Nerve, suprascapular, 1-174 (80, 365), 2-66 (117, 470)
Nerve, tibial, 2-96 (128, 505)
Nerve, ulnar, 1-8 (15, 180), 1-164 (77, 354)
Nerve, ulnar tunnel syndrome, 2-65 (116, 469)
Neuropathy, pudendal, 1-100 (51, 283)
Neuropathy, ulnar, 2-24 (99, 422), 2-75 (119, 480)
NSAIDs, pharmacology, 1-165 (77, 355)
Nursemaid's elbow, radial head dislocation, 2-22 (99, 420)
Nutrition, bodybuilders, 1-53 (31, 229)
Osteitis pubis, 1-170 (79, 360), 2-162 (156, 578)
Osteoarthritis, 2-145 (148, 557)
Osteochondritis dissecans, 1-128 (63, 316), 2-76 (120, 481)
Osteochondritis dissecans, patella, 2-76 (120, 481)
Osteoid osteoma, 1-112 (56, 297)
Osteonecrosis, Kienbock's disease, 2-71 (118, 475)
Overtraining syndrome, 1-142 (70, 332), 2-128 (141, 540), 2-189 (167, 607), 2-190 (167, 609), 2-195 (169, 614)
Overtraining syndrome, burnout, 2-196 (169, 615)
Overuse injuries, risk factors, 2-43 (108, 444)
Overuse injuries, sport specialization, 1-36 (26, 212)
Panner's disease (osteochondrosis capitellum), 2-73 (119, 478)
Parsonage-Turner syndrome, 1-25 (21, 198), 2-19 (97, 416)
Patellofemoral pain dysfunction, 1-4 (13, 176), 1-7 (15, 179), 1-94 (49, 277), 2-7 (93, 404)
Patellofemoral pain syndrome, rehabilitation, 2-7 (93, 404)
Pediatric, bone growth, 2-95 (128, 504)
Pediatric, heat acclimation, 2-194 (168, 613)
Pediatric, thermoregulation, 1-146 (71, 336)
Pediatric bone, 2-102 (130, 511)
Pediatric strength training, 1-92 (47, 274), 2-69 (117, 473), 2-193 (168, 612)
Performance-enhancing drugs, caffeine, 2-110 (134, 520)
Perilunate dissociation, 2-29 (101, 428)
Pharmacology, creatine, 1-166 (78, 356)
Pharmacology, hypertension, 2-91 (126, 500)
Pharmacology, NSAIDs, 1-165 (77, 355)
Piriformis syndrome, 1-167 (78, 357)
Plantar fasciitis, 1-120 (60, 306)

Plica syndrome, 1-95 (49, 278), 2-167 (159, 585)
Pneumothorax, 1-192 (87, 386), 2-56 (112, 459)
Popliteal artery entrapment syndrome, 1-158 (75, 348), 2-105 (131, 514)
Popliteus, tendinopathy, 1-161 (76, 351)
Posterior cruciate ligament, 1-97 (50, 280), 1-160 (76, 350)
Posterior tibialis tendon dysfunction, 1-109 (54, 292)
Pregnancy, exercise, 1-58 (33, 234), 1-150 (73, 340), 2-133 (143, 545)
Preparticipation exam, administration, 1-37 (26, 213), 1-44 (28, 220)
Preparticipation exam, cardiovascular, 1-74 (39, 252), 2-115 (136, 525), 2-116 (136, 526)
Preparticipation exam, Down syndrome, 1-45 (29, 221), 2-186 (166, 604), 2-187 (166, 605)
Preparticipation exam, Ehlers-Danlos clearance, 1-40 (27, 216)
Preparticipation exam, hypertension, 2-198 (170, 617)
Preparticipation exam, Marfan syndrome, 1-72 (38, 250), 2-120 (138, 531), 2-197 (169, 616)
Preparticipation exam, paired organs, 1-66 (35, 242), 2-177 (162, 595)
Preparticipation exam, paired organs, solitary kidney, 2-178 (163, 596)
Preparticipation exam, paired organs, solitary testicle, 2-176 (162, 594)
Preparticipation exam, scuba, 2-185 (165, 603)
Preparticipation exam, seizure disorder, 1-39 (27, 215), 2-174 (161, 592)
Preparticipation exam, splenic enlargement, 1-42 (28, 218)
Preparticipation exam, sport demands, 2-67 (117, 471)
Preparticipation exam, vision, 1-41 (27, 217), 2-26 (100, 424), 2-200 (170, 619)
Pubic rami stress fractures, 1-86 (45, 267)
Pudendal neuropathy, 1-100 (51, 283)
Pulmonary contusion, 1-14 (17, 186)
Radial head dislocation, nursemaid's elbow, 2-22 (99, 420)
Radial tunnel, 1-184 (84, 377)
Rectal bleeding, 1-91 (47, 273)
Rehabilitation, Achilles tendon, 2-5 (93, 402)
Rehabilitation, ACL, neuromuscular training, 2-72 (118, 477)
Rehabilitation, ankle, 2-3 (92, 400), 2-4 (92, 401)
Rehabilitation, patellofemoral pain syndrome, 2-7 (93, 404)
Rehabilitation, scapulothoracic dyskinesia, 2-6 (93, 403)
Relative energy deficiency in sport, 2-149 (150, 562)
Renal, proteinuria, 1-99 (50, 282)
Rhabdomyolysis, 2-60 (114, 463)
Role of the team physician, 1-88 (45, 270), 2-63 (115, 466), 2-64 (116, 467)
Role of the team physician, medico-legal concerns, 1-85 (44, 265)
Salter-Harris classification, 1-156 (74, 346), 2-97 (128, 506)
Scapulothoracic dyskinesia, rehabilitation, 2-6 (93, 403)
Scoliosis, 1-119 (59, 305), 2-14 (96, 411)
Scuba, 2-99 (129, 508)

Scuba, middle ear barotrauma, 1-153 (73, 343)
Scuba, preparticipation exam, 2-185 (165, 603)
Seizure disorder, preparticipation exam, 1-39 (27, 215), 2-174 (161, 592)
Seizure disorder, sport participation, 2-172 (160, 590)
Shoulder, dislocation, 1-26 (21, 199), 1-183 (83, 375)
Shoulder, dislocation, posterior, 2-17 (97, 414)
Shoulder, impingement syndrome, 2-20 (98, 417)
Shoulder, SLAP, 1-27 (22, 200)
Shoulder, sleeper stretch, 1-2 (13, 174)
Shoulder, supraspinatus, 2-18 (97, 415)
Sickle cell trait, 2-138 (145, 550), 2-140 (146, 552)
Sinding-Larsen-Johannson, 1-93 (48, 275)
Skull fracture, 2-9 (94, 406)
Slipped capital epiphysis, 1-126 (62, 312)
Snapping hip, 2-38 (105, 438)
Spleen, abdominal trauma, 1-18 (19, 191), 2-48 (109, 449)
Splenic enlargement, preparticipation exam, 1-42 (28, 218)
Spondylolisthesis, 1-20 (19, 193), 2-106 (132, 515)
Spondylolysis, 1-3 (13, 175), 1-21 (20, 194), 1-23 (20, 196)
Spontaneous pneumothorax, 2-52 (111, 455)
Sport hernia, 1-15 (17, 187), 2-1 (92, 398)
Sport psychology, 1-127 (63, 314)
Sport specialization, overuse injuries, 1-36 (26, 212)
Stener lesion, 2-35 (104, 434)
Sternoclavicular dislocation, 1-13 (17, 185)
Strain, hamstring, 1-87 (45, 269)
Stretching, 1-169 (78, 359)
Subdural hematoma, 1-190 (86, 384)
Subungual hematoma, 2-30 (102, 429)
Sudden cardiac death, 2-113 (135, 523), 2-151 (151, 564)
Syncope, 1-198 (89, 393)
Syndesmotic sprain, high ankle sprain, 1-121 (60, 307)
Tarsal coalition, 2-103 (130, 512)
Tarsal tunnel syndrome, 2-104 (131, 513)
Tendinopathy, De Quervain's tenosynovitis, 2-34 (103, 433)
Tendinopathy, intersection syndrome, 2-33 (103, 432), 1-178 (81, 369)
Tendinopathy, popliteus, 1-161 (76, 351)
Tendinopathy, posterior tibialis tendon dysfunction, 1-109 (54, 292)
Tendon, hamstring, 2-2 (92, 399)
Testicular torsion, 1-188 (85, 382), 2-51 (110, 453), 2-143 (148, 555)
Tibial plateau fracture, 1-163 (77, 353)

Tibial stress fracture, 1-102 (51, 285), 2-13 (95, 410)
Tinea capitis, 1-110 (54, 294)
Tinea corporis, 1-111 (55, 295)
Triangular fibrocartilage complex, 2-32 (103, 431)
Ulnar collateral ligament, Stener lesion, 2-35 (104, 434)
Urinary incontinence, 2-134 (144, 546)
Vitamin C, 1-51 (31, 227)
Vitamin D, 1-52 (31, 228), 1-131 (65, 319)
Vocal cord dysfunction, 1-83 (43, 263), 2-123 (140, 535)
Wolff-Parkinson-White (WPW) syndrome, 1-80 (42, 259), 2-122 (139, 533)

Image Index

Note: Question numbers are denoted using the test number (1 or 2) and sequence number (1 through 200), as follows: 1-1, 1-2, 2-1, 2-2, etc. Each question number is followed inparentheses by the page number(s) that the image(s) appear on.

Erythema chronicum migrans; image, 1-137 (68, 325)
External rotation test, syndesmosis sprain—ankle; image, 1-121 (307)
Fracture, avulsion ASIS; x-ray, 1-132 (66, 320)
Fracture, distal radius; x-ray, 2-81 (123, 488)
Fracture, hip, tension-side; x-ray, 1-1 (12, 172)
Fracture, metacarpal neck; x-ray, 1-32 (24, 206)
Fracture, phalanx, mallet finger; x-ray, 2-28 (426)
Fracture, radius bowing; x-ray, 2-21 (98, 418)
Fracture, Segond; x-ray, 2-163 (580)
Fracture, stress, hip, tension-side; x-ray and MRI, 2-158 (154, 572-573)
Fracture, tibial shaft; x-ray, 1-193 (87, 387)
Giant cell tumor, femur; x-ray and MRI, 2-39 (106, 439)
Hyphema; image, 1-186 (85, 379)
Impetigo; image, 1-118 (59, 304)
Iselin's foot; x-ray, 2-78 (121, 484)
Kienbock's disease; MRI, 2-71 (475-476)
Laceration, scalp; image, 2-154 (152, 567)
Laceration, thigh; image, 1-106 (53, 289)
Methicillin staph aureus resistant (MRSA) abscess; image, 2-142 (147, 554)
Mobitz II; ECG, 1-70 (248)
Molluscum contagiosum; image, 1-116 (58, 301)
Muscle insertion greater trochanter; ultrasound, 2-88 (497)
Osteitis pubis widening; x-ray, 2-162 (156, 578)
Osteoid osteoma; x-ray, 1-112 (56, 297)
Pneumothorax; x-ray, 2-56 (112, 459)

Right ventricular dysplasia; ECG, 1-69 (37, 245)
Shoulder, anterior dislocation; x-ray, 1-183 (83, 375)
Shoulder, biceps tendon; ultrasound, 2-77 (120, 482)
Shoulder, SLAP lesion; MRI, 1-27 (22, 200)
Sinding-Larsen-Johansson, OCD inferior pole; x-ray, 1-93 (48, 275)
Slipped capital femoral epiphysis; x-ray, 1-126 (62, 312)
Spondylolisthesis; x-ray, 2-106 (132, 515-516)
Subungual hematoma; image, 2-30 (102, 429)
Tinea corporus; image, 1-111 (55, 295)
Transient osteoporosis of hip; x-ray, 2-36 (104, 435)
Wolff-Parkinson-White (WPW) syndrome; ECG, 1-80 (42, 259), 2-122 (139, 533)

Case Study Index

Cervical neuropraxia, 622-624
Exertional compartment syndrome, 625-627
Fracture, ischial tuberosity, 628-630
Fracture, tarso-navicular, 631-634
Fracture, tibial stress, 635-637
Head injury, intracranial pathology, 638-641
Heat stroke, 642-645
Hypertrophic cardiomyopathy (HOCM), 646-651
Knee dislocation, 652-655
Knee, posterolateral complex, 656-659
Osteoid osteoma, 660-664
Overuse injury, pediatrics, 665-668
Patellofemoral pain dysfunction, 669-672
Peroneal neuropathy, 673-677
Pneumothorax, 678-680
Rhabdomyolysis, 681-683

AMSSM Sports Medicine CAQ Study Guide Test 1 Answer Sheet

1. Ⓐ Ⓑ Ⓒ Ⓓ Ⓔ
2. Ⓐ Ⓑ Ⓒ Ⓓ Ⓔ
3. Ⓐ Ⓑ Ⓒ Ⓓ Ⓔ
4. Ⓐ Ⓑ Ⓒ Ⓓ Ⓔ
5. Ⓐ Ⓑ Ⓒ Ⓓ Ⓔ
6. Ⓐ Ⓑ Ⓒ Ⓓ Ⓔ
7. Ⓐ Ⓑ Ⓒ Ⓓ Ⓔ
8. Ⓐ Ⓑ Ⓒ Ⓓ Ⓔ
9. Ⓐ Ⓑ Ⓒ Ⓓ Ⓔ
10. Ⓐ Ⓑ Ⓒ Ⓓ Ⓔ
11. Ⓐ Ⓑ Ⓒ Ⓓ Ⓔ
12. Ⓐ Ⓑ Ⓒ Ⓓ Ⓔ
13. Ⓐ Ⓑ Ⓒ Ⓓ Ⓔ
14. Ⓐ Ⓑ Ⓒ Ⓓ Ⓔ
15. Ⓐ Ⓑ Ⓒ Ⓓ Ⓔ
16. Ⓐ Ⓑ Ⓒ Ⓓ Ⓔ
17. Ⓐ Ⓑ Ⓒ Ⓓ Ⓔ
18. Ⓐ Ⓑ Ⓒ Ⓓ Ⓔ
19. Ⓐ Ⓑ Ⓒ Ⓓ Ⓔ
20. Ⓐ Ⓑ Ⓒ Ⓓ Ⓔ
21. Ⓐ Ⓑ Ⓒ Ⓓ Ⓔ
22. Ⓐ Ⓑ Ⓒ Ⓓ Ⓔ
23. Ⓐ Ⓑ Ⓒ Ⓓ Ⓔ
24. Ⓐ Ⓑ Ⓒ Ⓓ Ⓔ
25. Ⓐ Ⓑ Ⓒ Ⓓ Ⓔ
26. Ⓐ Ⓑ Ⓒ Ⓓ Ⓔ
27. Ⓐ Ⓑ Ⓒ Ⓓ Ⓔ
28. Ⓐ Ⓑ Ⓒ Ⓓ Ⓔ
29. Ⓐ Ⓑ Ⓒ Ⓓ Ⓔ
30. Ⓐ Ⓑ Ⓒ Ⓓ Ⓔ
31. Ⓐ Ⓑ Ⓒ Ⓓ Ⓔ
32. Ⓐ Ⓑ Ⓒ Ⓓ Ⓔ
33. Ⓐ Ⓑ Ⓒ Ⓓ Ⓔ
34. Ⓐ Ⓑ Ⓒ Ⓓ Ⓔ
35. Ⓐ Ⓑ Ⓒ Ⓓ Ⓔ
36. Ⓐ Ⓑ Ⓒ Ⓓ Ⓔ
37. Ⓐ Ⓑ Ⓒ Ⓓ Ⓔ
38. Ⓐ Ⓑ Ⓒ Ⓓ Ⓔ
39. Ⓐ Ⓑ Ⓒ Ⓓ Ⓔ
40. Ⓐ Ⓑ Ⓒ Ⓓ Ⓔ
41. Ⓐ Ⓑ Ⓒ Ⓓ Ⓔ
42. Ⓐ Ⓑ Ⓒ Ⓓ Ⓔ
43. Ⓐ Ⓑ Ⓒ Ⓓ Ⓔ
44. Ⓐ Ⓑ Ⓒ Ⓓ Ⓔ
45. Ⓐ Ⓑ Ⓒ Ⓓ Ⓔ
46. Ⓐ Ⓑ Ⓒ Ⓓ Ⓔ
47. Ⓐ Ⓑ Ⓒ Ⓓ Ⓔ
48. Ⓐ Ⓑ Ⓒ Ⓓ Ⓔ
49. Ⓐ Ⓑ Ⓒ Ⓓ Ⓔ
50. Ⓐ Ⓑ Ⓒ Ⓓ Ⓔ
51. Ⓐ Ⓑ Ⓒ Ⓓ Ⓔ
52. Ⓐ Ⓑ Ⓒ Ⓓ Ⓔ
53. Ⓐ Ⓑ Ⓒ Ⓓ Ⓔ
54. Ⓐ Ⓑ Ⓒ Ⓓ Ⓔ
55. Ⓐ Ⓑ Ⓒ Ⓓ Ⓔ
56. Ⓐ Ⓑ Ⓒ Ⓓ Ⓔ
57. Ⓐ Ⓑ Ⓒ Ⓓ Ⓔ
58. Ⓐ Ⓑ Ⓒ Ⓓ Ⓔ
59. Ⓐ Ⓑ Ⓒ Ⓓ Ⓔ
60. Ⓐ Ⓑ Ⓒ Ⓓ Ⓔ
61. Ⓐ Ⓑ Ⓒ Ⓓ Ⓔ
62. Ⓐ Ⓑ Ⓒ Ⓓ Ⓔ
63. Ⓐ Ⓑ Ⓒ Ⓓ Ⓔ
64. Ⓐ Ⓑ Ⓒ Ⓓ Ⓔ
65. Ⓐ Ⓑ Ⓒ Ⓓ Ⓔ
66. Ⓐ Ⓑ Ⓒ Ⓓ Ⓔ
67. Ⓐ Ⓑ Ⓒ Ⓓ Ⓔ
68. Ⓐ Ⓑ Ⓒ Ⓓ Ⓔ
69. Ⓐ Ⓑ Ⓒ Ⓓ Ⓔ
70. Ⓐ Ⓑ Ⓒ Ⓓ Ⓔ
71. Ⓐ Ⓑ Ⓒ Ⓓ Ⓔ
72. Ⓐ Ⓑ Ⓒ Ⓓ Ⓔ
73. Ⓐ Ⓑ Ⓒ Ⓓ Ⓔ
74. Ⓐ Ⓑ Ⓒ Ⓓ Ⓔ
75. Ⓐ Ⓑ Ⓒ Ⓓ Ⓔ
76. Ⓐ Ⓑ Ⓒ Ⓓ Ⓔ
77. Ⓐ Ⓑ Ⓒ Ⓓ Ⓔ
78. Ⓐ Ⓑ Ⓒ Ⓓ Ⓔ
79. Ⓐ Ⓑ Ⓒ Ⓓ Ⓔ
80. Ⓐ Ⓑ Ⓒ Ⓓ Ⓔ
81. Ⓐ Ⓑ Ⓒ Ⓓ Ⓔ
82. Ⓐ Ⓑ Ⓒ Ⓓ Ⓔ
83. Ⓐ Ⓑ Ⓒ Ⓓ Ⓔ
84. Ⓐ Ⓑ Ⓒ Ⓓ Ⓔ
85. Ⓐ Ⓑ Ⓒ Ⓓ Ⓔ
86. Ⓐ Ⓑ Ⓒ Ⓓ Ⓔ
87. Ⓐ Ⓑ Ⓒ Ⓓ Ⓔ
88. Ⓐ Ⓑ Ⓒ Ⓓ Ⓔ
89. Ⓐ Ⓑ Ⓒ Ⓓ Ⓔ
90. Ⓐ Ⓑ Ⓒ Ⓓ Ⓔ
91. Ⓐ Ⓑ Ⓒ Ⓓ Ⓔ
92. Ⓐ Ⓑ Ⓒ Ⓓ Ⓔ
93. Ⓐ Ⓑ Ⓒ Ⓓ Ⓔ
94. Ⓐ Ⓑ Ⓒ Ⓓ Ⓔ
95. Ⓐ Ⓑ Ⓒ Ⓓ Ⓔ
96. Ⓐ Ⓑ Ⓒ Ⓓ Ⓔ
97. Ⓐ Ⓑ Ⓒ Ⓓ Ⓔ
98. Ⓐ Ⓑ Ⓒ Ⓓ Ⓔ
99. Ⓐ Ⓑ Ⓒ Ⓓ Ⓔ
100. Ⓐ Ⓑ Ⓒ Ⓓ Ⓔ

A copy of this answer sheet can be downloaded at http://www.amssmstore.com/download/AnswerSheet.pdf

AMSSM Sports Medicine CAQ Study Guide Test 1 Answer Sheet

101. Ⓐ Ⓑ Ⓒ Ⓓ Ⓔ
102. Ⓐ Ⓑ Ⓒ Ⓓ Ⓔ
103. Ⓐ Ⓑ Ⓒ Ⓓ Ⓔ
104. Ⓐ Ⓑ Ⓒ Ⓓ Ⓔ
105. Ⓐ Ⓑ Ⓒ Ⓓ Ⓔ
106. Ⓐ Ⓑ Ⓒ Ⓓ Ⓔ
107. Ⓐ Ⓑ Ⓒ Ⓓ Ⓔ
108. Ⓐ Ⓑ Ⓒ Ⓓ Ⓔ
109. Ⓐ Ⓑ Ⓒ Ⓓ Ⓔ
110. Ⓐ Ⓑ Ⓒ Ⓓ Ⓔ
111. Ⓐ Ⓑ Ⓒ Ⓓ Ⓔ
112. Ⓐ Ⓑ Ⓒ Ⓓ Ⓔ
113. Ⓐ Ⓑ Ⓒ Ⓓ Ⓔ
114. Ⓐ Ⓑ Ⓒ Ⓓ Ⓔ
115. Ⓐ Ⓑ Ⓒ Ⓓ Ⓔ
116. Ⓐ Ⓑ Ⓒ Ⓓ Ⓔ
117. Ⓐ Ⓑ Ⓒ Ⓓ Ⓔ
118. Ⓐ Ⓑ Ⓒ Ⓓ Ⓔ
119. Ⓐ Ⓑ Ⓒ Ⓓ Ⓔ
120. Ⓐ Ⓑ Ⓒ Ⓓ Ⓔ
121. Ⓐ Ⓑ Ⓒ Ⓓ Ⓔ
122. Ⓐ Ⓑ Ⓒ Ⓓ Ⓔ
123. Ⓐ Ⓑ Ⓒ Ⓓ Ⓔ
124. Ⓐ Ⓑ Ⓒ Ⓓ Ⓔ
125. Ⓐ Ⓑ Ⓒ Ⓓ Ⓔ
126. Ⓐ Ⓑ Ⓒ Ⓓ Ⓔ
127. Ⓐ Ⓑ Ⓒ Ⓓ Ⓔ
128. Ⓐ Ⓑ Ⓒ Ⓓ Ⓔ
129. Ⓐ Ⓑ Ⓒ Ⓓ Ⓔ
130. Ⓐ Ⓑ Ⓒ Ⓓ Ⓔ
131. Ⓐ Ⓑ Ⓒ Ⓓ Ⓔ
132. Ⓐ Ⓑ Ⓒ Ⓓ Ⓔ
133. Ⓐ Ⓑ Ⓒ Ⓓ Ⓔ
134. Ⓐ Ⓑ Ⓒ Ⓓ Ⓔ

135. Ⓐ Ⓑ Ⓒ Ⓓ Ⓔ
136. Ⓐ Ⓑ Ⓒ Ⓓ Ⓔ
137. Ⓐ Ⓑ Ⓒ Ⓓ Ⓔ
138. Ⓐ Ⓑ Ⓒ Ⓓ Ⓔ
139. Ⓐ Ⓑ Ⓒ Ⓓ Ⓔ
140. Ⓐ Ⓑ Ⓒ Ⓓ Ⓔ
141. Ⓐ Ⓑ Ⓒ Ⓓ Ⓔ
142. Ⓐ Ⓑ Ⓒ Ⓓ Ⓔ
143. Ⓐ Ⓑ Ⓒ Ⓓ Ⓔ
144. Ⓐ Ⓑ Ⓒ Ⓓ Ⓔ
145. Ⓐ Ⓑ Ⓒ Ⓓ Ⓔ
146. Ⓐ Ⓑ Ⓒ Ⓓ Ⓔ
147. Ⓐ Ⓑ Ⓒ Ⓓ Ⓔ
148. Ⓐ Ⓑ Ⓒ Ⓓ Ⓔ
149. Ⓐ Ⓑ Ⓒ Ⓓ Ⓔ
150. Ⓐ Ⓑ Ⓒ Ⓓ Ⓔ
151. Ⓐ Ⓑ Ⓒ Ⓓ Ⓔ
152. Ⓐ Ⓑ Ⓒ Ⓓ Ⓔ
153. Ⓐ Ⓑ Ⓒ Ⓓ Ⓔ
154. Ⓐ Ⓑ Ⓒ Ⓓ Ⓔ
155. Ⓐ Ⓑ Ⓒ Ⓓ Ⓔ
156. Ⓐ Ⓑ Ⓒ Ⓓ Ⓔ
157. Ⓐ Ⓑ Ⓒ Ⓓ Ⓔ
158. Ⓐ Ⓑ Ⓒ Ⓓ Ⓔ
159. Ⓐ Ⓑ Ⓒ Ⓓ Ⓔ
160. Ⓐ Ⓑ Ⓒ Ⓓ Ⓔ
161. Ⓐ Ⓑ Ⓒ Ⓓ Ⓔ
162. Ⓐ Ⓑ Ⓒ Ⓓ Ⓔ
163. Ⓐ Ⓑ Ⓒ Ⓓ Ⓔ
164. Ⓐ Ⓑ Ⓒ Ⓓ Ⓔ
165. Ⓐ Ⓑ Ⓒ Ⓓ Ⓔ
166. Ⓐ Ⓑ Ⓒ Ⓓ Ⓔ
167. Ⓐ Ⓑ Ⓒ Ⓓ Ⓔ
168. Ⓐ Ⓑ Ⓒ Ⓓ Ⓔ

169. Ⓐ Ⓑ Ⓒ Ⓓ Ⓔ
170. Ⓐ Ⓑ Ⓒ Ⓓ Ⓔ
171. Ⓐ Ⓑ Ⓒ Ⓓ Ⓔ
172. Ⓐ Ⓑ Ⓒ Ⓓ Ⓔ
173. Ⓐ Ⓑ Ⓒ Ⓓ Ⓔ
174. Ⓐ Ⓑ Ⓒ Ⓓ Ⓔ
175. Ⓐ Ⓑ Ⓒ Ⓓ Ⓔ
176. Ⓐ Ⓑ Ⓒ Ⓓ Ⓔ
177. Ⓐ Ⓑ Ⓒ Ⓓ Ⓔ
178. Ⓐ Ⓑ Ⓒ Ⓓ Ⓔ
179. Ⓐ Ⓑ Ⓒ Ⓓ Ⓔ
180. Ⓐ Ⓑ Ⓒ Ⓓ Ⓔ
181. Ⓐ Ⓑ Ⓒ Ⓓ Ⓔ
182. Ⓐ Ⓑ Ⓒ Ⓓ Ⓔ
183. Ⓐ Ⓑ Ⓒ Ⓓ Ⓔ
184. Ⓐ Ⓑ Ⓒ Ⓓ Ⓔ
185. Ⓐ Ⓑ Ⓒ Ⓓ Ⓔ
186. Ⓐ Ⓑ Ⓒ Ⓓ Ⓔ
187. Ⓐ Ⓑ Ⓒ Ⓓ Ⓔ
188. Ⓐ Ⓑ Ⓒ Ⓓ Ⓔ
189. Ⓐ Ⓑ Ⓒ Ⓓ Ⓔ
190. Ⓐ Ⓑ Ⓒ Ⓓ Ⓔ
191. Ⓐ Ⓑ Ⓒ Ⓓ Ⓔ
192. Ⓐ Ⓑ Ⓒ Ⓓ Ⓔ
193. Ⓐ Ⓑ Ⓒ Ⓓ Ⓔ
194. Ⓐ Ⓑ Ⓒ Ⓓ Ⓔ
195. Ⓐ Ⓑ Ⓒ Ⓓ Ⓔ
196. Ⓐ Ⓑ Ⓒ Ⓓ Ⓔ
197. Ⓐ Ⓑ Ⓒ Ⓓ Ⓔ
198. Ⓐ Ⓑ Ⓒ Ⓓ Ⓔ
199. Ⓐ Ⓑ Ⓒ Ⓓ Ⓔ
200. Ⓐ Ⓑ Ⓒ Ⓓ Ⓔ

A copy of this answer sheet can be downloaded at http://www.amssmstore.com/download/AnswerSheet.pdf

AMSSM Sports Medicine CAQ Study Guide Test 2 Answer Sheet

AMSSM Sports Medicine CAQ Study Guide Test 2 Answer Sheet

101. Ⓐ Ⓑ Ⓒ Ⓓ Ⓔ	135. Ⓐ Ⓑ Ⓒ Ⓓ Ⓔ	169. Ⓐ Ⓑ Ⓒ Ⓓ Ⓔ
102. Ⓐ Ⓑ Ⓒ Ⓓ Ⓔ	136. Ⓐ Ⓑ Ⓒ Ⓓ Ⓔ	170. Ⓐ Ⓑ Ⓒ Ⓓ Ⓔ
103. Ⓐ Ⓑ Ⓒ Ⓓ Ⓔ	137. Ⓐ Ⓑ Ⓒ Ⓓ Ⓔ	171. Ⓐ Ⓑ Ⓒ Ⓓ Ⓔ
104. Ⓐ Ⓑ Ⓒ Ⓓ Ⓔ	138. Ⓐ Ⓑ Ⓒ Ⓓ Ⓔ	172. Ⓐ Ⓑ Ⓒ Ⓓ Ⓔ
105. Ⓐ Ⓑ Ⓒ Ⓓ Ⓔ	139. Ⓐ Ⓑ Ⓒ Ⓓ Ⓔ	173. Ⓐ Ⓑ Ⓒ Ⓓ Ⓔ
106. Ⓐ Ⓑ Ⓒ Ⓓ Ⓔ	140. Ⓐ Ⓑ Ⓒ Ⓓ Ⓔ	174. Ⓐ Ⓑ Ⓒ Ⓓ Ⓔ
107. Ⓐ Ⓑ Ⓒ Ⓓ Ⓔ	141. Ⓐ Ⓑ Ⓒ Ⓓ Ⓔ	175. Ⓐ Ⓑ Ⓒ Ⓓ Ⓔ
108. Ⓐ Ⓑ Ⓒ Ⓓ Ⓔ	142. Ⓐ Ⓑ Ⓒ Ⓓ Ⓔ	176. Ⓐ Ⓑ Ⓒ Ⓓ Ⓔ
109. Ⓐ Ⓑ Ⓒ Ⓓ Ⓔ	143. Ⓐ Ⓑ Ⓒ Ⓓ Ⓔ	177. Ⓐ Ⓑ Ⓒ Ⓓ Ⓔ
110. Ⓐ Ⓑ Ⓒ Ⓓ Ⓔ	144. Ⓐ Ⓑ Ⓒ Ⓓ Ⓔ	178. Ⓐ Ⓑ Ⓒ Ⓓ Ⓔ
111. Ⓐ Ⓑ Ⓒ Ⓓ Ⓔ	145. Ⓐ Ⓑ Ⓒ Ⓓ Ⓔ	179. Ⓐ Ⓑ Ⓒ Ⓓ Ⓔ
112. Ⓐ Ⓑ Ⓒ Ⓓ Ⓔ	146. Ⓐ Ⓑ Ⓒ Ⓓ Ⓔ	180. Ⓐ Ⓑ Ⓒ Ⓓ Ⓔ
113. Ⓐ Ⓑ Ⓒ Ⓓ Ⓔ	147. Ⓐ Ⓑ Ⓒ Ⓓ Ⓔ	181. Ⓐ Ⓑ Ⓒ Ⓓ Ⓔ
114. Ⓐ Ⓑ Ⓒ Ⓓ Ⓔ	148. Ⓐ Ⓑ Ⓒ Ⓓ Ⓔ	182. Ⓐ Ⓑ Ⓒ Ⓓ Ⓔ
115. Ⓐ Ⓑ Ⓒ Ⓓ Ⓔ	149. Ⓐ Ⓑ Ⓒ Ⓓ Ⓔ	183. Ⓐ Ⓑ Ⓒ Ⓓ Ⓔ
116. Ⓐ Ⓑ Ⓒ Ⓓ Ⓔ	150. Ⓐ Ⓑ Ⓒ Ⓓ Ⓔ	184. Ⓐ Ⓑ Ⓒ Ⓓ Ⓔ
117. Ⓐ Ⓑ Ⓒ Ⓓ Ⓔ	151. Ⓐ Ⓑ Ⓒ Ⓓ Ⓔ	185. Ⓐ Ⓑ Ⓒ Ⓓ Ⓔ
118. Ⓐ Ⓑ Ⓒ Ⓓ Ⓔ	152. Ⓐ Ⓑ Ⓒ Ⓓ Ⓔ	186. Ⓐ Ⓑ Ⓒ Ⓓ Ⓔ
119. Ⓐ Ⓑ Ⓒ Ⓓ Ⓔ	153. Ⓐ Ⓑ Ⓒ Ⓓ Ⓔ	187. Ⓐ Ⓑ Ⓒ Ⓓ Ⓔ
120. Ⓐ Ⓑ Ⓒ Ⓓ Ⓔ	154. Ⓐ Ⓑ Ⓒ Ⓓ Ⓔ	188. Ⓐ Ⓑ Ⓒ Ⓓ Ⓔ
121. Ⓐ Ⓑ Ⓒ Ⓓ Ⓔ	155. Ⓐ Ⓑ Ⓒ Ⓓ Ⓔ	189. Ⓐ Ⓑ Ⓒ Ⓓ Ⓔ
122. Ⓐ Ⓑ Ⓒ Ⓓ Ⓔ	156. Ⓐ Ⓑ Ⓒ Ⓓ Ⓔ	190. Ⓐ Ⓑ Ⓒ Ⓓ Ⓔ
123. Ⓐ Ⓑ Ⓒ Ⓓ Ⓔ	157. Ⓐ Ⓑ Ⓒ Ⓓ Ⓔ	191. Ⓐ Ⓑ Ⓒ Ⓓ Ⓔ
124. Ⓐ Ⓑ Ⓒ Ⓓ Ⓔ	158. Ⓐ Ⓑ Ⓒ Ⓓ Ⓔ	192. Ⓐ Ⓑ Ⓒ Ⓓ Ⓔ
125. Ⓐ Ⓑ Ⓒ Ⓓ Ⓔ	159. Ⓐ Ⓑ Ⓒ Ⓓ Ⓔ	193. Ⓐ Ⓑ Ⓒ Ⓓ Ⓔ
126. Ⓐ Ⓑ Ⓒ Ⓓ Ⓔ	160. Ⓐ Ⓑ Ⓒ Ⓓ Ⓔ	194. Ⓐ Ⓑ Ⓒ Ⓓ Ⓔ
127. Ⓐ Ⓑ Ⓒ Ⓓ Ⓔ	161. Ⓐ Ⓑ Ⓒ Ⓓ Ⓔ	195. Ⓐ Ⓑ Ⓒ Ⓓ Ⓔ
128. Ⓐ Ⓑ Ⓒ Ⓓ Ⓔ	162. Ⓐ Ⓑ Ⓒ Ⓓ Ⓔ	196. Ⓐ Ⓑ Ⓒ Ⓓ Ⓔ
129. Ⓐ Ⓑ Ⓒ Ⓓ Ⓔ	163. Ⓐ Ⓑ Ⓒ Ⓓ Ⓔ	197. Ⓐ Ⓑ Ⓒ Ⓓ Ⓔ
130. Ⓐ Ⓑ Ⓒ Ⓓ Ⓔ	164. Ⓐ Ⓑ Ⓒ Ⓓ Ⓔ	198. Ⓐ Ⓑ Ⓒ Ⓓ Ⓔ
131. Ⓐ Ⓑ Ⓒ Ⓓ Ⓔ	165. Ⓐ Ⓑ Ⓒ Ⓓ Ⓔ	199. Ⓐ Ⓑ Ⓒ Ⓓ Ⓔ
132. Ⓐ Ⓑ Ⓒ Ⓓ Ⓔ	166. Ⓐ Ⓑ Ⓒ Ⓓ Ⓔ	200. Ⓐ Ⓑ Ⓒ Ⓓ Ⓔ
133. Ⓐ Ⓑ Ⓒ Ⓓ Ⓔ	167. Ⓐ Ⓑ Ⓒ Ⓓ Ⓔ	
134. Ⓐ Ⓑ Ⓒ Ⓓ Ⓔ	168. Ⓐ Ⓑ Ⓒ Ⓓ Ⓔ	

A copy of this answer sheet can be downloaded at http://www.amssmstore.com/download/AnswerSheet.pdf